Basic ICD-10-CM and ICD-10-PCS Coding

2020

Lou Ann Schraffenberger, MBA, RHIA, CCS, CCS-P, FAHIMA
Brooke N. Palkie, EdD, RHIA

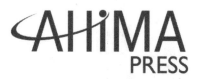

AHIMA PRESS

ISBN: **978-1-58426-744-7**

AHIMA Product No.: AC200519

AHIMA Staff:
Megan Grennan, Managing Editor
Kimberly Hooker, Production Development Editor
James Pinnick, Senior Director of Publications
Rachel Schratz, MA, Assistant Editor

Cover image: © iStock: Studio Pro

For more information, including updates, about AHIMA Press publications, visit http://www .ahima.org/education/press.

American Health Information Management Association
233 North Michigan Avenue, 21st Floor
Chicago, Illinois 60601-5809
ahima.org

Contents

Online Resources

Available at http://www.ahimapress.org/Schraffenberger7447/.

Appendix A   Glossary of Coding Terms

Appendix B   Case Studies

Appendix C   Answers to Odd-Numbered Check Your Understanding Questions

Appendix D   Answers to Odd-Numbered Review Exercises

Appendix E   Coding Self-Test Answer Key

Appendix F   ICD-10-CM Official Guidelines for Coding and Reporting FY 2020

Appendix G   ICD-10-PCS Official Guidelines for Coding and Reporting FY 2020

Appendix H   Microorganisms

Appendix I   Commonly Used Drugs

Appendix J   Morphology Terminology

Detailed Table of Contents

Online Resources

Available at http://www.ahimapress.org/Schraffenberger7447/.

About the Authors

Lou Ann Schraffenberger, MBA, RHIA, CCS, CCS-P, FAHIMA, is retired from Advocate Aurora Health as the manager of clinical data in their Center for Health Information Services based in Downers Grove, Illinois. Prior to her most recent position, Ms. Schraffenberger served as director of hospital health record departments, director of the Professional Practice Division of the American Health Information Management Association (AHIMA), and as a faculty member at the University of Illinois at Chicago and Moraine Valley Community College. Ms. Schraffenberger is an AHIMA-approved ICD-10-CM/PCS trainer. In 1997, Ms. Schraffenberger received the first AHIMA Volunteer Award, and in 2008 she received the AHIMA Legacy Award in recognition of her coding textbooks published by AHIMA. Ms. Schraffenberger graduated from the University of Illinois at the Medical Center with a bachelor's degree in health information management and received her MBA from the Loyola University Chicago Quinlan School of Business.

Brooke N. Palkie, EdD, RHIA, is the program director for the MS Health Care Administration and MS Health Informatics Programs at Charter Oak State College. She has a teaching focus on classifications, vocabularies, and clinical data standards, as well as assessing healthcare quality and corporate compliance. Dr. Palkie is an ICD-10-CM/PCS AHIMA-approved trainer and has been involved with several ICD-10 educational training programs and grant-funded projects. Prior to her higher education career, Dr. Palkie worked in management roles both within the hospital setting as well as for the State of Minnesota. Dr. Palkie graduated from the College of St. Scholastica with a bachelor's and a master's degree in health information management and received her EdD from Capella University with a focus on educational leadership.

Acknowledgments

This book on basic ICD-10-CM/PCS coding is built on the foundation of the *Basic ICD-9-CM Coding* textbook. Lou Ann Schraffenberger has written this text since 1999. The first *Basic ICD-9-CM Coding* textbook published in 1993. It was written by Toula Nicholas, RHIT, CCS, and Linda Ertl Bank, RHIA, CCS, and based on earlier ICD-9-CM instructional material authored by the late Rita M. Finnegan, MA, RHIA. Chapter 2 on ICD-10-PCS procedure coding was expanded by Therese M. Jorwic, MPH, RHIA, CCS, CCS-P, FAHIMA. Her expertise in ICD-10-PCS and authorship is acknowledged and appreciated. For an in-depth review of ICD-10-PCS principles and application of procedure coding rules, the reader is encouraged to examine *ICD-10-PCS: An Applied Approach* written by Lynn Kuehn, MS, RHIA, CCS-P, FAHIMA, and Therese M. Jorwic, MPH, RHIA, CCS, CCS-P, FAHIMA, published by AHIMA (AC201118). This is a comprehensive text for learning and mastering the procedure coding system, ICD-10-PCS. Coding practice exercises, case study coding, and a self-test are provided to reinforce the information in the text.

AHIMA Press and the authors would like to thank **Gretchen Jopp, MS, RHIA, CCS, CPC,** for her technical review and valuable feedback of this edition of this textbook. AHIMA Press would also like to acknowledge Jason Isley for providing medical illustrations.

Preface

Basic ICD-10-CM and ICD-10-PCS Coding, is a comprehensive text designed to help students master the range of coding skills, knowledge, and practice required to be successful. It introduces the basic principles and conventions of ICD-10-CM and ICD-10-PCS coding and illustrates the application of coding principles with examples and exercises based on actual case documentation.

The chapters are organized to cover each section of ICD-10-CM. A coding self-test is provided at the back of the text to allow for additional practice. Valuable information and resources are also available online.

This book must be used with the 2020 edition of ICD-10-CM and ICD-10-PCS code sets. The data files for the 2020 version of ICD-10-CM and ICD-10-PCS can be found at https://www.cdc.gov/nchs/icd/icd10cm.htm and https://www.cms.gov/Medicare/Coding /ICD10/2020-ICD-10-PCS.html.

Every effort has been made to include the most current coding information in this textbook. Because coding is so dynamic, there are continuous changes. To keep you informed about some of them, the following information is provided to you.

Official Coding Guidelines

The full 2020 *ICD-10-CM and ICD-10-PCS Official Guidelines for Coding and Reporting* are included as appendix F and appendix G, which are available on the AHIMA Press website, http://www.ahimapress.org/Schraffenberger7447/.

CG   The CG icon throughout the text displays coding guidelines that directly relate to the area of ICD-10-CM and ICD-10-PCS being discussed in the chapter, including the coding guideline number.

Key Concepts

 Throughout this edition of *Basic ICD-10-CM and ICD-10-PCS Coding* are the key concepts for students to know and areas of additional importance. These concepts are called out in the margins with an icon.

Additional Practice

In addition to the student review exercises throughout the chapters and at the end of each chapter, AHIMA Press also offers a student workbook, *Basic ICD-10-CM and ICD-10-PCS Coding Exercises*, Seventh Edition, by Lou Ann Schraffenberger, MBA, RHIA, CCS, CCS-P, FAHIMA, and Michelle Dionisio, MA, MSc, RHIA, CCS.

This resource contains ICD-10-CM coding exercises related to each chapter of *Basic ICD-10-CM and ICD-10-PCS Coding*. *Basic ICD-10-CM and ICD-10-PCS Coding Exercises* provides the student with the next level of coding practice—that is, coding from case studies or scenarios instead of one-line diagnostic or procedural statements. *Basic ICD-10-CM and ICD-10-PCS Coding Exercises* can be used as a student workbook in conjunction with this textbook for the lab portion of a coding course or as a text for a coding practicum or lab course, or can be used for independent study for skill building.

Readers who are interested in gaining more hands-on practice coding in ICD-10-CM and ICD-10-PCS should refer to the AHIMA bookstore at https://my.ahima.org/search/books for all the available ICD-10-CM and ICD-10-PCS publications.

Student and Instructor Online Resources

For Students

The resources listed below are available for students to help enhance their study and practice. Visit http://www.ahimapress.org/Schraffenberger7447/ and register your unique student access code that is provided on the inside front cover of this text to download the following files:

Appendix A	Glossary of Coding Terms
Appendix B	Case Studies
Appendix C	Answers to Odd-Numbered Check Your Understanding Questions
Appendix D	Answers to Odd-Numbered Review Exercises
Appendix E	Coding Self-Test Answer Key
Appendix F	ICD-10-CM Official Guidelines for Coding and Reporting FY 2020
Appendix G	ICD-10-PCS Official Guidelines for Coding and Reporting FY 2020
Appendix H	Microorganisms
Appendix I	Commonly Used Drugs
Appendix J	Morphology Terminology

For Instructors

Instructor materials for this book are provided only to approved educators. In addition to the materials listed above, instructor resources include full answer keys for all case studies, check your understanding questions, review exercises, and the self coding test at the back of this text. Please visit http://www.ahima.org/publications/educators.aspx for further instruction. If you have any questions regarding the instructor materials, please contact AHIMA Customer Relations at (800) 335-5535 or submit a customer support request at https://my.ahima.org/messages.

Introduction to Coding

Key Terms

Classification

Classification system

Coding

Diagnosis

Health Insurance Portability and
Accountability Act (HIPAA)

ICD-10-CM Coordination and Maintenance
(C&M) Committee

Medicare Prescription Drug,
Improvement, and Modernization
Act (MMA)

National Center for Health Statistics
(NCHS)

Official Addendum

Procedure

World Health Organization (WHO)

What Is Coding?

Coding is the transformation of verbal descriptions into numbers provided in a classification system. Codes are used every day to carry out simple business and personal transactions. For example, when a zip code is used in addressing a letter, a street address is transformed into numbers.

In the healthcare arena, specific codes describe diagnoses and procedures. A **diagnosis** is a word or phrase used by a physician to identify a disease from which an individual suffers or a condition for which the patient needs, seeks, or receives medical care. A surgical or therapeutic **procedure** is any single, separate, systematic process upon or within the body that can be complete in itself. A procedure is normally performed by a physician, dentist, or other licensed practitioner. A procedure can be performed with or without instrumentation. It is performed to restore disunited or deficient parts, remove diseased or injured tissues, extract foreign matter, assist in obstetrical delivery, or aid in diagnosis. Whereas assigning a zip code is a rather simple activity, the assignment of diagnostic and procedural codes requires a detailed thought process that is supported by a thorough knowledge of medical terminology, anatomy, and pathophysiology.

How Are Codes Assigned and What Systems Are Used?

Hospitals and other healthcare facilities index healthcare data by referring and adhering to a classification system maintained by the National Center for Health Statistics (NCHS) and Centers for Medicare and Medicaid Services (CMS). A **classification system** is a grouping of similar diseases and procedures organized for easy retrieval of related information. This type of system is used for coding or assigning numeric or alphanumeric code numbers to represent specific diseases or procedures. In the United States, the system that was implemented on October 1, 2015, is the *International Classification of Diseases, Tenth Revision, Clinical Modification* (ICD-10-CM) and the *International Classification of Diseases, Tenth Revision, Procedural Coding System* (ICD-10-PCS).

History of Coding

The notion of **classification** originated at the time of the ancient Greeks. In the seventeenth century, English statistician John Graunt developed the London Bills of Mortality, which provided the first documentation of the proportion of children who died before reaching age six years. In 1838, William Farr, the registrar general of England, developed a system to classify deaths. In 1893, a French physician, Jacques Bertillon, introduced the Bertillon Classification of Causes of Death at the International Statistical Institute in Chicago.

Several countries subsequently adopted Dr. Bertillon's system, and in 1898, the American Public Health Association (APHA) recommended that the registrars of Canada, Mexico, and the United States also adopt it. In addition, APHA recommended revising the system every 10 years to remain current with medical practice. As a result, the first international conference to revise the International Classification of Causes of Death convened in 1900; subsequent revisions occurred every 10 years. At that time, the classification system was contained in one book, which included an Alphabetic Index as well as a Tabular List. The book was quite small compared with current coding texts.

The revisions that followed contained minor changes; however, the sixth revision of the classification system brought drastic changes, as well as an expansion into two volumes. The sixth revision included morbidity and mortality conditions, and the Department of Health and Human Services (HHS) changed its title to reflect these changes: *Manual of International Statistical Classification of Diseases, Injuries and Causes of Death (ICD)*. Prior to the sixth revision, responsibility for ICD revisions fell to the Mixed Commission, a group composed of representatives from the International Statistical Institute and the Health Organization of the League of Nations. In 1948, the **World Health Organization (WHO)**, with headquarters in Geneva, Switzerland, assumed responsibility for preparing and publishing the revisions to ICD every 10 years. WHO sponsored the seventh and eighth revisions in 1957 and 1968, respectively.

The entire history of coding emphasizes the determination of many people to provide an international classification system for compiling and presenting statistical data. ICD has now become the most widely used statistical classification system in the world. Although some countries found ICD sufficient for hospital indexing purposes, many others believed it did not provide adequate detail for diagnostic indexing (WHO 2018a). In addition, the original revisions of ICD did not provide for classification of operative and diagnostic procedures. As a result, interested persons in the United States began to develop their own adaptation of ICD for use in this country.

In 1959, the US Public Health Service published the *International Classification of Diseases, Adapted for Indexing of Hospital Records and Operation Classification (ICDA)*.

Completed in 1962, a revision of this adaptation—considered to be the seventh revision of ICD—expanded a number of areas to more completely meet the indexing needs of hospitals. The US Public Health Service later published the *Eighth Revision, International Classification of Diseases, Adapted for Use in the United States*. Commonly referred to as ICDA-8, this classification system fulfilled its purpose to code diagnostic and operative procedural data for official morbidity and mortality statistics in the United States.

In 1978, WHO published the ninth revision of ICD (ICD-9). The US Public Health Service modified ICD-9 to meet the needs of American hospitals and called it *International Classification of Diseases, Ninth Revision, Clinical Modification* (ICD-9-CM). The ninth revision expanded the book to three volumes and introduced a fifth-digit subclassification. ICD-9-CM was the coding and classification system used in the United States to report diagnoses in all healthcare settings, inpatient procedures, and services for morbidity and mortality reporting starting in 1979. The ICD-9-CM system was discontinued in the United States on September 30, 2015 (WHO 2018a).

ICD-10-CM, ICD-10-PCS, and ICD-11

WHO published the 10th revision of ICD in 1990, and a number of countries subsequently adopted the system in either the original or an adapted form. The international version of the ICD-10 system has been used in the United States since January 1, 1999, for death certificate coding. This allows for collection of international mortality data.

A US clinical modification of the ICD-10 system was initiated in 1994 by **NCHS**. NCHS is the federal agency responsible for collecting and disseminating information on health services utilization and the health status of the population in the United States. NCHS is responsible for developing the clinical modifications for the United States to the ICD for the reporting of diseases. NCHS is also responsible for the development and the use of ICD-10 in the United States. The result, ICD-10-CM, was released in 1998 and updated several times since the initial version. ICD-10-CM is used for the reporting of diseases and conditions of patients treated in all settings in the US healthcare system effective October 1, 2015.

The ICD-10-CM system is more specific and contains significantly more codes than ICD-9-CM. It has the same hierarchical structure as ICD-9-CM, but the codes are alphanumeric with all letters except U used. The codes can extend to up to seven characters.

The 2020 version of ICD-10-CM is available on the NCHS website, at the Classifications of Diseases, Functioning, and Disability home page (CDC 2019). This version has been created by NCHS, under authorization by WHO.

On January 16, 2009, HHS published a final rule adopting ICD-10-CM (and ICD-10-PCS) to replace ICD-9-CM in HIPAA transactions, with an effective implementation date of October 1, 2013. The October 1, 2013, implementation date for ICD-10-CM and ICD-10-PCS was established in the original Final Rule of the HIPAA Administrative Simplification: Modifications to the Medical Data Code Set Standards to adopt ICD-10-CM and ICD-10-PCS, which was published in the *Federal Register* on January 16, 2009 (HHS 2009). The *Federal Register* is the daily publication of the federal government printed by the US Government Printing Office that announces all changes in regulations and federally mandated standards, including rules concerning prospective payment systems and code sets.

The Health Insurance Portability and Accountability Act (HIPAA) was federal legislation enacted to provide continuing health coverage, control fraud and abuse in healthcare, reduce healthcare costs, and guarantee the security and privacy of health information. HIPAA limits exclusions for pre-existing medical conditions, prohibits discrimination against employees and dependents based on health status, guarantees availability of health insurance to small employers, and guarantees renewability of insurance to all employees regardless of size. The law is also known as Public Law 104-191 and the Kassebaum-Kennedy Law.

On April 17, 2012, the secretary of HHS issued a proposed rule to change the compliance date for the ICD-10-CM and ICD-10-PCS code sets from October 1, 2013, to October 1, 2014. The comment period for the proposed rule closed in June 2012. The Final Rule published in the *Federal Register* on September 5, 2012, set the implementation date of October 1, 2014. On April 1, 2014, The Protecting Access to Medicare Act or PAMA (Pub. L. No. 113-93) was enacted, which stated the Secretary may not adopt ICD-10 prior to October 1, 2015. Accordingly, HHS released a final rule on July 31, 2014, that required a new compliance date for the use of ICD-10 beginning October 1, 2015. The rule also required HIPAA-covered entities to continue to use ICD-9-CM through September 30, 2015.

The Final Rule adopts modifications to two of the code set standards adopted in the Transactions and Code Sets Final Rule published in the *Federal Register* pursuant to certain provisions of the Administrative Simplification subtitle of HIPAA. Specifically, this Final Rule modifies the standard medical data code sets for coding diagnoses and inpatient hospital procedures by concurrently adopting the ICD-10-CM for diagnosis coding, including the *Official ICD-10-CM Guidelines for Coding and Reporting*, as maintained by the NCHS, and ICD-10-PCS for inpatient hospital procedure coding, including the *Official ICD-10-PCS Guidelines for Coding and Reporting*, as maintained and distributed by HHS. These new codes replace ICD-9-CM, Volumes 1, 2, and 3, including the *Official Guidelines for Coding and Reporting*.

ICD-10-PCS was developed by 3M Health Information Systems under contract with CMS. CMS is a division of HHS that is responsible for developing healthcare policy in the United States, administering the Medicare program and the federal portion of the Medicaid program, and maintaining the procedure portion of the ICD. On October 1, 2015, ICD-10-PCS replaced ICD-9-CM, Volume 3, for the reporting of hospital inpatient procedures. It is a significant improvement over ICD-9-CM, volume 3, in terms of its comprehensiveness and expandability. ICD-10-PCS is discussed in further detail in chapter 2, *Introduction to ICD-10-PCS*.

On June 18, 2018, the World Health Organization released the ICD-11 edition (WHO 2018b). Member states and stakeholders can now use ICD-11 to prepare for future implementations within different countries. This includes translations and modifications such as those needed within the US. According to WHO, ICD-11 includes more clinical detail, updates to scientific content, and links to other classifications and terminologies, and it is made for ready use in electronic environments. WHO identifies that ICD-11 has around 55,000 unique codes and will be presented at the World Health Assembly in May 2019 for an early implementation timeline of 2020 (WHO 2018b). It has yet to be identified when the United States will implement a clinically modified version of ICD-11.

HIPAA Electronic Transactions and Coding Standards Rule

In March 2009, the HHS published modifications (74 FR 3328) to the final regulations for electronic transactions and coding standards as established under HIPAA in the *Federal Register* (65 FR 50312). The final rule with the modifications designates the following medical code standards to be used under the current HIPAA rule. These included the following:

- *International Classification of Diseases, Tenth Revision, Clinical Modification (ICD-10-CM)*

- *International Classification of Diseases, Tenth Revision, Procedure Coding System (ICD-10-PCS)*

- *Current Procedural Terminology (CPT), Fourth Edition (CPT-4)*
- *Healthcare Common Procedure Coding System (HCPCS)*
- *Code on Dental Procedures and Nomenclatures, Second Edition (CDT-2)*
- *National Drug Codes (NDC)*

On February 20, 2003, the HHS published a final rule in the *Federal Register* (68 FR 8381) that repealed the adoption of the *National Drug Codes* (NDC) for institutional and professional claims. It did allow NDC to remain the standard medical data code set for reporting drugs and biologics for retail pharmacy claims. The intent of this decision was to give covered entities the choice in determining which code set to use with respect to payment of claims, including HCPCS and NDC codes. Hospitals and physicians are likely to continue using HCPCS. As a result of this repeal, there is no identified standard medical data code set in place for reporting drugs and biologics on nonretail pharmacy transactions. Covered entities could use HCPCS or NDC as the preferred and agreed-upon code set with their trading partners.

The *ICD-10-CM and ICD-10-PCS Official Guidelines for Coding and Reporting* were named as required components of the ICD-10-CM and ICD-10-PCS code set in the modified final rule for electronic transactions and coding standards This made adherence to the guidelines a requirement for compliance with the rule.

Although it is true that most of the code sets adopted are in current use, some changes were made regarding their use and context. It is important to note that, upon implementation, these medical code sets became the rule for nearly all insurance payers.

ICD-10-CM covers diseases, injuries, impairments, and other health problems and their manifestations, as well as causes of injury and disease impairment.

ICD-10-PCS is limited to procedures or other actions taken for diseases, injuries, and impairments of hospital inpatients reported by hospitals and related to prevention, diagnosis, treatment, and management. This means that nonacute facilities do not use ICD-10-PCS to report procedures but instead used HCPCS Level I (CPT® codes published by the American Medical Association) or HCPCS Level II codes as appropriate.

The CPT and HCPCS codes are used for physicians and other healthcare services, such as hospital outpatient services. These services include physician services, physical and occupational therapy services, radiological services, clinical laboratory tests, other medical diagnostic procedures, hearing and vision services, and transportation services, including ambulances. Physicians and other healthcare providers used the combination of CPT and HCPCS Level II codes to report procedures and services provided.

More information about the medical code sets and other facts about the HIPAA transactions and code sets final rule can be found on AHIMA's website or in the *Federal Register* may be accessed from the Government Printing Office website (GPO 2019).

Medicare Prescription Drug, Improvement, and Modernization Act of 2003

The **Medicare Prescription Drug, Improvement, and Modernization Act (MMA)** was signed into law on December 8, 2003. Section 503 of the bill includes language that opened up the possibility for code changes two times a year, on April 1 and October 1. Since this legislation took effect in 2005, there have not been any April 1 code changes. However, the potential for code changes twice a year still exists if a strong and convincing case is made by the requestor that the new code is needed to describe new technologies. Otherwise, the codes will be considered for the next October 1 implementation.

Official Addendum to ICD-10-CM and ICD-10-PCS

In contrast to international ICD updates that occur less frequently, ICD-10-CM and ICD-10-PCS undergo annual updates in the United States to remain current. Codes may be added, revised, or deleted. An *Official Addendum* documents the changes, which are effective April 1 and October 1 of each year. The addendum may be found at the NCHS website (CDC 2019). CMS and NCHS publish the ICD-10-CM/PCS annual addenda with the approval of the WHO. NCHS is responsible for maintaining the diagnosis classification; CMS is responsible for maintaining the procedure classification. AHIMA and AHA give advice and assistance, as do HIM practitioners, physicians, and other users of ICD-10-CM and ICD-10-PCS.

Coordination and Maintenance Committee

The **ICD-10-CM Coordination and Maintenance (C&M) Committee** is chaired by a representative from the NCHS and a representative from CMS. The ICD-10-CM Coordination and Maintenance Committee is responsible for maintaining the United States' clinical modification version of the ICD-10-CM and ICD-10-PCS code sets. The Coordination and Maintenance Committee holds two open meetings each year that serve as a public forum for discussing (but not making decisions) proposed revisions to ICD-10-CM and ICD-10-PCS. Information about the ICD-10-CM and ICD-10-PCS Coordination and Maintenance Committee, including meeting minutes, can be found on the CDC and CMS websites (CDC 2017; CMS 2018).

A point to remember: To ensure accurate coding, all ICD-10-CM and ICD-10-PCS code books must be updated yearly with the revisions published. In addition, all coding software (encoders) must be updated to reflect the new revisions. As a general rule, new ICD-10-CM and ICD-10-PCS codes will be effective October 1 of each year.

ICD-10-CM Review Exercises: Introduction to Coding

1. Identify the difference between assigning a number to a verbal description such as for a zip code and the activity of assigning a diagnosis or procedure code to medical documentation.

2. How often must the ICD-10-CM and ICD-10-PCS code books be updated and when do the updates go into effect?

3. What did the statistician John Graunt develop in the seventeenth century that is considered an early classification system?

4. Between 1838 and 1893, what other early classification systems were developed?

(Continued on next page)

ICD-10-CM Review Exercises: Introduction to Coding (Continued)

5. What did the American Public Health Association recommend to countries to do in 1898, and what occurred in 1900 as a result of the recommendation?

   _____

6. How did the World Health Organization become involved with the classification system in 1948?

   _____

7. What organization released the 11th version of the International Classification of Diseases? What are the main benefits that differentiate it from the current edition?

   _____

8. How do the Electronic Transaction and Coding Standards correlate to coding and why are they important?

   _____

9. What is the main difference between the ICD-10 annual revision released by the WHO and the ICD-10-CM and ICD-10-PCS annual revisions released by CMS and NCHS? Identify which addenda CMS publishes and which addenda NCHS publishes along with the overall connection to the WHO.

   _____

10. What is the importance of having the Official Guidelines as a required component of the ICD-10-CM and ICD-10-PCS code set in the final rule of the electronic transactions and coding standards?

   _____

11. What is the purpose of the *Official Addendum for ICD-10-CM and ICD-10-PCS?*

   _____

12. What government agencies provide the representatives to chair the ICD-10-CM Coordination and Maintenance Committee, and what is the committee's responsibility?

   _____

Reference

Centers for Disease Control and Prevention (CDC). 2017. ICD-10 Coordination and Maintenance Committee. http://www.cdc.gov/nchs/icd/icd10_maintenance.htm.

Centers for Disease Control and Prevention (CDC). 2019. International Classification of Diseases, Tenth Revision, Clinical Modification (ICD-10-CM). https://www.cdc.gov/nchs/icd/icd10cm.htm.

Centers for Medicare and Medicaid Services (CMS). 2018. ICD-10 Coordination and Maintenance Committee. https://www.cms.gov/medicare/coding/icd9providerdiagnosticcodes/meetings.html.

Government Printing Office (GPO). 2019. http://www.gpo.gov/fdsys/browse/collection.action?collectionCode=FR.

Department of Health and Human Services (HHS). HIPAA Administrative Simplification: Modifications to Medical Data Code Set Standards to Adopt ICD-10-CM and ICD-10-PCS. *Federal Register*. 2009 Jan 16; 74(11):3328–62.

World Health Information (WHO). 2018a. International Classification of Diseases (ICD) Information Sheet. http://www.who.int/classifications/icd/factsheet/en/.

World Health Organization (WHO). 2018b. Classifications. http://www.who.int/classifications/icd/en/.

Chapter 1

Introduction to ICD-10-CM

Learning Objectives

At the conclusion of this chapter, you should be able to do the following:

- Indicate the characteristics of the ICD-10-CM classification system
- Describe the format of the Tabular List of Diseases and Injuries
- Identify and define the chapters and subchapters or blocks used in ICD-10-CM
- Identify and define the main terms, subterms, carryover lines, nonessential modifiers, and eponyms used in ICD-10-CM
- Recognize the contents of the Appendices of ICD-10-CM
- Explain the format of the Alphabetic Index to Diseases in ICD-10-CM
- Identify and define the main terms, subterms, nonessential modifiers, and eponyms used in ICD-10-CM
- Identify and define the cross-reference terms and instructional notes used in ICD-10-CM
- Describe the rules for multiple coding
- Explain how connecting words are used in the Alphabetic Index
- Apply the symbols, punctuations, and abbreviations used in ICD-10-CM
- List the basic steps in ICD-10-CM coding
- Assign diagnosis codes using the Alphabetic Index and Tabular List

Key Terms

Alphabetic Index to Diseases and Injuries
"And"
Carryover lines

Category
"Code also" note
"Code first" note

"Code, if applicable, a causal
condition first"
Colon
Connecting words
Default code
Eponyms
Etiology
Excludes notes
Excludes1 notes
Excludes2 notes
Includes notes
Inclusion term
Indiscriminate multiple coding
Main Terms
Manifestation
NEC: Not elsewhere classified

Nonessential modifiers
NOS: Not otherwise specified
Other or other specified codes
Parentheses
Placeholder
"See" note
"See also" note
Sequela
Slanted brackets
Square brackets
Subcategory
Subterms
Tabular List
Unspecified codes
"Use additional code" note
"With"

Characteristics of ICD-10-CM

The ICD-10-CM system is used for all diagnosis coding and began on October 1, 2015. ICD-10-CM is divided into the Alphabetic Index, which is an alphabetic listing of terms and codes, and the Tabular List, which is a numerical list of the codes divided by chapters.

Conventions for ICD-10-CM

To assign ICD-10-CM codes accurately, a thorough understanding of the ICD-10-CM conventions is necessary. These coding conventions are located within the *ICD-10-CM Official Guidelines for Coding and Reporting*. They address the structure and format of the coding system, including how to use the Alphabetic Index and the Tabular List, as well as the rules and instructions that the coder must follow.

Alphabetic Index

According to the *ICD-10-CM Official Guidelines for Coding and Reporting*, the **Alphabetic Index to Diseases and Injuries** is an alphabetic listing of terms and their corresponding codes (CDC 2019). The Alphabetic Index is divided into two parts—the Index to Diseases and Injury and the Index to External Causes of Injury. Within the Index of Diseases and Injury, there is a Neoplasm Table and a Table of Drugs and Chemicals.

Main Terms

The Alphabetic Index to Diseases and Injuries in ICD-10-CM is formatted with main terms set in boldface and listed in alphabetical order. **Main terms** are entries printed in boldface type and flush with the left margin of each column in the Alphabetic Index. Main terms represent the following:

- Diseases such as influenza or bronchitis

- Conditions such as fatigue, fracture, or injury

- Nouns such as disease, disorder, or syndrome

- Adjectives such as double, kink, or large

The Alphabetic Index is the first place the coder uses to locate the ICD-10-CM code for the patient's disease or condition. Instead of a listing of sites where diseases may occur, ICD-10-CM provides anatomical terms with a cross-reference that directs the coder to reference the condition. For example, bronchial asthma is found under the disease term "asthma" rather than the anatomical term or site of "bronchial." However, if the anatomical term is part of the disease title, the anatomical term may be the main term. For example, the diagnosis of "acute abdomen" is found in the Alphabetic Index under the main term of "abdomen."

Many conditions are found in more than one place in the Alphabetic Index. For example:

- Complications of medical and surgical care are indexed under the name of the condition as well as under the main term "Complications." For example, kidney transplant failure is found under "complication, transplant, kidney" and "failure, transplant, kidney."

- Obstetrical conditions are found under the name of the condition and under the main terms such as "Delivery," "Pregnancy," or "Puerperal." For example, preterm delivery is found under "Delivery, preterm" and "Pregnancy, complicated by, preterm."

- Conditions that include the term "disease" or "syndrome" in their titles or descriptions may be found under "Disease" or "Syndrome" as well as under the disease or syndrome's name. For example, "chronic obstruction lung disease" may be found in the Alphabetic Index under "Disease, lung, obstructive" as well as under "Obstructive, lung, disease."

Check Your Understanding 1.1

Using the Alphabetic Index, underline the main term in each of the following diagnoses.

1. Breast Mass
2. Primary hydronephrosis
3. Deviation of nasal septum
4. Inguinal adenopathy
5. Gastric pouch
6. Tension headache
7. Acute pancreatitis
8. Mild persistent asthma
9. Otitis externa
10. Major Depressive Disorder

Alphabetic Index Subterms

Indented beneath the main term, any applicable **subterms**, also called essential modifiers are shown in their own alphabetic list. The indented subterm is always read in combination with the main term. The subterms form individual line entries arranged in alphabetical order and printed in regular type beginning with a lowercase letter. Subterms are indented one standard indentation to the right under the main term. Subterms describe essential differences in the site, cause, or the clinical type of the condition. More specific subterms are indented farther to the right as needed, indented one standard indentation after the preceding subterm, and listed in alphabetic order. The dash (-) at the end of an Index entry indicates that additional characters are required.

Prior to selecting a code, all subentries following the main term should be reviewed to determine the appropriate code. Note that the terms "with" or "without" are listed at the beginning of all the subterms, rather than in alphabetic order.

Actinomycosis, actinomycotic A42.9   ← Main term
- with pneumonia A42.0   ← "with" appears at the beginning
- abdominal A42.1   ← Subterms identify specific site or type
- cervicofacial A42.2
- cutaneous A42.89
- gastrointestinal A42.1
- pulmonary A42.0
- sepsis A42.7
- specified site NEC A42.89

Incontinence R32   ← Main term
- anal sphincter R15.9   ← Site
- coital N39.491
- feces R15.9
- - nonorganic origin F98.1
- insensible (urinary) N39.42
- overflow N39.490
- postural (urinary) N39.492
- psychogenic F45.8
- rectal R15.9
- reflex N39.498
- stress (female) (male) N39.3   ← Cause
- - and urge N39.46
- urethral sphincter R32
- urge N39.41
- - and stress (female) (male) N39.46
- urine (urinary) R32
- - continuous N39.45
- - due to cognitive impairment, or severe physical disability or immobility R39.81   ← Clinical type
- - functional R39.81
- - insensible N39.42
- - mixed (stress and urge) N39.46
- - nocturnal N39.44
- - nonorganic origin F98.0
- - overflow N39.490
- - post dribbling N39.43
- - postural N39.492
- - reflex N39.498

- - specified NEC N39.498
- - stress (female) (male) N39.3
- - - and urge N39.46
- - total N39.498
- - unaware N39.42
- - urge N39.41
- - - and stress (female) (male) N39.46

Carryover Lines

Carryover lines are needed on occasion in the Alphabetic Index because the number of words that can fit on a single line of print is limited. They are two indents from the preceding line. Coders must be careful to avoid confusing the carryover line with the subterm entries. For example, the diagnosis of "Cesarean delivery occurring after 37 weeks of gestation but before 39 completed weeks of gestation due to spontaneous onset of labor" is found in the Alphabetic Index under the main term "delivery" with the subterm "cesarean" with a carryover line starting with the phrase "occurring after 37 completed weeks." The following is an example of a carryover line as it appears in the Alphabetic Index:

> **Delivery (childbirth) (labor)**
> cesarean (for)
> occurring after 37 completed weeks of gestation but before 39 completed
> weeks of gestation due to (spontaneous) onset of labor O75.82

Check Your Understanding 1.2

Using the Alphabetic Index, underline the subterm in each of the following diagnoses.

1. Atrial septal defect
2. Reflux esophagitis
3. Blood loss anemia
4. High arch, of foot
5. Bullous impetigo
6. Lactose intolerance
7. Spontaneous delivery
8. Cerebrospinal meningitis
9. Nausea with vomiting
10. Capillary nevus
11. Aortoiliac occlusion
12. Accessory nerve paralysis
13. Low basal metabolic rate
14. Q fever with pneumonia

(Continued)

(Continued)

15. Congenital scoliosis

16. Traumatic shock

17. Venous stasis

18. Pulmonary tuberculosis

19. Giant urticaria

20. Joint xanthoma

Nonessential Modifiers

A term or a series of terms that appear in parentheses following a main term or subterm are known as **nonessential modifiers**. The presence or absence of these parenthetical terms in the diagnosis statement has no effect on the selection of the codes listed for that main term or subterm. The words in parentheses are not considered important descriptors of the diagnosis or condition in the ICD-10-CM classification system.

The nonessential modifiers apply to the main term and to subterms following the main term. However, there is an exception to this rule when a nonessential modifier term and a subterm are mutually exclusive. In this instance, the subterm takes precedence for the code assigned. For example, the subterms of "acute" and "chronic" are mutually exclusive descriptors. In the Alphabetic Index, under the main term "enteritis," there is a nonessential modifier of "acute." There is also a subterm of "chronic" under enteritis in the Alphabetic Index. In this example, the nonessential modifier of acute does not apply to the subterm chronic for enteritis.

Pneumonia (acute) (double) (migratory) (purulent) (septic) (unresolved) **J18.9**

For example, if the patient was discharged from the hospital after treatment of acute pneumonia, the diagnosis code assigned is J18.9. The term "acute" is a nonessential modifier and does not describe the specific type of pneumonia the patient had, such as bacterial or viral.

For example, if the patient was seen in the emergency department and a diagnosis of "pneumonia" was made, the appropriate code assignment would be J18.9. No essential modifier is included in the diagnostic statement.

Check Your Understanding 1.3

Using the Alphabetic Index, underline the nonessential modifier in each of the following diagnoses.

1. Chronic alcoholism

2. Angina pectoris

3. Animal bite to hand

4. Benign hypertension

5. Congestive systolic heart failure

6. Acquired deafness

(Continued)

(Continued)

7. Diabetes mellitus
8. Tropical dysentery
9. Pulmonary emphysema
10. Fever of unknown origin
11. Dry gangrene
12. Recurrent hernia
13. Large-for-dates infant
14. Malignant mesothelioma
15. Blindness, both eyes
16. Pericarditis with effusion
17. Background retinopathy
18. Generalized sepsis
19. Secondary polycythemia
20. Migratory pneumonia

Eponyms

Many diseases and operations carry the name of a person, or an eponym. An **eponym** is a name, as in a drug or disease, based on or derived from the name of a person (Mosby 2017, 471). As a proper name, the eponym name is capitalized, such as Dupuytren's contraction or disease. The main terms for eponyms are located in the Alphabetic Index as follows:

- Under the eponym itself, such as Barrett's

  Barrett's
  ulcer K22.10

- Under main terms of the disease or condition, such as ulcer

  Ulcer
  Barrett's (esophagus) K22.10

- For other eponyms, the Alphabetic Index entry may include the description of the disease or syndrome, usually enclosed in parentheses but sometimes following the eponym

  Chiari's
  disease or syndrome (hepatic vein thrombosis) I82.0

- For some eponyms, the eponym may be found in the Alphabetic Index under the main terms of disease, syndrome, disorder, deformity, as well as other words used in the diagnostic statement.

  Disease
  Alzheimer's G30.9 *[F02.80]*

Check Your Understanding 1.4

Using the Alphabetic Index only, assign codes to the following.

1. Huntington's disease
2. Sprengel's deformity
3. Stokes-Adams syndrome
4. Briquet's disorder
5. Costen's complex
6. Christmas disease
7. Cushing's syndrome
8. Colles' fracture of right radius
9. Bell's palsy
10. Aarskog's syndrome

"See" and "See Also" Instructions

The Alphabetic Index in ICD-10-CM includes both "see" and "see also" instructions following a main term to indicate that another term should be referenced.

The **"see" note** is a cross-reference term in the Alphabetic Index to Diseases and Injuries that provides direction to the coder to look elsewhere in the Index before assigning a code. The "see" cross-reference points to an alternative term. This is a mandatory instruction that must be followed to ensure accurate ICD-10-CM code assignment.

The **"see also" note** in the Alphabetic Index to Disease and Injuries provides direction to the coder to look elsewhere in the Index. It requires the review of another term in the Index if all the needed information cannot be found under the first main term. However, it is not necessary to follow the *see also* note when the original main term provides the necessary code.

> **EXAMPLE:** **Aberrant (congenital)—see also Malposition, congenital**
> -adrenal gland Q89.1
> -artery (peripheral) Q27.8
> ---basilar NEC Q28.1
> ---cerebral Q28.3

"Code Also" Note

The **"code also" note** appears in ICD-10-CM, meaning that two codes may be required to fully describe a condition, but this note does not provide sequencing direction. The sequencing depends on the circumstances of the encounter.

The ICD-10-CM Alphabetic Index includes manifestation of disease codes by including the manifestation code as the second code, shown in brackets, directly after the underlying or etiology code, which should always be reported first.

EXAMPLES: **Dementia**
-with
    –Parkinson's disease G20 *[F02.80]*
Retinitis
-renal N18.9 *[H32]*
-syphilitic
    –congenital (early) A50.01 *[H32]*

Default Code

ICD-10-CM refers to the code listed next to a main term in the Alphabetic Index as a **default code**. The default code represents the condition that is most commonly associated with the main term, or is the unspecified code for the condition. If a condition is documented in the health record without any additional information, such as whether it is acute or chronic, the default code should be assigned.

Check Your Understanding 1.5

Review each diagnostic statement. Underline the appropriate main term to use in the Alphabetic Index. Locate the main term and follow all cross-reference instructions or identify the default code provided. Confirm the code in the Tabular List and enter it in the space provided.

1. Subacute endomyometritis

2. Rheumatic pneumonia

3. Osteoarthrosis, both hips

4. Cervical intervertebral disc prolapse

5. Stenosis of cerebral artery

6. Early-onset Alzheimer's disease

7. Meningitis in bacterial disease

8. Aspiration pneumonia

9. Nutritional polyneuritis

10. Ankylosing spondylitis with lung involvement

11. Acute sigmoiditis

12. Abdominal hernia

13. Cholesteatoma, left ear

14. Idiopathic dystonia

15. Acute necrotizing myopathy

Tabular List

The ICD-10-CM **Tabular List** is a structured list of codes divided into chapters based on body system or condition. The Tabular List is divided into 21 chapters. For some chapters, the body or organ system is the axis of the classification. This means in this example that the body system is the focal point of that chapter. Other chapters, such as Chapter 1: Certain Infectious and Parasitic Diseases, group together conditions by etiology or nature of the disease process.

The 21 chapters of the ICD-10-CM classification system are as follows:

1. Certain Infectious and Parasitic Diseases (A00–B99)

2. Neoplasms (C00–D49)

3. Diseases of the Blood and Blood-Forming Organs and Certain Disorders Involving the Immune Mechanism (D50–D89)

4. Endocrine, Nutritional and Metabolic Disorders (E00–E89)

5. Mental, Behavioral and Neurodevelopmental Disorders (F01–F99)

6. Diseases of the Nervous System (G00–G99)

7. Diseases of the Eye and Adnexa (H00–H59)

8. Diseases of the Ear and Mastoid Process (H60–H95)

9. Diseases of the Circulatory System (I00–I99)

10. Diseases of the Respiratory System (J00–J99)

11. Diseases of the Digestive System (K00–K95)

12. Diseases of the Skin and Subcutaneous Tissue (L00–L99)

13. Diseases of the Musculoskeletal System and Connective Tissue (M00–M99)

14. Diseases of the Genitourinary System (N00–N99)

15. Pregnancy, Childbirth and the Puerperium (O00–O9A)

16. Certain Conditions Originating in the Perinatal Period (P00–P96)

17. Congenital Malformations, Deformations and Chromosomal Abnormalities (Q00–Q99)

18. Symptoms, Signs and Abnormal Clinical and Laboratory Findings, Not Elsewhere Classified (R00–R99)

19. Injury, Poisoning and Certain Other Consequences of External Causes (S00–T88)

20. External Causes of Morbidity (V00–Y99)

21. Factors Influencing Health Status and Contact with Health Services (Z00–Z99)

Each chapter in the Tabular List of ICD-10-CM begins with a summary of the blocks to provide an overview of the categories within the chapter.

Code Format and Structure

ICD-10-CM contains chapters, categories, subcategories, and codes. Chapters are further subdivided into subchapters (blocks) and subcategories that contain three-character categories and form the foundation of the code.

Categories, Subcategories, and Codes

The characters for categories, subcategories, and codes may contain either letters or numbers. A **category** is composed of three characters that represent a single disease or a group of similar or closely related conditions. A three-character category that has no further subdivision is equivalent to a code.

Most three-character categories are further subdivided into four- or five-character sub-categories. Codes can be three, four, five, six, or seven characters. Each level of subdivision after a category is a **subcategory**. Five- and six-character codes provide greater specificity or additional information about the condition being coded. The subcategory codes add more specificity to the description of the disease in terms of the etiology (cause of the disease), site (anatomic location), severity, or the manifestation of the disease. A manifestation may be a complication of the disease or characteristics, signs, symptoms, or secondary processes that occur with the disease or illness.

The final level of subdivision of a category is a code. Certain categories have an additional seventh character. The seventh character must always be the final character of the code. When the code contains fewer than seven characters, yet a 7th character is required by the Tabular, the placeholder X must be used to fill the empty character(s) spaces.

The fourth character 8, when placed after a decimal point (.8), is used to indicate some "other" specified category. The fourth character 9, when placed after a decimal point (.9), is usually reserved for an unspecified condition. In ICD-10-CM, the "other specified" and "unspecified" conditions each have their own code and are not combined into one code.

First Character

The first character of an ICD-10-CM code is always an alphabetic letter. All the letters of the alphabet are utilized with the exception of the letter U. The letter U has been reserved by the World Health Organization (WHO) for the provisional assignment of new diseases of uncertain etiology (U00–U49) and for bacterial agents resistant to antibiotics (U80–U89). No codes from categories U00–U49 and U80–U89 are valid for use in the United States. ICD-10-CM codes may consist of up to seven characters and are formatted as shown in figure 1.1.

Figure 1.1.   **ICD-10-CM code format**

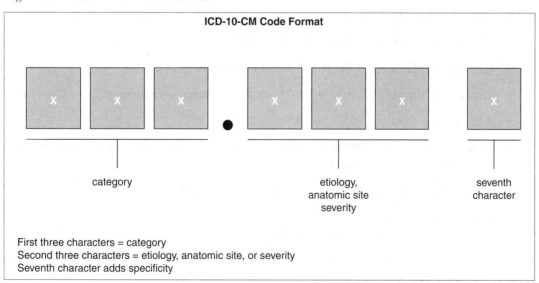

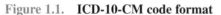

Placeholder Character

ICD-10-CM utilizes a **placeholder** character, which is always the letter X, and it has two uses:

1. The X provides for future expansion without disturbing the overall code structure.

    EXAMPLE: T42.3X1A, Poisoning by barbiturates, accidental, initial encounter

2. It is also used when a code has fewer than six characters and a seventh character extension is required. The X is assigned for all characters less than six in order to meet the requirement of coding to the highest level of specificity.

    EXAMPLE: T58.11XA, Toxic effect of carbon monoxide from utility gas, accidental, initial encounter

Seventh (7th) Character

Certain ICD-10-CM categories have applicable seventh characters. The applicable seventh character is required for all codes within the category, or as the notes in the Tabular List instruct. The seventh character must always be the seventh character in the data field. If a code that requires a seventh character does not contain six characters, a placeholder X must be used to fill in the empty characters.

EXAMPLES: O40.1XX1, Polyhydramnios, first trimester, fetus 1
S05.01XA, Injury of conjunctiva and corneal abrasion without foreign body, right eye, initial encounter

Code Format and Structure

To summarize the code format and structure of ICD-10-CM, the following facts are presented:

*   ICD-10-CM codes consist of three to seven characters.

*   The first character of an ICD-10-CM code is always an alphabetic character.

*   All letters are used except U in the ICD-10-CM codes.

*   The second character of the ICD-10-CM code is always numeric.

*   Characters 3 through 7 of ICD-10-CM can be alphabetic or numeric.

*   Characters 4 through 7 add specificity to the code.

*   A decimal is placed after the first three characters of an ICD-10-CM code. The first three characters are considered the category.

*   Alpha characters used in the ICD-10-CM codes are not case-sensitive.

*   Only complete ICD-10-CM codes are used for reporting purposes, not categories (unless it is a valid three-character code) or subcategories.

*   When a seventh character is required but there are fewer than six characters, the X must be used as a placeholder for the ICD-10-CM code to be valid.

Check Your Understanding 1.6

Answer the following questions about the ICD-10-CM code format and structure.

1. Turn to the code B05, Measles, listed in the Tabular List for ICD-10-CM to answer the following questions:
   a. Is code B05, Measles, a category code or a subcategory code?
   b. In what chapter and within what block or section of codes does category B05 appear?
   c. Are the subcategories B05.0–B05.9 codes identifying manifestations, sites, or the etiology or causes of the disease?
   d. What do the subcategory codes represent?
   e. What is the subcategory code for measles without complications?

2. Turn to the code J20, Acute bronchitis, listed in the Tabular List for ICD-10-CM to answer the following questions:
   a. Is code J20, Acute bronchitis, a category code or a subcategory code?
   b. In what chapter and within what block or section of codes does category J20 appear?
   c. Are the subcategories J20.0–J20.9 codes identifying manifestations, sites, or causes of the acute bronchitis?
   d. What do the subcategory codes represent?
   e. What is the subcategory code for acute bronchitis with no organism identified as responsible for the infection?

3. Turn to the code L89.51, listed in the Tabular List for ICD-10-CM to answer the following questions:
   a. Is code L89.51, Pressure ulcer of right ankle, a category code or a subcategory code?
   b. In what chapter and within what block or section of codes do the codes under L89.51 appear?
   c. Are the subcategories L89.51 codes identifying manifestations, sites, severity, or causes of the measles disease?
   d. What do the subcategory codes represent?
   e. What is the subcategory code for the pressure ulcer of the right ankle that is not identified with a stage?

4. Turn to subcategory code O09.0, Supervision of pregnancy with history of infertility. What does the fifth character represent in the codes O09.00–O09.03?

5. Turn to subcategory code M06.21, Rheumatoid bursitis, shoulder. What does the sixth character represent in the codes M06.211–M06.219?

6. Turn to category code S05, Injury of eye and orbit. What does the seventh character represent for the codes in category S05?

7. Would a placeholder of X be required for the diagnosis of "abrasion of scalp" with code S00.01 when the patient is seen at the initial encounter for care? What would be the complete code?

8. Would a placeholder of X be required for the diagnosis of "nondisplaced traumatic trapezoid fracture of the left wrist" with code S62.185 when the patient is seen at the initial encounter for closed fracture? What would be the complete code?

9. What chapters in ICD-10-CM include codes that have the first character of H?

10. What is the only alphabetic character that is not used as the first character of an ICD-10-CM code and why?

Abbreviations

Two abbreviations are used in ICD-10-CM: Not Elsewhere Classifiable and Not Otherwise Specified.

NEC: Not Elsewhere Classifiable

An abbreviation of **not elsewhere classifiable (NEC)** is used in ICD-10-CM. This abbreviation appears in the Alphabetic Index. When NEC appears in the Alphabetic Index, it will direct the coder to the Tabular List showing an "other specified" codes description. The NEC entry appears when a specific code is not available. The NEC code usually directs the coder to an "other specified" code in the Tabular List that includes the number 8 after the decimal point.

> **EXAMPLES:**   K65.8, Other peritonitis
> N30.80, Other cystitis without hematuria

NOS: Not Otherwise Specified

The abbreviation of **not otherwise specified (NOS)** is the equivalent of unspecified. The abbreviation NOS appears in the Alphabetic Index and the Tabular List. The unspecified or NOS codes are available for use when the documentation of the condition identified by the provider in the health record does not provide enough information to assign a more specific code.

> **EXAMPLES:**   I50.9, Heart failure, unspecified
> L02.93, Carbuncle, unspecified

Punctuation

The punctuation used in ICD-10-CM is brackets, parentheses, and colons.

Brackets [ ]

Square brackets [ ] are a punctuation mark used in the Tabular List to enclose synonyms, abbreviations, alternative wording, or explanatory phrases. The terms within the brackets are presented for informational purposes. The words within the square brackets are not required to be part of the diagnostic statement to use the code.

Slanted brackets [ ] are used in the Alphabetic Index to identify manifestation codes. Manifestation codes represent the secondary condition that is present in addition to the underlying or primary disease that caused the secondary condition. Two codes are required when the patient has both the underlying disease and the secondary condition. The use of the slanted bracket in the Alphabetic Index provides sequencing direction. The code that appears in the slanted bracket is listed in the second position or follows the disease code listed directly after the diagnosis term in the Index. The diagnosis in the slanted brackets is not entered into a computer or data entry system in the italicized font. The italicized font is used to emphasize the presence of the second code that is required.

EXAMPLES: Tabular List:
> **B20, Human immunodeficiency virus [HIV] disease**

The HIV that appears in the brackets is an abbreviation for human immunodeficiency virus.
> Alphabetic Index:
> **Amyloid heart (disease) E85.4 *[I43]***

For amyloid heart disease, two codes are required in the following order or sequence:
> E85.4 Organ-limited amyloidosis
> I43 Cardiomyopathy in diseases classified elsewhere

Parentheses ( )

Parentheses are a punctuation mark that encloses supplementary words or explanatory information that may or may not be present in the statement of a diagnosis. The words within the parentheses do not affect the code assigned to the condition. Terms in parentheses are considered nonessential modifiers and appear in both the Alphabetic Index and the Tabular List.

EXAMPLE: Alphabetic Index:
> Amputee (bilateral) (old) Z89.9

The diagnosis statement could be amputee, bilateral amputee, old amputee, or old bilateral amputee, and the code would be the same for all: Z89.9.

EXAMPLE: Tabular List:
> C83.5 Lymphoblastic (diffuse) lymphoma

The diagnosis statement could be lymphoblastic lymphoma or lymphoblastic diffuse lymphoma, and the code would be the same for both: C83.5.

Colon (:)

The **colon** (:) is a punctuation mark that is used in the Tabular List after an incomplete term that needs one or more additional terms in order to be assigned to a particular code.

In the official ICD-10-CM electronic version, the colon is used with "includes" and "excludes" notes, in which the words that precede the colon are not considered complete terms and must be appended by one of the modifiers indented under the statement before the condition can be assigned the correct code. Other publishers of the printed version of the ICD-10-CM codes have not used the colon punctuation with the "includes" and "excludes" notes.

EXAMPLE: F02 Dementia in other diseases classified elsewhere
> Code first the underlying physiological condition, such as:
> > Alzheimer's (G30.-)
> > cerebral lipidosis (E75.4)
> > Creutzfeldt-Jakob disease (A81.0-)

Check Your Understanding 1.7

Answer the following questions about abbreviations and punctuations.

1. Using the Alphabetic Index and the Tabular List, what is the ICD-10-CM code for the following diagnoses? Underline the code if the code is an NEC or not elsewhere classifiable.
   a. Poxvirus
   b. Enterovirus enteritis
   c. Pyrexia

(Continued)

(Continued)

2. Using the Alphabetic Index and the Tabular List, what is the ICD-10-CM code for the following diagnoses? Underline the code if the code is an unspecified or not otherwise specified (NOS) code.
   a. Repeated falls
   b. Chronic respiratory disease
   c. Dental caries

3. What word is included in [square brackets] in the title of the code B06, and why is it included?

4. What are the two codes required to classify the diagnosis of "frontal lobe dementia," and which code is the underlying disease and which code is the manifestation?

5. What does the abbreviation NOS stand for, and what is its intent within the classification?

Other and Unspecified Codes

ICD-10-CM provides codes to be used when the documentation in the health record is more specific than any code available to be used. On the other hand, ICD-10-CM has codes that can be used when the documentation in the health record is insufficient to assign a specific code that is available in ICD-10-CM. Coders must appreciate the differences in these codes that include the terminology of other, other specified, and unspecified in the code title and know when these codes are appropriate to be used.

Other or Other Specified Codes

The terms **"other"** or **"other specified"** codes are used when the information in the health record is more descriptive than the available codes in ICD-10-CM. Alphabetic Index entries with NEC in the line designate "other" codes in the Tabular List. These Alphabetic Index entries represent specific conditions or facts about the patient for which no specific code exists, so the term is included with an "other" code.

> **EXAMPLE:**
> Alphabetic Index entry:
> Abnormal radiological examination of genitourinary organs—*see* Abnormal, diagnostic imaging
>
> Tabular List entry:
> R93.89 Abnormal finding on diagnostic imaging of other specified body structures

Unspecified Codes

A code that includes the term "**unspecified**" in the title of the code is used when the information in the health record is insufficient to assign a more specific code. For example, if the physician instead had documented mild intermittent asthma in place of simply "asthma," the use of a more specific code for the type of asthma (J45.20) could have been assigned. When the physician documents only "asthma," the unspecified asthma code (J45.909) would have been assigned.

EXAMPLE:

Alphabetic Index entry:

Asthma, asthmatic J45.909

Asthma, intermittent (mild) J45.20

Tabular List entry:

J45.909 Unspecified asthma, uncomplicated

J45.20 Mild intermittent asthma, uncomplicated

Instructional Notes

Instructional notes are included in the Tabular List to clarify information and provide additional directions for the coder. The following paragraphs describe the various types of instructional notes.

Beginning of Chapter Note

At the beginning of many chapters of ICD-10-CM, the chapter starts with a "note." The note introduces the content of the chapter and the intended use of the categories and codes within the chapter. Instructions on how to apply the codes from a particular chapter are also explained in the beginning of chapter note.

At the start of Chapter 2: Neoplasms (C00–D49), there are four beginning of chapter notes. The "Functional Activity" note explains that "all neoplasms are classified in this chapter, whether they are functionally active or not, and that an additional code from Chapter 4 may be used to identify functional activity associated with any neoplasm" (CDC 2019). Additional notes explain the concepts of morphology or histology, primary malignant neoplasms overlapping site boundaries, and malignant neoplasm of ectopic tissue.

The note at the start of Chapter 16: Certain Conditions Originating in the Perinatal Period (P00–P96), is a one-sentence statement: "codes from this chapter are for use on newborn records only, never on maternal records" (CDC 2019).

The note at the beginning of Chapter 18: Symptoms, Signs and Abnormal Clinical and Laboratory Findings, Not Elsewhere Classified is a lengthy note explaining the intent of the codes within the chapter. It further describes when the coder can expect to use one of the categories R00–R94 for

- Cases for which no more specific diagnosis can be made even after all the facts bearing on the case have been investigated

- Signs or symptoms existing at the time of initial encounter that proved to be transient and whose causes could not be determined

- Provisional diagnosis in a patient who failed to return for further investigation or care

- Cases referred elsewhere for investigation or treatment before the diagnosis was made

- Cases in which a more precise diagnosis was not available for any other reason

- Certain symptoms, for which supplementary information is provided, that represent important problems in medical care in their own right (CDC 2019)

Coders must take the opportunity to read the beginning of chapter notes to understand the intent and content of the chapters within ICD-10-CM.

Inclusion Terms

Inclusion terms are lists of medical diagnoses under some codes in the Tabular List. These are conditions for which that code is to be used. The terms may be synonyms of the code title or the terms are a list of various conditions assigned to "other specified" codes. The inclusion terms are not an exhaustive list of terms. Additional terms found only in the Alphabetic Index may also be assigned to a code.

> **EXAMPLE:** I51.7 Cardiomegaly
> Cardiac dilatation
> Cardiac hypertrophy
> Ventricular dilatation

Includes Notes

Another type of inclusion term is the **includes note** used in the ICD-10-CM Tabular List. Includes notes appear immediately under a three-character code title to further define, or give examples of, the content of the category.

> **EXAMPLE:** J44 Other chronic obstructive pulmonary disease
> Includes: asthma with chronic obstructive pulmonary disease
> chronic asthmatic (obstructive) bronchitis
> chronic bronchitis with airways obstruction
> chronic bronchitis with emphysema
> chronic emphysematous bronchitis
> chronic obstructive asthma
> chronic obstructive bronchitis
> chronic obstructive tracheobronchitis

Excludes Notes

ICD-10-CM has two types of excludes notes. Each type of note has a different definition for use. However, they are similar in intent. The **excludes note** indicates that codes excluded from each other are independent of each other. In ICD-10-CM, there are two types of excludes notes designated as either Excludes1 or Excludes2 in their title. Either or both may appear under a category, subcategory, or code.

The Excludes1 Note

The **Excludes1 note** indicates that the conditions listed after it cannot ever be used at the same time as the code above the Excludes1 note. The conditions listed in the code and in the Excludes1 note are mutually exclusive. A patient cannot have both conditions at the same time. The coder must determine, based on the documentation in the health record, which condition the patient actually has in order to assign the correct code.

> **EXAMPLE:** E06 Thyroiditis
> Excludes1: postpartum thyroiditis (O90.5)

In this example, a patient who is in the postpartum period and has thyroiditis would have the diagnosis code O90.5 assigned. Other patients who have thyroiditis and are not in the postpartum period would have the disease coded as E06.-. This is an either/or situation. Both codes could not be used on the same patient during the same episode of care.

An exception to the Excludes1 definition is the circumstance when the two conditions are unrelated to each other. If it is not clear whether the two conditions involving an Excludes1 note are related or not, query the provider. For example, code F45.8, Other somatoform disorders, has an Excludes1 note for "sleep related teeth grinding (G47.63)," because "teeth grinding" is an inclusion term under F45.8. Only one of these two codes should be assigned for teeth grinding. However psychogenic dysmenorrhea is also an inclusion term under F45.8, and a patient could have both this condition and sleep related teeth grinding. In this case, the two conditions are clearly unrelated to each other, and so it would be appropriate to report F45.8 and G47.63 together.

The Excludes2 Note

The **Excludes2 note** means that two codes are applied when both conditions are present. The conditions that appear as an Excludes2 note are not part of the code that is listed above it. A patient may have both conditions at the same time. One code does not include both conditions. When both conditions are present, two codes are applied. A coder can think of it as 2 codes are required when there is documentation for a condition present in the Excludes 2 note.

> **EXAMPLE:** G47 Sleep disorders
> Excludes2: nightmares (F51.5)
> nonorganic sleep disorders (F51.-)
> sleep terrors (F51.4)
> sleepwalking (F51.3)

In this example, a patient can have sleep disorders and nightmares at the same time. The Excludes2 note means that code G47 for sleep disorders does not include the condition of nightmares. When the patient has both a sleep disorder and nightmares, two codes must be used: a code from the category G47 and the code F51.4.

Check Your Understanding 1.8

Answer the following questions about instructional notes within ICD-10-CM.

1. In the ICD-10-CM Tabular List, locate code E78.2, Mixed hyperlipidemia. What are the additional diagnosis terms listed beneath the code title and what would they be considered?

2. Locate category N01, Rapidly progressive nephritic syndrome, in the ICD-10-CM Tabular List. What other diagnosis statements are considered included under the three-character code title N01 as examples of the content of the category?

3. Under code R00.0, Tachycardia, unspecified in the ICD-10-CM Tabular List, are the three diagnosis statements of rapid heartbeat, Sinoauricular tachycardia NOS, and Sinus [sinusal] tachycardia NOS considered inclusion terms or an includes note?

4. Under the three-character code title A23, Brucellosis, in the ICD-10-CM Tabular List, are the three diagnosis statements of malta fever, Mediterranean fever, and undulant fever considered inclusion terms or an includes note?

(Continued)

(Continued)

5. What are the chapter notes for Chapter 16: Certain Conditions Originating in the Perinatal Period (P00–P96) and what do they mean?

6. What is the intent of the two types of Excludes Notes that appear in the Tabular List of ICD-10-CM?

7. What is the intent of the Excludes1 notes in ICD-10-CM?

8. What is the intent of the Excludes2 notes in ICD-10-CM?

9. Review category code Q61, Cystic kidney disease, in the Tabular List of ICD-10-CM. Can the diagnosis of acquired cyst of kidney (code N28.1) be used with a code from category Q61? Why or why not?

10. Review category I42, Cardiomyopathy, in the Tabular List of ICD-10-CM. Can the diagnosis of ventricular hypertrophy (I51.7) be coded with the diagnosis of cardiomyopathy? Why or why not?

Etiology and Manifestation Convention

Some diseases produce another disease or a condition the patient would not have without the underlying disease. In ICD-10-CM, there is a coding convention that requires two codes for situations when one disease produces another condition. The first disease is considered the **etiology,** and the second condition that it produces is called the **manifestation**. The etiology or the first disease must be coded first. The manifestation(s) are listed as additional codes.

Code First and Use Additional Code Notes

The coding convention used in ICD-10-CM that directs the coder as to which condition is coded first is known as a **"code first" note**. The "code first" note appears in the Tabular List under the manifestation code to identify the condition usually considered the etiologic condition. The title of the manifestation code usually includes the phrase "in diseases classified elsewhere" in the title. It is important to remember that the "in diseases classified elsewhere" or "in other specified diseases classified elsewhere" codes are never first-listed or principal diagnosis codes, nor can these codes be listed as a single code. These manifestation codes also appear in *italicized fonts*. These instructions make sure the proper sequencing of codes is followed, that is, the etiology condition is coded first, followed by the manifestation code. "Code first" notes also appear under codes that are not specifically manifestation codes but may be due to an underlying cause. When there is a "code first" note and underlying cause, the underlying cause should be sequenced, if known.

There are also diseases that require two codes to completely describe the condition because all the facts of the disease are not expressed in one code. When such a condition exists, the coding convention in ICD-10-CM will remind the coder to **"use additional code"** to fully describe the condition. This also indicates the sequencing required with the code identified as the "use additional code" listed as an additional code, if known.

The etiology and manifestation conventions appear in both the Alphabetic Index and the Tabular List. In the Alphabetic Index, both conditions may be listed on one line with the etiology code listed first and the manifestation code appearing in slanted brackets after it. The code in the brackets is never listed first or used as a single code. The manifestation code must be listed second. In the Tabular List, there are notes the coder must read at the category or at the code level, that is, "code first" a certain condition or "use additional code" as an additional code to the code it appears with.

An example of the etiology or manifestation convention is dementia in Alzheimer's disease. The main term is disease, subterm is Alzheimer's, with an indent term for early onset.

> **EXAMPLE:** Early-onset Alzheimer's disease with dementia without behavioral
> disturbance
> G30.0, Alzheimer's disease with early onset
> F02.80, Dementia in other diseases classified elsewhere, without
> behavioral disturbance

In the above example, Alzheimer's disease with early onset is coded to G30.0. Under category G30, there is a directive to "use additional code to identify" dementia without behavioral disturbance (F02.80). If the patient had early-onset Alzheimer's disease with dementia without behavioral disturbance, two codes would be required: G30.0 with F02.80. Under category F02, Dementia in other diseases classified elsewhere, there is a "code first the underlying physiological condition, such as" note directing the coder to first assign a code for the type of Alzheimer's disease present with a code from category G30.

Code First

"Code first" notes appear under certain codes that are not specifically manifestation codes. But certain conditions may be due to an underlying cause. When there is a code first note and an underlying condition present, the underlying condition should be sequenced first, if known. In the following example, a patient with malignant ascites suffers from the ascites because the patient also has a malignant condition that should be coded first as it is the underlying cause of the ascites.

> **EXAMPLE:** R18.0, Malignant ascites
> Code first malignancy, such as:
> malignant neoplasm of ovary (C56.-)
> secondary malignant neoplasm of retroperitoneum and
> peritoneum (C78.6)

Code, If Applicable, a Causal Condition First

A "**Code, if applicable, a causal condition first**" note indicates that this code may be assigned as a first-listed or principal diagnosis when the causal condition is unknown or not applicable. If a causal condition is known, then the code for that condition should be sequenced as the principal or first-listed diagnosis. In the following example, if a patient has urinary retention and the cause of the urinary retention, such as an enlarged prostate, is known, the code for the enlarged prostate is coded first followed by a second code for the urinary retention.

> **EXAMPLE:** R33.8, Other retention of urine
> Code first, if applicable, any causal condition, such as:
> Enlarged prostate (N40.1)

Code Also

A "Code also" note indicates that two codes may be required to fully describe a condition. This note does not provide sequencing direction, that is, either code may be listed first depending on the circumstances of the medical visit or admission. In the following example, a patient may be seen for the purpose of receiving renal dialysis. The fact that the patient has end-stage renal disease that requires the patient to have renal dialysis is an important fact that is reported with an additional code.

> **EXAMPLE:** Z49, Encounter for care involving renal dialysis
> Code also associated end stage renal disease (N18.6)

Indiscriminate Multiple Coding

Indiscriminate multiple coding rules identify when multiple codes should or should not occur. For example, multiple codes should not be used to code irrelevant medical information, such as certain signs and symptoms that are integral to a condition. The signs and symptoms that are characteristic of an illness are not coded when the cause of the signs and symptoms are known. For example, abdominal pain is integral to acute pancreatitis and thus is not coded.

Another rule is that indiscriminate coding of conditions listed in diagnostic test reports should be avoided. When a laboratory test, x-ray, electrocardiogram, or other diagnostic test includes a finding, that condition is not coded unless the diagnosis is confirmed by the physician.

Coders must follow the Uniform Hospital Discharge Data Set (UHDDS) criteria when reporting additional diagnosis and how to avoid indiscriminate multiple coding. That is, other diagnoses are those defined as all conditions that coexist at the time of admission, that develop subsequently, or that affect the treatment received or the length of stay (LOS). Diagnoses are to be excluded that relate to an earlier episode that has no bearing on the current hospital stay. Other diagnostic reports mention conditions like atelectasis, hiatal hernia, or nonspecific cardiac arrhythmias with no other information in the record as to treatment of evaluation of these conditions. Assigning a code for such conditions would be inappropriate without first consulting with the physician for the relevance of these conditions to the present healthcare visit.

Finally, coding both a specified and an unspecified type of condition is usually not done to describe the same general condition in the same healthcare visit. For example, if the patient's diagnosis is recurrent maxillary sinusitis, code J01.01 would be assigned. It would not be necessary to also code sinusitis with code J32.9 as the type (recurrent) and the site (maxillary) are best described with the code J01.01.

Check Your Understanding 1.9

Answer the following questions related to multiple coding.

1. What is the difference between two conditions with one disease considered the *etiology* and a disease considered the *manifestation,* and how would the two conditions be coded?

2. What is the purpose of the "code also" instruction in ICD-10-CM?

3. If a code appears in an *italicized font*, what is the coder expected to know about that code?

4. In the example provided, which code is the etiology code and which code is the manifestation code? Dementia with Parkinson's disease G20 *[F02.80]*

(Continued)

(Continued)

5. Look at code A48.3, Toxic shock syndrome, in the ICD-10-CM Tabular List. What is the purpose of the note below the code title that states "Use additional code to identify the organism (B95, B96)"?

6. Under category B39, Histoplasmosis, two instructional notes appear. What are the instructions given in the two notes?

7. Look at category code R35, Polyuria, in the ICD-10-CM Tabular List. What is the purpose of the note below the code title that states "code first, if applicable, any causal condition, such as enlarged prostate (N40.1)?"

8. Look at category code S04, Injury of cranial nerve, in the ICD-10-CM Tabular List. What is the intent of the instructional note that appears under the category heading for S04?

9. Look at code C80.2, Malignant neoplasm associated with transplanted organ and the two instructional notes that appear below it. What are the instructions provided under code C80.2?

10. Look at code E10.22, Type 1 diabetes mellitus with diabetic chronic kidney disease. What is the instruction provided in the note below code E10.22?

Cross-References and Other Terms Used in ICD-10-CM

Cross-references such as « see » and « see also » are used as directions for the coder to look elsewhere in the Alphabetic Index before assigning a code. Other terms are used to explain the relationships between the diagnoses and conditions included in both the Alphabetic Index and the Tabular List. To assign diagnosis codes accurately, a thorough understanding of the ICD-10-CM cross-references and other terms is essential.

And

The term **"and"** is interpreted to mean "and" or "or" when it appears in a code title. The term "and" means the patient may have one or the other of the statements included in the code title. In the following example, code Z51.1 is used if the patient's encounter is for the purpose of receiving antineoplastic chemotherapy or for the purpose of receiving antineoplastic immunotherapy. If the patient is receiving both chemotherapy and immunotherapy, the code is also appropriate to use.

> **EXAMPLE:** Z51.1, Encounter for antineoplastic chemotherapy and immunotherapy

With

The term **"with"** or "in" in a diagnostic statement means that there are two conditions present. The term "with" or "in" may be used by the physician to acknowledge two conditions exist, but the physician may also use other phrases such as "associated with" or "due to" to describe the presence of the two conditions. The classification presumes a causal relationship between the two conditions linked by these terms in the Alphabetic Index or Tabular List.

The ICD-10-CM phrase of "with" or "in" also applies in the Alphabetic Index or in the Tabular List in an instructional note. For conditions not specifically linked by these relational terms in the classification or when a guideline requires that a linkage between two conditions be explicitly documented, provider documentation must link the conditions in order to code them as related.

In the Alphabetic Index, the term "with" will appear immediately following the main term or subterm.

In the Tabular List, the term "with" appearing in a code title means that two conditions (condition A with condition B) must be present in the patient to use that particular code.

> **EXAMPLE:** Tabular List:
> B15.0, Hepatitis A with hepatic coma

In this example, code B15.0 presents the fact that the patient has two conditions: hepatitis A and hepatic coma. Here, "with" means both conditions exist at the same time.

> **EXAMPLE:** Alphabetic Index:
> Bronchiolitis
> with
> bronchospasm or obstruction J21.9
> influenza, flu, grippe—see Influenza, with, respiratory manifestations NEC
> chemical (chronic) J68.4
> acute J68.0
> chronic (fibrosing)(obliterative) J44.9
> due to
> external agent—see Bronchitis, acute, due to

In this example, the condition of bronchiolitis with bronchospasm is found in the Alphabetic Index under the main term "bronchiolitis." The "with" connecting term, to identify that bronchospasm also exists, appears immediately under the main term and before the other terms that appear in alphabetic order such as chemical, chronic, or due to.

See and See Also

In ICD-10-CM, the "see" direction is used to instruct the coder to reference another term in the Alphabetic Index that provides more complete information about the condition to be coded. The "see" note also appears with an anatomical site main term to direct the coder to locate the disease present at that anatomic site in the Alphabetic Index.

> **EXAMPLE:** Angina with atherosclerotic heart disease—see Arteriosclerosis, coronary (artery)

This "see" direction advises the coder to use the term of arteriosclerosis to find more complete listing of the options for coding angina with atherosclerotic heart disease.

> **EXAMPLE:** Leg—see (the) condition

The anatomic term "leg" is not a medical diagnosis. Therefore, if the main term of "leg" is located in the Alphabetic Index, the same line includes the phrase "see condition." Instead, a condition affecting the leg, such as traumatic fracture, should be sought out.

The cross-reference note "see also" in the Alphabetic Index follows a main term if the coder should reference another term in the Index for additional information. The instruction is intended to help the coder find the most information available in the Alphabetic Index when the coder may not identify all the options that could be used. However, it is not necessary to follow the "see also" note when the original main term provides all the necessary information to assign a complete code. The sequencing of codes with a "see also" note depends on the circumstances of the encounter.

> **EXAMPLE:** Alphabetic Index:
> Bruise (skin surface intact) (see also Contusion)

In this example, no codes are available under the main term of bruise that occurs on the skin. The more appropriate medical term of contusion should be referenced to identify the many anatomic sites on which a bruise may be found.

Connecting Words

Connecting words or connecting terms are subterms in the Alphabetic Index that appear after a main term to indicate a relationship between the main term and an associated condition or etiology.

- Associated with
- Complicated by
- Due to
- During
- Following
- In
- Secondary to
- With
- With mention of
- Without

Code Assignment and Clinical Criteria

The connecting words "with" and "without" appear in both the Alphabetic Index and in the Tabular List in code titles. "With" and "without" connecting terms are sequenced before all other subterms in the Alphabetic Index but may also appear with the other subterms in alphabetic order.

The assignment of a diagnosis code is based on the provider's diagnostic statement that the condition exists. The provider's statement that the patient has a particular condition is sufficient. Code assignment is not based on the clinical criteria used by the provider to establish the diagnosis.

Check Your Understanding 1.10

Answer the following questions regarding cross-reference and other terms used in ICD-10-CM.

1. What is the purpose of the cross-reference terms in ICD-10-CM, and where is the coder likely to find the cross-reference terms?

2. How should the word "and" used in a diagnosis code title be interpreted by the coder?

3. How is the term "with" used in ICD-10-CM for diagnosis coding, and where does the term "with" appear in the classification system?

4. Refer to the diagnosis of Asthma in the ICD-10-CM Alphabetic Index. What other condition must be present with Asthma in order to assign the diagnosis code of J44.9?

5. What is the purpose of the cross-reference terms of "see" and "see also" in ICD-10-CM, and where will the coder find the terms of "see" and "see also"?

6. Using the Alphabetic Index to ICD-10-CM, what cross-reference is included for the coding of the diagnosis of buttonhole deformity of the finger?

7. The main term of "dysplasia" appears in the ICD-10-CM Alphabetic Index with a cross-reference note of "see also Anomaly." If the provider documented the diagnosis of perinatal bronchopulmonary dysplasia, would the coder be obligated to refer to the main term of anomaly in the Alphabetic Index in order to code perinatal bronchopulmonary dysplasia?

8. The coder is provided with the diagnosis of enchondroma to code. Using the main term of enchondroma, how is the coder directed to locate the appropriate code for this condition?

9. What is the purpose of connecting terms in ICD-10-CM, such as associated with, complicated by, or due to?

10. Locate the diagnosis of "female infertility" in the ICD-10-CM Alphabetic Index. What two connecting terms appear as subterms under the main term of infertility in the Alphabetic Index, and what is the purpose of including the connecting terms to code these conditions?

General Coding Guidelines

There are basic concepts and rules that a coder must understand in order to assign ICD-10-CM codes accurately and completely. These general coding guidelines describe how to locate a code in ICD-10-CM and how to apply all the necessary codes to fully describe a patient's condition and reason for health services.

Locating a Code in ICD-10-CM

The coder must use both the Alphabetic Index and Tabular List when locating and assigning a code. The first step in coding is to locate the main term and applicable subterms in the Alphabetic Index. Then, the code found in the Alphabetic Index is verified in the Tabular List. The coder must read and be guided by the instructional notations that appear in both the Alphabetic Index and the Tabular List.

The Alphabetic Index does not always provide the complete code or applicable notes. Every code listed in the Alphabetic Index must be reviewed in the Tabular List. Selection of the complete code, including laterality and any applicable seventh character, can only be done in the

Tabular List. If additional characters are required, a dash (-) at the end of the Alphabetic Index entry is present. The coder then uses the Tabular List to identify what additional characters are necessary to complete the code to fully describe the patient's condition. Even if it appears that a complete code is included in the Alphabetic Index, it is mandatory for the coder to review the code in the Tabular List for all the instructional notes that may require additional coding.

Level of Detail in Coding

Diagnosis codes are to be used and reported with the highest number of characters available. Codes with three characters are included in ICD-10-CM as the heading of a category of codes. A category may be further subdivided by the use of fourth, fifth, or sixth characters to provide greater detail. A seventh character may be applicable for certain codes. A three-character code is to be used only if it is not further subdivided, that is, there are no applicable fourth, fifth, sixth, or seventh characters to be used. A code is invalid if it is not coded to the full number of characters required for that code. Remember, the use of the placeholder X can be utilized in situations where a seventh character is required.

Code or codes from A00.0 through T88.9, Z00–Z99.8

The appropriate code or codes from A00.0 through T88.9, Z00-Z99.8 must be used to identify diagnoses, symptoms, conditions, problems, complaints or other reason(s) for the encounter/visit.

Signs and Symptoms

Codes that describe symptoms and physical signs are perfectly acceptable for reporting when the sign or symptom is what the physician knows for certain about the patient at the conclusion of the encounter. There are occasions when no definitive diagnosis can be made, even after investigation or study of the patient's presenting signs and symptoms. Signs and symptoms may be transient and disappear before the physician can identify their cause. A patient may come to a physician for treatment of a sign or symptom but fail to return for further investigation and it is not determined what caused the problem. Patients with certain signs and symptoms may be referred to another physician or treatment center for investigation before the physician can identify the cause of the symptom or sign. In all of these situations and the other scenarios described at the start of Chapter 18: Symptoms, Signs and Abnormal Clinical Findings, Not Elsewhere Classified (R00–R99), the assignment of a sign or symptom code is appropriate. Most but not all signs and symptoms appear in Chapter 18. Signs and symptoms applicable to certain body systems appear in the body system chapter of ICD-10-CM, for example, ear pain is assigned a code from ICD-10-CM Chapter 8: Diseases of the Ear and Mastoid Process.

Conditions That Are an Integral Part of a Disease Process

Signs and symptoms that are associated routinely with a disease process should not be assigned as additional codes, unless other instructions exist. Once the reason for the signs and symptoms are known and these complaints routinely occur with that particular disease process, the signs and symptoms are not coded. For example, abdominal pain is a common symptom of acute appendicitis and is not coded when the reason for abdominal pain is attributed to the appendicitis. The coder's knowledge of disease processes is essential to coding, especially to avoid coding the unnecessary signs and symptoms codes.

Conditions That Are Not an Integral Part of a Disease Process

Additional signs and symptoms that may not be associated routinely with a disease process should be coded when present. Again, the coder's knowledge of disease pathology is essential to coding. The coder needs to know when the physician describes accompanying signs and symptoms with a disease whether to code these conditions or not. For example, if a patient with a skull fracture is in a coma, the coma is assigned an additional code. Not every patient with a skull fracture will be in a coma. This additional detail about the patient's condition that is not present routinely with the injury or disease is valuable information concerning the patient's severity of their illness.

Multiple Coding for a Single Condition

Multiple codes may be required to code a disease that includes multiple disease processes or factors. As noted in the prior section, ICD-10-CM uses such conventions as "use additional code" in the Tabular List to identify a condition that is not part of the code it appears with. Another example when a "use additional code" note appears is with an infectious disease code that does not identify the specific bacterial or viral organism that caused it, but that organism can be identified with another code.

Other requirements for multiple coding of a single condition or a condition that includes multiple parts can be identified in ICD-10-CM with such notes as "code first," code, if applicable, a causal condition first, and "code also."

Acute and Chronic Conditions

If a patient has both the acute form and the chronic form of one disease, the coder must identify in the Alphabetic Index if there are separate entries at the same indentation level. If there are two separate lines in the Alphabetic Index for acute and chronic forms, then both codes are assigned. The acute or subacute code is sequenced first, followed by the chronic code for the disease. For example, the physician may describe the patient's condition as acute and chronic pancreatitis. The Alphabetic Index includes but is not limited to the following entries:

```
Pancreatitis
Acute (without necrosis or infections) K85.90
  with necrosis K85.91
  alcoholic induced K85.20
  biliary K85.10
  drug induced K85.30
  gallstone K85.10
  idiopathic K85.00
  specified NEC K85.80
Chronic (infectious) K86.1
  alcohol induced K86.0
  recurrent K86.1
  relapsing K86.1
```

The code for acute pancreatitis, K85.90, is listed first with an additional code for chronic pancreatitis, K86.1, as both conditions are listed in the Alphabetic Index at the same indentation level.

Combination Codes

A combination code is a single code used to classify two diagnoses. A combination code may also represent a diagnosis with an associated secondary process or manifestation. Finally, a combination code can be a diagnosis with an associated complication.

Combination codes are identified by referring to subterm entries in the Alphabetic Index that identify conditions that are associated with or due to each other. Combination codes are also identified by reading all the includes and excludes notes in the Tabular List. Combination codes are only assigned when the one code fully identifies the condition.

Multiple coding should not occur when the classification provides a combination code that clearly identifies all of the elements documented in the diagnosis. An additional code should be used as a secondary code only when the combination code lacks necessary specificity in describing the manifestation or complication. There may be a third condition that exists with two other conditions that requires an additional code. For example, a patient may have acute bronchitis with bronchiectasis and tobacco use. Two codes are required: J47.0, a combination code for bronchiectasis with acute bronchitis, and Z72.0, the code for tobacco use.

Check Your Understanding 1.11

Answer the following questions concerning general coding guidelines.

1. What is the first step a coder must take to assign a diagnosis code in ICD-10-CM?

2. If diagnosis codes are to be used and reported with the highest number of characters available, are there any instances where the three character category codes are considered valid codes?

3. Which of the five diagnosis codes listed below are valid ICD-10-CM diagnosis codes with the level of detail provided to describe the condition?
   a. K80.8, Other cholelithiasis
   b. O82, Encounter for cesarean delivery without indication
   c. P05.0, Newborn light for gestational age
   d. B20, Human immunodeficiency virus [HIV] disease
   e. I63.21, Cerebral infarction due to unspecified occlusion or stenosis of vertebral arteries

4. True or false: ICD-10-CM diagnosis codes for physical signs and symptoms are acceptable for reporting when the sign or symptom is what the physician knows for certain about the patient at the conclusion of the encounter. Provide an explanation for your answer.

5. True or false: Signs and symptoms that are associated routinely with a disease process should be assigned as additional codes, unless other instructions exist. Provide and explanation for your answer.

6. True or false: Additional signs and symptoms that may not be routinely associated with a disease process should be coded when present. Provide an explanation for your answer.

(Continued)

(Continued)

7. Which of the following diagnosis statements would likely require the additional coding of the signs or symptoms present with the disease?
   a. Abdominal pain due to acute appendicitis
   b. Burning with urination due to a urinary tract infection
   c. Respiratory failure due to heroin overdose
   d. Headache due to a classical migraine
   e. Cardiac arrest due to underlying cardiac condition

8. Can a condition be coded as both acute and chronic? If no, why not. If yes, when is it considered appropriate, and which code should be sequenced first?

9. True or False: Multiple coding should still occur when the classification provides a combination code that clearly identifies all of the elements documented in the diagnosis. Provide an explanation for your answer.

10. Examine the following diagnosis codes (A–E) in the Alphabetic Index of ICD-10-CM. Which of the following diagnosis statements represents a combination code?
    a. J03.00, Acute streptococcal tonsillitis, unspecified
    b. K40.41, Unilateral inguinal hernia, with gangrene, recurrent
    c. L10.5, Drug-induced pemphigus
    d. N80.3, Endometriosis of pelvic peritoneum
    e. Q05.2, Lumbar spina bifida with hydrocephalus and paraplegia

Sequela or Late Effects

A condition that is produced by another illness or an injury and remains after the acute phase of the illness or injury is referred to as a **sequela**. There is no time period as to when a sequela must appear or be present. The condition can be identified at the same time as the original disease, such as dysphagia that occurs with a cerebral infarction. Other conditions may occur a period of time after the acute phase of the illness is over, for example, the scar that remains after a burn heals.

Two codes are required for coding sequela conditions. The first reported code is the condition that exists at present or the sequela. The second code is the original condition identified as the cause of the present condition. However, the code for the acute phase of an illness that led to the sequela is never used with a code for the late effect.

There are exceptions to the above guideline:

- The code for the sequela is followed by a manifestation code identified in the Tabular List and title.

- The sequela code has been expanded at the fourth, fifth, or sixth character levels to include the manifestations.

The main term "sequela" must be referenced in the Alphabetic Index to identify if a combination code for the sequela and the underlying cause exists. In the Tabular List, an instructional note may appear under these category codes to "code first condition resulting from (sequela of)" that particular category. In the Alphabetic Index, following the main term "sequela," is the direction term "see also condition" to remind the coder that other entries in the Alphabetic Index are also applicable to coding of these conditions.

The following is a step-by-step example of how to accurately code a sequela and the underlying condition:

EXAMPLE: A physician documents the following condition: scar of the skin on the face due to previous third-degree burn of the face. The coder must recognize the condition present today is the scar and the cause of the scar was the previous third-degree burn on the face.

First the coder accesses the term "scar" in the Alphabetic Index as follows:

> Alphabetic Index:
> Scar, scarring (see also Cicatrix) L90.5
> Cicatrix, skin L90.5

Then, the coder must confirm the code in the Tabular List as L90.5. There are no further instructions in the Tabular List. The code does not include any anatomic locations so all scars of the skin are coded here. However, the coder must know to identify the cause of the scar having been stated as due to a previous burn on the face.

The coder must translate that fact to the word "sequela" to identify the burn and use the Alphabetic Index again as follows:

> Alphabetic Index:
> Sequela, burn and corrosion—code to injury with seventh character S
> Burn, face—see Burn, head
> Burn, head, third degree, T20.30

Again, the coder must access the Tabular List to review the entry of code T20.30 to determine if more characters are required to complete the coding assignment. T20.30 requires a seventh character of S for sequela; therefore, a placeholder character of X is needed in the sixth position, that is, T20.30XS.

After following these steps, the coder concludes that the coding of scar of the skin of the face due to previous third-degree burn of the face is coded as L90.5 and T20.30XS.

Impending or Threatened Condition

Physicians may describe a patient's condition as impending or threatened, such as impending delirium tremens or threatened abortion. The coder needs to determine if the condition actually did or did not occur. The ICD-10-CM classification and guidelines give directions to the coder on how to interpret this terminology used by physicians. According to the *ICD-10-CM Official Guidelines for Coding and Reporting*, Guideline I.B.11, impending or threatened conditions are coded as follows:

If a condition described at the time of discharge as "impending" or "threatened," it should be coded as follows:

1. If the condition did occur, code as a confirmed diagnosis.

2. If the condition did not occur, reference the Alphabetic Index to determine if the condition has a subentry term for "impending" or "threatened" and also reference main term entries for "Impending" and for "Threatened."

   a. If the subterms are listed, assign the given code.
   b. If the subterms are not listed, code the existing underlying condition(s) and not the condition described as impending or threatened (CDC 2019).

Reporting Same Diagnosis Code More Than Once

According to the *ICD-10-CM Official Guidelines for Coding and Reporting*, Guideline I.B.12, "each unique ICD-10-CM diagnosis code may be reported only once for an encounter. This applies to bilateral conditions when there are no distinct codes identifying laterality or two different conditions classified to the same ICD-10-CM diagnosis code" (CDC 2019). For example, if a patient had cellulitis on both sides on the face, the diagnosis code of L03.211, Cellulitis of face, would be reported once as there are no distinct codes for cellulitis of the right face or left face.

Laterality

 Some ICD-10-CM diagnosis codes include laterality or whether the condition exists on the right or left side of the body. For bilateral sites, the final character of the code indicates laterality. An unspecified side code is available for use if the side of the body is not identified in the health record. If no bilateral code is provided and the condition is bilateral, the coder must assign separate codes for both the left and right side. For example, if a patient had a right ovarian carcinoma, then code C56.1, Malignant neoplasm of right ovary would be used. Separate codes exist of the left ovary (C56.2) and unspecified ovary (C56.9). Another example of laterality indicated by the codes occurs when ICD-10-CM includes the option of unilateral, bilateral, or unspecified. For example, if the physician documents small kidney of unknown origin on the left side, code N27.0, Small kidney, unilateral, would be assigned. Other options in category N27 include code N27.1, small kidney, bilateral, and N27.9, small kidney, unspecified. The *ICD-10-CM Official Guidelines for Coding and Reporting* addresses the subject of laterality in the code in Guideline I.B.13.

Documentation by Clinicians Other Than the Patient's Provider

In the *ICD-10-CM Official Guidelines for Coding and Reporting*, Guideline I.B.14 describes code assignment based on the documentation by patient's provider with a few exceptions, such body mass index (BMI) and depth of non-pressure chronic ulcers:

> For the body mass index (BMI), depth of non-pressure chronic ulcers and pressure ulcer stage codes, coma scale, and NIH stroke scale (NIHSS) codes, the code assignment may be made based on the medical record documentation from clinicians who are not the patient's provider (such as a physician or other qualified healthcare practitioner legally accountable for establishing the patient's diagnosis). This information is typically documented by other clinicians involved in the care of the patient, for example, a dietitian documents the BMI and nurses often document the pressure ulcer stages. However, the associated diagnosis (such as overweight, obesity or pressure ulcer) must be documented by the patient's provider. If there is conflicting medical record documentation, either from the same clinician or different clinicians, the patient's attending provider should be queried for clarification.

> Guideline I.B.14 is guidance for social determinants of health, such as information found in categories Z55-Z65:

> Persons with potential health hazards related to socioeconomic and psychosocial circumstances, code assignment may be based on medical record documentation from clinicians involved in the care of the patient who are not the patient's provider since this information represents social information, rather than medical diagnosis (CDC 2019).

The BMI, coma scale, and NIHSS codes **and categories Z55–Z65** should only be reported as secondary diagnoses. As with all other secondary diagnosis codes, the BMI codes should only be assigned when they meet the definition of a reportable additional diagnosis (CDC 2019).

Syndromes

Guideline I.B.15 in the *ICD-10-CM Official Guidelines for Coding and Reporting* describes the coding of named syndromes.

> The coder should follow the Alphabetic Index guidance when coding named syndromes. In the absence of Alphabetic Index guidance, the coder should assign codes for the documented manifestations of the syndrome. Additional codes for manifestations that are not an integral part of the disease process may also be assigned when the condition does not have a unique code (CDC 2019).

For example, ICD-10-CM diagnosis code I82.0, Budd-Chiari syndrome, is a known disorder of hepatic circulation marked by occlusion of the hepatic veins that leads to liver enlargement, ascites, extensive development of collateral vessels, and severe portal hypertension (*Dorland's Medical Dictionary* 2018). One code identified the multiple conditions that are known as Budd-Chiari syndrome, and the individual problems are not coded separately. However, another example of named syndrome is the CHARGE syndrome that the ICD-10-CM Alphabetic Index presents the code Q89.8, Other specified congenital malformations. However, in the Tabular List, there is a "use additional" code note to identify all associated manifestation. CHARGE syndrome is a syndrome of associated defects, including coloboma of the eye, heart anomaly, choanal atresia, growth retardation, and genital and ear anomalies. Facial palsy, cleft palate, and dysphagia are often present (*Dorland's Medical Dictionary* 2018). Because code Q89.8 is not strictly "CHARGE syndrome" but instead "other specified congenital malformations," the coder must assign individual codes for each of the conditions or malformations present in the patient diagnosed with CHARGE syndrome.

Documentation of Complications of Care

In Guideline I.B.16 of the *ICD-10-CM Official Guidelines for Coding and Reporting*, the coder is given direction on how and when to assign complication codes:

> Code assignment is based on the provider's documentation of the relationship between the condition and the care or procedure, unless otherwise instructed by the classification. The guideline extends to any complication of care, regardless of the chapter the code is located in. It is important to note that not all conditions that occur during or following medical care or surgery are classified as complications. There must be a cause-and-effect relationship between the care and the condition, and an indication in the documentation that it is a complication. The physician should be queried or asked for clarification if the complication is not clearly documented (CDC 2019).

The important message here is that the physician must document the cause-and-effect relationship between the medical and surgical care provided and the condition that exists after the care is provided. For example, the surgeon may document the patient has a fever the day after a surgical procedure. The coder cannot assume the diagnosis of "postoperative fever" should be coded because the fever is present during the postoperative period. Fever is often expected for a time period after a surgical procedure. The physician would have to identify the fever as a complication with the documentation of fever due to the procedure.

Borderline Diagnosis

When the physician uses the adjective of « borderline » with a diagnosis, the coder must consider the meaning of the word borderline by the physician. If the physician documents a "borderline" diagnosis at the time of discharge, the physician is likely to mean the patient has the condition but possibly a milder form of the disease than most people would likely experience. A "borderline" diagnosis documented at discharge should be coded as a confirmed condition, such as borderline hyperlipidemia. The coder should confirm that the Alphabetic Index entry for hyperlipidemia does not include a subterm "borderline" that provides a specific code. On the other hand, the term "borderline" may be a specific type of a condition, for example, borderline personality disorder. This is a specific type of a personality disorder. The Alphabetic Index includes an entry of "disorder, personality, borderline" with a specific code of F60.3 provided. In general, the classification system does not represent the severity of a condition present in the patient but rather that the condition is present. There are exceptions to this statement. For example, the diagnosis codes for asthma specify mild, moderate, and severe states. Whenever the coder is uncertain as to the intent of the term "borderline" used by a physician in the documentation of diagnoses, the coder should query the physician to clarify the diagnosis. Guideline I.B.17 of the *ICD-10-CM Official Guidelines for Coding and Reporting*, addresses the coding of diagnoses labeled as "borderline" by the physician in the patient's health documentation.

Use of Sign, Symptom, and Unspecified Codes

In Guideline I.B.18 of the *ICD-10-CM Official Guidelines for Coding and Reporting*, a statement is made that sign, symptom, and unspecified codes have acceptable, even necessary, uses in coding today. There are occasions when the best information known about a patient is the physical sign or subjective symptom that he or she describes. Every encounter should be coded to the highest level of certainty known about the patient. If the most certain information is the patient complains of abdominal pain but the source of the abdominal pain has not been determined, the best description of that patient at the time is to assign the diagnosis code of abdominal pain for that visit.

The guideline continues by stating, "If a definitive diagnosis has not been established at the end of the encounter, it is appropriate to report codes for sign(s) and/or symptom(s) in lieu of a definitive diagnosis" (CDC 2019). In addition, the guideline states, "When sufficient clinical information isn't known or available about a particular health condition to assign a more specific code, it is acceptable to report the appropriate 'unspecified' code."

The guideline also states, "Unspecified codes should be reported when they are the codes that most accurately reflect what is known about the patient's condition at the time of the encounter. It would be inappropriate to select a specific code that is not supported by the health record documentation or conduct medically unnecessary diagnostic testing in order to determine a more specific code" (CDC 2019).

Coding for Healthcare Encounters in Hurricane Aftermath

In Guideline I.B.19 of the *ICD-10-CM Official Guidelines for Coding and Reporting*, guidance has been added for use of external cause of morbidity codes, sequencing of external causes of morbidity codes, uses of other external causes of morbidity codes, and Z code use for healthcare encounters in a hurricane aftermath. An external cause of morbidity code should be assigned to identify the causes of the injury(ies) incurred as a result of the hurricane. These are considered supplemental to the other ICD-10-CM codes and are not considered as a principal diagnosis; the appropriate injury code should be sequenced first. These codes are not to be assigned to medical conditions when no injury, adverse effect, or poisoning is involved. For the purpose of capturing complete and accurate ICD-10-CM data in the aftermath of the hurricane, a healthcare setting should be considered as any location where medical care is provided by licensed health professionals (CDC 2019). The guideline further identifies that codes for cataclysmic events, such as a hurricane, take priority over all other external cause codes except for child and adult abuse and terrorism and should be sequenced before other external cause injury codes (CDC 2019). Z codes may further explain the reasons for presenting for healthcare services such as transfers between healthcare facilities.

Check Your Understanding 1.12

Answer the following questions.

1. Are codes assigned to conditions described as "impending" or "threatened"? Explain your answer in detail.

2. How is a condition referred to as a sequela coded in ICD-10-CM?

3. Code the following condition: Mild protein–calorie malnutrition due to the late effects of rickets.

4. Code the following condition: Borderline hypertension

5. How often can the same diagnosis code be reported for a patient's condition?

6. If a patient has a bilateral condition, that is, the same condition that occurs on the right and left side of the body, how is this condition coded?

7. What three conditions can be coded based on the documentation of clinicians who are not the patient's physician or provider according to the *ICD-10-CM Official Guidelines for Coding and Reporting*, Guideline I.B.14?

8. Code the following conditions as documented by the physician (morbid obesity) and the dietitian (BMI of 45.0) in an adult.

9. When a patient receives an encounter for care in a hurricane aftermath for the maintenance of a chronic condition only, are external cause of morbidity codes applied?

10. True or false: A coder can assume the diagnosis of "postoperative fever" when the documentation identifies a fever occurred a short period of time after a surgical procedure. Explain your answer.

Basic Steps in ICD-10-CM Coding

Chapter 1 has explained the characteristics of ICD-10-CM, how the ICD-10-CM classification system is organized, and how to use the *ICD-10-CM Official Guidelines for Coding and Reporting*. In order to take the first step toward becoming an accurate and complete coder of diagnoses, follow the basic steps in this chapter when assigning a code in ICD-10-CM. To code each disease or condition completely and accurately, the coder should:

1. Identify all main terms included in the diagnostic statement

2. Locate each main term in the Alphabetic Index

3. Refer to any subterms indented under the main term. The subterms form individual line entries and describe essential differences by site, etiology, or clinical type

4. Follow the instructions (see, see also) provided in the Alphabetic Index if the needed code is not located under the first main entry consulted

5. Verify the code selected in the Tabular List

6. Read and be guided by any instructional terms in the Tabular List

7. Assign codes to their highest level of specificity, up to a total of seven characters if applicable

8. Continue coding the diagnostic statement until all the component elements are fully identified

ICD-10-CM Review Exercises: Chapter 1

Assign the correct ICD-10-CM diagnosis codes to the following exercises.

1. Acute recurrent nonsuppurative otitis media of the left ear

_____

2. Morbid obesity with a BMI of 44 in an adult male

_____

3. Cervical spine pain

_____

4. Left eye moderate stage primary open-angle glaucoma

_____

5. Streptococcal pneumonia

_____

6. Toxic nodular goiter

_____

7. Extra thyroid gland

_____

8. Osteoarthrosis, primary of right ankle

_____

9. Acute tracheobronchitis with bronchospasm (age 16)

_____

10. Arteriosclerotic heart disease of native coronary artery with angina pectoris

_____

ICD-10-CM Review Exercises: Chapter 1 *(continued)*

11. Angiodysplasia of the colon with hemorrhage

    _____

12. Prenatal care, normal first pregnancy, second trimester

    _____

13. Traumatic comminuted fracture (non-displaced fracture) of left femur involving the intertrochanteric section, initial visit (Use 7th character option for correct coding)

    _____

14. Nephritis due to systemic lupus erythematosus

    _____

15. Hypertensive systolic heart failure

    _____

16. Acute hepatitis C with hepatic coma

    _____

17. Irregular astigmatism of both eyes

    _____

18. Benign carcinoid tumor of the appendix

    _____

19. Enlarged prostate with urinary obstruction

    _____

20. Acute lymphoblastic leukemia in remission

    _____

References

Centers for Disease Control and Prevention (CDC), National Center for Health Statistics (NCHS). 2019. *International Classification of Diseases, Tenth Revision, Clinical Modification (ICD-10-CM).* http://www.cdc.gov/nchs/icd/icd10cm.htm.

Dorland's Elsevier. 2018. *Dorland's Medical Dictionary Online.* https://www.dorlandsonline.com/dorland/definition?id=100103943&searchterm=Budd-Chiarisyndrome.

Mosby. 2017. *Mosby's Pocket Dictionary of Medicine, Nursing, and Health Professions*, 8th ed. St. Louis: Mosby, Inc.

Chapter 2

Introduction to ICD-10-PCS

Learning Objectives

At the conclusion of this chapter, you should be able to do the following:

- Identify the design characteristics of ICD-10-PCS

- Define the general design principles of ICD-10-PCS

- Describe the code structure of the ICD-10-PCS codes

- Explain how the ICD-10-PCS Index is organized and used

- Illustrate the general organization of the ICD-10-PCS code tables

- Describe how a code is constructed using the Index and Tables

- Identify the seven characters that compose an ICD-10-PCS code

- List the 16 sections in the Medical and Surgical and Medical and Surgical–related section of codes

- Apply the concept of the root operation used in ICD-10-PCS

- Specify the options to describe the approach used to perform a procedure

- Identify the 9 groups and 31 root operations

- Apply the seven different approaches used in the root operations

- Demonstrate how to code multiple procedures

- Assign procedure codes using the ICD-10-PCS system

Key Terms

Characters
Completeness
Expandability
ICD-10-PCS
Index

Multiaxial
Standardized terminology
Tables
Values

Introduction to ICD-10-PCS

ICD-10-PCS was implemented on October 1, 2015, and is used for reporting inpatient procedures on electronic healthcare claims transactions. **ICD-10-PCS** stands for *International Classification of Diseases, Tenth Revision, Procedure Coding System.*

ICD-10-PCS is a unique procedure classification system used in the United States. In 1992, CMS began the process of replacing ICD-9-CM Volume 3 by funding a research project to design a new procedure coding system. In 1995, CMS awarded 3M Health Information Systems a three-year contract to complete the development of the new ICD-10-PCS procedure coding system. The most recent version of the ICD-10-PCS can be located on the CMS website.

Characteristics of the ICD-10 Procedure Coding System

ICD-10-PCS is a multiaxial seven-character alphanumeric code structure. ICD-10-PCS provides a unique code for all substantially different procedures and allows new procedures to be easily incorporated as new codes. It is exclusively designed for the United States.

Development of ICD-10-PCS

The report *Development of the ICD-10 Procedure Coding System (ICD-10-PCS)* identified four attributes that were included in the development of ICD-10-PCS: Completeness, Expandability, Multiaxial, and Standardized Terminology (Averill et al. 2016).

Completeness

The objective of **completeness** means there should be a unique code for all substantially different procedures. Different procedures performed on different body parts with differing approaches will have a unique code. To meet this objective, there are more than 78,000 ICD-10-PCS codes (CMS 2018). For example, the ICD-10-PCS code 0SR9049 completely describes the procedure of a right hip replacement performed through an open approach using a ceramic on polyethylene synthetic substitute for the hip joint that was cemented in place.

Expandability

When new procedures are developed, the structure of ICD-10-PCS should allow a code for the new procedure to be easily identified. The concept of **expandability** means the structure of the codes allows for changes to be made easily by adding values as needed or using existing values to identify new procedures. For example, if a procedure is developed in the future to place a drainage device in the subcutaneous tissue and fascia of the pelvic region, the character of 0 could be added to the device column on table 0JX, transfer procedures on subcutaneous tissue and fascia.

Multiaxial

ICD-10-PCS consists of independent characters. **Multiaxial** is a term to describe the ability of a nomenclature to express the meaning of a concept across several axes. Each individual axis retains its meaning across broad ranges of codes as much as possible. For example, the third character is the root operation to describe the objective of the procedure. In some sections, the title of the third character changes; for example, in radiology, the third character is "root type" but it still reflects the objective of the procedure.

Standardized Terminology

ICD-10-PCS includes singular definitions of the terminology used. The **standardized terminology** in ICD-10-PCS means each term has a specific meaning or definition. The coding system tries to be as specific as possible with only limited options for "not elsewhere classified" (NEC) procedures. There are limited NEC options to allow for updates to the system as needed between updates. If the coder finds there is a new device being used during the year and there is not a device value for that particular procedure, the coder can use the value of "other device" until a possible update for that device is added when the coding system is updated on an annual basis.

General Development Principles

Four principles were incorporated in the development of ICD-10-PCS according to the report *2016 Development of the ICD-10 Procedure Coding System (ICD-10-PCS):*

- The first principle is there is *no diagnosis or reason for the procedure* included in the ICD-10-PCS procedure code description. The reason the procedure is being performed is not important for coding of the procedures. The ICD-10-CM diagnosis code identifies the diagnosis being treated. The ICD-10-PCS code identifies what procedure is being performed according to the objective of the procedure, the approach, device used, and so forth.

- A second principle was to limit the *"not otherwise specified" (NOS) codes* available in ICD-10-PCS. The coder needs facts about the procedure in order to code it. There is no option for the coder to use an unspecified value for a character in the ICD-10-PCS code in the event the documentation about the procedure is incomplete. The operative report prepared by the physician is essential; in fact, it is hard to imagine how a procedure would be coded without an operative report. The coder needs, at a minimum, the objective or root operation of the procedure, the body system and body part involved, the approach, and any device left in place to perform the procedure.

- Similarly, there is a *limited use of NEC codes* in ICD-10-PCS as the third stated principle in the development of the procedure coding system. NEC values in the PCS Tables are identified as the "other" specified type. For example, in the Medical and Surgical section, there is a value for "other" for the device character when another type of device is used than specified by the device values listed on the table. In the Imaging section, there is a value for "other" for the type of contrast used that is not high osmolar or low osmolar contrast material. In the Physical Rehabilitation section, there is a value for "other equipment" to identify when something different than the specified type of equipment is used. Otherwise, the values specifically identify the significant components of the procedure in the ICD-10-PCS codes.

- Finally, as the fourth principle states, *the system allows for all procedures to be coded* with ICD-10-PCS. Each variation of a procedure can be identified with the specific values available for the body part involved, the approach used, any devices left in place, and such. Some of the combination of values that create a code may not be performed frequently or even at all at this time, yet a procedure code is available if needed (Averill et al. 2016).

A summary of the characteristics of the ICD-10-PCS structure is found in table 2.1.

Table 2.1. **Characteristics of ICD-10-PCS codes**

ICD-10-PCS	
Overall attributes	Completeness Expandability Multiaxial Standardized terminology
Development principles	No diagnostic information included Limited NOS and NEC codes Specificity included
Codes are alphanumeric	Seven characters using digits 0–9 and letters A–H, J–N, P–Z
Consistent number of characters	All codes are seven characters long

Check Your Understanding 2.1

Answer the following questions about the development of ICD-10-PCS.

1. What company was awarded a contract in 1995 by CMS to develop a new procedure coding system for ICD-10 in the United States?

2. When was ICD-10-PCS officially implemented in the United States?

3. ICD-10-PCS is intended for use in reporting procedures on electronic healthcare claim transactions for what group of patients?

4. The attribute of ICD-10-PCS that retains its meaning across a broad range of codes as much as possible for a procedure within the coding system is known as? How is this objective met?

5. How can the ICD-10-PCS coding system be expanded to allow the coding of new procedures?

6. How should a coder handle coding a new device used for a procedure however no device value option is available for that procedure?

7. True or false: The terminology used in ICD-10-PCS has multiple meanings for the same term depending on the type of procedure performed. Explain why you think the answer is true or false.

8. True or false: ICD-10-PCS does not include the diagnosis or reason for the procedure within the PCS code description.

9. True or false: ICD-10-PCS includes the reason the procedure was performed in the procedure code description. Explain why you think the answer is true or false.

10. True or false: ICD-10-PCS contains numeric character values only.

Code Structure

The ICD-10-PCS code is constructed by the coder using the Alphabetic Index and the Code Tables. On occasion, a complete seven-character code may be found in the Alphabetic Index. However, many Alphabetic Index entries contain the first three or four characters of the ICD-10-PCS code. The complete seven-character code is constructed using the Code Tables. The process of constructing codes in ICD-10-PCS is intended to be logical and consistent and uses individual letters and numbers called **values** to occupy the seven characters (digits or letters) of the codes. Each value is a specific option for each character; for example, upper esophagus is a body part within the gastrointestinal system. Each of the seven digits or letters of a code are called **characters**, for example, in the Medical Surgical Section: section, body system, root operation, body part, approach, device, and qualifier.

Each character has 1 of 34 possible values. A value can be a number from 0 to 9 or a letter from A–H, J–N, and P–Z. An important fact in ICD-10-PCS, the alphabetic letters O and I are not used so the letters are not confused with the numbers zero (0) and one (1). An example of a complete code is 0DB68ZX for esophagogastroduodenoscopy with gastric diagnostic biopsy.

Each code is constructed by choosing a specific value for each of the seven characters. Based on the details of the procedure documented, values are assigned for each character specifying the section, the body system, root operation, body part, approach, device, and qualifier.

Because the definition of each character is a function of its physical position in the code, the same value placed in a different position means something different. For example, a drainage procedure performed in the central nervous system could have the value of 0 (zero), while the value of 0 in the fourth character would represent the body part of the brain:

First character 0	= Medical and Surgical
Second character 0	= Central Nervous System
Fourth character 0	= Brain
Fifth character 0	= Open approach
Sixth character 0	= Drainage device

All codes in ICD-10-PCS are seven characters long. Each character in the seven-character code represents a particular aspect of the procedure. For the example in figure 2.1, in the main section of ICD-10-PCS, Medical and Surgical, the characters are used as follows:

Figure 2.1. **The seven characters of the ICD-10-PCS code**

> Character 1 = Section of ICD-10-PCS
>
> Character 2 = Body System
>
> Character 3 = Root Operation
>
> Character 4 = Body Part
>
> Character 5 = Approach
>
> Character 6 = Device
>
> Character 7 = Qualifier

An ICD-10-PCS code is best understood as being the result of a process rather than an isolated fixed process of accessing the Alphabetic Index to locate a code. The process consists of assigning values from among the value choices for that part of the system according to the design of the system.

More information about the specifics of the seven characters of the ICD-10-PCS code is discussed later in this chapter.

Check Your Understanding 2.2

Answer the following questions about the code structure of ICD-10-PCS.

1. What is the difference between "characters" and "values" in the ICD-10-PCS code structure?

2. How many possible values does each character have in the ICD-10-PCS code?

3. Identify the value letters that are *not* used in an ICD-10-PCS code.

4. How many characters are used for all ICD-10-PCS codes, and what do the characters represent in the Medical and Surgical section?

The ICD-10-PCS Format: Index and Tables

The ICD-10-PCS coding system is composed of two parts: the Index and the Tables.

The **Index** provides an alphabetic listing of procedure titles, root operations, body parts, and devices. A reference to the Code Tables can be found in the Index based on the root operation for a procedure, for example, excision or resection. In addition, the Index contains entries for more commonly used procedure titles, such as cholecystectomy or percutaneous endoscopic gastrostomy (PEG).

When the term is located in the Index, the Index specifies the first three or four characters of the code, for example, 0DT, or directs the coder to see another term. Each **Table** also identifies the first three characters of the code. Based on the first three characters of the code, the corresponding Table can be located. The Table is then used to obtain the complete code by specifying the last four characters. Even when the Index provides a seven-character code next to the Index entry, the coder must examine that code in the appropriate code Table to verify the complete code has been provided.

Each Table is composed of rows that specify the valid combinations of code values. In ICD-10-PCS, the upper portion of each Table specifies the values for the first three characters of the codes in that Table. In the Medical and Surgical section, the first three characters are the section, the body system, and the root operation.

In table 2.2, the values 0DT specify that Section = Medical and Surgical (0); Body System = Gastrointestinal System (D); and Root Operation = Resection (T).

Table 2.2. 0DT: Medical and surgical, Gastrointestinal system, Resection

Section:	0	Medical and Surgical
Body System:	D	Gastrointestinal System
Root Operation:	T	Resection—Cutting out or off, without replacement, all of a body part

Body Part Character 4	Approach Character 5	Device Character 6	Qualifier Character 7
1 Esophagus, Upper 2 Esophagus, Middle 3 Esophagus, Lower 4 Esophagogastric Junction 5 Esophagus 6 Stomach 7 Stomach, Pylorus 8 Small Intestine 9 Duodenum A Jejunum B Ileum C Ileocecal Valve E Large Intestine F Large Intestine, Right H Cecum J Appendix K Ascending Colon P Rectum Q Anus	0 Open 4 Percutaneous Endoscopic 7 Via Natural or Artificial Opening 8 Via Natural or Artificial Opening Endoscopic	Z No Device	Z No Qualifier
G Large Intestine, Left L Transverse Colon M Descending Colon N Sigmoid Colon	0 Open 4 Percutaneous Endoscopic 7 Via Natural or Artificial Opening 8 Via Natural or Artificial Opening Endoscopic F Via Natural or Artificial Opening with Percutaneous Endoscopic Assistance	Z No Device	Z No Qualifier
R Anal Sphincter U Omentum	0 Open 4 Percutaneous Endoscopic	Z No Device	Z No Qualifier

Source: CMS 2019

In Table 0DT, for the root operation, Resection, the root operation definition is provided. The lower portion of the Table specifies all the valid combinations of the remaining characters four through seven. The four columns in the table specify the last four characters. In the Medical and Surgical section, the columns are labeled as Body Part, Approach, Device, and Qualifier respectively. Each row in the table specifies the valid combination of values for characters four through seven. The Tables contain only the combinations of values that result in a valid procedure code. Also, the coder must stay on one row of a Table to select a valid procedure code.

The following is an example of how to use the ICD-10-PCS Index and Tables. The procedure to be coded is an open appendectomy:

EXAMPLE: The coder accesses the Index using the term "appendectomy" and finds two entries under Appendectomy—see Excision, Appendix 0DBJ and see Resection, Appendix

0DTJ. The coder must know the definition of the root operations "excision" and "resection" for this example. Because an appendectomy is the cutting out or off of the entire appendix, the entry for "resection" should be used. Using the first three characters, the coder locates Table 0DT in the ICD-10-PCS code book.

There are four columns to be considered with values that are appropriate with 0DT. The Index has given the code the fourth character J for appendix. The coder needs to select the fifth, sixth, and seventh characters to complete the code. The coder must stay on the same row where the fourth character J for appendix is located. The choice for approach for an open appendectomy is 0 for open. There are no choices for the device and the qualifier, so the sixth and seventh characters are Z and Z.

By collecting the seven characters together, the coder uses 0DTJ0ZZ for coding an open appendectomy as shown in table 2.3.

The code for a laparoscopic appendectomy has one character different for the approach. The laparoscopic appendectomy would be coded 0DTJ4ZZ, as shown in table 2.4.

Table 2.3. Open appendectomy 0DTJ0ZZ

Character	Code	Explanation
Section	0	Medical and Surgical
Body System	D	Gastrointestinal
Root Operation	T	Resection
Body Part	J	Appendix
Approach	0	Open
Device	Z	No Device
Qualifier	Z	No Qualifier

INDEX: Appendectomy, see Resection, Appendix 0DTJ

Table 2.4. Laparoscopic appendectomy 0DTJ4ZZ

Character	Code	Explanation
Section	0	Medical and Surgical
Body System	D	Gastrointestinal
Root Operation	T	Resection
Body Part	J	Appendix
Approach	4	Percutaneous Endoscopic
Device	Z	No Device
Qualifier	Z	No Qualifier

INDEX: Appendectomy, see Resection, Appendix 0DTJ

The ICD-10-PCS Code

All codes in ICD-10-PCS have seven characters. Each character represents an aspect of the procedure. For example, in the first section of ICD-10-PCS, Medical and Surgical, the characters represent the following:

1	2	3	4	5	6	7
Section	Body System	Root Operation	Body Part	Approach	Device	Qualifier

Each of the characters has a defined meaning:

- Character 1: Section—The first character of a code determines the broad procedure category, or section, where the code is located. The first section of ICD-10-PCS includes the vast majority of codes. Codes in the first section, the Medical and Surgical Section, all begin with the 0 (zero) character. Other sections will be covered in the next portion of this discussion.

- Character 2: Body System—The second character defines the body system that is the general physiological system or anatomical region involved. Examples of body systems in the Medical and Surgical section include central nervous system, upper arteries, respiratory system, tendons, muscles, and upper joints. Note that in some of the Sections of ICD-10-PCS, the second character may have an alternate meaning. For example, in the Physical Rehabilitation and Diagnostic Audiology section (F), the second character indicates whether this is Rehabilitation or Diagnostic Audiology.

- Character 3: Root Operation—The third character defines the root operation, or the objective of the procedure being performed. Examples of root operations are excision, bypass, division, and fragmentation. In some sections, the root operation is known as the root type. For example, in the Imaging section (B), the third character indicates the root type, not the root operation.

- Character 4: Body Part—The fourth character generally defines the body part or specific anatomical site where the procedure was performed. Character three is considered the axis of the code tables. The body system, second character, provides only a general indication of the procedure site, and the body part, fourth character, indicates the precise body part. This can vary in some sections of ICD-10-PCS. As in the Physical Rehabilitation and Diagnostic Audiology section example, in this section, the fourth character represents the body system or region rather than the body part.

- Character 5: Approach—The fifth character defines the approach, or the technique used to reach the operative site. Seven different approach values are used in the Medical and Surgical section of ICD-10-PCS. The meaning of the fifth character can vary in sections other than the Medical and Surgical section. For example, in the Imaging section (B), the fifth character indicates Contrast used in the Imaging Procedure.

- Character 6: Device—The sixth character defines the device. Depending on the procedure performed, there may or may not be a device left in place at the end of the procedure. If no device applies to the procedure, the Z value is used in character 6. If a device is used, the values fall into four basic categories:

○ Grafts and Prostheses

○ Implants

○ Simple or Mechanical Appliances

○ Electronic Appliances

Again, not all sections in ICD-10-PCS include Device as the sixth character. For example, in the Radiation Therapy section (D), the sixth character represents the Isotope used, if applicable.

- Character 7: Qualifier—The seventh character defines a qualifier for a particular code. A qualifier specifies an additional attribute of the procedure, if applicable. Not every ICD-10-PCS code will have options for a qualifier value to be used with the code. In fact, more codes will not offer an option for a qualifier other than the value of Z for no qualifier. There is no value for "none" as qualifier. Instead, the Z value is used to represent no option for the reporting of a qualifier for a particular procedure.

   In the code Tables, if a given character does not have a value assigned, the Z value is used. This is particularly frequent for the seventh character, qualifier, and the sixth character, generally for the device.

Overall Organization of ICD-10-PCS

ICD-10-PCS is composed of 16 sections, represented by the numbers 0–9 and the letters B–D and F–H. Reminder, the letters I and O are not used in ICD-10-PCS so as not to confuse letters with numbers of 0 and 1. The broad procedure categories contained in these sections range from surgical procedures to substance abuse treatment. The 16 sections are contained in three main sections: Medical and Surgical section, Medical and Surgical–related sections, and Ancillary sections.

   The first section, Medical and Surgical section, contains the majority of procedures typically reported in an inpatient setting. All procedure codes in this section begin with the section value of 0 (zero.)

Section Value	Description
0	Medical and Surgical

Sections 1–9 of ICD-10-PCS comprise the Medical and Surgical–related sections. These sections include the following:

Section Value	Description
1	Obstetrics
2	Placement
3	Administration
4	Measurement and Monitoring
5	Extracorporeal or Systemic Assistance and Performance

Section Value	Description
6	Extracorporeal or Systemic Therapies
7	Osteopathic
8	Other Procedures
9	Chiropractic

Codes in Sections 1–9 are structured for the most part like their counterparts in the Medical and Surgical section, with a few exceptions. For example, in Sections 5 and 6, the fifth character is defined as the duration instead of approach.

Additional differences include these uses of the sixth character:

- Section 3 defines the sixth character as substance

- Sections 4 and 5 define the sixth character as function

- Sections 7–9 define the sixth character as method

Sections B–D and F–H constitute the Ancillary sections of ICD-10-PCS that include the following sections:

Section Value	Description
B	Imaging
C	Nuclear Medicine
D	Radiation Therapy
F	Physical Rehabilitation and Diagnostic Audiology
G	Mental Health
H	Substance Abuse Treatment
X	New Technology

Section X constitutes the New Technology section of ICD-10-PCS. The definitions of some characters in the Ancillary New Technology sections also differ from those seen in the previous sections. For example, in the Imaging section, the third character is defined as the root type, and the fifth and sixth characters define contrast and contrast or qualifier, respectively. The New Technology Section (Section X) codes are standalone codes and are not to be considered supplemental codes. In this section, the sixth characters define device, substance, and technology and the seventh character qualifier identifies the new technology group.

Check Your Understanding 2.3

Answer the following questions about the ICD-10-PCS Index, Tables, and the overall organization of ICD-10-PCS.

1. Should a coder select a code directly from the Index in ICD-10-PCS?

2. The top of each code Table includes what three characters in the Medical and Surgical Section?

(Continued)

(Continued)

3. What are the four characters that appear in the columns of Tables in the Medical and Surgical Section?

4. Many code Tables include multiple rows of values for the body part, approach, device, and qualifier. Can the coder use any value from multiple rows to construct a valid code? Explain your answer.

5. Given the example in the chapter for coding an open appendectomy and a laparoscopic appendectomy, what value changed for which of the seven characters in the codes for both procedures? Explain your answer.

6. What are the descriptions of the sections within the Medical and Surgical–related sections?

7. Describe what the 3rd character of the ICD-10-PCS Table is considered and why is this important?

8. Explain the intent of the 5th character Approach for the Medical and Surgical section, and identify the different approach values via the ICD-10-PCS online code set.

9. What are the four basic categories of device values that can be used in an ICD-10-PCS code?

10. True or false: Section X: New Technology is a component of the Ancillary Section.

The Medical and Surgical Section (0)

The Medical and Surgical section is the largest in ICD-10-PCS. The first character of the codes in the Medical and Surgical section is always the number 0. The second through seventh characters will be the concentration of this section.

Body Systems

The meaning of the second character in the Medical and Surgical section is general body system. The way in which ICD-10-PCS defines a body system, however, is a bit different than the usual meaning of the term. Table 2.5 shows how some customary body systems are given multiple body-system values. For example, note the circulatory system does not have a single value but instead is identified as 2—Heart and Great Vessels, 3—Upper Arteries, 4—Lower Arteries, 5—Upper Veins, and 6—Lower Veins.

Table 2.5. **ICD-10-PCS body system values**

Values	ICD-10-PCS body systems
0	Central Nervous System
1	Peripheral Nervous System
2	Heart and Great Vessels
3	Upper Arteries
4	Lower Arteries
5	Upper Veins
6	Lower Veins
7	Lymphatic and Hemic System
8	Eye
9	Ear, Nose, Sinus

Values	ICD-10-PCS body systems
B	Respiratory System
C	Mouth and Throat
D	Gastrointestinal System
F	Hepatobiliary System and Pancreas
G	Endocrine System
H	Skin and Breast
J	Subcutaneous Tissue and Fascia
K	Muscles
L	Tendons
M	Bursae and Ligaments
N	Head and Facial Bones
P	Upper Bones
Q	Lower Bones
R	Upper Joints
S	Lower Joints
T	Urinary System
U	Female Reproductive System
V	Male Reproductive System
W	Anatomic Regions, General
X	Anatomical Regions, Upper Extremities
Y	Anatomic Regions, Lower Extremities

Root Operations

The third character in the Medical and Surgical section is the root operation. There are 31 root operations in the Medical and Surgical section, each representing the specific objective of the procedure. Each root operation has a precise definition that must be applied to assign the ICD-10-PCS code. There is a clear distinction between the definitions of the root operations. To make it easier to understand the intent of each root operation, they can be divided into nine groups of root operations that share similar attributes. It is the coder's responsibility to translate the physician's description of the procedure performed into one of the 31 root operations. The physician is not required to use the ICD-10-PCS root operation terminology in the procedure report.

The nine groups of root operations are as follows:

1. Root operations that take out some or all of a body part
2. Root operations that take out solids or fluids or gases from a body part
3. Root operations involving cutting or separation only
4. Root operations that put in or put back or move some or all of a body part
5. Root operations that alter the diameter or route of a tubular body part
6. Root operations that always involve a device
7. Root operations involving examination only
8. Root operations that define other repairs
9. Root operations that define other objectives (Kuehn and Jorwic 2018, 9–10)

Table 2.6 is from the *ICD-10-PCS Reference Manual* (CMS 2016a) and lists these nine groups and the root operations within each group.

Table 2.6.   **Nine groups of root operations**

Root operation	What operation does	Objective of procedure	Procedure site	Example
Root operations that take out some or all of a body part				
Excision (B)	Takes out some or all of a body part	Cutting out or off without replacement	Some of a body part	Breast lumpectomy
Resection (T)	Takes out some or all of a body part	Cutting out or off without replacement	All of a body part	Total mastectomy
Detachment (6)	Takes out some or all of a body part	Cutting out or off without replacement	Extremity only, any level	Amputation above elbow
Destruction (5)	Takes out some or all of a body part	Eradicating without replacement	Some or all of a body part	Fulguration of endometrium
Extraction (D)	Takes out some or all of a body part	Pulling out or off without replacement	Some or all of a body part	Suction D&C
Root operations that take out solids or fluids or gases from a body part				
Drainage (9)	Takes out solids or fluids or gases from a body part	Taking or letting out fluids or gases	Within a body part	Incision and drainage
Extirpation (C)	Takes out solids or fluids or gases from a body part	Taking or cutting out solid matter	Within a body part	Thrombectomy
Fragmentation (F)	Takes out solids or fluids or gases from a body part	Breaking solid matter into pieces	Within a body part	Lithotripsy
Root operations involving cutting or separation only				
Division (8)	Involves cutting or separation only	Cutting into or separating a body part	Within a body part	Neurotomy
Release (N)	Involves cutting or separation only	Freeing a body part from constraint	Around a body part	Adhesiolysis
Root operations that put in or put back or move some or all of a body part				
Transplantation (Y)	Puts in or puts back or moves some or all of a body part	Putting in a living body part from a person or animal	Some or all of a body part	Kidney transplant
Reattachment (M)	Puts in or puts back or moves some or all of a body part	Putting back a detached body part	Some or all of a body part	Reattach severed finger
Transfer (X)	Puts in or puts back or moves some or all of a body part	Moving, to function for a similar body part	Some or all of a body part	Skin tissue transfer
Reposition (S)	Puts in or puts back or moves some or all of a body part	Moving, to normal or other suitable location	Some or all of a body part	Reduction of a displace fracture of a bone

Root operation	What operation does	Objective of procedure	Procedure site	Example
Root operations that alter the diameter or route of a tubular body part				
Restriction (V)	Alters the diameter or route of a tubular body part	Partially closing orifice or lumen	Tubular body part	Gastroesophageal fundoplication
Occlusion (L)	Alters the diameter or route of a tubular body part	Completely closing orifice or lumen	Tubular body part	Fallopian tube ligation
Dilation (7)	Alters the diameter or route of a tubular body part	Expanding orifice or lumen	Tubular body part	Percutaneous transluminal coronary angioplasty (PTCA)
Bypass (1)	Alters the diameter or route of a tubular body part	Altering route of passage	Tubular body part	Coronary artery bypass graft (CABG)
Root operations that always involve a device				
Insertion (H)	Always involves a device	Putting in nonbiological device	In or on a body part	Central line insertion
Replacement (R)	Always involves a device	Putting in device that replaces a body part	Some or all of a body part	Total hip replacement
Supplement (U)	Always involves a device	Putting in device that reinforces or augments a body part	In or on a body part	Abdominal wall herniorrhaphy using mesh
Change (2)	Always involves a device	Exchanging a device without cutting or puncturing	In or on a body part	Drainage tube change
Removal (P)	Always involves a device	Taking out device	In or on a body part	Central line removal
Revision (W)	Always involves a device	Correcting a malfunctioning or displaced device	In or on a body part	Revision of pacemaker insertion
Root operations involving examination only				
Inspection (J)	Involves examination only	Visual or manual exploration	Some or all of a body part	Diagnostic cystoscopy
Map (K)	Involves examination only	Locating electrical impulses or functional areas	Brain or cardiac conduction mechanism	Cardiac mapping
Root operations that include other repairs				
Repair (Q)	Includes other repairs	Restoring body part to its normal structure	Some or all of a body part	Suture laceration
Control (3)	Includes other repair	Stopping or attempting to stop postprocedural bleed	Anatomical region	Postprostatectomy bleeding

(Continued)

Root operation	What operation does	Objective of procedure	Procedure site	Example
Root operations that include other objectives				
Fusion (G)	Includes other objectives	Rending joint immobile	Joint	Spinal fusion
Alteration (0)	Includes other objectives	Modifying body part for cosmetic purposes without affecting function	Some or all of a body part	Face lift
Creation (4)	Includes other objectives	Making new structure for sex change operation	Perineum	Artificial vagina or penis

Source: CMS 2018

Objective of the Procedure

In ICD-10-PCS, each component of a procedure is defined separately. The objective of the procedure, for example, to resect a part of the colon, is specified by the root operation. The precise anatomical site operated on is identified as the body part. The method to reach and visualize the operative site is identified as the approach with the fifth character. If the objective of the procedure includes the use of a device to accomplish the desired outcome, the device remaining in the body is identified by the sixth character, such as a stent. Together, the seven characters are intended to describe the complete procedure performed. The coder must analyze all of the documentation contained in the operative report to identify the objective of the procedure.

The procedure is coded in ICD-10-PCS as the procedure that was actually performed. If the procedure performed completed was not what was intended when the procedure started, that does not matter. The intended procedure may not always be completed. When the intended or anticipated procedure is changed or discontinued, the root operation is coded based on the actual procedure that was performed.

Multiple Procedures

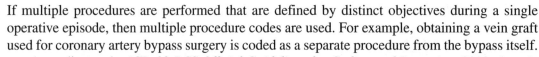

If multiple procedures are performed that are defined by distinct objectives during a single operative episode, then multiple procedure codes are used. For example, obtaining a vein graft used for coronary artery bypass surgery is coded as a separate procedure from the bypass itself.

According to the *ICD-10-PCS Official Guidelines for Coding and Reporting*, 2020, there is direction on how and when to code multiple procedures. Guideline B.3.2, Multiple procedures states during the same operative episode, multiple procedures are coded if

a. The same root operation is performed on different body parts as defined by distinct values of the body part character. For example, excision of lesion in the ascending colon and excision of lesion in the transverse colon are coded separately.

b. The same root operation is repeated in multiple body parts, and those body parts are separate and distinct body parts classified to a single ICD-10-PCS body part value. For example, excision of the sartorius muscle and excision of the gracilis muscle are both included in the upper leg muscle body part value, and multiple procedures are coded.

c. Multiple root operatives with distinctive objectives are performed on the same body part. For example, destruction of sigmoid lesion and bypass of sigmoid colon are coded separately.

d. The intended root operation is attempted using one approach but is converted to a different approach. For example, a laparoscopic cholecystectomy converted to an open cholecystectomy is coded as percutaneous endoscopic Inspection and open Resection (CMS 2019).

Redo of Procedures

If the procedure performed is a complete or partial redo of a previous procedure, the root operation that identifies the redo procedure that was performed is what is coded rather than the root operation of revision. For example, a complete redo of a knee replacement procedure that requires taking out the original prosthesis and putting in a new prosthesis is coded to the root operations of Removal and Replacement instead of Revision. The physician is likely to describe this procedure as a "revision arthroplasty," but the coder must use the definitions of the root operations to identify the objective of a revision.

The correction of complications arising from the original procedure other than device complications as defined in the root operation Revision are also coded to the procedure performed. For example, a procedure to add mesh to the abdominal wall to repair a postoperative ventral hernia is coded to Supplement rather than Revision.

Check Your Understanding 2.4

Answer the following questions about the Medical and Surgical section, body systems, and root operations.

1. Using the list of ICD-10-PCS body systems provided in table 2.5, what values would likely be used to represent parts of the musculoskeletal body system?

2. Using the list of ICD-10-PCS body systems provided in table 2.5, what values would likely be used to represent parts of the genitourinary body system?

3. Name the root operation for correcting a malfunctioning or displaced device.

4. Name the root operations that involve cutting or separation only and identify the objective of each procedure.

5. True or false: Only one code is selected for the extraction of multiple toenails. Explain why you think the answer is true or false.

6. Matching: Match the procedure title with the likely root operation from the group of procedures for taking out some or all of a body part.
   A. Total Mastectomy
   B. Prostate biopsy
   C. Amputation below knee
   D. Cryoablation of a colon polyp
   E. Dilatation and curettage

   1. Destruction
   2. Detachment
   3. Excision
   4. Extraction
   5. Resection

(Continued)

(Continued)

7. Match the procedure title with the likely root operation from the group of procedures for altering the diameter or route of a tubular body part
   A. Coronary artery bypass graft
   B. Percutaneous transluminal coronary angioplasty
   C. Ligation of inferior vena cava
   D. Uterine cervix cerclage

   1. Occlusion
   2. Restriction
   3. Dilation
   4. Bypass

8. If the patient had a traumatic amputation of the right index finger in an industrial accident and the physician was able to put the finger back to its original location, what would likely be the root operation for this procedure?

9. If the patient had a dual chamber pacemaker system implanted into his body, what would likely be the root operation for this procedure?

10. If the patient had a laparoscopic cholecystectomy converted to an open cholecystectomy, which part of the procedure is coded?

Body Part

The fourth character in the Medical and Surgical section is body part. The value chosen for this character represents the specific part of the body system (character 2) on which the surgery was performed. Body parts may specify laterality. It is very important that the coder understands the body part values are defined in ICD-10-PCS in character 4 for each of the body systems and root operations. What the coder interprets as a body part and what ICD-10-PCS defines as a body part may not be the same thing.

Some examples of body parts and their body systems in ICD-10-PCS are shown in table 2.7.

Table 2.7. **Body systems and parts**

Body System	Body Part
Lower extremities	Left foot
Central nervous	Trigeminal nerve
Upper veins	Right cephalic vein
Gastrointestinal	Stomach

ICD-10-PCS does not provide a specific value for every body part. In those instances, the body part value selected would be either the whole body part value (for example, alveolar process is part of the mandible) or, in the instance of nerves and vessels, the body part value is coded to the closest proximal branch.

ICD-10-PCS originally included an appendix titled the Body Part Key. Now the entries of the Body Part Key have been incorporated into the Alphabetic Index. However, PCS still provides the Body Part Key for the purpose of translating specific anatomical sites that could be found in a health record or operative report, such as a specific named muscle or tendon, to the body part term or description used in ICD-10-PCS. For example, the adductor brevis muscle does not have its own body part value identified in ICD-10-PCS. The Body Part Key has an entry for the adductor muscle that instructs the coder to use "upper leg muscle" as the equivalent for the body part in the ICD-10-PCS code.

Since ICD-10-PCS was first published by CMS, yearly revisions have added the body part key entries to the Alphabetic Index of ICD-10-PCS for ease of reference. For this reason, a new coder should also reference the body part named in the operative report to the Alphabetic Index to determine the PCS body part terminology. Any coder having difficulty identifying the body part value should use the Alphabetic Index and reference the anatomic site there to verify the correct PCS body part used. Using the example above, in the ICD-10-PCS Index, there is an entry for "adductor hallucis muscle" that states "use foot muscle, left" or "use foot muscle, right."

Approach

ICD-10-PCS defines approach as the technique used to reach the site of the procedure. It is important to know the differences between the different approaches in order to correctly assign the fifth character value in the Medical and Surgical section (CMS 2019).

There are seven different approaches as shown with the approach value used in the tables. Table 2.8 defines each approach.

Table 2.8.   **The seven approaches and definitions**

Approach	Definition	Examples
Open (0)	Cutting through the skin or mucous membrane and any other body layers necessary to expose the site of the procedure	Open cholecystectomy, open appendectomy
Percutaneous (3)	Entry, by puncture or minor incision, of instrumentation through the skin or mucous membrane and/or any other body layers necessary to reach the site of the procedure	Needle biopsy of breast
Percutaneous Endoscopic (4)	Entry, by puncture or minor incision, of instrumentation through the skin or mucous membrane and/or any other body layers necessary to reach and visualize the site of the procedure	Laparoscopic cholecystectomy, laparoscopic appendectomy
Via Natural or Artificial Opening (7)	Entry of instrumentation through a natural or artificial external opening to reach the site of the procedure	Insertion of Foley urinary catheter, endotracheal intubation
Via Natural or Artificial Opening Endoscopic (8)	Entry of instrumentation through a natural or artificial external opening to reach and visualize the site of the procedure	Colonoscopy, cystoscopy, esophagogastroduodenoscopy
Via Natural or Artificial Opening Endoscopic with Percutaneous Endoscopic Assistance (F)	Entry of instrumentation through a natural or artificial external opening to reach and visualize the site of the procedure, and entry, by puncture or minor incision, of instrumentation through the skin or mucous membrane and any other body layers necessary to aid in the performance of the procedure	Laparoscopic-assisted vaginal hysterectomy (This is the only current procedure that uses this approach)
External (X)	Procedures performed directly on the skin or mucous membrane and procedures performed indirectly by the application of external force through the skin or mucous membrane	Closed reduction of fracture of radius, extraction of upper or lower teeth

Source: CMS 2019

Figures 2.2 through 2.7 are examples of the types of procedures that are described in the seven approaches used in ICD-10-PCS.

Figure 2.2. **Comparison of open and percutaneous endoscopic approach**

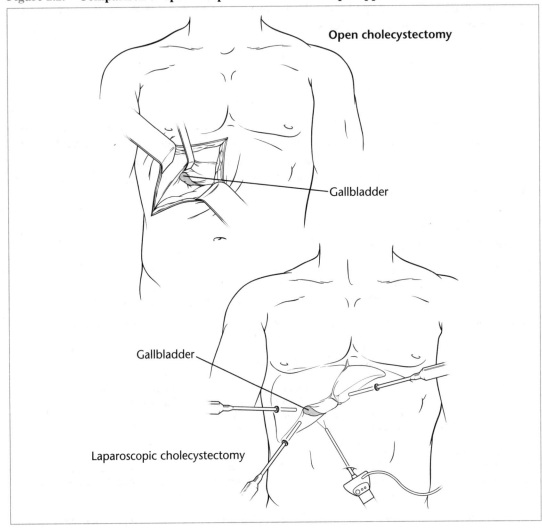

Open cholecystectomy

Gallbladder

Gallbladder

Laparoscopic cholecystectomy

© AHIMA

Two approaches that enter the body through the skin or mucous membrane are the open and percutaneous endoscopic approach (see figure 2.2). The open approach requires cutting through the skin or mucous membrane to expose the anatomical site. With the open approach, the surgeon is able to visualize the site where the procedure is being performed. The percutaneous approach also allows the surgeon to visualize the site where the procedure is being performed but not directly. The surgeon can see the anatomical site through the endoscope that is inserted through a puncture of minor incision, not by cutting through skin or mucous membranes.

Figure 2.3. Percutaneous approach

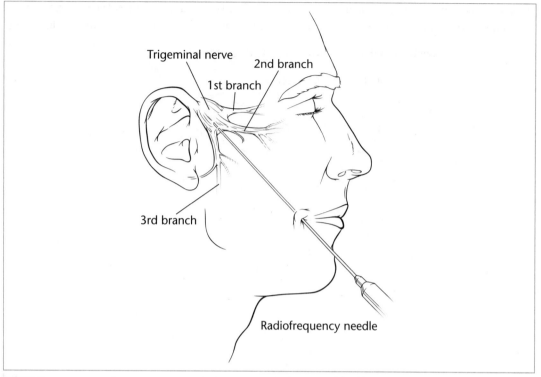

Trigeminal nerve

2nd branch

1st branch

3rd branch

Radiofrequency needle

© AHIMA

The third approach that involves entry through skin or mucous membrane or other body layers is the percutaneous approach, as identified in figure 2.3. By using this type of approach, the physician is able to reach the site of the procedure with an instrument that is inserted through the puncture of minor incision. The physician is not able to visualize the site but may use radiology imaging to perform the procedure with the instrument inserted.

Figure 2.4. Approach via natural or artificial opening

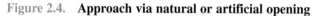
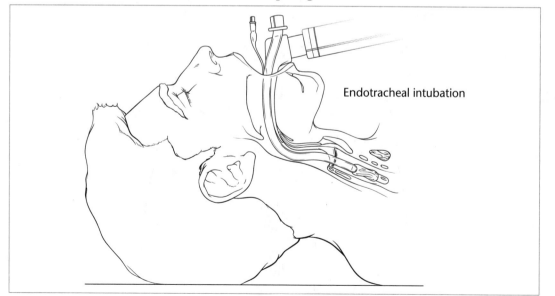

Endotracheal intubation

© AHIMA

Figure 2.4 shows approach via natural or artificial opening. With this approach, the physician inserts an instrument through a natural opening or artificial external opening to reach the anatomical site in order to perform the procedure, such as the endotracheal intubation shown in the illustration.

Figure 2.5. **Approach via natural or artificial opening endoscopic**

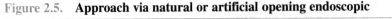
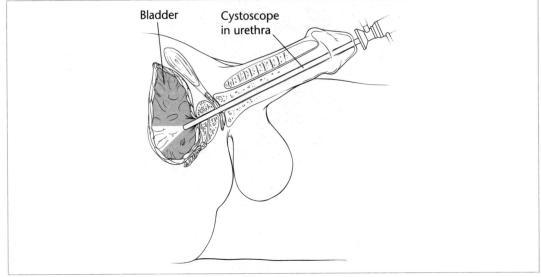

© AHIMA

In the approach via natural or artificial opening endoscopic, an endoscopic instrument is inserted via a natural opening or an artificial opening to reach and visualize the site of the procedure. The physician can see the anatomical site where the procedure is performed through the endoscope. A cystoscopic examination of the bladder is shown in figure 2.5.

Figure 2.6. **Approach via natural or artificial opening with percutaneous endoscopic assistance**

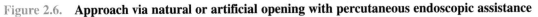
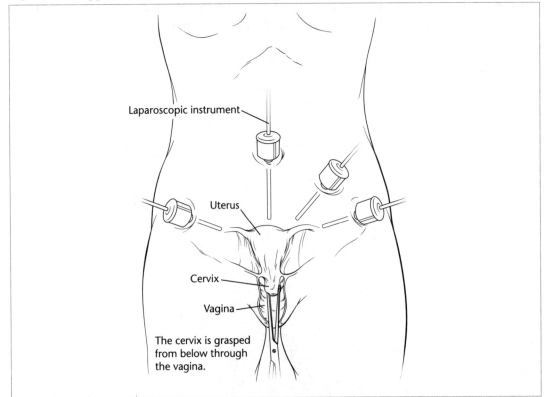

© AHIMA

The approach via natural or artificial opening with percutaneous endoscopic assistance is limited at this time to one procedure, that is, a laparoscopic-assisted vaginal hysterectomy (see figure 2.6). The procedure is performed through the vagina, the natural opening, with a laparoscopic instrument inserted by puncture or minor incision through the pelvic region. The laparoscope is used to visualize the internal organs during the procedure, but the organs are removed through the vagina.

Figure 2.7.   External approach

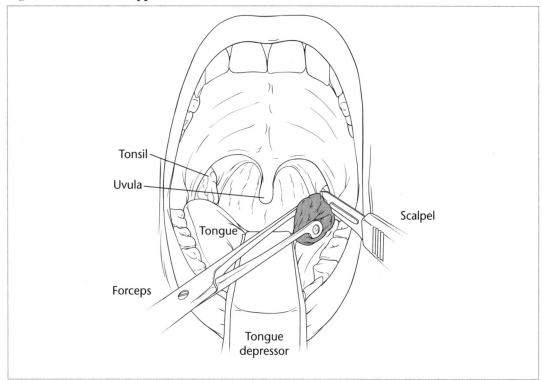

Tonsil

Uvula

Tongue

Forceps

Tongue depressor

Scalpel

© AHIMA

The external approach is used for procedures that are performed directly on the skin or mucous membrane and with procedures that are performed by the application of external force through the skin or mucous membranes. The external approach is also used when a procedure is performed through a natural orifice or structure that is visible to the physician without the use of any instrumentation, such as a tonsillectomy performed through the patient's mouth, shown in figure 2.7.

The approach is composed of three components: the access location, method, and type of instrumentation.

Access Location

For procedures performed on an internal organ, the access location specifies the external site through which the internal organ is reached. There are two types of access locations: skin or mucous membrane and external orifices. Except for the external approach, every other approach value includes one of these two access locations. The skin or mucous membrane can be incised or punctured to reach the procedure site. All open and percutaneous approach values use skin or mucous membrane as the access location. The site of a procedure can also be reached through an external opening. External openings can be natural (for example, mouth) or artificial (for example, nephrostomy stoma).

Method

The method of approach specifies how the internal or external part of the body is accessed so that the procedure can be performed on a body part. An open approach requires cutting through the skin or mucous membrane and other body layers to expose the site of the procedure. An instrumental approach uses instrumentation placed into the body through the access location to the internal procedure site. The instrument can be introduced by puncture or minor incision into the body's skin or subcutaneous tissue or through a natural external opening. The puncture or minor incision should not be interpreted as an open approach. An operative approach can involve multiple methods of access. For example, the approach through a natural or artificial orifice with percutaneous endoscopic assistance uses both the orifice and the percutaneous endoscopic approach to reach the procedure site (Averill et al. 2016).

Type of Instrumentation

The physician may use instrumentation or specialized equipment to perform a procedure on an internal body part. Other than the basic open approach where the physician has direct visual access to the body part being operated on, instrumentation is used in all other approaches to reach an internal body part. The instrument, such as an endoscope, may or may not be used to visualize the procedure site. For example, the bronchoscope is the instrument used to perform a bronchoscopy that permits the internal site of the procedure to be visualized. The term "endoscopic" as used in approach values refers to instrumentation that permits a procedure site to be visualized by the physician during the procedure. An instrument such as a needle, for example, used to perform a needle biopsy of the pancreas, does not give the physician visualization of the operative site, instead the needle is used to reach the operative site (Averill et al. 2016).

External Approaches

 The external approach is used when procedures are performed directly on the skin or mucous membrane. External procedures may be performed indirectly by the application of external force. Examples of procedures using external approaches are skin lesion excision, closed reduction of a fracture, and tonsillectomy (because the tonsils can be reached through the mouth) (CMS 2019).

Device and Qualifier

In the Medical and Surgical section, the sixth character specifies devices that remain after the procedure is completed. The seventh character, qualifier, is used with certain procedures to define an additional attribute of the procedure. The tables 2.9 and 2.10 illustrate examples of the sixth and seventh characters available in the Urinary system.

Table 2.9. **Character 6—Device**

0	Drainage Device
2	Monitoring Device
3	Infusion Device
7	Autologous Tissue Substitute
C	Extraluminal Device
D	Intraluminal Device
J	Synthetic Substitute
K	Nonautologous Tissue Substitute
L	Artificial Sphincter
M	Stimulator Lead
Y	Other Device
Z	No Device

Table 2.10.   **Character 7—Qualifier**

0	Allogeneic
1	Syngeneic
2	Zooplastic
3	Kidney Pelvis, Right
4	Kidney Pelvis, Left
6	Ureter, Right
7	Ureter, Left
8	Colon
9	Colocutaneous
A	Ileum
B	Bladder
C	Ileocutaneous
D	Cutaneous
X	Diagnostic
Z	No Qualifier

Device

A device is specified in the sixth character and is only used to specify devices that remain after the procedure is completed. There are four general types of devices:

- Grafts and prostheses are biological or synthetic material that takes the place of all or a portion of a body part (that is, skin graft or joint prosthesis).

- Implants are therapeutic material made of biological or synthetic material that is not absorbed by, eliminated by, or incorporated into a body part (that is, radioactive implant). The therapeutic implants can be retained permanently in the body or removed when no longer needed. Examples of implants are internal fixation devices, an intramedullary nail, or a tissue expander implanted under the skin or muscle.

- Simple or mechanical appliances are therapeutic biological or synthetic material that assists or prevents a physiological function. Examples of these appliances are a tracheostomy airway device, a monoplanar external fixation device, or an intraluminal device such as a vascular graft.

- Mechanical or electronic appliances are used to assist, monitor, take the place of, or prevent a physiological function. Examples of electronic appliances are a cardiac pacemaker generator, cochlear implant hearing device, or a neurostimulator (CMS 2019).

The instrument used to visualize the procedure site in order to perform the procedure is not specified in the device value. This use of an instrument is specified in the approach value.

The objective of the root operation Insertion is to put in a device. If the device is put in to meet another objective, such as dilation of a tubular body part, the root operation defining the underlying objective of the procedure is used, with the device specified in the sixth character. For example, if the surgeon performs a joint replacement on the hip joint, the root operation Replacement is coded and the prosthetic device used to replace the joint is specified as the sixth character. Materials incidental to a procedure such as clips, ligatures, and sutures are not specified in the device character (Averill et al. 2016).

Qualifier

The qualifier is specified in the seventh character as appropriate. The values listed as an option for a qualifier are unique to individual procedures. A qualifier specifies a particular attribute about a procedure. For example, the qualifier for a bypass procedure identifies the destination site of the bypass. There is an option of a qualifier of "diagnostic" to be used with excision procedures to identify when an excision of a body part was done as a biopsy for diagnostic purposes.

Device Key

ICD-10-PCS includes Device and Substance Classification Keys. Names of devices are also included in the Alphabetic Index to allow the coder to have easy access to the ICD-10-CM device terminology. The Device Key translates specific device terms to an equivalent PCS description for the sixth character of an ICD-10-PCS code. The device terms may be general device descriptions, such as nontunneled central venous catheter, or a device by a specific trade name, such as Kirschner wire. Using the later example, if "Kirschner wire" is located in the Device Key, the coder is instructed to use "internal fixation device" in the bone or joint it is inserted.

As ICD-10-PCS has been updated by CMS over the past few years, the Device Key entries have been added to the Index for ICD-10-PCS for ease of reference. When the coder is uncertain what PCS description should be used for the sixth character of a code, the coder should access the Index to see if the device is located there. For example, in the ICD-10-PCS Index, an entry for Kirschner wire is included and instructs the coder to "use internal fixation device" as the description of the device in the ICD-10-PCS code.

Root Operations and Devices

Devices can be removed from the body, but some devices cannot be removed without being replaced with another nonbiological appliance or another substitute for the body part.

The following root operations may or may not have specific devices as part of the procedure:

> Alteration
> Bypass
> Creation
> Destruction
> Dilation
> Division
> Drainage
> Excision
> Extirpation
> Fragmentation
> Fusion
> Map
> Occlusion
> Release
> Repair
> Reposition
> Resection
> Restriction
> Transfer

The following root operations must have specific devices coded with these procedures:

Change
Insertion
Removal
Replacement
Revision
Supplement

The approach includes the fact that instrumentation was used to visualize the procedure site. This information is not specified in the device value.

The root operation of Insertion is used when the procedure's objective is to put in a device. If the device is put in to meet a procedure's objective other than insertion, then the root operation defining the underlying objective of the procedure is used. The device used is identified with the device specified in the device character. For example, if the procedure is to replace the shoulder joint, the root operation is Replacement, and the prosthetic device is specified in the device character. The device is being inserted to replace the joint so the objective of the procedure is Replacement. Otherwise, materials incidental to a procedure such as clips, ligatures, and sutures are not what is meant by a device and is not specified in the device character.

Because new devices can be developed at any time, the value Other Device is provided as an option for use until a specific device value may be added to the system. With this option, a procedure that involves a new device can be coded as soon as the device is available instead of waiting until the coding system is updated in the future.

Table 2.11 provides examples of the sixth character available for the Skeletal system.

Table 2.11.   **Sixth characters available in the Skeletal system**

Device—Character 6	
4	Internal Fixation Device
5	External Fixation Device
6	Internal Fixation Device, Intramedullary
B	External Fixation Device, Monoplanar
C	External Fixation Device, Ring
D	External Fixation Device, Hybrid
Z	No Device

Qualifier

The seventh character is the qualifier to add more information to describe the procedure. Individual procedures have unique values for the qualifier in the seventh character position. The qualifiers may have a narrow application to a specific root operation, body system or body part. For example, the qualifier can be used to identify the destination site in a bypass procedure. Other qualifiers identify the type of transplant performed such as allogeneic, syngeneic, and zooplastic. Allogeneic is the transplant of a living organ taken from a different individual of the same species. Syngeneic is a transplant from a genetically identical person such as an identical twin. Zooplastic is the transfer of living tissue to humans from an animal of another species for transplant purposes. The more common qualifier that is expected to be used is the qualifier X for diagnostic to identify when a biopsy procedure is performed.

Table 2.12 illustrates examples of the seventh character available in the Heart and Great Vessels system.

Table 2.12. **Example qualifier characters used in the Heart and Great Vessels—Character 7**

2	Common Atrioventricular Valve
3	Coronary Artery
4	Coronary Vein
5	Coronary Circulation
6	Bifurcation
7	Atrium, Left
8	Internal Mammary, Right
9	Internal Mammary, Left
A	Innominate Artery
B	Subclavian
C	Thoracic Artery
D	Carotid
F	Abdominal Artery
J	Truncal Valve
K	Left Atrial Appendage
P	Pulmonary Trunk
Q	Pulmonary Artery, Right
R	Pulmonary Artery, Left
S	Pulmonary Vein, Right
T	Pulmonary Vein, Left
U	Pulmonary Vein, Confluence
W	Aorta

Check Your Understanding 2.5

Answer the following questions about the body part, approach, device, and qualifier characters used in the ICD-10-PCS codes.

1. True or false: ICD-10-PCS provides a specific value for every body part. Explain your answer.

2. What are the seven values identified as approaches for Medical and Surgical procedures in ICD-10-PCS?

3. In addition to the external approach, what are the two types of access locations for procedures performed on an internal organ?

4. Matching: Match the medical and surgical procedure with the likely approach using the approach definitions within ICD-10-PCS.

   A. Closed reduction of a fracture
   B. Coronary artery bypass graft through a sternotomy
   C. Arthroscopy
   D. Colonoscopy opening
   E. Needle biopsy of breast
   F. Insertion of endotracheal tube
   G. Laparoscopic-assisted vaginal hysterectomy

   1. Open
   2. Percutaneous
   3. Percutaneous endoscopic
   4. Via natural or artificial opening
   5. Via natural or artificial opening endoscopic
   6. External
   7. Via natural or artificial opening with percutaneous endoscopic assistance

5. Name examples of three electronic appliances that are considered devices that can remain in the body after the procedure is completed.

(Continued)

(Continued)

6. The term "endoscopic" used in approach values refers to instrumentation that allows what to occur during a medical and surgical procedure?

7. Identify the root operations that require specific devices coded with the procedure.

8. When is it appropriate to capture a device character for a procedure? Provide three examples of types of device options in ICD-10-PCS.

9. What is the purpose of the "qualifier" used as the seventh character in certain Medical and Surgical procedures in ICD-10-PCS?

10. What does the term "allogeneic" mean when used as a value for the qualifier character in ICD-10-PCS?

ICD-10-PCS Official Guidelines for Coding and Reporting

Two departments within the Federal Government's Department of Health and Human Services provide the *ICD-10-PCS Official Guidelines for Coding and Reporting*. The guidelines were developed by CMS and the National Center for Health Statistics (NCHS). The guidelines were approved by the four organizations that comprise the Cooperating Parties for ICD-10-PCS, that is, American Hospital Association (AHA), AHIMA, CMS, and NCHS.

The guidelines are intended to accompany and assist in the interpretation of the official conventions and instructions within the ICD-10-PCS coding system. It is important to note that the conventions and instructions in the ICD-10-PCS coding system take precedence over the guidelines, that is, they are the most important rules for coding. The guidelines are based on the coding instructions and definitions found in ICD-10-PCS. Adherence to the guidelines is required under the Health Insurance Portability and Accountability Act (HIPAA) as the ICD-10-PCS codes are required for hospital inpatient healthcare settings under HIPAA.

The 2020 edition of the *ICD-10-PCS Official Guidelines for Coding and Reporting* can be located in appendix G on the website accompanying this text. In addition, the guidelines can be accessed on the CMS website (CMS 2019).

The guidelines consist of six parts:

A. Conventions

B. Medical and Surgical Section Guidelines including directions for body system, root operations, body part, approach, and device characters in the ICD-10-PCS code

C. Obstetrics Section Guidelines

D. Radiation Therapy Section Guidelines

E. New Technology Section Guidelines

F. Selection of Principal Procedure

Overview of the ICD-10-PCS Guidelines

The entire set of *ICD-10-PCS Official Guidelines for Coding and Reporting* is required reading for coders. The following table is intended to be a synopsis of the information contained within the guidelines:

Table 2.13. Overview of *ICD-10-PCS Official Guidelines for Coding and Reporting*

Section	Summary of instruction
Conventions	
A1	ICD-10-PCS codes are composed of seven characters. Each character is an axis of classification that specifies information about the procedure performed. Within a defined code range, a character specifies the same type of information in that axis of classification.
A2	One of 34 possible values can be assigned to each axis in the seven-character code. Values are numbers 0–9 and letters A–Z without using letters I and O so not to confuse with numbers 1 and 0. The number of unique values used in an axis of classification differs as needed.
A3	Valid values for an axis of classification can be added as needed.
A4	As with words in their context, the meaning of any single value is a combination of its axis of classification and any preceding values on which it may be dependent.
A5	As the system is expanded to become increasingly detailed, over time more values will depend on preceding values for their meaning.
A6	The purpose of the alphabetic index is to locate the appropriate table that contains all the information necessary to construct a procedure code. The PCS Tables should always be consulted to find the most appropriate valid code.
A7	It is not required to consult the index first before proceeding to the tables to complete the code. A valid code may be chosen directly from the tables.
A8	All seven characters must be specified to be a valid code. If the documentation is incomplete for coding purposes, the physician should be queried for the necessary information.
A9	Within a PCS table, valid codes include all combinations of choices in characters 4 through 7 contained in the same row of the table.
A10	"And," when used in a code description, means "and/or," except when used to describe a combination of multiple body parts for which separate values exist for each body part (e.g. Skin and Subcutaneous Tissue used as a qualifier, where there are separate body part values for "Skin" and "Subcutaneous Tissue").
A11	Many of the terms used to construct PCS codes are defined within the system. It is the coder's responsibility to determine what the documentation in the health record equates to in the PCS definitions. The physician is not expected to use the terms used in PCS code descriptions, nor is the coder required to query the physician when the correlation between the documentation and the defined PCS terms is clear.
Medical and Surgical Section Guidelines (section 0)	
B2 Body System	
B2.1a Body System General Guidelines	The procedure codes in Anatomical Regions, General, Anatomical Regions, Upper Extremities and Anatomical Regions, Lower Extremities can be used when the procedure is performed on an anatomical region rather than a specific body part (e.g., root operations Control and Detachment, Drainage of a body cavity) or on the rare occasion when no information is available to support assignment of a code to a specific body part.
B2.1b Upper and Lower	Where the general body part values "upper" and "lower" are provided as an option in the Upper Arteries, Lower Arteries, Upper Veins, Lower Veins, Muscles and Tendons body systems, "upper" or "lower" specifies body parts located above or below the diaphragm respectively.

Section	Summary of instruction
B3 Root Operations	
B3.1a Root operations General Guidelines	In order to determine the appropriate root operation, the full definition of the root operation as contained in the PCS Tables must be applied.
B3.1b Components of a Procedure	Components of a procedure specified in the root operation definition or explanation as integral to that root operation are not coded separately. Procedural steps necessary to reach the operative site and close the operative site, including anastomosis of a tubular body part, are also not coded separately.
B3.2 Multiple Procedures	During the same operative episode, multiple procedures are coded if: a. Same root operation is performed on different body parts as defined by distinct values of the body part character b. Same root operation is repeated in multiple body parts, and those body parts are separate and distinct body parts classified to a single ICD-10-PCS body part value. c. Multiple root operations with distinct objectives are performed on the same body part. d. The intended root operation is attempted using one approach but is converted to a different approach.
B3.3 Discontinued Procedures	If the intended procedure is discontinued or otherwise not completed, code the procedure to the root operation performed. If a procedure is discontinued before any other root operation is performed, code the root operation Inspection of the body part or anatomical region inspected.
B3.4a Biopsy Procedures	Biopsy procedures are coded with root operations Excision, Extraction, or Drainage and the qualifier Diagnostic.
B3.4b Biopsy Followed by More Definitive Treatment	If a diagnostic Excision, Extraction, or Drainage procedure (Biopsy) is followed by a more definitive procedure, such as Destruction, Excision, or Resection at the same procedure site, both the biopsy and the more definitive treatment are coded.
B3.5 Overlapping Body Layers	If root operations such as Excision, Extraction, Repair, or Inspection are performed on overlapping layers of the musculoskeletal system, the body part specifying the deepest layer is coded.
B3.6a Bypass Procedures	Bypass procedures are coded by identifying the body part bypassed "from" and the body part bypassed "to." The fourth character body part specifies the body part bypassed from, and the qualifier specifies the body part bypassed to.
B3.6b Coronary Arteries	Coronary artery bypass procedures are coded differently than other bypass procedures as described in the previous guideline. Rather than identifying the body part bypassed from, the body part identifies the number of coronary arteries bypassed to, and the qualifier specifies the vessel bypassed from.
B3.6c Multiple Sites Bypassed	If multiple coronary arteries are bypassed, a separate procedure is coded for each coronary artery site that uses a different device and/or qualifier.
B3.7 Control vs. more definitive root operations	The root operation Control is defined as, "Stopping, or attempting to stop, postprocedural or other acute bleeding." If an attempt to stop postprocedural or other acute bleeding is initially unsuccessful, and to stop the bleeding requires performing a more definitive root operation, such as Bypass, Detachment, Excision, Extraction, Reposition, Replacement, or Resection, then the more definitive root operation is coded instead of Control.
B3.8 Excision versus Resection as Root Operation	PCS contains specific body parts for anatomical subdivisions of a body part, such as lobes of the lungs or liver and regions of the intestine. Resection of the specific body part is coded whenever all of the body part is cut out or off, rather than coding Excision of a less specific body part.

(Continued on next page)

Section	Summary of instruction
B3.9 Excision for Graft	If an autograft is obtained from a different procedure site in order to complete the objective of a procedure, a separate procedure is coded. Exception when the seventh character qualifier value in the ICD-10-PCS table fully specifies the site from which the autograft was obtained.
B3.10a Fusion Procedures of the spine	The body part coded for a spinal vertebral joint(s) rendered immobile by a spinal fusion procedure is classified by the level of the spine (e.g. thoracic). There are distinct body part values for a single vertebral joint and for multiple vertebral joints at each spinal level.
B3.10B Fusion Procedures Using Different Device and/or Qualifier	If multiple vertebral joints are fused, a separate procedure is coded for each vertebral joint that uses a different device and/or qualifier.
B3.10c Fusion Procedures— Combinations of Devices and Materials Hierarchy	Combinations of devices and materials are often used on a vertebral joint to render the joint immobile. When combinations of devices are used on the same vertebral joint, the device value coded for the procedure is as follows: • If an interbody fusion device is used to render the joint immobile (alone or containing other material like bone graft), the procedure is coded with the device value Interbody Fusion Device • If bone graft is the *only* device used to render the joint immobile, the procedure is coded with the device value Nonautologous Tissue Substitute or Autologous Tissue Substitute • If a mixture of autologous and nonautologous bone graft (with or without biological or synthetic extenders or binders) is used to render the joint immobile, code the procedure with the device value Autologous Tissue Substitute
B3.11a Inspection procedures as Root Operation	Inspection of a body part(s) performed in order to achieve the objective of a procedure is not coded separately.
B3.11b Inspection of Most Distal Body Part	If multiple tubular body parts are inspected, the most distal body part inspected (the body part furthest from the starting point of the inspection) is coded. If multiple nontubular body parts in the region are inspected, the body part that specifies the entire area inspected is coded.
B3.11c Inspection Done by Different Approach	When both an Inspection procedure and another procedure are performed on the same body part during the same episode, if the Inspection procedure is performed using a different approach than the other procedure, the Inspection procedure is coded separately.
B3.12 Occlusion versus Restriction as Root Operation	If the objective of an embolization procedure is to completely close a vessel, the root operation Occlusion is coded. If the objective is to narrow the lumen of a vessel, the root operation Restriction is coded.
B3.13 Release Procedures as Root Operation	In the root operation Release, the body part value is the body part being freed and not the tissue being manipulated or cut to free the body part.
B3.14 Release versus Division Procedures as Root Operation	If the sole objective of the procedure is freeing a body part without cutting the body part, the root operation is Release. If the sole objective is separating or transecting a body part, the root operation is Division.
B3.15 Reposition for fracture treatment	Reduction of a displaced fracture is coded to the root operation Reposition and the application of a cast or splint with the reposition procedure is not coded separately. The treatment of a nondisplaced fracture is coded to the procedure performed.

Section	Summary of instruction
B3.16 Transplantation versus Administration	Putting in a mature and functioning living body part taken from another individual or animal is coded to the root operation Transplantation. Putting in autologous or nonautologous cells is coded to the Administration section.
B3.17 Transfer procedures using multiple tissue layers	The root operation Transfer contains qualifiers that can be used to specify when a transfer flap is composed of more than one tissue layer, such as a musculocutaneous flap. For procedures involving transfer of multiple tissue layers including skin, subcutaneous tissue, fascia or muscle, the procedure is coded to the body part value that describes the deepest tissue layer in the flap, and the qualifier can be used to describe the other tissue layer(s) in the transfer flap.
B4 Body Part	
B4.1a Portion of a Body Part	If the procedure is performed on a portion of a body part that does not have a separate body part value, code the body part value corresponding to the whole body part.
B4.1b Prefix "Peri" used with a Body part	If the prefix "peri" is combined with a body part to identify the site of the procedure, and the site of the procedure is not further specified, then the procedure is coded to the body part named. This guideline only applies when a more specific body part value is not available.
B4.1c Continuous section of tubular body part	If a procedure is performed on a continuous section of a tubular body part, code the body part value corresponding to the furthest anatomical site from the point of entry.
B4.2 Branches of a Body Part	Where a specific branch of a body part does not have its own body part value in PCS, the body part is typically coded to the closest proximal branch that has a specific body part value. In the cardiovascular body systems, if a general body part is available in the correct root operation table, and coding to a proximal branch would require assigning a code in a different body system, the procedure is coded using the general body part value.
B4.3 Bilateral Body Parts	Bilateral body part values are available for a limited number of body parts. If the identical procedure is performed on contralateral body parts, and a bilateral body part value exists for that body part, a single procedure is coded using the bilateral body part value. If no bilateral body part value exists, each procedure is coded separately using the appropriate body part value.
B4.4 Coronary Arteries	The coronary arteries are classified as a single body part that is further specified by number of arteries treated. One procedure code specifying multiple arteries is used when the same procedure is performed, including the same device and qualifier values.
B4.5 Tendons, Ligaments, Bursae and Fascia Near a Joint	Procedures performed on tendons, ligaments, bursae and fascia supporting a joint are coded to the body part in the respective body system that is the focus of the procedure. Procedures performed on joint structures are coded to the body part in the joint body systems.
B4.6 Skin, Subcutaneous Tissue and Fascia Overlying a Joint	If a procedure is performed on the skin, subcutaneous tissue or fascia overlying a joint, the procedure is coded to the following body part: • Shoulder is coded to Upper Arm • Elbow is coded to Lower Arm • Wrist is coded to Lower Arm • Hip is coded to Upper Leg • Knee is coded to Lower Leg • Ankle is coded to Foot
B4.7 Fingers and Toes	If a body system does not contain a separate body part value for fingers, procedures performed on the fingers are coded to the body part value for the hand. If a body system does not contain a separate body part value for toes, procedures performed on the toes are coded to the body part value for the foot.

(Continued on next page)

Section	Summary of instruction
B4.8 Upper and Lower Intestinal Tract	In the Gastrointestinal body system, the general body part values Upper Intestinal Tract and Lower Intestinal Tract are provided as an option for the root operations Change, Inspection, Removal and Revision. Upper Intestinal Tract includes the portion of the gastrointestinal tract from the esophagus down to and including the duodenum, and Lower Intestinal Tract includes the portion of the gastrointestinal tract from the jejunum down to and including the rectum and anus.
B5 Approach	
B5.2 Open Approach with Percutaneous Endoscopic Assistance	Procedures performed using the open approach with percutaneous endoscopic assistance is coded to the approach Open.
B5.3a External Approach	Procedures performed within an orifice on structures that are visible without the aid of any instrumentation are coded to the approach External.
B5.3b External Approach through Body Layers	Procedures performed indirectly by the application of external force through the intervening body layers are coded to the approach External.
B5.4 Percutaneous Procedure via Device	Procedures performed percutaneously via a device placed for the procedure are coded to the approach percutaneous.
B6 Device	
B6.1a General Guidelines	A device is coded only if a device remains after the procedure is completed. If no device remains, the device value No Device is coded. In limited root operations, the classification provides the qualifier values Temporary and Intraoperative, for specific procedures involving clinically significant devices, where the purpose of the device is to be utilized for a brief duration during the procedure or current inpatient stay. If a device that is intended to remain after the procedure is completed requires removal before the end of the operative episode in which it was inserted (for example, the device size is inadequate or a complication occurs), both the insertion and removal of the device should be coded.
B6.1b What is Not Considered a Device	Materials such as sutures, ligatures, radiological markers, and temporary postoperative wound drains are considered integral to the performance of the procedure and not coded as devices.
B6.1c Procedures Performed on a Device Only	Procedures performed on a device only, and not on a body part, specified in the root operations Change, Irrigation, Removal, and Revision are coded to the procedure performed.
B6.2 Drainage Device	A separate procedure to put in a drainage device is coded to the root operation Drainage with the device value Drainage Device.
C. Obstetric Section Guidelines	
C1 Products of Conception	Procedures performed on the products of conception are coded to the Obstetrics section. Procedures performed on the pregnant female other than the products of conception are coded to the root operation in the Medical and Surgical section.
C2 Procedures Following Delivery or Abortion	Procedure performed following a delivery or abortion for curettage of the endometrium or evacuation of retained products of conception are all coded in the Obstetrics section, to the root operation Extraction and the body part Products of Conception, retained. Diagnostic or therapeutic D&C performed during times other than postpartum or post-abortion are coded to the Medical and Surgical section, to the root operation Extraction and the body part Endometrium.

Section	Summary of instruction
D. Radiation Therapy Section	
D1.a Brachytherapy	Brachytherapy is coded to the modality Brachytherapy in the Radiation Therapy section. When a radioactive brachytherapy source is left in the body at the end of the procedure, it is coded separately to the root operation Insertion with the device value Radioactive Element. Exception : implantation of Cesium-131 brachytherapy seeds embedded in a collagen matrix to the treatment site after resection of brain tumor is coded to the root operation Insertion with the device value Radioactive Element, Cesium-131 Collagen Implant.
D1.b Separate procedure	A separate procedure to place a temporary applicator for delivering the brachytherapy is coded to the root operation Insertion and the device value Other Device.
E. New Technology Section (Section X)	
E1.a General Guidelines	Section X codes fully represent the specific procedure described in the code title, and do not require additional codes from other sections of ICD-10-PCS. When section X contains a code title which fully describes a specific new technology procedure, and it is the only procedure performed, only the section X code is reported for the procedure. There is no need to report an additional code in another section of ICD-10-PCS.
E1.b Multiple procedures	When multiple procedures are performed, New Technology section X codes are coded following the multiple procedures guideline.
F. Section of Principal Procedure	The following instructions should be applied in the selection of principal procedure and clarification on the importance of the relation to the principal diagnosis when more than one procedure is performed.
1. Procedure performed for Definitive Treatment for Both Principal Diagnosis and Secondary Diagnosis	Sequence procedure performed for definitive treatment most related to principal diagnosis as principal procedure.
2. Procedure performed for Definitive Treatment and Diagnostic Procedure performed for Both Principal Diagnosis and Secondary Diagnosis	Sequence procedure performed for definitive treatment most related to principal diagnosis as principal procedure.
3. Diagnostic Procedure performed for the Principal Diagnosis and Procedure performed for Definitive Treatment of a Secondary Diagnosis	Sequence diagnostic procedure as principal procedure, since the procedure most related to the principal diagnosis takes precedence.
4. No Procedure Performed for Principal Diagnosis. Procedure performed for Definitive Treatment and Diagnostic Procedure performed for Secondary Diagnosis.	Sequence procedure performed for definitive treatment of secondary diagnosis as principal procedure, since there are no procedures (definitive or nondefinitive treatment) related to principal diagnosis.

Source: CMS 2019

ICD-10-PCS New Technology Section Codes

Section X New Technology is a section added to ICD-10-PCS that began October 1, 2015. This section provides a place for codes that uniquely identify procedures requested via the New Technology Application Process or that capture other new technologies not currently classified in ICD-10-PCS. This section may include codes for medical and surgical procedures, medical and surgical-related procedures, or ancillary procedures designated as new technology.

In Section X, the seven characters are defined as follows:

First character = Section (X)
Second character = Body system
Third character = Operation
Fourth character = Body part
Fifth character = Approach
Sixth character = Device, Substance, Technology
Seventh character = Qualifier: new technology group

The New Technology section includes new technology drug infusions and can potentially include a wide range of other new technology in medical, surgical, and ancillary procedures (CMS 2019).

Section X codes are similar to codes within other sections of ICD-10-PCS by using some of the same root operations and body parts as in other sections of ICD-10-PCS. For example, two codes for the infusion of a new technology antibiotic use the same root operation (Introduction) and body part values (Central Vein and Peripheral Vein) in Section X as the infusion codes in Section 3 Administration, which are their closest counterparts in the other sections of ICD-10-PCS. In Section X, the seventh character is used exclusively to indicate the new technology group.

The New Technology Group is a number or letter that can change each year as new technology codes are added to the system. For example, the seventh character of 1 is used for codes added the first year. 2019 Section X codes added the seventh character value 3 New Technology Group 3, and so on.

Changing the seventh character New Technology Group to a unique value every year when new codes are added to this section allows the ICD-10-PCS to reuse the values in the third, fourth, and sixth characters as needed. This avoids the creation of duplicate codes. Having a unique code for the New Technology Group creates the flexibility and capacity of Section X over time and allows it to evolve as medical technology develops.

The body system values are the second character for the new technology codes. These values do not change from year to year. Body system values, however, are broader values in New Technology than in other parts of ICD-10-PCS to allow the values to be as general or as specific as necessary to describe the procedure.

The third character is the root operation. For 2020, the root operations include Dilation, Assistance, Extirpation, Replacement, Reposition, Introduction, Measurement, Monitoring, Destruction, and Fusion (CMS 2019).

Extirpation

Definition: Taking or cutting out solid matter from a body part
Explanation: The solid matter may be an abnormal by-product of a biological function or a foreign body; it may be imbedded in a body part or in the lumen of a tubular body part.

The solid matter may or may not have been previously broken into pieces. As an example, table 2.14 is the X2C table for new technology.

Table 2.14.   **New Technology table X2C**

Section	X	New Technology
Body System	2	Cardiovascular System
Operation	C	Extirpation: Taking or cutting out solid matter from a body part

Body Part	Approach	Device/Substance/Technology	Qualifier
0 Coronary artery, one artery 1 Coronary artery, two arteries 2 Coronary artery, three arteries 3 Coronary artery, four or more arteries	3 Percutaneous	6 Orbital atherectomy technology	1 New Technology Group 1

Source: CMS 2019

Introduction

Definition: Putting in or on a therapeutic, diagnostic, nutritional, physiological, or prophylactic substance except blood or blood products. The new technology procedures could be done by intravenous infusions via a peripheral or central vein as shown in table 2.15, the XY0 table, below.

Table 2.15.   **New Technology table XY0**

Section	X	New Technology
Body System	Y	Extracorporeal
Operation	0	Introduction: Putting in or on a therapeutic, diagnostic, nutritional, physiological, or prophylactic substance except blood or blood products

Body Part	Approach	Device/Substance/Technology	Qualifier
V Vein Graft	X External	8 Endothelial Damage Inhibitor	3 New Technology Group 3

Source: CMS 2019

Monitoring

Definition: Determining the level of a physiological or physical function repetitively over a period of time. This new technology uses an intraoperative knee replacement sensor that is used during the knee replacement surgery to assess the function of the joint within the knee. As an example, table 2.16 is the XR2 table for new technology.

Table 2.16.   **New Technology table XR2**

Section	X	New Technology
Body System	R	Joints
Operation	2	Monitoring: Determining the level of a physiological or physical function repetitively over a period of time

Body Part	Approach	Device/Substance/Technology	Qualifier
G Knee joint right H Knee joint left	0 Open	2 Intraoperative knee replacement sensor	1 New Technology Group 1

Source: CMS 2019

The body part value is the fourth character in Section X. The body part values do not change from year to year but rather combine the uses of body system, body region, and physiological system as specified in other sections of ICD-10-PCS. For this reason, the second character body system values are more broad values. This allows the body part values to be as general or as specific as needed to represent the body part applicable to the new technology.

New Technology Section Guidelines for Section X

Section X codes are standalone codes. They are not used as a second code with another ICD-10-PCS code to describe the procedure. Section X codes fully represent the specific procedure described in the code title. When Section X contains a code title that describes a specific new technology procedure, only that X code is reported for the procedure. There is no need to report a broader, nonspecific code in another section of ICD-10-PCS (CMS 2016b). Additionally, when multiple procedures are performed, New Technology section X codes are coded following the multiple procedures guideline.

For example, code XW04321 Introduction of Ceftazidime-Avibactam Anti-infective into Central Vein, Percutaneous Approach, New Technology Group 1, would be reported to indicate that Ceftazidime-Avibactam Anti-infective was administered via central vein. A separate code from table 3E0 in the Administration section of ICD-10-PCS would not be reported in addition to this code. The X section code fully identifies the administration of the ceftazidime-avibactam antibiotic, and no additional code is needed.

Alphabetic Index for New Technology Codes

The New Technology section codes are located by using the ICD-10-PCS Index or the Tables. In the Index, the name of the new technology device, substance or technology for a Section X code is included as a main term. The codes in Section X are also listed under the main term New Technology. An example of the index entry for MIRODERM is shown below.

> **EXAMPLE:** MIRODERM™ Biologic Wound Matrix
> *use* Skin Substitute, Porcine Liver Derived in New Technology
> XHR

In the Tables, New Technology codes are displayed like other ICD-10-PCS tables with a separate table for each root operation and body system.

Selection of Principal Procedure

According to the *ICD-10-PCS Official Guidelines for Coding and Reporting*, the following instructions should be applied in the selection of principal procedure and clarification on the importance of the relation to the principal diagnosis when more than one procedure is performed:

1. Procedure performed for definitive treatment of both principal diagnosis and secondary diagnosis

   a. Sequence procedure performed for definitive treatment most related to principal diagnosis as principal procedure (CMS 2019).

      EXAMPLE: The patient was admitted with coronary artery disease with angina and is later found to have pulmonary hypertension scheduled for a coronary artery bypass graft. The principal procedure is the coronary artery bypass graft as it is the definitive treatment most related to the principal diagnosis of coronary artery disease with angina.

2. Procedure performed for definitive treatment and diagnostic procedures performed for both principal diagnosis and secondary diagnosis.

   a. Sequence procedure performed for definitive treatment most related to principal diagnosis as principal procedure (CMS 2019).

      EXAMPLE: The patient was admitted with known coronary artery disease with angina and is later found to have mitral valve stenosis. A diagnostic cardiac catheterization and coronary angiography is performed for both of the patient's cardiac conditions, coronary artery disease and mitral valve stenosis. A coronary artery bypass graft is immediately performed based on the severity of the findings of the coronary angiography procedure. The principal procedure is the coronary artery bypass procedure as it is performed for definitive treatment most related to the principal diagnosis of the known coronary artery disease with angina.

3. A diagnostic procedure was performed for the principal diagnosis, and a procedure is performed for definitive treatment of a secondary diagnosis (CMS 2019).

   a. Sequence diagnostic procedure as principal procedure, since the procedure most related to the principal diagnosis takes precedence.

      EXAMPLE: The patient is admitted to the hospital for known coronary artery disease with angina and has a diagnostic cardiac catheterization and coronary angiography procedure performed. Once the patient was stabilized for his cardiac condition, the patient complains of urinary symptoms and has a transurethral resection of his prostate for his known enlarged prostate. The principal procedure is the diagnostic cardiac catheterization procedure as it is most related to the principal diagnosis of coronary artery disease with angina even though the patient had a definitive procedure of a secondary diagnosis.

4. No procedures performed that are related to principal diagnosis; procedures performed for definitive treatment and diagnostic procedures were performed for secondary diagnosis.

   a. Sequence procedure performed for definitive treatment of secondary diagnosis as principal procedure, since there are no procedures (definitive or nondefinitive treatment) related to principal diagnosis (CMS 2019).

      EXAMPLE: The patient is admitted to the hospital for known coronary artery disease with angina. He was treated with medications. Once the patient was stabilized for his cardiac condition, the patient complains of urinary symptoms and has a transurethral resection of his prostate for his known enlarged prostate. The principal procedure is the transurethral resection of his prostate as it is a definitive procedure performed for a secondary diagnosis when there are no procedures (definitive or nondefinitive <u>treatment</u>) related to his principal diagnosis of coronary artery disease with angina.

ICD-10-PCS References

The Centers for Medicare and Medicaid Services (CMS) website discontinued publishing general equivalence mappings (GEMS) following the 2018 ICD-10-PCS code set release. The files on the website for the current version of ICD-10-PCS contain the actual coding system as well as background material, references, and ICD-10-PCS guidelines. The coder should thoroughly review all the downloadable files on the site for daily use. The *ICD-10-PCS Official Guidelines for Coding and Reporting* is referenced throughout this chapter, and a complete document is available in appendix G.

Assigning an ICD-10-PCS Code

An ICD-10-PCS code is constructed by assigning values for each of the characters. The procedural term is referenced in the Index. The main terms listed in the Index can be either the root operation phrase, such as Resection, with the subterm gallbladder, or occasionally a common procedure term, such as cholecystectomy.

According to the *ICD-10-PCS Official Guidelines for Coding and Reporting*, the purpose of the Alphabetic Index is to locate the appropriate table to construct an ICD-10-PCS procedure code. The PCS tables should also be consulted for the most appropriate valid code (guideline A6.) However, the coder does not have to use the Index before proceeding to the tables to construct a code. A coder may choose the appropriate code directly from the code tables (guideline A7). A coder experienced with ICD-10-PCS may perform ICD-10-PCS coding directly from the tables after becoming confident with the definitions of the root operations and the body systems. For new coders, the normal process would likely be to locate the procedure first in the Index and then move to the code tables as directed (CMS 2019).

As an example, to code a laparoscopic total cholecystectomy, the coder could access the root operation Resection in the Index and find:

> Resection
>> Gallbladder, 0FT4

Alternatively, the coder could access the common procedure term "Cholecystectomy" in the Index and find:

> Cholecystectomy
>> See Excision, Gallbladder 0FB4
>> See Resection, Gallbladder 0FT4

It is important to note that in order to choose the appropriate cross reference, the coder must know the definitions of the root operations Excision and Resection. *Excision* is defined as cutting out or off, without replacement, a portion of a body part. *Resection* is defined as cutting out or off, without replacement, all of a body part. A cholecystectomy would be a resection of the gallbladder, as the entire gallbladder is removed during a cholecystectomy.

The next step in the process is to access the 0FT code table. The remaining four characters are assigned based on this table. The values for each of the characters must be from the same row.

For example, using the table that follows, the code for a cholecystectomy performed through a laparoscopic approach would be 0FT44ZZ. Each of the seven characters of the procedure code describes the procedure of a laparoscopic total cholecystectomy:

0 = Medical and Surgical Section

F = Hepatobiliary system and pancreas body system

T = Resection

4 = Gallbladder body part

4 = Percutaneous endoscopic approach

Z = No device

Z = No qualifier

Table 2.17. shows an example of an ICD-10-PCS table. This table is for 0FT, the first three characters for a surgical procedure in the hepatobiliary system and pancreas that is a resection.

Table 2.17. **Resection within the hepatobiliary system and pancreas, 0FT**

0 Medical and Surgical
F Hepatobiliary System and Pancreas
T Resection—Cutting out or off, without replacement, all of a body part

Body Part Character 4	Approach Character 5	Device Character 6	Qualifier Character 7
0 Liver **1** Liver, Right Lobe **2** Liver, Left Lobe **4** **Gallbladder** **G** Pancreas	**0** Open **4** **Percutaneous Endoscopic**	**Z** No Device	**Z** No Qualifier
5 Hepatic Duct, Right **6** Hepatic Duct, Left **7** Hepatic Duct, Common **8** Cystic Duct **9** Common Bile Duct **C** Ampulla of Vater **D** Pancreatic Duct **F** Pancreatic Duct, Accessory	**0** Open **4** Percutaneous Endoscopic **7** Via Natural or Artificial Opening **8** Via Natural or Artificial Opening Endoscopic	**Z** No Device	**Z** No Qualifier

Source: CMS 2019

ICD-10-PCS Review Exercises: Chapter 2

Assign the appropriate ICD-10-PCS codes to the following statements:

1. Esophagogastroduodenoscopy (EGD)

2. Complete bilateral mastectomy

3. Open left femoral-popliteal artery bypass using cadaver vein graft

4. Laparoscopy with lysis of adhesions of bilateral ovaries and bilateral fallopian tubes

(*Continued on next page*)

ICD-10-PCS Review Exercises: Chapter 2 *(continued)*

5. Posterior approach spinal fusion of the anterior column at L2–L4 with Bak cage interbody fusion device, open

6. Right-sided craniotomy for evacuation of subacute subdural hematoma

7. Percutaneous surgical pinning and casting of nondisplaced fracture of left ulna

8. Diagnostic percutaneous paracentesis for ascites in peritoneal cavity

9. Transmetatarsal amputation of foot at right big toe

10. Endoscopic polypectomy conducted at the splenic flexure and biopsy obtained at the transverse colon to evaluate for colitis

11. Percutaneous repositioning of cardiac pacemaker right ventricular electrode via fluoroscopy

12. Administration of Bezlotoxumab Monoclonal Antibody via peripheral vein

13. Mitral valve replacement using porcine tissue, open

14. Percutaneous transluminal coronary angioplasty of right coronary artery

15. Endoscopic fulguration of sigmoid colon polyp

16. Coronary artery bypass, one site from thoracic artery with autologous venous tissue, percutaneous endoscopic approach

17. Revision of left knee replacement with readjustment of prosthesis, open

18. Hysteroscopy with diagnostic D&C

19. Extracorporeal shockwave lithotripsy (EWSL) of right ureter

20. Esophagogastroduodenoscopy with esophagomyotomy of esophagogastric junction

References

Averill, R. F., R. L. Mullin, B. A. Steinbeck, N. I. Goldfield, T. M. Grant, and R. R. Butler. 2016. Development of the ICD-10 Procedure Coding System (ICD-10-PCS). https://www.cms.gov/Medicare/Coding/ICD10/Downloads/2016-Developmentofthe-ICD-10-Procedure-Coding-System.pdf.

Centers for Medicare and Medicaid Services (CMS). 2016a. ICD-10-PCS Reference Manual. https://www.cms.gov/Medicare/Coding/ICD10/downloads/pcs_refman.pdf.

Centers for Medicare and Medicaid Services (CMS). 2016b. Using the ICD-10-PCS New Technology Section X Codes. MLN Matters. https://www.cms.gov/Outreach-and-Education/Medicare-Learning-Network-MLN/MLNMattersArticles/downloads/SE1519.pdf.

Centers for Medicare and Medicaid Services (CMS). 2019. *ICD-10-PCS Official Guidelines for Coding and Reporting*, 2019. https://www.cms.gov/Medicare/Coding/ICD10/2019-ICD-10-PCS-and-GEMs.html.

Kuehn, L. and T. Jorwic. 2018. *ICD-10-PCS: An Applied Approach,* 2018. Chicago: AHIMA.

Chapter 3

Introduction to the Uniform Hospital Discharge Data Set and Official ICD-10-CM Coding Guidelines

Learning Objectives

At the conclusion of this chapter, you should be able to do the following:

- Describe the purpose of the Uniform Hospital Discharge Data Set and identify its data elements

- Apply the *ICD-10-CM Official Guidelines for Coding and Reporting* for selecting the principal diagnosis for inpatient care and reporting of additional diagnoses

- Apply the *ICD-10-CM Official Guidelines for Coding and Reporting* for coding of diagnoses for outpatient services

Key Terms

Comorbidity
Complication
Diagnosis
Disposition of patient
Expected payer
Hospital identification
Other diagnosis

Personal identification
Physician identification
Principal diagnosis
Principal procedure
Significant procedure
Uniform Hospital Discharge Data Set
    (UHDDS)

Uniform Hospital Discharge Data Set

There are many uses for the data that are created by coding activity, including compiling statistical data. In order for these data to be useful, everyone gathering the data must collect the same data the same way. The **Uniform Hospital Discharge Data Set (UHDDS)** was promulgated by the US Department of Health, Education, and Welfare in 1974 as a minimum, common core of data on individual acute care short-term hospital discharges in Medicare and Medicaid programs. It sought to improve the uniformity and comparability of hospital discharge data.

In 1985, the data set was revised to improve the original version in light of timely needs and developments. These data elements and their definitions can be found in the July 31, 1985, *Federal Register* (50 FR 31038, Vol. 50, No. 147, 31038–31040). Since that time, the application of the UHDDS definitions has been expanded to include all nonoutpatient settings (acute care, short-term care, long-term care, and psychiatric hospitals; home health agencies; rehabilitation facilities; nursing homes; and so forth).

Part of the current UHDDS includes the following specific items pertaining to patients and their episodes of care:

- **Personal identification:** The unique number assigned to each patient that distinguishes the patient and his or her health record from all others

- **Date of birth**

- **Sex**

- **Race**

- **Ethnicity (Hispanic–Non-Hispanic)**

- **Residence:** The zip code or code for foreign residence

- **Hospital identification:** The unique number assigned to each institution

- **Admission and discharge dates**

- **Physician identification:** The unique number assigned to each physician within the hospital (the attending physician and the operating physician [if applicable] are both to be identified)

- **Disposition of patient:** The destination of the patient upon leaving the hospital—discharged to home, left against medical advice, discharged to another short-term hospital, discharged to a long-term care institution, died, or other

- **Expected payer:** The single major source expected by the patient to pay for this bill (for example, Blue Cross/Blue Shield, Medicare, Medicaid, workers' compensation)

In keeping with UHDDS standards, medical data items for the following diagnoses and procedures also are reported:

- **Diagnoses:** All diagnoses affecting the current hospital stay must be reported as part of the UHDDS.

- **Principal diagnosis:** The principal diagnosis is designated and defined as the condition established after study to be chiefly responsible for occasioning the admission of the patient to the hospital for care.

- **Other diagnoses:** These are designated and defined as all conditions that coexist at the time of admission, that develop subsequently, or that affect the treatment received or the length of stay (LOS). Diagnoses are to be excluded that relate to an earlier episode that has no bearing on the current hospital stay. Within the Medicare Acute Care Inpatient Prospective Payment System (IPPS), other diagnoses may qualify as a major complication or comorbidity (MCC), or other complication or comorbidity

(CC). The terms complication and comorbidity are not part of the UHDDS definition set but were developed as part of the diagnosis-related group (DRG) system. The presence of the complication or comorbidity may influence the MS-DRG assignment and produce a higher-valued DRG with a higher payment for the hospital.

- **Complication:** This is defined as an *additional* diagnosis that describes a condition arising after the beginning of hospital observation and treatment and then modifying the course of the patient's illness or the medical care required.

- **Comorbidity:** This is defined as a *pre-existing* condition that, because of its presence with a specific principal diagnosis, will likely cause an increase in the patient's length of stay in the hospital.

- **Procedures and dates:** All significant procedures are to be reported. For significant procedures, both the identity (by unique number within the hospital) of the person performing the procedure and the date of the procedure must be reported.

- **Significant procedure:** A procedure is identified as significant when it

  - Is surgical in nature
  - Carries a procedural risk
  - Carries an anesthetic risk
  - Requires specialized training

Deciding whether a procedure performed is a significant procedure is often the determinant if the coder assigns a procedure code to identify the procedure. Nonsignificant procedures are usually not coded.

- **Principal procedure:** This type of procedure is performed for definitive treatment rather than for diagnostic or exploratory purposes, or when it is necessary to take care of a complication. If two procedures appear to be principal, the one most related to the principal diagnosis should be selected as the principal procedure.

Check Your Understanding 3.1

Answer the following questions about the Uniform Hospital Discharge Data Set.

1. How is the individual patient identified according to the data elements in the UHDDS?

2. What is the difference between a complication and comorbidity as identified according to the MS-DRG and why are they important to capture as a code?

3. How does the coder determine if a procedure is significant to code?

4. How does the coder determine if they should capture "other diagnoses?"

5. In addition to the UHDDS specific items collected pertaining to patient demographics and their episode of care (personal identification, DOB, sex, race, ethnicity, residence, hospital identification, admission and discharge dates, physician identification, disposition of patient and expected payer); what other specific medical data items are reported?

Selection of Principal Diagnosis

As the UHDDS definition states, a principal diagnosis is the condition "established after study to be chiefly responsible for occasioning the admission of the patient to the hospital for care" (the UHDDS data elements and definitions can be found in the July 31, 1985, *Federal Register* (50 FR 31038, Vol. 50, No. 147, 31038–31040)). Selecting the principal diagnosis depends on the circumstances of the admission, or why the patient was admitted. The admitting diagnosis has to be determined through diagnostic tests and studies. Therefore, the words "after study" serve as an integral part of this definition. During the course of hospitalization, the admitting diagnosis, which may be a symptom or ill-defined condition, could change substantially based on the results of further study.

> **EXAMPLE:** Patient was admitted through the emergency department with an admitting diagnosis of seizure disorder. During hospitalization, diagnostic tests and studies revealed carcinoma of the brain, which explained the seizures.
>
> The principal diagnosis was the carcinoma of the brain, which was the condition determined after study.

At times, however, it may be difficult to distinguish between the *principal* diagnosis and the *most significant* diagnosis. The most significant diagnosis is defined as the condition having the most impact on the patient's health, LOS, resource consumption, and the like. However, the most significant diagnosis may or may not be the principal diagnosis.

> **EXAMPLE:** Patient was admitted with a fractured hip due to an accident. The fracture was reduced and the patient discharged home.
>
> In this case, the principal diagnosis was fracture of the hip.

> **EXAMPLE:** Patient was admitted with a fractured hip due to an accident. While hospitalized, the patient suffered a myocardial infarction.
>
> In this case, the principal diagnosis was still the fracture of the hip, with the myocardial infarction coded as an additional diagnosis. Although the myocardial infarction may be the most significant diagnosis in terms of the patient's health and resource consumption, it was not the reason, after study, for the admission; therefore, it was not the principal diagnosis.

Another important consideration in determining principal diagnosis is the fact that the coding conventions and instructions of the classification in ICD-10-CM take precedence over the Official Coding Guidelines. See Section I Conventions for the ICD-10-CM.

ICD-10-CM Official Guidelines for Coding and Reporting

The *ICD-10-CM Official Guidelines for Coding and Reporting* is available from the Centers for Disease Control and Prevention website (CDC 2019). All coding students are strongly encouraged to read the guidelines and become familiar with the rules in order to put them into practice. The application of the guidelines in everyday practice helps to ensure data accuracy in both coding and reporting for all healthcare encounters. Reporting is the process of communicating the patient's diagnoses and procedures in codes to third-party payers for reimbursement purposes and to other internal or facility databases and other external required databases for financial, quality measurement, public data, and other purposes.

The *ICD-10-CM Official Guidelines for Coding and Reporting* is referenced throughout this book. The complete document can be found in appendix F.

Selecting Principal Diagnosis for Inpatient Care

The following information on selecting the principal diagnosis and additional diagnoses should be reviewed carefully to ensure appropriate coding and reporting of hospital claims.

The circumstances of inpatient admission always govern selection of the principal diagnosis in keeping with the UHDDS definition of the term as "that condition established after study to be chiefly responsible for occasioning the admission of the patient to the hospital for care" (50 FR 31038, Vol. 50, No. 147, 31038–31040) and included in the Section II. Selection of the Principal Diagnosis, *ICD-10-CM Official Guidelines for Coding and Reporting* FY 2020. The UHDDS definitions also include all non-outpatient settings including hospice services.

In determining the principal diagnosis, the coding directives in ICD-10-CM, the Tabular List, and Alphabetic Index take precedence over all other guidelines.

The importance of consistent, complete documentation in the medical record cannot be overemphasized. Without such documentation, the application of all coding guidelines is a difficult, if not impossible, task.

Section II of the *ICD-10-CM Official Guidelines for Coding and Reporting* addresses the selection of the principal diagnosis:

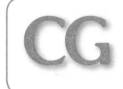

Guideline II.A. Codes for symptoms, signs, and ill-defined conditions: Codes for symptoms, signs, and ill-defined conditions from chapter 18 are not to be used as the principal diagnosis when a related definitive diagnosis has been established.

EXAMPLE: Patient was admitted to the hospital with chest pain to rule out myocardial infarction. After study, myocardial infarction was ruled out; the cause of the chest pain was undetermined.

Code R07.9, Chest pain, unspecified, was assigned. Although the code for chest pain (R07.9) is located in Chapter 18, Symptoms, Signs and Abnormal Clinical and Laboratory Findings, Not Elsewhere Classified, a definitive diagnosis could not be made, so chest pain was coded as the principal diagnosis.

EXAMPLE: Patient was admitted to the hospital with dysphagia secondary to malignant neoplasm of the esophagus. A PEG tube was inserted.

Code C15.9, Malignant neoplasm of the esophagus, unspecified, was selected as the principal diagnosis, with code R13.10 as an additional diagnosis to describe the dysphagia. Because the dysphagia was related to the malignancy and code R13.10 is from Chapter 18, the principal diagnosis was the definitive diagnosis rather than the symptom.

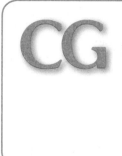

Guideline II.B. Two or more interrelated conditions, each potentially meeting the definition for principal diagnosis: When there are two or more interrelated conditions (such as diseases in the same ICD-10-CM chapter, or manifestations characteristically associated with a certain disease) potentially meeting the definition of principal diagnosis, either condition may be sequenced first, unless the circumstances of the admission, the therapy provided, the Tabular List, or the Alphabetic Index indicates otherwise.

EXAMPLE: Patient was admitted for initial treatment for a closed fracture of the right femur lower end and fracture of the right tibia upper end.

The following diagnosis codes were assigned: S72.401A, Fracture of femur, right, lower end, closed; S82.101A, Fracture of tibia, right, upper end, closed. Both fractures potentially met the definition of principal diagnosis; therefore, either code could be sequenced first.

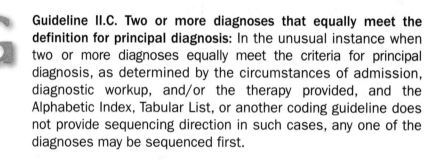

Guideline II.C. Two or more diagnoses that equally meet the definition for principal diagnosis: In the unusual instance when two or more diagnoses equally meet the criteria for principal diagnosis, as determined by the circumstances of admission, diagnostic workup, and/or the therapy provided, and the Alphabetic Index, Tabular List, or another coding guideline does not provide sequencing direction in such cases, any one of the diagnoses may be sequenced first.

EXAMPLE: Patient was admitted for elective surgery. A lesion on the left breast was excised and revealed fibroadenosis of breast. In addition, a right recurrent inguinal hernia was repaired.

The following diagnosis codes were assigned: N60.22, Fibroadenosis of left breast and K40.91, Unilateral inguinal hernia, without mention of obstruction or gangrene, recurrent. Both the fibroadenosis of left breast and the right recurrent inguinal hernia met the criteria for principal diagnosis. Therefore, either condition could be selected as the principal diagnosis.

Guideline II.D. Two or more comparative or contrasting conditions: In those rare instances when two or more contrasting or comparative diagnoses are documented as "either/or" (or similar terminology), they are coded as if confirmed and sequenced according to the circumstances of the admission. If no further determination can be made as to which diagnosis is principal, either diagnosis may be sequenced first.

EXAMPLE: Diverticulosis of large intestine versus angiodysplasia of colon

Codes K57.30, Diverticulosis of large intestine without perforation or abscess without bleeding and K55.20, Angiodysplasia of colon without hemorrhage are assigned.

Either unconfirmed diagnosis, diverticulosis or angiodysplasia of colon, may be sequenced as the principal diagnosis.

Note: Guidelines II.A through II.D reveal that designation of the principal diagnosis is not always an exact and easy task. At times, more than one condition may have occasioned the admission. In such cases, the actual circumstances of the case dictate designation of the principal diagnosis.

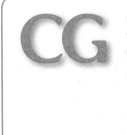

Guideline II.E. A symptom(s) followed by contrasting or comparative diagnoses:
GUIDELINE HAS BEEN DELETED EFFECTIVE OCTOBER 1, 2014

Guideline II.F. Original treatment plan not carried out: Sequence as the principal diagnosis the condition which after study occasioned the admission to the hospital, even though treatment may not have been carried out due to unforeseen circumstances.

EXAMPLE: Patient with ulcerated internal hemorrhoids was admitted for hemorrhoidectomy. Prior to the beginning of surgery, the patient developed bradycardia and the surgery was canceled.

The following codes were assigned: K64.8, Ulcerated internal hemorrhoids; R00.1, Bradycardia; and Z53.09, Procedure not carried out because of contraindication. The code for ulcerated internal hemorrhoids (K64.8) was listed as the principal diagnosis because it was the reason for admission. An additional code for bradycardia (R00.1) was reported, as well as code Z53.09, Procedure not carried out because of contraindication, to indicate that the procedure was not carried out due to the complication of bradycardia.

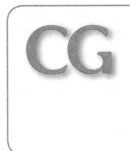

Guideline II.G. Complications of surgery and other medical care: When the admission is for treatment of a complication resulting from surgery or other medical care, the complication code is sequenced as the principal diagnosis. If the complication is classified to T80-T88 series, and the code lacks the necessary specificity in describing the complication, an additional code for the specific complication should be assigned.

EXAMPLE: Patient was being treated for an atelectasis due to recent cardiovascular surgery. The diagnosis codes would include J95.89, Other postprocedural complications and disorders of respiratory system, not elsewhere classified, and J98.11, Atelectasis.

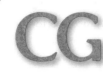

Guideline II.H. Uncertain diagnosis: If the diagnosis documented at the time of discharge is qualified as "probable," "suspected," "likely," "questionable," "possible," or "still to be ruled out," «compatible with,» «consistent with,» or other similar terms indicating uncertainty, code the condition as if it existed or was established. The bases for these guidelines are the diagnostic workup, arrangements for further workup or observation, and initial therapeutic approach that correspond most closely with the established diagnosis. Note: This guideline is applicable only to inpatient admissions to short-term, acute care, long-term care, and psychiatric hospitals.

Guideline II.I. Admission from observation unit:

1. Admission Following Medical Observation.

   When a patient is admitted to an observation unit for a medical condition, which either worsens or does not improve, and is subsequently admitted as an inpatient of the same hospital for this same medical condition, the principal diagnosis would be the medical condition that led to the hospital admission.

2. Admission Following Postoperative Observation.

   When a patient is admitted to an observation unit to monitor a condition (or complication) that develops following outpatient surgery, and then is subsequently admitted as an inpatient of the same hospital, hospitals should apply the UHDDS definition of principal diagnosis as "that condition established after study to be chiefly responsible for occasioning the admission of the patient to the hospital for care."

Guideline II.J. Admission from outpatient surgery: When a patient receives surgery in the hospital's outpatient surgery department and is subsequently admitted for continuing inpatient care at the same hospital, the following guidelines should be followed in selecting the principal diagnosis for the inpatient admission:

- When the reason for the inpatient admission is a complication, assign the complication as the principal diagnosis.

- When the reason for the inpatient admission is another condition unrelated to the surgery, assign the unrelated condition as the principal diagnosis.

Guideline II.K. Admissions/Encounters for Rehabilitation: When the purpose for the admission/encounter is rehabilitation, sequence first the code for the condition for which the service is being performed.

For example, for an admission/encounter for rehabilitation for right-sided dominant hemiplegia following a cerebrovascular infarction, report code I69.351, Hemiplegia and hemiparesis following cerebral infarction affecting right dominant side, as the first-listed or principal diagnosis.

If the condition for which the rehabilitation service is no longer present, report the appropriate aftercare code as the first-listed or principal diagnosis, unless the rehabilitation service is being provided following an injury. For rehabilitation services following active treatment of an injury, assign the injury code with the appropriate seventh character for subsequent encounter as the first-listed or principal diagnosis.

For example, if a patient with severe degenerative osteoarthritis of the hip, underwent hip replacement and the current encounter/admission is for rehabilitation, report code Z47.1, Aftercare following joint replacement surgery, as the first-listed or principal diagnosis. If the patient requires rehabilitation post hip replacement for right intertrochanteric femur fracture, report code S72.141D, Displaced intertrochanteric fracture of right femur, subsequent encounter for closed fracture with routine healing, as the first-listed or principal diagnosis.

See Section I.C.21.c.7, Factors influencing health states and contact with health services, Aftercare.

See Section I.C.19.a for additional information about the use of 7th characters for injury codes.

Check Your Understanding 3.2

Answer the following questions about the official coding guidelines regarding the selection of the principal diagnosis.

1. According to Guideline II.A., can diagnosis codes for symptoms, signs, and ill-defined conditions be assigned as a principal diagnosis and in what circumstance?

2. According to Guideline II.F., how would a coder capture the principal diagnosis when the original treatment plan was not carried out?

3. What is the difference between the admitting diagnosis, the principle diagnosis, and the most significant diagnosis?

4. According to Guideline II.H., when the diagnosis documented at the time of discharge is qualified as "probable," "suspected," "likely," "questionable," Possible, or "still to be ruled out," how should the coder proceed with coding?

5. According to Guideline II.J., how is the principal diagnosis assigned when a patient is admitted to the hospital from outpatient surgery?

Reporting of Additional Diagnoses

Deciding what else to code can be a challenge for coders. Physicians write many facts about the patient in terms of diagnoses and conditions that are present in the patient. However, not everything a physician includes in a record is something to be coded. The *ICD-10-CM Official Guidelines for Coding and Reporting* help the coder decide what else to code in addition to the principal diagnosis.

In the definition of "other diagnoses," conditions that require clinical evaluation are to be coded. Clinical evaluation usually means the physician has taken the condition into consideration when examining the patient. An evaluation can mean the physician is considering testing of the condition or closely observing the condition to decide if new treatment is necessary or if the current treatment is sufficient. Frequently when a condition is being evaluated, there also will be treatment or diagnostic procedures performed for it.

The sequencing of the additional diagnoses is not mandated by a particular coding guideline. Generally, the diagnoses that were more significant in terms of what received the most attention during the patient's hospital stay are listed first in the list of all additional diagnoses. This is a style that many coders follow but again, not a specific coding guideline.

Section III of the *ICD-10-CM Official Guidelines for Coding and Reporting* addresses the general rules for reporting other or additional diagnoses. For example, the guidelines in Section III A through Section III C identify when previous conditions and abnormal findings of diagnostic tests are coded and how to code uncertain diagnoses as described by the physician as possible, probable, or similar terminology.

For reporting purposes, the definition for "other diagnoses" is interpreted as additional conditions that affect patient care in terms of requiring one of the five factors about the patient care:

- clinical evaluation;

- therapeutic treatment;

- diagnostic procedures;

- extended length of hospital stay; or

- increased nursing care or monitoring.

The UHDDS item #11-B defines other diagnoses as "all conditions that coexist at the time of admission, that develop subsequently, or that affect the treatment received or the length of stay. Diagnoses that relate to an earlier episode that have no bearing on the current hospital stay are to be excluded." UHDDS definitions apply to inpatients in acute care, short- and long-term care, and psychiatric hospital settings. The UHDDS definitions are used by acute care short-term hospitals to report inpatient data in a standardized manner. These data elements and their definitions can be found in the July 31, 1985 *Federal Register* (Vol. 50, No. 147, 31038–31040).

Since that time, the application of the UHDDS definitions has been expanded to include all nonoutpatient settings (acute care, short- and long-term care, and psychiatric hospitals; home health agencies; rehab facilities; nursing homes, and such). The UHDDS definitions also apply to hospice services (all levels of care).

The following guidelines are to be applied in designating "other diagnoses" when neither the Alphabetic Index nor the Tabular List in ICD-10-CM provide directions. The listing of the diagnoses in the patient record is the responsibility of the attending provider.

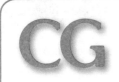 **Guideline III.A. Previous conditions:** If the provider has included a diagnosis in the final diagnostic statement, such as the discharge summary or the face sheet, it should ordinarily be coded. Some providers include in the diagnostic statement resolved conditions or diagnoses and status post procedures from a previous admission that have no bearing on the current stay. Such conditions are not to be reported and are coded only if required by hospital policy.

However, history codes (categories Z80–Z87) may be used as secondary codes if the historical condition or family history has an impact on current care or influences treatment.

EXAMPLE: The face sheet states the following diagnoses: acute diverticulitis, congestive heart failure, status post cholecystectomy, status post hysterectomy.

All are coded except the status post cholecystectomy and hysterectomy. The heart failure and the diverticulitis affect the current hospitalization and thus are coded.

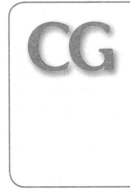 **Guideline III.B. Abnormal findings:** Abnormal findings (laboratory, x-ray, pathologic, and other diagnostic results) are not coded and reported unless the provider indicates their clinical significance. If the findings are outside the normal range and the attending provider has ordered other tests to evaluate the condition or prescribed treatment, it is appropriate to ask the provider whether the abnormal finding should be added. Note: this differs from the coding practices in the outpatient setting for coding encounters for diagnostic tests that have been interpreted by a provider.

EXAMPLE: In the inpatient setting, coders should not assign codes for conditions described in a pathology report alone without the provider's input. The provider or physician should be asked for clarification of the pathological findings if the provider has not documented the same condition in the health record.

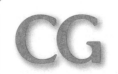 **Guideline III.C. Uncertain diagnosis:** If the diagnosis documented at the time of discharge is qualified as "probable," "suspected," "likely," "questionable," "possible," or "still to be ruled out," « compatible with, » « consistent with, » or other similar terms indicating uncertainty, code the condition as if it existed or was established. The bases for these guidelines are the diagnostic workup, arrangements for further workup or observation, and initial therapeutic approach that correspond most closely with the established diagnosis.

Note: This guideline is applicable only to inpatient admissions to short-term, acute, long-term care, and psychiatric hospitals.

Check Your Understanding 3.3

Answer the following questions about the official coding guidelines regarding the selection of the additional diagnosis codes.

1. What is the UHDDS's definition of "Other Diagnoses"?

2. To determine if an additional diagnosis should be reported, what five factors should the coder consider for "other diagnoses" when defined as conditions that affect patient care?

3. According to Guideline III.A., is it appropriate to code for documented resolved conditions or status-post procedures from previous admissions?

4. Reflecting on Guideline III.B., what should a coder do if they notice findings outside of the normal ranges (such on a lab or other diagnostic report) and the attending provider has ordered other tests to evaluate the condition?

5. According to Guideline III.C., can uncertain diagnoses be reported as additional diagnosis?

Section IV: Diagnostic Coding and Reporting Guidelines for Outpatient Services

The coding of healthcare services in an outpatient setting is different from the coding of patients' diagnoses provided in an inpatient setting. Outpatient encounters are often short visits, and there is not a lot of time to study the patient's condition in depth. For the outpatient visit, the goal of coding is to code what is known for certain about the patient's diagnosis, problem, or condition at that point in time and what was the focus of the healthcare attention at that time. The coding guidelines listed below direct the coder on how to code patient visits in a hospital outpatient setting, physician's office, or other ambulatory care center.

Section IV of the *ICD-10-CM Official Guidelines for Coding and Reporting* address the general rules for diagnostic coding and reporting guidelines for outpatient services:

Note: The most recent complete version of the *ICD-10-CM Official Guidelines for Coding and Reporting* can be found on the CDC website (CDC 2019) and are also included in appendix F.

CG These coding guidelines for outpatient diagnoses have been approved for use by hospitals/providers in coding and reporting hospital-based outpatient services and provider-based office visits. Guidelines in Section I, Conventions, general coding guidelines and chapter-specific guidelines, should also be applied for outpatient services and office visits.

Information about the use of certain abbreviations, punctuation, symbols, and other conventions used in the ICD-10-CM Tabular List (code numbers and titles) can be found in Section IA of these guidelines, under "Conventions Used in the Tabular List." Information about the correct sequence to use in finding a code is also described in Section I.

The terms encounter and visit are often used interchangeably in describing outpatient service contacts and, therefore, appear together in these guidelines without distinguishing one from the other.

Though the conventions and general guidelines apply to all settings, coding guidelines for outpatient and provider reporting of diagnoses will vary in a number of instances from those for inpatient diagnoses, recognizing that:

The Uniform Hospital Discharge Data Set (UHDDS) definition of principal diagnosis does not apply to hospital-based outpatient services and provider-based office visits.

Coding guidelines for inconclusive diagnoses (probable, suspected, rule out, etc.) were developed for inpatient reporting and do not apply to outpatients.

A. **Selection of first-listed condition**

In the outpatient setting, the term first-listed diagnosis is used in lieu of principal diagnosis.

In determining the first-listed diagnosis the coding conventions of ICD-10-CM, as well as the general and disease specific guidelines take precedence over the outpatient guidelines.

Diagnoses often are not established at the time of the initial encounter/visit. It may take two or more visits before the diagnosis is confirmed.

The most critical rule involves beginning the search for the correct code assignment through the Alphabetic Index. Never begin searching initially in the Tabular List as this will lead to coding errors.

1. **Outpatient Surgery**

When a patient presents for outpatient surgery (same day surgery), code the reason for the surgery as the first-listed diagnosis (reason for the encounter), even if the surgery is not performed due to a contraindication.

2. **Observation Stay**

When a patient is admitted for observation for a medical condition, assign a code for the medical condition as the first-listed diagnosis.

(Continued)

(Continued)

When a patient presents for outpatient surgery and develops complications requiring admission to observation, code the reason for the surgery as the first-reported diagnosis (reason for the encounter), followed by codes for the complications as secondary diagnoses.

B. **Codes from A00.0 through T88.9, Z00–Z99**

The appropriate code(s) from A00.0 through T88.9, Z00–Z99 must be used to identify diagnoses, symptoms, conditions, problems, complaints, or other reason(s) for the encounter/visit.

C. **Accurate reporting of ICD-10-CM diagnosis codes**

For accurate reporting of ICD-10-CM diagnosis codes, the documentation should describe the patient's condition, using terminology that includes specific diagnoses as well as symptoms, problems, or reasons for the encounter. There are ICD-10-CM codes to describe all of these.

D. **Codes that describe symptoms and signs**

Codes that describe symptoms and signs, as opposed to diagnoses, are acceptable for reporting purposes when a diagnosis has not been established (confirmed) by the provider. Chapter 18 of ICD-10-CM, Symptoms, Signs, and Abnormal Clinical and Laboratory Findings Not Elsewhere Classified (codes R00–R99) contain many, but not all codes for symptoms.

E. **Encounters for circumstances other than a disease or injury**

ICD-10-CM provides codes to deal with encounters for circumstances other than a disease or injury. The Factors Influencing Health Status and Contact with Health Services codes (Z00–Z99) are provided to deal with occasions when circumstances other than a disease or injury are recorded as diagnosis or problems.

See Section I.C.21. Factors influencing health status and contact with health services.

F. **Level of Detail in Coding**

1. **ICD-10-CM codes with 3, 4, 5, 6 or 7 characters**

ICD-10-CM is composed of codes with 3, 4, 5, 6 or 7 characters. Codes with three characters are included in ICD-10-CM as the heading of a category of codes that may be further subdivided by the use of fourth, fifth, sixth or seventh characters to provide greater specificity.

2. **Use of full number of *characters* required for a code**

   A three-character code is to be used only if it is not further subdivided. A code is invalid if it has not been coded to the full number of characters required for that code, including the 7th character, if applicable.

G. **ICD-10-CM code for the diagnosis, condition, problem, or other reason for encounter/visit**

   List first the ICD-10-CM code for the diagnosis, condition, problem, or other reason for encounter/visit shown in the medical record to be chiefly responsible for the services provided. List additional codes that describe any coexisting conditions. In some cases the first-listed diagnosis may be a symptom when a diagnosis has not been established (confirmed) by the provider.

H. **Uncertain diagnosis**

   Do not code diagnoses documented as "probable," "suspected," "questionable," "rule out," « compatible with, » « consistent with, » or "working diagnosis" or other similar terms indicating uncertainty. Rather, code the condition(s) to the highest degree of certainty for that encounter/visit, such as symptoms, signs, abnormal test results, or other reason for the visit.

   Note: This differs from the coding practices used by short-term, acute care, long-term care and psychiatric hospitals.

I. **Chronic diseases**

   Chronic diseases treated on an ongoing basis may be coded and reported as many times as the patient receives treatment and care for the condition(s).

J. **Code all documented conditions that coexist**

   Code all documented conditions that coexist at the time of the encounter/visit and require or affect patient care treatment or management. Do not code conditions that were previously treated and no longer exist. However, history codes (categories Z80–Z87) may be used as secondary codes if the historical condition or family history has an impact on current care or influences treatment.

K. **Patients receiving diagnostic services only**

   For patients receiving diagnostic services only during an encounter/visit, sequence first the diagnosis, condition, problem, or other reason for encounter/visit shown in the medical record to be chiefly responsible for the

   (Continued)

105

(Continued)

outpatient services provided during the encounter/visit. Codes for other diagnoses (e.g., chronic conditions) may be sequenced as additional diagnoses.

For encounters for routine laboratory/radiology testing in the absence of any signs, symptoms, or associated diagnosis, assign Z01.89, Encounter for other specified special examinations. If routine testing is performed during the same encounter as a test to evaluate a sign, symptom, or diagnosis, it is appropriate to assign both the Z code and the code describing the reason for the non-routine test.

For outpatient encounters for diagnostic tests that have been interpreted by a physician, and the final report is available at the time of coding, code any confirmed or definitive diagnosis(es) documented in the interpretation. Do not code related signs and symptoms as additional diagnoses.

Note: This differs from the coding practice in the hospital inpatient setting regarding abnormal findings on test results.

L. **Patients receiving therapeutic services only**

For patients receiving therapeutic services only during an encounter/visit, sequence first the diagnosis, condition, problem, or other reason for encounter/visit shown in the medical record to be chiefly responsible for the outpatient services provided during the encounter/visit. Codes for other diagnoses (e.g., chronic conditions) may be sequenced as additional diagnoses.

The only exception to this rule is that when the primary reason for the admission/encounter is chemotherapy or radiation therapy, the appropriate Z code for the service is listed first, and the diagnosis or problem for which the service is being performed listed second.

M. **Patients receiving preoperative evaluations only**

For patients receiving preoperative evaluations only, sequence first a code from subcategory Z01.81, Encounter for pre-procedural examinations, to describe the pre-op consultations. Assign a code for the condition to describe the reason for the surgery as an additional diagnosis. Code also any findings related to the pre-op evaluation.

N. **Ambulatory surgery**

For ambulatory surgery, code the diagnosis for which the surgery was performed. If the postoperative diagnosis is known to be different from the preoperative diagnosis at the time the diagnosis is confirmed, select the postoperative diagnosis for coding, since it is the most definitive.

O. **Routine outpatient prenatal visits**

See Guidelines for Coding and Reporting Section I.C.15. Routine outpatient prenatal visits.

P. **Encounters for general medical examinations with abnormal findings**

The subcategories for encounters for general medical examinations, Z00.0- and encounter for routine child health examination, Z00.12-, provide codes for with and without abnormal findings. Should a general medical examination result in an abnormal finding, the code for general medical examination with abnormal finding should be assigned as the first-listed diagnosis. An examination with abnormal findings refers to a condition/diagnosis that is newly identified or a change in severity of a condition (such as uncontrolled hypertension, or an acute exacerbation of chronic obstructive pulmonary disease) during a routine physical examination. A secondary code for the abnormal finding should also be coded.

Q. **Encounters for routine health screenings**

See Guidelines for Coding and Reporting Section I.C.21. Factors influencing health status and contact with health services, Screening

Check Your Understanding 3.4

Answer the following questions about the official coding guidelines regarding the diagnostic coding and reporting of outpatient services.

1. According to Guideline IV.G, what should be listed as the first diagnosis code for the outpatient visit?

2. According to Guideline IV.H, can uncertain diagnosis be assigned diagnosis codes for outpatient visits?

3. Can a coder code for medical encounters other than those for treatment of a disease or injury?

4. According to Guideline IV.A, when a patient is admitted for observation, what two options does a coder have for assigning the appropriate code?

5. According to Guideline IV.L., what is reported as the diagnosis when the patient is receiving therapeutic services and is there an exception to this rule?

Review Exercises: Chapter 3

Answer the following questions or assign the correct ICD-10-CM diagnosis codes to the following exercises.

1. What is the purpose of the Uniform Hospital Discharge Data Set? What healthcare organizations collect UHDDS?

2. What is the UHDDS definition of principal diagnosis?

3. What is the UHDDS definition of principal procedure?

4. Can codes for symptoms, signs, and ill-defined conditions (Chapter 18) be sequenced as a principal diagnosis? If no, why not? If yes, when is it appropriate?

5. Do the official ICD-10-CM guidelines take precedence over the coding directives within the code set (that is, index/tabular) when determining the principal diagnosis?

6. According to the Section IV: Diagnostic coding and reporting guideline for Outpatient Services, how does the first listed diagnosis in the outpatient setting differ from the selection of the principal diagnosis in the Inpatient Setting?

For exercises 7–16: Apply the *ICD-10-CM Official Guidelines for Coding and Reporting* of the Principal Diagnosis for Inpatient Care (Guidelines II A–J) to identify the *principal diagnosis* in the following scenarios.

7. Patient was admitted to the hospital after having a seizure at work. The admitting diagnosis was to rule out epilepsy. After testing was performed, the cause of the seizure was not determined, as the physician stated the patient did not have epilepsy.

8. Patient was admitted to the hospital with acute pyelonephritis and acute cystitis. Both infections were evaluated and treated with intravenous antibiotic therapy. The patient was discharged home to continue taking oral medications.

9. Patient was admitted to the hospital with acute exacerbation of chronic obstructive pulmonary disease and acute low back pain. Both conditions were evaluated, and the patient received medical treatment. The patient was discharged home to continue to receive physical therapy for the back pain and pulmonary rehabilitation therapy for his chronic lung disease.

Review Exercises: Chapter 3 *(continued)*

10. The patient was admitted to the hospital with a multitude of gastrointestinal symptoms. After diagnostic tests were performed, the physician was unable to determine exactly what was causing the patient's symptoms. The physician's final diagnosis was "acute pancreatitis versus acute cholangitis."

    _____

11. The patient was admitted to the hospital with left lower quadrant abdominal pain. After study, the physician concluded the patient's abdominal pain could have been due to either of two conditions. Her final diagnosis was abdominal pain due to either a ruptured ovarian cyst or acute salpingitis.

    _____

12. The patient was admitted to the hospital for a total right knee replacement for osteoarthritis of the knee. During the patient's preoperative preparation, the patient began having chest pain. The patient's knee surgery was cancelled, and the patient had extensive testing to determine the source of the chest pain, which was determined to be due to hypertensive heart disease.

    _____

13. The patient was readmitted to the hospital for a postoperative wound infection. The patient had been discharged from the hospital five days ago, after having colon surgery for ruptured diverticulitis. During this hospital stay, the patient was treated for the wound infection and monitored for the remaining diverticulitis in his colon.

    _____

14. The patient was admitted to the hospital with fever, cough, and shortness of breath. After study, the physician could not identify the exact cause of these symptoms but felt the most likely cause was pneumonia. The physician's final diagnosis was "possible viral pneumonia now resolving."

    _____

15. The patient comes to the Emergency Department complaining of an asthma attack. The patient is placed into the observation unit to monitor his response to the asthma treatment. During the observation time, the patient is determined to have status asthmaticus and is admitted for treatment of this condition. After a three-day hospital stay, the patient's asthma is better controlled, and he is discharged.

    _____

16. The patient was registered as an outpatient for a left-sided cataract extraction, which was performed successfully. While the patient was preparing to leave the hospital after surgery, the patient felt faint, and it was determined the patient's blood pressure was much lower than earlier in the day. The patient was admitted to the hospital to monitor the low blood pressure. The next day, the patient felt well again and was discharged. The physician described the patient's condition as "orthostatic hypotension."

    _____

(Continued on next page)

Review Exercises: Chapter 3 *(continued)*

For exercises 17–20: Apply the *ICD-10-CM Official Guidelines for Coding and Reporting* for Reporting Additional Diagnoses (Guideline Section III), along with the ICD-10-CM Classification, to identify the other diagnosis/diagnoses in the following scenarios.

17. The physician's discharge summary includes the final diagnoses of (1) acute cholecystitis, with additional diagnosis of (2) cholelithiasis, (3) type 2 diabetes, (4) history of pneumonia last year, and (5) status post bunionectomy three months ago.

_____

18. The physician's discharge summary includes the final diagnoses of (1) coronary artery disease, (2) hypertension, and (3) benign prostatic hypertrophy. The coder notes in the patient's laboratory reports that the patient has an elevated cholesterol level and an elevated PSA positive finding.

_____

19. The physician's discharge summary includes the final diagnoses of (1) acute hemorrhagic gastritis, (2) acute duodenitis, and (3) possible acute pancreatitis.

_____

20. The physician's discharge summary includes the final diagnoses of (1) Congestive heart failure, with additional diagnosis of (2) with hypertension, and (3) status post cholecystectomy.

_____

References

50 FR 31038, Vol. 50, No. 147, pp. 31038–31040.

Centers for Disease Control and Prevention (CDC), National Center for Health Statistics (NCHS). 2019. *ICD-10-CM Official Guidelines for Coding and Reporting*, 2020. https://www.cdc.gov/nchs/data/icd/10cmguidelines_fy2019_final.pdf.

Chapter 4

Certain Infectious and Parasitic Diseases (A00–B99)

Learning Objectives

At the conclusion of this chapter, you should be able to do the following:

- Describe the organization of the conditions and codes Infectious in Chapter 1 of ICD-10-CM, Certain Infectious and Parasitic Diseases (A00–B99)

- Apply the chapter-specific coding guidelines for Chapter 1 of ICD-10-CM

- Explain how and when the sequelae of infectious and parasitic disease codes are applied

- Explain the circumstances in which codes from ICD-10-CM categories B95–B97 are used

- Summarize the coding guidelines for human immunodeficiency infection (HIV) disease reporting

- Explain how methicillin-resistant *Staphylococcus aureus* (MRSA) conditions are coded

- Assign diagnosis codes for infectious and parasitic diseases

- Assign procedure codes related to treatment of infectious and parasitic diseases

Key Terms

Acquired immune deficiency syndrome (AIDS)

Combination codes

Human immunodeficiency virus (HIV)

Methicillin-resistant *Staphylococcus aureus* (MRSA)

Methicillin-susceptible *Staphylococcus aureus* (MSSA)

Residual condition

Sepsis

Septic shock

Severe sepsis

Overview of ICD-10-CM Chapter 1: Certain Infectious and Parasitic Diseases

Chapter 1 of ICD-10-CM includes categories A00–B99 arranged in the following blocks:

A00–A09	Intestinal infectious diseases
A15–A19	Tuberculosis
A20–A28	Certain zoonotic bacterial diseases
A30–A49	Other bacterial diseases
A50–A64	Infections with a predominantly sexual mode of transmission
A65–A69	Other spirochetal diseases
A70–A74	Other diseases caused by *Chlamydiae*
A75–A79	Rickettsioses
A80–A89	Viral and prion infections of the central nervous system
A90–A99	Arthropod-borne viral fevers and viral hemorrhagic fevers
B00–B09	Viral infections characterized by skin and mucous membrane lesions
B10	Other human herpes viruses
B15–B19	Viral hepatitis
B20	Human immunodeficiency virus [HIV] disease
B25–B34	Other viral diseases
B35–B49	Mycoses
B50–B64	Protozoal diseases
B65–B83	Helminthiases
B85–B89	Pediculosis, acariasis and other infestations
B90–B94	Sequelae of infectious and parasitic diseases
B95–B97	Bacterial and viral infectious agents
B99	Other infectious diseases

In ICD-10-CM Chapter 1, a separate subchapter, or block, has been created and appropriate conditions have been grouped together for infections with a predominantly sexual mode of transmission (A50–A64). Two additional examples of separate blocks with the appropriate conditions grouped together are viral hepatitis (B15–B19) and other viral diseases (B25–B34).

 The term sepsis is used throughout ICD-10-CM Chapter 1. The medical term septicemia may be found in medical records. Physicians may use septicemia as an equivalent term for sepsis. Category A41, Other sepsis, includes a code first note, and Excludes1 and Excludes2 notes to indicate how particular types of sepsis are coded as well.

Many of the codes in ICD-10-CM Chapter 1 reflect manifestations of the disease with the use of fourth or fifth characters allowing the infectious disease and manifestation to be captured in one **combination code**. Combination codes capture facts about a patient's condition. For example, in Chapter 1, the combination codes for localized salmonella infections identify the infectious disease (salmonella) and the manifestation of the disease (meningitis, pneumonia, and so on).

> **EXAMPLES:** **A02.2, Localized salmonella infections**
> A02.20, Localized salmonella infection, unspecified
> A02.21, Salmonella meningitis
> A02.22, Salmonella pneumonia
> A02.23, Salmonella arthritis
> A02.24, Salmonella osteomyelitis
> A02.25, Salmonella pyelonephritis
> A02.29, Salmonella with other localized infection

Coding Guidelines and Instructional Notes for ICD-10-CM Chapter 1

The NCHS has published chapter-specific guidelines for Chapter 1 in the *ICD-10-CM Official Guidelines for Coding and Reporting*. The coding student should review all of the coding guidelines for Chapter 1 of ICD-10-CM, which appear in an ICD-10-CM code book or at the CDC website (CDC 2019) or in appendix F.

CG

Chapter 1 : Certain Infectious and Parasitic Diseases (A00-B99)

Guideline I.C.1.a. Human Immunodeficiency Virus [HIV] Infections

1. Code only confirmed cases

   Code only confirmed cases of HIV infection/illness. This is an exception to the hospital inpatient guideline Section II, H. In this context, "confirmation" does not require documentation of positive serology or culture for HIV; the provider's diagnostic statement that the patient is HIV positive, or has an HIV-related illness is sufficient.

2. Selection and sequencing of HIV codes

   a. Patient admitted for HIV-related condition
      If a patient is admitted for an HIV-related condition, the principal diagnosis should be B20, Human immunodeficiency virus [HIV] disease followed by additional diagnosis codes for all reported HIV-related conditions.

   b. Patient with HIV disease admitted for unrelated condition
      If a patient with HIV disease is admitted for an unrelated condition (such as a traumatic injury), the
      (Continued)

(Continued)

code for the unrelated condition (e.g., the nature of injury code) should be the principal diagnosis. Other diagnoses would be B20 followed by additional diagnosis codes for all reported HIV-related conditions.

c. Whether the patient is newly diagnosed
Whether the patient is newly diagnosed or has had previous admissions/encounters for HIV conditions is irrelevant to the sequencing decision.

d. Asymptomatic human immunodeficiency virus
Z21, Asymptomatic human immunodeficiency virus [HIV] infection status, is to be applied when the patient without any documentation of symptoms is listed as being "HIV positive," "known HIV," "HIV test positive," or similar terminology. Do not use this code if the term "AIDS" is used or if the patient is treated for any HIV-related illness or is described as having any condition(s) resulting from his/her HIV positive status; use B20 in these cases.

e. Patients with inconclusive HIV serology
Patients with inconclusive HIV serology, but no definitive diagnosis or manifestations of the illness, may be assigned code R75, Inconclusive laboratory evidence of human immunodeficiency virus [HIV].

f. Previously diagnosed HIV-related illness
Patients with any known prior diagnosis of an HIV-related illness should be coded to B20. Once a patient has developed an HIV-related illness, the patient should always be assigned code B20 on every subsequent admission/encounter. Patients previously diagnosed with any HIV illness (B20) should never be assigned to R75 or Z21, Asymptomatic human immunodeficiency virus [HIV] infection status.

g. HIV Infection in Pregnancy, Childbirth and the Puerperium
During pregnancy, childbirth or the puerperium, a patient admitted (or presenting for a health care encounter) because of an HIV-related illness should receive a principal diagnosis code of O98.7-, Human immunodeficiency [HIV] disease complicating pregnancy, childbirth and the puerperium, followed by B20 and the code(s) for the HIV-related illness(es). Codes from Chapter 15 always take sequencing priority. Patients with asymptomatic HIV infection

status admitted (or presenting for a health care encounter) during pregnancy, childbirth, or the puerperium should receive codes of O98.7- and Z21.

h. Encounters for testing for HIV

If a patient is being seen to determine his/her HIV status, use code Z11.4, Encounter for screening for human immunodeficiency virus [HIV]. Use additional codes for any associated high risk behavior. If a patient with signs or symptoms is being seen for HIV testing, code the signs and symptoms. An additional counseling code Z71.7, Human immunodeficiency virus [HIV] counseling, may be used if counseling is provided during the encounter for the test.

When a patient returns to be informed of his/her HIV test results and the test result is negative, use code Z71.7, Human immunodeficiency virus [HIV] counseling. If the results are positive, see previous guidelines and assign codes as appropriate.

Guideline I.C.1.b. Infectious Agents as the Cause of Diseases Classified to Other Chapters

Certain infections are classified in chapters other than Chapter 1 and no organism is identified as part of the infection code. In these instances, it is necessary to use an additional code from Chapter 1 to identify the organism. A code from category B95, Streptococcus, Staphylococcus, and Enterococcus as the cause of diseases classified to other chapters, B96, Other bacterial agents as the cause of diseases classified to other chapters, or B97, Viral agents as the cause of diseases classified to other chapters, is to be used as an additional code to identify the organism. An instructional note will be found at the infection code advising that an additional organism code is required.

Guideline I.C.1.c. Infections Resistant to Antibiotics

Many bacterial infections are resistant to current antibiotics. It is necessary to identify all infections documented as antibiotic resistant. Assign a code from category Z16, Resistance to antimicrobial drugs, following the infection code only if the infection code does not identify drug resistance.

Guideline I.C.1.d. Sepsis, Severe Sepsis, and Septic Shock

1. Coding of sepsis and severe sepsis

   a. Sepsis

   For a diagnosis of sepsis, assign the appropriate code for the underlying systemic infection. If the

(Continued)

(Continued)

type of infection or causal organism is not further specified, assign code A41.9, Sepsis, unspecified organism.

A code from subcategory R65.2, Severe sepsis, should not be assigned unless severe sepsis or an associated acute organ dysfunction is documented.

i. Negative or inconclusive blood cultures and sepsis
    Negative or inconclusive blood cultures do not preclude a diagnosis of sepsis in patients with clinical evidence of the condition, however, the provider should be queried.

ii. Urosepsis
    The term urosepsis is a nonspecific term. It is not to be considered synonymous with sepsis. It has no default code in the Alphabetic Index. Should a provider use this term, he/she must be queried for clarification.

iii. Sepsis with organ dysfunction
    If a patient has sepsis and associated acute organ dysfunction or multiple organ dysfunction (MOD), follow the instructions for coding severe sepsis.

iv. Acute organ dysfunction that is not clearly associated with the sepsis
    If a patient has sepsis and an acute organ dysfunction, but the medical record documentation indicates that the acute organ dysfunction is related to a medical condition other than the sepsis, do not assign a code from subcategory R65.2, Severe sepsis. An acute organ dysfunction must be associated with the sepsis in order to assign the severe sepsis code. If the documentation is not clear as to whether an acute organ dysfunction is related to the sepsis or another medical condition, query the provider.

b. Severe sepsis
    The coding of severe sepsis requires a minimum of 2 codes: first a code for the underlying systemic infection, followed by a code from subcategory R65.2, Severe sepsis. If the causal organism is not documented, assign code A41.9, Sepsis, unspecified organism, for the infection. Additional code(s) for the associated acute organ dysfunction are also required. Due to the complex nature of severe sepsis, some cases may require querying the provider prior to assignment of the codes.

2. Septic shock

a. Septic shock generally refers to circulatory failure associated with severe sepsis, and therefore, it represents a type of acute organ dysfunction. For cases of septic shock, the code for the systemic infection should be sequenced first, followed by code R65.21, Severe sepsis with septic shock or code T81.12, Postprocedural septic shock. Any additional codes for the other acute organ dysfunctions should also be assigned. As noted in the sequencing instructions in the Tabular List, the code for septic shock cannot be assigned as a principal diagnosis.

3. Sequencing of severe sepsis

If severe sepsis is present on admission, and meets the definition of principal diagnosis, the underlying systemic infection should be assigned as principal diagnosis followed by the appropriate code from subcategory R65.2 as required by the sequencing rules in the Tabular List. A code from subcategory R65.2 can never be assigned as a principal diagnosis.

When severe sepsis develops during an encounter (it was not present on admission) the underlying systemic infection and the appropriate code from subcategory R65.2 should be assigned as secondary diagnoses.

Severe sepsis may be present on admission but the diagnosis may not be confirmed until sometime after admission. If the documentation is not clear whether severe sepsis was present on admission, the provider should be queried.

4. Sepsis or severe sepsis with a localized infection

If the reason for admission is both sepsis or severe sepsis and a localized infection, such as pneumonia or cellulitis, a code(s) for the underlying systemic infection should be assigned first and the code for the localized infection should be assigned as a secondary diagnosis. If the patient has severe sepsis, a code from subcategory R65.2 should also be assigned as a secondary diagnosis. If the patient is admitted with a localized infection, such as pneumonia, and sepsis/severe sepsis doesn't develop until after admission, the localized infection should be assigned first, followed by the appropriate sepsis/severe sepsis codes.

(Continued)

(Continued)

5. Sepsis due to a postprocedural infection

   a. Documentation of causal relationship
   As with all postprocedural complications, code assignment is based on the provider's documentation of the relationship between the infection and the procedure.

   b. Sepsis due to a postprocedural infection
   For infections following a procedure, a code from T801.40 to T81.43, Infection following a procedure, or a code from O86.00 to O86.03, Infection of obstetric surgical wound, that identifies the site of the infection should be coded first, if known. Assign an additional code for sepsis following a procedure (T81.44) or sepsis following an obstetrical procedure (O86.04). Use an additional code to identify the infectious agent. If the patient has severe sepsis, the appropriate code from subcategory R65.2 should also be assigned with the additional code(s) for any acute organ dysfunction.

   For infections following infusion, transfusion, therapeutic injection, or immunization, a code from subcategory T80.2, Infections following infusion, transfusion, and therapeutic injection, or code T88.0-, Infection following immunization, should be coded first, followed by the code for the specific infection. If the patient has severe sepsis, the appropriate code from subcategory R65.2 should also be assigned, with the additional code(s) for any acute organ dysfunction.

   c. Postprocedural infection and postprocedural septic shock
   If a postprocedural infection has resulted in postprocedural septic shock, assign the codes indicated above for sepsis due to a postprocedural infection, followed by code T81.12-, Postprocedural septic shock. Do not assign code R65.21, Severe sepsis with septic shock. Additional code(s) should be assigned for any acute organ dysfunction.

6. Sepsis and severe sepsis associated with a noninfectious process (condition)

   In some cases a noninfectious process (condition), such as trauma, may lead to an infection which can result in sepsis or severe sepsis. If sepsis or severe sepsis is documented as associated with a noninfectious condition, such as a burn or serious injury, and this condition meets the definition for principal diagnosis, the code for the noninfectious condition should be sequenced first, followed by the code for the resulting infection. If severe sepsis is present a code from subcategory R65.2 should also be assigned with any associated organ dysfunction(s) codes. It is not necessary to assign a code from subcategory R65.1, Systemic inflammatory response syndrome (SIRS) of non-infectious origin, for these cases.

If the infection meets the definition of principal diagnosis it should be sequenced before the non-infectious condition. When both the associated non-infectious condition and the infection meet the definition of principal diagnosis either may be assigned as principal diagnosis.

Only one code from category R65, Symptoms and signs specifically associated with systemic inflammation and infection, should be assigned. Therefore, when a non-infectious condition leads to an infection resulting in severe sepsis, assign the appropriate code from subcategory R65.2, Severe sepsis. Do not additionally assign a code from subcategory R65.1, Systemic inflammatory response syndrome (SIRS) of non-infectious origin.

See Section I.C.18. SIRS due to non-infectious process

7. Sepsis and septic shock complicating abortion, pregnancy, childbirth, and the puerperium

See Section I.C.15. Sepsis and septic shock complicating abortion, pregnancy, childbirth and the puerperium

8. Newborn sepsis

See Section I.C.16.f. Bacterial sepsis of Newborn

Guidelines I.C.1.e. Methicillin Resistant *Staphylococcus aureus* (MRSA) Conditions

1. Selection and sequencing of MRSA codes

    a. Combination codes for MRSA infection
    When a patient is diagnosed with an infection that is due to methicillin resistant *Staphylococcus aureus* (MRSA), and that infection has a combination code that includes the causal organism (e.g., sepsis, pneumonia) assign the appropriate combination code for the condition (e.g., code A41.02, Sepsis due to Methicillin resistant Staphylococcus aureus or code J15.212, Pneumonia due to Methicillin resistant Staphylococcus aureus). Do not assign code B95.62, Methicillin resistant Staphylococcus aureus infection as the cause of diseases classified elsewhere, as an additional code because the combination code includes the type of infection and the MRSA organism. Do not assign a code from subcategory Z16.11, Resistance to penicillins, as an additional diagnosis.

    (Continued)

(Continued)

> *See Section C.1. for instructions on coding and sequencing of sepsis and severe sepsis*

b. Other codes for MRSA infection

When there is documentation of a current infection (e.g., wound infection, stitch abscess, urinary tract infection) due to MRSA, and that infection does not have a combination code that includes the causal organism, assign the appropriate code to identify the condition along with code B95.62, Methicillin resistant Staphylococcus aureus infection as the cause of diseases classified elsewhere for the MRSA infection. Do not assign a code from subcategory Z16.11, Resistance to penicillins.

c. Methicillin susceptible Staphylococcus aureus (MSSA) and MRSA colonization

The condition or state of being colonized or carrying MSSA or MRSA is called colonization or carriage, while an individual person is described as being colonized or being a carrier. Colonization means that MSSA or MSRA is present on or in the body without necessarily causing illness. A positive MRSA colonization test might be documented by the provider as "MRSA screen positive" or "MRSA nasal swab positive."

Assign code Z22.322, Carrier or suspected carrier of Methicillin resistant Staphylococcus aureus, for patients documented as having MRSA colonization. Assign code Z22.321, Carrier or suspected carrier of Methicillin susceptible Staphylococcus aureus, for patients documented as having MSSA colonization. Colonization is not necessarily indicative of a disease process or as the cause of a specific condition the patient may have unless documented as such by the provider.

d. MRSA colonization and infection

If a patient is documented as having both MRSA colonization and infection during a hospital admission, code Z22.322, Carrier or suspected carrier of Methicillin resistant Staphylococcus aureus, and a code for the MRSA infection may both be assigned.

Guidelines I.C.1.f. Zika virus infections

1. Code only confirmed cases.

Code only a confirmed diagnosis of Zika virus (A92.5, Zika virus disease) as documented by the provider. This is an exception to the hospital inpatient guidelines Section II, H. In this context, "confirmation" does not require documentation of the type of test performed;

the provider's diagnostic statement that the condition is confirmed is sufficient. This code should be assigned regardless of the stated mode of transmission. If the provider documents "suspected", "possible" or "probable" Zika, do not assign code A92.5. Assign a code(s) explaining the reason for encounter (such as fever, rash, or joint pain) or Z20.821, Contact with and (suspected) exposure to Zika virus.

Coding Certain Infectious and Parasitic Diseases in ICD-10-CM Chapter 1

The following notes are available at the beginning of ICD-10-CM Chapter 1 in the Tabular List of Diseases and Injuries and tell the coder what is included in the diseases classified to Chapter 1 and what diseases are excluded and assigned codes from other chapters in ICD-10-CM:

Includes: Diseases generally recognized as communicable or transmissible

Use additional code to identify resistance to antimicrobial drugs (Z16.-).

Excludes1:   Certain localized infections—see body system–related chapters

Excludes2:   Carrier or suspected carrier of infectious disease (Z22.-)

              Infectious and parasitic diseases complicating pregnancy, childbirth and the puerperium (O98.-)

              Infectious and parasitic diseases specific to the perinatal period (P35–P39)

              Influenza and other acute respiratory infections (J00–J22)

In coding certain infectious and parasitic diseases, the entire health record must be reviewed to identify the following:

- Body site; for example, eye, intestine, or blood

- Specific organism responsible; for example, bacteria, virus, or fungus

- Etiology of disease; for example, parasite or food poisoning

- Severity of the disease; for example, acute or chronic

Combination Codes and Multiple Coding

Chapter 1 of ICD-10-CM includes combination codes to identify both the condition and the causative organism.

        EXAMPLE: B30.1, Conjunctivitis due to adenovirus

                          B37.0, Candidal stomatitis

                          A06.1, Chronic intestinal amebiasis

All three of these examples of combination codes describe the location of the condition (eye, stomach, intestine) and the causal organism or parasite (adenovirus, candida, and ameba).

Mandatory multiple coding is required to describe etiology and manifestation when infectious and parasitic diseases produce a manifestation within another body system. The Alphabetic Index identifies when the etiology and manifestation convention or mandatory multiple coding is required by listing two codes after the main term with the second code listed in brackets. The first code identifies the underlying infectious or parasitic condition. The second code identifies the manifestation that occurs as a result of it.

EXAMPLE: Schistosomiasis with muscle disorder B65.9 *[M63.80]*
The underlying cause and first listed code is B65.9. The second code describes the muscle disorder caused by the Schistosomiasis, M63.80.

Sepsis, Severe Sepsis, and Septic Shock

When coding sepsis, it is important to review the coding guidelines and the notes at the category level of ICD-10-CM.

Sepsis is a serious medical condition caused by the body's immune response to an infection. The body's immune system releases chemicals into the blood to fight the infection and triggers widespread inflammation. This inflammation causes blood clots and other complications in the vascular system. This impairs blood flow and damages the body organs by depriving the structures of oxygen and nutrients. Sepsis does not occur without another reason, especially in the lungs, abdomen, urinary tract, or skin. Surgical and invasive medical procedures can cause sepsis by introducing bacteria into the bloodstream. The pathologic organisms in the blood or tissue may include bacteria, viruses, fungi, or other organisms that produce a systemic disease (National Institute of General Medical Sciences 2018).

Sepsis due to *Streptococcus* group A and B, and *Streptococcus pneumoniae* are classified to category A40, Streptococcal sepsis. Because streptococcal sepsis may occur after a procedure, immunization, or infusion as well as during labor or following an abortion or ectopic or molar pregnancy, a "code first" note exists to remind the coder that other codes should be assigned first to reflect those conditions.

Sepsis caused by other organisms than *Streptococcus* is classified to Category A41, Other sepsis. This category contains numerous codes to identify sepsis caused by a particular organism, such as *Staphylococcus aureus*, *Haemophilus influenzae*, anaerobes, other gram-negative organisms, and such. An unspecified type of sepsis is coded A41.9, Sepsis, unspecified organism, in cases where a specific underlying systemic infection is not further specified.

To code sepsis, the coder must review the physician's documentation to determine if the causative organism is known. By accessing the Alphabetic Index under the main term, sepsis, the coder can find the type of organism documented and its corresponding code in the list of subterms. If only the term "sepsis" is documented, code A41.9, Sepsis, unspecified organism is the appropriate code.

Severe sepsis is an infection with associated acute organ dysfunction. It may also be referred to as systemic inflammatory response syndrome due to an infectious process with acute organ dysfunction (Chang 2010).

In severe sepsis, one or more of the body's organs fail. In the extreme situation, the patient suffers from very low blood pressure and heart failure. This situation advances to **septic shock**, which is potentially deadly. It causes circulatory failure and the failure of organs such as lungs, kidneys, and the liver.

Two codes at a minimum are required for the coding of severe sepsis. The first code is for the underlying infection, which may be categories A40 or A41 or codes for obstetric, puerperal, or postprocedural sepsis. A second code is from subcategory R65.2-, Severe sepsis. If septic shock is present, additional codes are required to identify the specific acute organ dysfunction, such as acute kidney failure (N17.-) or acute respiratory failure (J96.0-). The Tabular List reminds the coder that code R65.20 or R65.21 for severe sepsis without or with septic shock cannot be used as the principal, first listed, or the only code. A "code first underlying infection" note appears to direct the coder to code first the particular infection that produced the severe sepsis.

When severe sepsis is present on admission, and meets the definition of principal diagnosis, the underlying systemic infection is assigned as the principal diagnosis followed by the appropriate code from subcategory R65.2- as required by the sequencing rules in the Tabular List.

If the patient is admitted to the hospital for treatment of the sepsis and severe sepsis develops that was not present on admission, the underlying systemic infection is coded first and the appropriate code from subcategory R65.2- should be assigned as secondary diagnoses with the present on admission indicator of "no" reported.

It is possible that a patient has an infection in a particular body system that advances to a systemic infection. If this patient is admitted to the hospital for treatment of a body system or localized infection, such as pneumonia, as well as sepsis or severe sepsis, the code for the systemic infection is sequenced first. The sepsis would be the first-reported or principal diagnosis. Another code would be assigned for the localized infection, such as the pneumonia. If the patient has severe sepsis, an additional code from category R65.2- would be assigned depending on whether the patient had septic shock or not.

In a different situation, a patient can be admitted to the hospital for treatment of pneumonia or another localized infection and the condition worsens while the patient is in the hospital to the extent of having sepsis or severe sepsis. In this situation, the localized infection would be coded and reported as the first code, followed by the appropriate sepsis or severe sepsis codes.

Check Your Understanding 4.1

When applicable, assign the following diagnosis codes according to the Guideline I.C.1.d. Sepsis, Severe Sepsis, and Septic Shock.

1. Methicillin-resistant *Staphylococcus aureus* sepsis

2. Borderline tuberculoid leprosy

3. Severe gram-negative sepsis with septic shock and acute hepatic failure

4. E. coli septicemia with severe sepsis and acute renal failure

5. Postprocedural sepsis, severe (initial encounter for treatment)

Human Immunodeficiency Virus (HIV) Disease

HIV is the medical abbreviation for **human immunodeficiency virus**. It is the virus that can lead to acquired immune deficiency syndrome (AIDS). There are two types of HIV: HIV-1 and HIV-2. In the United States, unless otherwise noted, the term "HIV" primarily refers to HIV-1. The virus damages a person's body by destroying specific blood cells called CD4+ T cells, which are essential in helping the body fight diseases (NLM 2019a).

Within a few weeks of being infected with HIV, people may develop flu-like symptoms that last for a week or two, but others have no symptoms at all. People living with HIV may appear and feel healthy for several years. However, even if they feel healthy, HIV is still affecting their bodies. Many people with HIV, including those who feel healthy, can benefit greatly from current medications used to treat HIV infection. These medications can limit or slow down the destruction of the immune system, can improve the health of people living with HIV, and may reduce their ability to transmit HIV. Untreated early HIV infection is also associated with many diseases including cardiovascular disease, kidney disease, liver disease, and cancer. Figure 4.1 shows a human T cell that is under attack by HIV virus cells that appear as the tiny specks on the surface of the T cell. The HIV virus specifically targets the T cells, which play a critical role in the body's immune response against invaders like bacteria and viruses. As the HIV virus destroys the T cells, the body is less capable of resisting infections and succumbs to AIDS-related illnesses as a result of the body's diminished immune defenses. The number of T cells present in the blood can be measured by laboratory testing. The lower the T-cell count, the more likely the person will become ill as it is a measure of the health of the person's immune system. Anyone who has fewer than 200 T cells or a percentage of less than 14 percent is considered to have AIDS (AIDS.org 2019).

Acquired immune deficiency syndrome (AIDS) is the late stage of HIV infection, when a person's immune system is severely damaged and has difficulty fighting diseases and certain cancers. Before the development of antiviral medications, people with HIV could progress to AIDS in a short period of time. Today, people can live much longer with HIV before they develop AIDS. This is because of antiviral medications that a person can tolerate over an indefinite period of time. Another treatment is to prevent opportunistic infections that can prove fatal in a person with the HIV infection.

Figure 4.1. Human T cell under attack by HIV virus

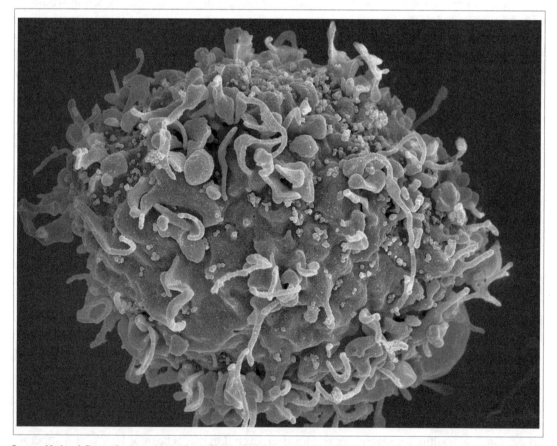

Source: National Cancer Institute. 2014. VisualsOnline. Seth Pincus, Elizabeth Fischer, and Austin Athman, creators. https://visualsonline.cancer.gov/details.cfm?imageid=9849

The HIV classification includes the following categories and codes:

- B20, Human immunodeficiency virus [HIV] disease. Patients with HIV-related illness should be coded to B20. Category B20 includes acquired immune deficiency syndrome [AIDS], AIDS-related complex [ARC], and HIV infection, symptomatic. This code is located under the Alphabetic Index entries of AIDS and Disease, human immunodeficiency virus [HIV], Human, immunodeficiency virus [HIV] disease.

- Z21, Asymptomatic human immunodeficiency virus [HIV] infection status. Patients with physician-documented asymptomatic HIV infection who have never had an HIV-related illness should be coded to Z21. This code is located under the Alphabetic Index entries of HIV, positive, seropositive or Human, immunodeficiency virus [HIV], asymptomatic.

- R75, Inconclusive laboratory evidence of human immunodeficiency virus [HIV]. This code should be used for patients, including infants, with nonconclusive HIV-test finding. This code is located under the Alphabetic Index entry of Human, immunodeficiency virus, laboratory evidence (Casto 2019).

Coding guidelines direct that only confirmed cases of HIV infection or illness be coded. The instruction to code only confirmed cases of HIV infection or HIV-related illness represents an exception to the general ICD-10-CM inpatient coding guidelines that state that diagnoses identified as suspected, possible, or other terms that reflect uncertainty as to whether or not the condition exists should be coded as if they had been established. In this context, a confirmation does not mean a positive serology or culture for HIV is in the record. The physician's statement of the patient's diagnosis of AIDS or HIV-related illness is sufficient.

However, if the diagnosis of AIDS or HIV-related illness is suspected, likely, possible, probable, questionable, or another term that reflects uncertainty, it should not be coded with code B20. Instead, the physician should be asked to clarify what is known for certain about the patient, which may be symptoms of the disease or an inconclusive test result.

Patients who are diagnosed and treated for an HIV-related illness should be assigned a minimum of two codes in the following order:

1. Code B20 to identify the HIV disease

2. Additional codes to identify all manifestations of HIV infection as directed by the "use additional code" note that appears under code B20

> **EXAMPLE:** Disseminated candidiasis secondary to AIDS
> B20, Human immunodeficiency virus [HIV] disease
> B37.7, Candidal sepsis

> **EXAMPLE:** Acute lymphadenitis with HIV infection
> B20, Human immunodeficiency virus [HIV] disease
> L04.9, Acute lymphadenitis, unspecified

During pregnancy, childbirth, or puerperium, a patient admitted because of HIV-related illness or asymptomatic HIV positive status should receive a principal diagnosis of human immunodeficiency virus [HIV] complicating pregnancy, childbirth, and the puerperium (O98.7-). See Guideline 1.C.15.f. An additional code is assigned to identify the type of HIV disease. Guideline 1.C.15.a.3 states whenever delivery occurs during current admit and there is a childbirth option, assign the in childbirth code. This is an exception to the sequencing rule discussed above.

EXAMPLE: Pregnancy, delivered, 38 weeks, single liveborn infant in a patient with AIDS
O98.72, Human immunodeficiency virus (HIV) complicating childbirth
B20, Human immunodeficiency virus [HIV] disease
Z37.0, Single live birth
Z3A.38, Weeks of gestation pregnancy, 38 weeks

When a patient with HIV disease is admitted for an unrelated condition (such as a traumatic injury or a disease that was not caused by the HIV disease, such as an inguinal hernia), the code for the unrelated condition (that is, the nature of injury code) should be the principal diagnosis. Other diagnoses would be B20 followed by additional diagnosis codes for all reported HIV-related conditions.

EXAMPLE: Patient with AIDS admitted with traumatic comminuted fracture femur shaft, right leg, initial encounter
S72.351A, Displaced comminuted fracture of shaft of right femur
B20, Human immunodeficiency virus [HIV] disease

Code Z21, Asymptomatic human immunodeficiency virus [HIV] infection status, is used when the patient has the HIV virus in the blood but does not have any documented symptoms of the infection. The patient may be reported as being HIV positive or known HIV positive. Code Z21 is not used if the terms AIDS or HIV-related illness are used to describe the patient. Code Z21 is not used if the patient is being treated for any HIV-related illness or is described as having any condition resulting from his HIV positive status. Instead, code B20 is used for symptomatic patients. Once a patient has conditions related to the HIV infection, even if the condition is resolved, the patient's HIV-related illness is coded as B20.

If a woman is pregnant and has HIV positive status but has no HIV-related illness, code O98.71- is used as the first-listed or principal diagnosis followed with an additional code for the HIV positive status, that is, Z21. The codes from the pregnancy chapter take sequencing priority over any other ICD-10-CM body system chapter.

Code R75, Inconclusive laboratory evidence of human immunodeficiency virus [HIV], is reported for patients who have healthcare services because of their inconclusive HIV serology. This code means the patient's HIV status has not been determined and he or she is likely to have additional testing in the future. This code is usually used on a short-term basis until the additional testing is completed.

It is important to remember that a patient with any known prior diagnosis of an HIV-related illness should be assigned code B20. After a patient has developed an HIV-related illness, the patient should always be assigned code B20 on every subsequent visit or admission.

Testing for HIV

Patients requesting testing for HIV should be assigned code Z11.4, Encounter for screening for human immunodeficiency virus [HIV]. In addition, code Z72.5-, High risk sexual behavior, may be assigned to identify patients who are in a known high-risk group. The code for screening is used for patients who have no signs or symptoms of HIV disease. Code Z71.7, Human immunodeficiency virus [HIV] counseling, may also be assigned if these services are provided during the screening encounter.

If the results of the test are positive and the patient is asymptomatic, code Z21, Asymptomatic human immunodeficiency virus [HIV] infection status, should be assigned. If the results are positive and the patient is symptomatic with an HIV-related illness, such as Kaposi's sarcoma, the coder should assign code B20, human immunodeficiency virus [HIV] disease.

Check Your Understanding 4.2

Assign the following diagnosis codes according to the Guideline I.C.1.a. Human Immunodeficiency Virus [HIV] Infections.

1. The patient was discharged from the hospital with the final diagnosis of "Probable AIDS."

2. The patient was discharged from the hospital with the final diagnoses of (1) Initial treatment of a traumatic greenstick fracture of the shaft of the right ulna and (2) AIDS. List the diagnosis codes in the appropriate sequence.

3. The patient was seen in the outpatient Infectious Disease clinic for continued management of his HIV positive condition.

4. The patient was discharged from the hospital with the final diagnoses of (1) AIDS and (2) Pneumocystis carinii pneumonia.

5. The 3-month-old infant was seen in the pediatrician's office for further testing for his nonconclusive laboratory evidence of HIV status.

Sequelae of Infectious and Parasitic Diseases (B90–B94)

There is an important note in the Sequelae of Infectious and Parasitic Diseases (B90–B94) section that must be reviewed to understand how the codes are intended to be used. Certain infectious and parasitic diseases leave long-lasting effects after the infection is cured, which may be called a **residual condition**.

The codes in categories B90–B94 are to be used to identify the original infection that produced the problem or condition the patient has as a result of it. The categories B90–B94 are not used if the original condition is still present or if the condition is identified as a chronic infection. These categories represent the sequelae of the disease. If the patient has a current chronic infection, the coder must assign codes for an active infectious disease. There is a "code first" note above the category codes B90–B94 that instructs the coder that the condition resulting from the original infectious and parasitic condition, the condition the patient has today, is coded first.

> **EXAMPLE:** A 60-year-old female patient has a shortened right leg that is of unequal length compared to her left leg. The deformity of her right lower extremity is a result of the fact that she had acute poliomyelitis when she was 3 years old.
>
> The residual condition is the deformity of her right tibia that is an unequal length compared to the left tibia. The deformity is the result

or sequela of the past polio that she had as a child. The codes, in the correct sequence, to be assigned are

M21.761, Unequal limb length (acquired), right tibia

B91, Sequelae of poliomyelitis

Bacterial and Viral Infectious Agents (B95–B97)

ICD-10-CM contains a series of codes to identify the infective agents causing diseases. The note that appears in the Tabular List under this block heading states "These categories are provided for use as supplementary or additional codes to identify the infectious agent(s) in diseases classified elsewhere" (CMS 2019).

The infective agents are as follows:

- B95.0–B95.8, *Streptococcus*, *Staphylococcus*, and *Enterococcus*, as the cause of diseases classified elsewhere; for example, Methicillin-resistant *Staphylococcus aureus* (MRSA) with code B95.62

- B96.0–B96.89, Other bacterial agents, as the cause of diseases classified elsewhere; for example, *Escherichia coli* (*E. coli*) with code B96.20

- B97.0–B97.89, Viral agents, as the cause of diseases classified elsewhere; for example, respiratory syncytial virus with code B97.4

 The codes from B95–B97 will most likely be used with another code that identifies the site of an infection but does not include the causative organism. For example, to code "urinary tract infection due to *E. coli*" would require two codes:

N39.0, Urinary tract infection, site not specified

B96.20, Unspecified *Escherichia coli* [*E. coli*] as the cause of diseases classified elsewhere

The following are examples of how these conditions appear in the Alphabetic Index:

- Infection, infected, infective; bacterial as cause of disease classified elsewhere; *Streptococcus* group A—B95.0

- *Streptococcus*, streptococcal; group A, as cause of disease classified elsewhere—B95.0

To locate these bacterial and viral infectious agent codes that are used in addition to the site of the infection code, the coder must access the Alphabetic Index as follows:

1. Main term of "Infection"

2. Subterm of the name of the bacterial or viral agent, for example, adenovirus

3. Next subterm under the name of the bacterial or viral agent "as cause of disease classified elsewhere"

For example, if the patient had an acute upper respiratory infection that was caused by an adenovirus, first the localized infection would be coded.

For the first-listed code, the coder would follow the path in the Alphabetic Index of

Infection, respiratory, upper, viral, J06.9

Next, for the causative adenovirus infectious agents, the coder would follow the path in the Alphabetic Index of

Infection, adenovirus, as cause of disease classified elsewhere, B97.0

Check Your Understanding 4.3

Assign the following diagnosis codes that describe sequelae of infectious and parasitic diseases and bacterial and viral infectious agents.

1. Attention and concentration deficit as a result of past viral encephalitis

2. Portal cirrhosis as a result of previous viral hepatitis

3. Acute pyelonephritis due to *group B streptococci*

4. Right-dominant spastic paralysis due to old bacterial meningitis

5. Acute maxillary sinusitis due to rhinovirus

Infection with Drug-Resistant Microorganisms

ICD-10-CM allows for the coding of bacterial infections that are resistant to current antibiotics. This specificity is necessary to identify all infections documented as antibiotic resistant. The ICD-10-CM code Z16, Infection with drug-resistant microorganisms, is assigned following the infection code for such cases. The Alphabetic Index entry to locate the drug-resistant organisms is the word "resistance, resistant." Under the entry for resistance are the "subterm organism(s), to, drug" followed by a list of drugs that identify what drug the bacterial organism is resistant to or not effectively treated by. For example, if the patient had an infection that was resistant to the drug amoxicillin, that fact would be coded as Z16.11, resistance, organism(s), to, drug, amoxicillin.

Methicillin-Resistant *Staphylococcus aureus* (MRSA) Conditions

Coding of conditions due to **methicillin-resistant *Staphylococcus aureus* (MRSA)** bacteria are coded in one of two ways: with a combination code that identifies the infection is due to MRSA or with the use of an additional code to identify the MRSA as the causative organism with a code for the site of the infection. MRSA is called a "staph" germ that is not cured with the typical antibiotic that usually cures *Staphylococcus* infections. When the typical antibiotic does not cure the infection, the organism is considered "resistant" to the antibiotic. The MRSA organism is resistant to several common antibiotics such as methicillin or penicillins. There are two types of infection. "Hospital-associated MRSA happens to people in healthcare settings. Community-associated MRSA happens to people who have close skin-to-skin contact with others, such as athletes involved in football and wrestling" (NLM 2019b).

Examples of combination codes that identify the site of the infection and the MRSA causative organism are:

A41.02, Sepsis due to methicillin-resistant *Staphylococcus aureus*
J15.212, Pneumonia due to methicillin-resistant *Staphylococcus aureus*

An example of a condition that require two codes to identify the site of the infection and the MRSA causative organism is an infectious endocarditis due to MRSA:

I33.0, Acute and subacute infective endocarditis
B95.62, Methicillin-resistant *Staphylococcus aureus* infection as cause of diseases classified elsewhere

To locate the additional code to identify MRSA or other bacteria that causes a disease, the coder must access the main term "infection" in the Alphabetic Index as follows:

Infection, infected, infective
bacterial
as cause of disease classified elsewhere
Staphylococcus
aureus
methicillin resistant (MRSA) B95.62

Another entry that may be used in the Alphabetic Index is:

Infection, infected, infective
Staphylococcal, unspecified site
as cause of disease classified elsewhere
aureus
methicillin resistant (MRSA) B95.62

However, if the coder did not follow the subterm "as cause of disease classified elsewhere," the coder would have accessed code A49.02, Methicillin-resistant *Staphylococcus aureus*, unspecified site. This code would not be used with another code that identifies the site of the infection. The A49.02 code is used when the site of the infection is not identified by the physician and there is no other information in the record, nor is there the opportunity to ask the physician a question to clarify the patient's condition.

Additional codes are available to capture *Staphylococcus aureus* that is susceptible to methicillin. These codes, A49.01 and B95.61, **Methicillin-susceptible *Staphylococcus aureus*,** identify that the organism can be treated with methicillin antibiotics.

Check Your Understanding 4.4

Assign the following diagnosis codes that describe drug-resistant infections.

1. Multiple drug resistant (tuberculostatics) pulmonary tuberculosis

2. Bronchopneumonia due to multiple antibiotic resistant *Pseudomonas aeruginosa*

3. Urinary tract infection (UTI) due to MRSA

4. Acute bacterial prostatitis

5. Acute recurrent tonsillitis due to *Streptococcus*

ICD-10-PCS Coding for Infectious and Parasitic Diseases

Commonly, sepsis and other infections are treated with long-term antibiotic therapy through a central venous access catheter. This long-term therapy usually requires the insertion of a peripherally inserted central catheter, also known as a PICC line. The correct coding of a venous catheter of this type depends on the end placement of the catheter, that is, the internal site where the catheter tip is located. A PICC line may be inserted in the right internal jugular and then inserted through the vein into the superior vena cava that qualifies it as a central line. The ICD-10-PCS code for a PICC line insertion is 02HV33Z, insertion of infusion device into superior vena cava by a percutaneous approach.

Table 4.1 shows the ICD-10-PCS Index main term "Insertion of device in" and subterm "Vena cava" superior, code 02HV.

Table 4.1.   Insertion of device in Vena cava, 02HV

0 Medical and Surgical **2 Heart and Great Vessels** **H Insertion—putting in a nonbiological appliance that monitors, assists, performs, or prevents a physiological function but does not physically take the place of a body part**			
Body Part (4th)	**Approach (5th)**	**Device (6th)**	**Qualifier (7th)**
P Pulmonary trunk Q Pulmonary Artery, right R Pulmonary Artery, left S Pulmonary Vein, right T Pulmonary Vein, left **V Superior vena cava** W Thoracic aorta, Descending	0 Open **3 Percutaneous** 4 Percutaneous endoscopic	0 Monitoring Device, Pressure Sensor 2 Monitoring Device **3 Infusion Device** D Intraluminal Device Y Other Device	**Z No Qualifier**

Source: CMS 2019

The complete code for insertion of the PICC line or other central infusion device with the catheter end tip in the superior vena cava is 02HV33Z.

Other forms of therapy may require the insertion of a totally implantable central venous access device, also known as a port-a-cath. The port-a-cath is actually two devices and requires two ICD-10-PCS codes: one for the implantable infusion device and one for the central line catheter into the vascular system. A subcutaneous pocket is created, usually in the chest sub-cutaneous tissue, by incision or by an open approach. The second code is the threading of the catheter tip through a central vein in the upper chest or neck to its end placement of the superior vena cava by a percutaneous approach. The two codes for a totally implantable central venous access device (VAD) would be

1. 02HV33Z, Insertion of infusion device into superior vena cava, percutaneous approach as demonstrated above; and

2. 0JH60XZ, Insertion of vascular access device into chest, subcutaneous tissue and fascia, open approach.

The ICD-10-PCS Index main term entry to code the insertion of the port or reservoir into subcutaneous tissue, for example, into the chest wall, would be "Insertion of device in" and subterm of "Subcutaneous tissue and fascia, chest" with the first four characters of 0JH6, as seen in table 4.2.

Table 4.2. **Insertion of device in Subcutaneous tissue and fascia, 0JH**

0 Medical and Surgical J Subcutaneous Tissue and Fascia H Insertion—putting in a nonbiological appliance that monitors, assists, performs, or prevents a physio- logical function but does not physically take the place of a body part			
Body Part (4th)	**Approach (5th)**	**Device (6th)**	**Qualifier (7th)**
6 Subcutaneous Tissue and Fascia, chest 8 Subcutaneous Tissue and Fascia, Abdomen	**0 Open** 3 Percutaneous	0 Monitoring Device, Hemodynamic 2 Monitoring Device 4 Pacemaker, Single Chamber 5 Pacemaker, Single Chamber rate responsive 6 Pacemaker, Dual Chamber 7 Cardiac Resynchronization Pacemaker Pulse Generator 8 Defibrillator Generator 9 Cardiac Resynchronization Defibrillator Pulse Generator A Contractility Modulation Device B Stimulator Generator, Single Array C Stimulator Generator, Single Array Rechargeable D Stimulator Generator, Multiple Array E Stimulator Generator, Multiple Array Rechargeable H Contraceptive Device M Stimulator Generator N Tissue Expander P Cardiac Rhythm Related Device V Infusion Device, Pump W Vascular Access Device, Reservoir **X Vascular Access Device**	**Z No Qualifier**

Source: CMS 2019

The complete code for insertion of the vascular access device into the chest subcutaneous tissue and fascia by open approach is 0JH60XZ.

When a device is no longer needed, the root operation Removal would be the ICD-10-PCS code applied. A Removal procedure takes out or takes off a device from a body part. In the case of a port-a-cath, it is removal of two devices: one from the subcutaneous tissue of the trunk and one from the superior vena cava or a great vessel.

The ICD-10-PCS Index entry would be
> Removal of device from, great vessel, 02PY
> Removal of device from, subcutaneous tissue, trunk (chest) 0JPT

The following ICD-10-PCS Table (table 4.3) would be used for the removal of both devices:

Table 4.3. **Removal of device from, 02P**

0 Medical and Surgical 2 Heart and Great Vessels P Removal: Taking out or off a device from a body part			
Body Part (4th)	**Approach (5th)**	**Device (6th)**	**Qualifier (7th)**
Y Great Vessel	0 Open **3 Percutaneous** **4 Percutaneous Endoscopic**	2 Monitoring Device **3 Infusion Device** 7 Autologous Tissue Substitute 8 Zooplastic Tissue C Extraluminal Device D Intraluminal Device J Synthetic Device K Nonautologous Tissue Substitute Y Other Device	**Z No Qualifier**

Source: CMS 2019

The complete code for removal of the central infusion device with the catheter end tip in the superior vena cava is 02PY33Z.

The following ICD-10-PCS Table (table 4.4) would be used for the removal of both devices:

Table 4.4.   **Removal of device from, 0JP**

0 Medical and Surgical J Subcutaneous Tissue and Fascia P Removal: Taking out or off a device from a body part			
Body Part (4th)	**Approach (5th)**	**Device (6th)**	**Qualifier (7th)**
T Subcutaneous Tissue and Fascia, Trunk	**0 Open** 3 Percutaneous	0 Drainage Device 1 Radioactive Device 2 Monitoring Device 3 Infusion Device 7 Autologous Tissue Substitute H Contraceptive Device J Synthetic Device K Nonautologous Device M Stimulator Generator N Tissue Expander P Cardiac Rhythm Related Device V Infusion Device, Pump W Vascular Access Device, Totally Implantable **X Vascular Access Device, Tunneled** Y Other Device	**Z No Qualifier**

Source: CMS 2019

The complete code for removal of the implanted port-a-cath in the subcutaneous tissue of the chest is 0JPT0XZ

A patient may acquire sepsis from a disease in the digestive system, especially if there is a rupture or perforation of the intestine that allows organisms to escape and contaminate the internal cavity. Repairing the intestine likely will involve taking out some or all of a body part. The root operation Excision would be used for cutting out or off without replacement a part of the intestine as identified by the body part values in the Table. The root operation Resection would be used for cutting out or off without replacement all of a body part, as identified by one of the values of the body parts for the gastrointestinal system. For example, excision by laparotomy of a portion of the ascending colon would be 0DBK0ZZ. In comparison, if the entire ascending colon was removed by laparotomy the procedure would be coded as a resection with 0DTK0ZZ. The Index entries for either of these intestinal procedures would be "excision, colon, ascending" and "resection, colon, ascending."

Intestinal procedures may include a bypass procedure to completely treat the condition. The root operation Bypass is the altering of the route of passage of the contents of a tubular body party. A bypass can be considered a "rerouting" procedure, thereby, redirecting the contents of a tubular body part, such as an intestine, to travel through a different path. The bypass can send contents in a downstream route or to a similar body part or route. A bypass can also send contents to an abnormal route and different body parts such as to an external location other than a natural orifice. For non–coronary artery bypass, the body part values (character 4) indicate where the bypass originates or starts and the qualifier content indicates where the bypass goes to or ends (character 7). The Index entry is "Bypass" with the subterm for the anatomic location when the bypass originates. For example, a bypass of the ascending colon as a colostomy would be coded as 0D1K0Z4. The Index entry in this example would be "Bypass, ascending colon" as this is where the bypass originated. The documentation of this procedure would likely describe the open procedure as directing the contents of the ascending colon to come out of the body through the skin as a stoma. For this example, Table 0D1 would include the fourth character K for ascending colon, fifth character 0 for open, sixth character device Z for no device used, and seventh character 4 for cutaneous, which is the skin level of a colostomy.

ICD-10-CM and ICD-10-PCS Review Exercises: Chapter 4

Assign the correct ICD-10-CM diagnosis codes and ICD-10-PCS procedure codes to the following diagnoses.

1.   Urinary tract infection due to *Proteus mirabilis*

2.   *Clostridium difficile* (C. diff) colitis. This organism was resistant to multiple drugs, antibiotics

3.   Acute bacterial food poisoning with gastroenteritis due to *Salmonella*

4.   Gonococcal urethritis

5.   Chronic (viral) hepatitis B without delta-agent

6.   Sepsis due to *Enterococcus* from perforated diverticulitis of the small and large intestine

7.   Severe sepsis due to *Haemophilus influenzae* with septic shock with acute renal failure

8.   Whooping cough due to *Bordetella parapertussis* with pneumonia

9.   Acute hepatitis C with hepatic coma

10.   Candidal esophagitis

11.   Insertion of central venous catheter, multilumen, via left subclavian vein for intravenous infusion

(Continued on next page)

ICD-10-CM and ICD-10-PCS Review Exercises: Chapter 4 (continued)

12. Introduction of anti-inflammatory medication via peripheral vein for treatment of ulcerative colitis

   _____

13. Insertion of venous access device (percutaneous port) via subclavian vein, advanced to the superior vena cava with a subcutaneous pocket for port place in chest wall. Device was placed for future chemotherapy to treat colon carcinoma and required an incision to create the subcutaneous pocket.

   _____

14. Low anterior resection of sigmoid colon, 30 cm removed, with end-to-end anastomosis of sigmoid colon

   _____

15. Patient has a malfunction with a right internal jugular tunneled catheter. The old catheter was removed and a new one placed. The new catheter was tunneled through the subcutaneous tissue from the chest wall up into the neck. Fluoroscopy confirmed the catheter tip was in the Superior Vena Cava. Code for both the removal and insertion of the internal jugular tunneled catheter.

   _____

References

AIDS.org. 2019. CD4 (T-Cell Counts). http://www.aids.org/topics/aids-factsheets/aids-background-information/what-is-aids/hiv-testing/cd4-t-cell-tests/.

Casto, A.B. 2019. *ICD-10-CM Code Book,* 2019. Chicago: AHIMA.

Centers for Disease Control and Prevention (CDC), National Center for Health Statistics (NCHS). 2019. *ICD-10-CM Official Guidelines for Coding and Reporting*, 2020. https://www.cdc.gov/nchs/data/icd/10cmguidelines_fy2019_final.pdf.

Centers for Medicare and Medicaid Services (CMS). 2019. 2020 ICD-10. https://www.cms.gov/medicare/Coding/ICD10/index.html.

Chang, H.J. 2010. Sepsis. *Journal of American Medical Association.* 304(16):1856. http://jama.jamanetwork.com/article.aspx?articleid=186795.

National Cancer Institute. 2014. VisualsOnline. Seth Pincus, Elizabeth Fischer, and Austin Athman, creators. https://visualsonline.cancer.gov/details.cfm?imageid=9849.

National Institute of General Medical Sciences. 2018. Sepsis Fact Sheet, January 2018. http://www.nigms.nih.gov/Education/pages/factsheet_sepsis.aspx.

U.S. National Library of Medicine, MedlinePlus (NLM). 2019a. HIV/AIDS. https://www.nlm.nih.gov/medlineplus/hivaids.html.

U.S. National Library of Medicine, MedlinePlus (NLM). 2019b. MRSA. https://www.nlm.nih.gov/medlineplus/mrsa.html.

Chapter 5

Neoplasms (C00–D49)

Learning Objectives

At the conclusion of this chapter, you should be able to do the following:

- Describe the organization of the conditions and codes included in Chapter 2 of ICD-10-CM, Neoplasms

- Review and apply the chapter-specific guidelines for Chapter 2

- Define the seven specific types of neoplasm behavior

- Describe the organization of the Table of Neoplasms

- Explain the purpose of morphology codes

- Apply the guidelines for using ICD-10-CM for Z codes to describe patients with neoplasms

- Describe how to use the Alphabetic Index and Tabular List to locate a neoplasm code

- Identify the purpose of the dash (-) in the ICD-10-CM Table of Neoplasms

- Explain how ICD-10-CM accommodates the coding of contagious sites

- Describe how to code a primary malignant neoplasm according to its site

- Describe how to code a secondary malignant neoplasm according to its site

- Assign ICD-10-CM codes for neoplasms

- Assign ICD-10-PCS codes for procedures related to treating neoplasms

Key Terms

Benign
Biopsy
Carcinoma *in situ*
Histology

Laterality
Malignant
Malignant primary
Malignant secondary

Metastasis	Secondary site
Metastatic cancer	Table of Neoplasms
Morphology	Topography
Neoplasm	Uncertain behavior
Overlapping lesion	Unspecified behavior
Primary site	

Overview of ICD-10-CM Chapter 2: Neoplasms (C00–D49)

Chapter 2 includes categories C00–D49 arranged in the following blocks:

C00–C75	Malignant neoplasms stated or presumed to be primary (of specific sites) and certain specified histologies, except neuroendocrine, and of lymphoid, hematopoietic, and related tissues
C00–C14	Malignant neoplasms of lip, oral cavity, and pharynx
C15–C26	Malignant neoplasms of digestive organs
C30–C39	Malignant neoplasms of respiratory and intrathoracic organs
C40–C41	Malignant neoplasms of bone and articular cartilage
C43–C44	Melanoma and other malignant neoplasms of skin
C45–C49	Malignant neoplasms of mesothelial and soft tissue
C50	Malignant neoplasms of breast
C51–C58	Malignant neoplasms of female genital organs
C60–C63	Malignant neoplasms of male genital organs
C64–C68	Malignant neoplasms of urinary tract
C69–C72	Malignant neoplasms of eye, brain, and other parts of central nervous system
C73–C75	Malignant neoplasms of thyroid and other endocrine glands
C7A	Malignant neuroendocrine tumors
C7B	Secondary neuroendocrine tumors
C76–C80	Malignant neoplasms of ill-defined, other secondary, and unspecified sites
C81–C96	Malignant neoplasm of lymphoid, hematopoietic, and related tissue
D00–D09	*In situ* neoplasms
D10–D36	Benign neoplasms, except benign neuroendocrine tumors
D3A	Benign neuroendocrine tumors
D37–D48	Neoplasms of uncertain behavior, polycythemia vera, and myelodysplastic syndromes
D49	Neoplasms of unspecified behavior

To properly code a neoplasm, it is necessary to determine from the health record if the neoplasm is benign, *in situ*, malignant, or of uncertain histologic behavior. If malignant, any secondary (metastatic) sites should be determined. Neoplasms of uncertain behavior are defined as tumors whose histologic cell type cannot determine whether the tumor is malignant or benign. Neoplasms of unspecified behavior include terms such as growth NOS (not otherwise specified), neoplasm NOS, new growth NOS, or tumor NOS. The term "mass," unless otherwise stated, is not to be regarded as a neoplastic growth.

Chapter 2 classifies neoplasms primarily by site or by topography. Included in the site codes are broad groupings for behavior (malignant, *in situ*, benign, and such). The Table of Neoplasms should be used to identify the correct topography code. For malignant melanoma and certain neuroendocrine tumors, the morphology (histologic type) is included in the category and codes.

Neoplasm Behavior

The term **neoplasm** refers to any new or abnormal growth of body tissue. Definitions describing the behavior of the specific neoplasms include the following:

- **Malignant:** Malignant neoplasms are collectively referred to as cancers. A malignant neoplasm can invade and destroy adjacent structures, as well as spread to distant sites to cause death.

  - **Malignant primary:** A primary neoplasm is the site where a neoplasm originated.

  - **Malignant secondary:** A secondary neoplasm may be described as a metastatic site. **Metastasis** is the movement or spreading of cancer cells from one organ or tissue to another.

    A secondary neoplasm is the site(s) to which the neoplasm has spread via

    - Direct extension, in which the primary neoplasm infiltrates and invades adjacent structures
    - Metastasis to local lymph vessels by tumor cell infiltration
    - Invasion of local blood vessels
    - Implantation in which tumor cells shed into body cavities

  - **Carcinoma *in situ*:** In an *in situ* neoplasm, the tumor cells undergo malignant changes but are still confined to the point of origin without invasion of surrounding normal tissue. The following terms also describe *in situ* malignancies: noninfiltrating, intracystic, intraepithelial carcinoma, and such.

- **Benign:** In benign neoplasms, growth does not invade adjacent structures or spread to distant sites but may displace or exert pressure on adjacent structures.

- **Uncertain behavior:** Neoplasms of uncertain behavior are tumors that a pathologist cannot determine as being either benign or malignant because some features of each are present.

- **Unspecified behavior:** Neoplasms of unspecified behavior include tumors in which neither the behavior nor the histological type is specified in the diagnosis (NLM 2019).

The illustration in figure 5.1 is a comparison of carcinoma *in situ* and carcinoma tumors. In the panel on the left, the carcinoma *in situ* occurs when abnormal tissue cells collect in a body part but remain in place in the inner tissue layer and do not invade other tissue layers. In the panel on the right, a carcinoma tumor is shown. The carcinoma tumor is also composed of abnormal cells but spreads into nearby local issue invading connective tissue, muscle, and other layers within an organ (NCI 2019a).

Figure 5.1. **Carcinoma** *in situ* **and cancer**

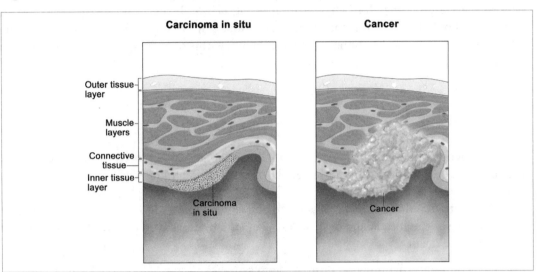

© 2014 Terese Winslow LLC, U.S. Govt. has certain rights

Coding Guidelines for ICD-10-CM Chapter 2

The NCHS has published chapter-specific guidelines for Chapter 2 in the *ICD-10-CM Official Guidelines for Coding and Reporting*. The coding student should review all of the coding guidelines for Chapter 2 of ICD-10-CM, which appear in an ICD-10-CM code book or on the CDC website (CDC 2019).

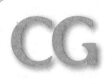

I. C. 2 General guidelines

Chapter 2 of the ICD-10-CM contains the codes for most benign and all malignant neoplasms. Certain benign neoplasms, such as prostatic adenomas, may be found in the specific body system chapters. To properly code a neoplasm it is necessary to determine from the record if the neoplasm is benign, in-situ, malignant, or of uncertain histologic behavior. If malignant, any secondary (metastatic) sites should also be determined.

Primary malignant neoplasms overlapping site boundaries

A primary malignant neoplasm that overlaps two or more contiguous (next to each other) sites should be classified to the subcategory/code 8 ('overlapping lesion'), unless the combination is specifically indexed elsewhere. For multiple neoplasms of the same site that are not contiguous such as tumors of different quadrants of the same breast, codes for each site should be assigned.

Malignant neoplasm of ectopic tissue

Malignant neoplasms of ectopic tissue are to be coded to the site of origin mentioned, e.g., ectopic pancreatic malignant neoplasm involving the stomach are coded to malignant neoplasm of pancreas, unspecified (C25.9).

The Neoplasm Table in the Alphabetic Index should be referenced first. However, if the histological term is documented, that term should be referenced first rather than going immediately to the Neoplasm Table in order to determine which column in the Neoplasm Table is appropriate. For example, if the documentation indicates "adenoma," the coder must refer to that term in the Alphabetic Index to review the entries under this term and the instructional note to "see also neoplasm, by site, benign." The table provides the proper code based on the type of neoplasm and the site. It is important to select the proper column in the table that corresponds to the type of neoplasm. The Tabular List should then be referenced to verify that the correct codes have been selected from the table and that a more specific site codes does not exist.

See Section I.C.21. Factors influencing health status and contact with health services, Status, for information regarding Z15.0, codes for genetic susceptibility to cancer.

Guideline I.C.2.a. Treatment directed at the malignancy: If the treatment is directed at the malignancy, designate the malignancy as the principal diagnosis. The only exception to this guideline is if a patient admission/encounter is solely for the administration of chemotherapy, immunotherapy or external beam radiation therapy, assign the appropriate Z51.– code as the first-listed or principal diagnosis and the diagnosis or problem for which the service is being performed as a secondary diagnosis.

Guideline I.C.2.b. Treatment of secondary site: When a patient is admitted because of a primary neoplasm with metastasis and treatment is directed toward the secondary site only, the secondary neoplasm is designated as the principal diagnosis even though the primary malignancy is still present.

Guideline I.C.2.c. Coding and sequencing of complications: Coding and sequencing of complications associated with the malignancies or with the therapy thereof are subject to the following guidelines:

1. Anemia associated with malignancy: When admission/ encounter is for management of an anemia associated with the malignancy, and the treatment is only for the

(Continued)

(Continued)

anemia, the appropriate code for the malignancy is sequenced as principal or first-listed diagnosis followed by the appropriate code for the anemia, such as code D63.0, Anemia in neoplastic disease.

2. Anemia associated with chemotherapy, immunotherapy, and radiation therapy: When the admission/encounter is for management of an anemia associated with an adverse effect of the administration of chemotherapy or immunotherapy and the only treatment is for the anemia, the anemia code is sequenced first followed by the appropriate codes for the neoplasm and the adverse effect (T45.1X5, Adverse effect of antineoplastic and immunosuppressive drugs). When the admission/encounter is for management of an anemia associated with an adverse effect of radiotherapy, the anemia code should be sequenced first, followed by the appropriate neoplasm and code Y84.2, Radiological procedure and radiotherapy as the cause of the abnormal reaction of the patient, or of later complication, without mention of misadventure at the time of the procedure.

3. Management of dehydration due to the malignancy: When the admission/encounter is for management of dehydration due to the malignancy and only the dehydration is being treated (intravenous hydration), the dehydration is sequenced first, followed by the code(s) for the malignancy.

4. Treatment of a complication resulting from a surgical procedure: When the admission/encounter is for treatment of a complication resulting from a surgical procedure, designate the complication as the principal or first-listed diagnosis if the treatment is directed at resolving the complication.

Guideline I.C.2.d. Primary malignancy previously excised: When a primary malignancy has been previously excised and eradicated from its site and there is no further treatment directed to that site and there is no evidence of any existing primary malignancy at that site, a code from category Z85, Personal history of malignant neoplasm, should be used to indicate the former site of the malignancy. Any mention of extension, invasion, or metastasis to another site is coded as a secondary malignant neoplasm to that site. The secondary site may be the principal or first-listed diagnosis with the Z85 code used as a secondary code.

Guideline I.C.2.e Admissions/Encounters involving chemotherapy, immunotherapy and radiation therapy

1. Episode of care that involves the surgical removal of a neoplasm: When an episode of care involves the surgical removal of a neoplasm, primary or secondary site, followed by adjunct chemotherapy or radiation treatment during the same episode of care, the code for the neoplasm should be assigned as principal or first-listed diagnosis.

2. Patient admission/encounter solely for administration of chemotherapy, immunotherapy, and radiation therapy: If the patient admission/encounter is solely for the administration of chemotherapy, immunotherapy or external beam radiation therapy assign code Z51.0, Encounter for antineoplastic radiation therapy, or Z51.11, Encounter for antineoplastic chemotherapy, or Z51.12, Encounter for antineoplastic immunotherapy as the first-listed or principal diagnosis. If a patient receives more than one of these therapies during the same admission more than one of these codes may be assigned, in any sequence. The malignancy for which the therapy is being administered should be assigned as a secondary diagnosis.

   If a patient admission/encounter is for the insertion or implantation of radioactive elements (e.g., brachytherapy) the appropriate code for the malignancy is sequenced as the principal or first-listed diagnosis. Code Z51.0 should not be assigned.

3. Patient admitted for radiation therapy, chemotherapy, or immunotherapy and develops complications: When a patient is admitted for the purpose of radiotherapy, immunotherapy or chemotherapy and develops complications such as uncontrolled nausea and vomiting or dehydration, the principal or first-listed diagnosis is Z51.0, Encounter for antineoplastic radiation therapy, of Z51.11, Encounter for antineoplastic chemotherapy, or Z51.12, Encounter for antineoplastic immunotherapy followed by any codes for the complications.

   When a patient is admitted for the purpose of insertion or implantation of radioactive elements (e.g., brachytherapy) and develops complications such as uncontrolled nausea and vomiting or dehydration, the principal or first-listed diagnosis is the appropriate code for the malignancy followed by any codes for the complications.

(Continued)

(Continued)

Guideline I.C.2.f. Admission/encounter to determine extent of malignancy: When the reason for admission/encounter is to determine the extent of the malignancy, or for a procedure such as paracentesis or thoracentesis, the primary malignancy or appropriate metastatic site is designated as the principal or first-listed diagnosis, even though chemotherapy or radiotherapy is administered.

Guideline I.C.2.g. Symptoms, signs, and abnormal findings listed in Chapter 18 associated with neoplasm: Symptoms, signs, and ill-defined conditions listed in Chapter 18 characteristic of, or associated with, an existing primary or secondary or first-listed diagnosis cannot be used to replace the malignancy as principal or first-listed diagnosis, regardless of the number of admissions or encounters for treatment and care of the neoplasm. *See section I.C.21, Factors influencing health status and contact with health services, Encounter for prophylactic organ removal.*

Guideline I.C.2.h. Admission/encounter for pain control/management

See Section I.C.6 for information on coding admission/encounter for pain control management.

Guideline I.C.2.i. Malignancy in two or more contiguous site: A patient may have more than one malignant tumor in the same organ. These tumors may represent different primaries or metastatic disease, depending on the site. Should the documentation be unclear, the provider should be queried as to the status of each tumor so that the correct codes can be assigned.

Guideline I.C.2.j. Disseminated malignant neoplasm, unspecified: Code C80.0, Disseminated malignant neoplasm, unspecified, is for use only in those cases where the patient has advanced metastatic disease and no known primary or secondary sites are specified. If should not be used in place of assigning codes for the primary site and all know secondary sites.

Guideline I.C.2.k. Malignant neoplasm without specification of site: Code C80.1, Malignant (primary) neoplasm, unspecified, equates to Cancer, unspecified. This code should only be used when no determination can be made as to the primary site of a malignancy. This code should rarely be used in the inpatient setting.

Guidelines I.C.2.l. Sequencing of neoplasm codes:

1. Encounter for treatment of primary malignancy: If the reason for the encounter is for treatment of a primary malignancy, assign the malignancy as the principal/

first-listed diagnosis. The primary site is to be sequenced first, followed by any metastatic sites.

2. Encounter for treatment of secondary malignancy: When an encounter is for a primary malignancy with metastasis and treatment is directed toward the metastatic (secondary) site(s) only, the metastatic site(s) is designated as the principal/first-listed diagnosis. The primary malignancy is coded as an additional code.

3. Malignant neoplasm in a pregnant patient: When a pregnant woman has a malignant neoplasm, a code from subcategory O9A.1-, Malignant neoplasm complicating pregnancy, childbirth, and the puerperium, should be sequenced first, followed by the appropriate code from Chapter 2 to indicate the type of neoplasm.

4. Encounter for complication associated with a neoplasm: When an encounter is for management of a complication associated with a neoplasm, such as dehydration, and the treatment is only for the complication, the complication is coded first, followed by the appropriate code(s) for the neoplasm. The exception to this guideline is anemia. When the admission/encounter is for management of an anemia associated with the malignancy, and the treatment is only for anemia, the appropriate code for the malignancy is sequenced as the principal or first-listed diagnosis followed by code D63.0, Anemia in neoplastic disease.

5. Complication from surgical procedure for treatment of an neoplasm: When an encounter is for treatment of a complication resulting from a surgical procedure performed for the treatment of the neoplasm, designate the complication as the principal/first-listed diagnosis. See the guideline regarding coding of a current malignancy versus personal history to determine if the code for the neoplasm should also be assigned.

6. Pathologic fracture due to a neoplasm: When an encounter is for a pathologic fracture due to a neoplasm, and the focus of treatment is the fracture, a code from subcategory M84.5, Pathological fracture in neoplastic disease, should be sequenced first, followed by the code for the neoplasm. If the focus of the treatment is the neoplasm with an associated pathological fracture, the neoplasm code should be sequenced first, followed by a code from M84.5 for the pathological fracture.

(Continued)

(Continued)

Guideline I.C.2.m. Current malignancy versus personal history of malignancy: When a primary malignancy has been excised but further treatment, such as an additional surgery for the malignancy, radiation therapy or chemotherapy is directed to that site, the primary malignancy code should be used until treatment is completed.

When a primary malignancy has been previously excised or eradicated from its site, there is no further treatment (of the malignancy) directed to that site, and there is no evidence of any existing primary malignancy at that site, a code from category Z85, Personal history of malignant neoplasm, should be used to indicate the former site of the malignancy.

Subcategories Z85.0–Z85.7 should only be assigned for the former site of a primary malignancy, not the site of a secondary malignancy. Codes from subcategory Z85.8-, may be assigned for the former site(s) of either a primary or secondary malignancy included in this subcategory. *See Section I.C.21. Factors influencing health status and contact with health services, History (of)*

Guideline I.C.2.n. Leukemia, Multiple Myeloma, and Malignant Plasma Cell Neoplasms in remission versus personal history: The categories for leukemia, and category C90, Multiple myeloma and malignant plasma cell neoplasms, have codes indicating whether or not the leukemia has achieved remission. There are also codes Z85.6, Personal history of leukemia, and Z85.79, Personal history of other malignant neoplasms of lymphoid, hematopoietic and related tissues. If the documentation is unclear as to whether the leukemia has achieved remission, the provider should be queried. *See Section I.C.21. Factors influencing health status and contact with health services, History (of)*

Guideline I.C.2.o Aftercare following surgery for neoplasm: *See Section I.C.21. Factors influencing health status and contact with health services, Aftercare*

Guideline I.C.2.p Follow-up care for completed treatment of a malignancy: *I.C.21. Factors influencing health status and contact with health services, Follow-up*

Guideline I.C.2.q Prophylactic organ removal for prevention of malignancy: *I.C.21. Factors influencing health status and contact with health services, Prophylactic organ removal*

Guideline I.C.2.r Malignant neoplasm associated with transplanted organ: A malignant neoplasm of a transplanted organ should be coded as a transplant complication. Assign first the appropriate code from category T86.-, Complications of transplanted organs and tissue, followed by code C80.2, Malignant neoplasm associated with transplanted organ. Use an additional code for the specific malignancy.

Coding Neoplasms in ICD-10-CM Chapter 2

The coding of neoplasms requires understanding of the organization of the ICD-10-CM Table of Neoplasms as well as the Index to Diseases and Injuries and the Tabular List to completely code the malignant, benign, and other neoplasms described by physicians in patients' records.

ICD-10-CM Table of Neoplasms

The ICD-10-CM **Table of Neoplasms** is a listing of codes that follows the ICD-10-CM Index of Diseases and Injuries. The ICD-10-CM Table of Neoplasms is organized into seven columns. The first or the left column lists the anatomic site for the neoplasm. The next six columns provide codes for malignant primary, malignant secondary, carcinoma (CA) *in situ*, benign, uncertain behavior, and unspecified behavior for each anatomic site. Malignant tumor codes start with the alphabetic character C in the range of C00–C96. Benign, *in situ*, and neoplasms of uncertain behavior and unspecified behavior are listed in the range of D00–D49. An example of the ICD-10-CM Table of Neoplasms is shown in table 5.1 with the anatomic site in the first column with the next six columns specifying the ICD-10-CM diagnosis code based on the behavior of the neoplasm.

Table 5.1. **Example of ICD-10-CM Table of Neoplasms**

	Malignant Primary	Malignant Secondary	Ca *in situ*	Benign	Uncertain Behavior	Unspecified Behavior
Neoplasm, neoplastic	C80.1	C79.9	D09.9	D36.9	D48.9	D49.9
- Abdomen, abdominal	C76.2	C79.8-	D09.8	D36.7	D48.7	D49.89
-- cavity	C76.2	C79.8-	D09.8	D36.7	D48.7	D49.89
-- organ	C76.2	C79.8-	D09.8	D36.7	D48.7	D49.89
-- viscera	C76.2	C79.8-	D09.8	D36.7	D48.7	D49.89
-- wall—see also Neoplasm, abdomen, wall, skin	C44.509	C79.2-	D04.5	D23.5	D48.5	D49.2
--- connective tissue	C49.4	C79.8-	-	D21.4	D48.1	D49.2
--- skin	C44.509	-	-	-	-	-
---- basal cell carcinoma	C44.519	-	-	-	-	-
---- specified type NEC	C44.599	-	-	-	-	-
---- squamous cell carcinoma	C44.529	-	-	-	-	-

Source: CMS 2019

Topography and Histology

ICD-10-CM classifies neoplasms by topography. **Topography** is a description of the site, region, or a special part of the body (see table 5.1 Abdomen, cavity). The ICD-10-CM Table of Neoplasms does not include neoplasms by histology. **Histology** is the study of the cell structures under the microscope. Certain neoplasms are identified by the histologic name of the cell structures, for example, oat cell carcinoma of the lung. For certain neoplasms, such as for malignant melanoma and certain neuroendocrine tumors, the histology is included in the category and codes. The term **morphology** is the study of the physical shape or size of a specimen, plant, or animal (Mosby 2017, 867). In medicine, the term morphology is also used to describe neoplasms, that is, the form and structure of the tumor in the organ.

The description of the neoplasm will usually indicate which of the six columns is appropriate for coding, for example, basal cell carcinoma of the skin, benign fibroadenoma of the breast, or carcinoma *in situ* of the larynx. When the name of the neoplasm does not readily identify the behavior of the neoplasm as malignant or benign, the coder should use the remainder of the Index to identify which column to use on the Table of Neoplasms to assign the code. For example, giant cell glioblastoma of the brain is included in the Index to Diseases and Injuries with the following entry: see Neoplasm, malignant, by site (brain). The next step for the coder is to reference the Table of Neoplasms under the anatomic site, brain, malignant, primary, to assign the code.

Laterality

A feature in ICD-10-CM is the concept of **laterality**. Codes listed in the ICD-10-CM Table of Neoplasms with a dash (-) following the code have a required fifth character for laterality, that is, right or left side. The Tabular List must be reviewed for the complete code. Neoplasm codes are specific as to whether the location is the right or left organ when a tumor is present in an organ that exists bilaterally. Examples of laterality would be a malignant neoplasm of the upper-outer quadrant of the right female breast (C50.411) and a benign neoplasm of the left kidney (D30.02). Codes also exist for an unspecified side of bilateral locations.

Check Your Understanding 5.1

Using the Table of Neoplasms and the Tabular List, assign codes to the following.

1. Encounter for brachytherapy for carcinoma of the prostate

2. Secondary malignant neoplasm of small intestine

3. Benign neoplasm of the small intestine

4. Neoplasm of the cerebrum, behavior uncertain

5. Carcinoma *in situ* of the cervix

6. Secondary malignant neoplasm involving the lower lobe of the right lung

---

ICD-10-CM Chapter 2 Index Instructions

If the coder can identify the behavior and site of the neoplasm, the usual first step is to access the ICD-10-CM Table of Neoplasms. However, the main terms and subterms in the ICD-10-CM Alphabetic Index to Diseases and Injuries assists the coder in locating the morphological type of neoplasms. When a specific code or site is not listed in the Index, cross-references direct the coder to the Table of Neoplasms. It is essential to validate the code identified in the Table of Neoplasms in the Tabular List. The assignment of the code should not be used without this step. The following instructions for classifying neoplasms should be followed:

1. If the morphology is stated, the coder must locate the morphology of the tumor in the Alphabetic Index to Diseases and Injuries. For example, entries exist for lipoma,

melanoma, sarcoma, and such, and specific codes for these types of neoplasms are included in the Index; the coder does not need to reference the Table of Neoplasms at all.

2. If the morphology is stated, the coder must locate the morphology of the tumor in the Alphabetic Index to Diseases and Injuries. However, not every entry in the Index will include codes. For example, if the physician writes "subependymal glioma of the brain" as the diagnosis, the Index entry of glioma, subependymal, brain (specified site) is referenced and a cross-reference directs the coder to the following entry: see Neoplasm, uncertain behavior, by site (brain).

3. If the morphology is stated but the physician does not include an anatomic site, the coder should locate the morphology of the tumor in the Alphabetic Index to Diseases and Injuries. Certain types of morphology indicate the anatomic site as the only possible site where the tumor would develop. The physician would consider writing both the morphology and the site as redundant terminology. For example, the physician documents "serous papillary carcinoma" but the site is not stated. The Index entry of carcinoma, papillary, serous or carcinoma, serous, papillary is referenced and the coder will note that an entry exists for "unspecified site" and code C56.9. C56.9 is the code for malignant neoplasm of ovary, unspecified side. The coder can trust that entry because serous papillary carcinoma will only occur in an ovary.

4. If the coder is certain about the behavior of the neoplasm, for example, carcinoma is always a malignant primary tumor, the coder should reference the ICD-10-CM Table of Neoplasms as the first step. The site of the neoplasm is located and the code is selected based on the behavior of the neoplasm from the appropriate column.

Check Your Understanding 5.2

Using Alphabetic Index and Tabular List, assign codes to the following.

1. Hurthle cell carcinoma

2. Choriocarcinoma of left testis (male patient, age 31)

3. Acute monocytic leukemia

4. Relapse of multiple myeloma

5. Wilms' tumor, left

6. A patient was admitted with diagnosis of bone metastasis originating from right upper lobe of the lung. Pathology was consistent with oat cell carcinoma. This admission was for the purpose of chemotherapy administration.

7. Carcinoma *in situ* of endocervix

8. Female patient was admitted with history of right breast carcinoma with mastectomy performed two years ago and no treatment currently given for breast carcinoma. Patient presents with complaints of vision disturbances. Workup revealed metastasis to the brain.

ICD-10-CM Chapter 2 Tabular List Instructions

 In ICD-10-CM, instructional notes are found under many of the categories for malignant neoplasms. Instructional notes unique to ICD-10-CM direct coding professionals to use an additional code to identify such conditions as alcohol abuse and dependence, history of tobacco use, tobacco dependence, history of tobacco use, exposure to environmental tobacco smoke, and other facts.

All neoplasms are classified in this chapter, whether they are functionally active or not. An additional code from Chapter 4, Endocrine, nutritional and metabolic diseases, may be used to identify functional activity associated with any neoplasm. Functional activity, such as increased or decreased hormone production, may occur when a neoplasm is present in a glandular organ. For example, when a patient has carcinoma of the ovary, she may also experience hyperestrogenism that produces excessive or frequent menstruation.

> **EXAMPLE:** C73, Malignant neoplasm of thyroid gland
>
> Use additional code to identify any functional activity

An instructional note under category D3A, Benign neuroendocrine tumor and C7A, Malignant neuroendocrine tumors instructs the coding professional to code additional disorders.

> **EXAMPLE:** D3A, Benign neuroendocrine tumors
>
> Code also any associated multiple endocrine neoplasia [MEN] syndromes (E31.2-)
>
> Use additional code to identify any associated endocrine syndrome, such as: carcinoid syndrome (E34.0)

> **EXAMPLE:** C7A, Malignant neuroendocrine tumors
>
> Code also any associated multiple endocrine neoplasia [MEN] syndromes (E31.2-)
>
> Use additional code to identify any associated endocrine syndrome, such as: carcinoid syndrome (E34.0)

Check Your Understanding 5.3

Using the Alphabetic Index and Tabular List, assign codes to the following.

1. Malignant melanoma of skin of scalp

2. Benign melanoma of skin of shoulder, left

3. Glioma of the occipital lobe of the brain

4. Benign carcinoid tumor of the cecum with carcinoid syndrome

5. Ewing's sarcoma of pelvis

6. Hypoglycemia due to islet cell adenoma of pancreas

7. Carcinoma of the right ovary with hyperestrogenism

8. Galactorrhea due to pituitary adenoma

9. Adenoma of adrenal cortex, right with Conn's syndrome

10. Carcinoma *in situ* of larynx

ICD-10-CM Coding of the Anatomical Site

ICD-10-CM provides guidelines for coding the anatomical site of a neoplasm to the highest degree of specificity. These guidelines are discussed in the following sections.

Classification of Malignant Neoplasms

Malignant neoplasms are separated into primary sites (C00–C75, C7A, C76–C80) and secondary or metastatic sites (C7B, C77–C79), with further subdivisions by anatomic sites.

Neoplasms of the lymphatic and hematopoietic system are always coded to categories C81–C96, regardless of whether the neoplasm is stated as primary or secondary. Neoplasms of the lymphatic and hematopoietic system, such as leukemias and lymphomas, are considered widespread and systemic in nature and, as such, do not metastasize. Therefore, they are not coded to category C77, Secondary and unspecified malignant neoplasms of lymph nodes, which includes codes identifying secondary or metastatic neoplasms of the lymphatic system.

Neuroendocrine tumors include both malignant (C7A) and benign tumors (D3A) that arise from endocrine or neuroendocrine cells scattered throughout the body. Neuroendocrine tumors are classified into two types: carcinoid tumors and pancreatic endocrine tumors. Many of these tumors are associated with the multiple endocrine neoplasia syndromes identified by ICD-10-CM subcategory codes E31.20–E31.23. There is a note under subcategory E31.2- to code first any associated malignancies and other conditions associated with the syndromes. Under category C7A, Malignant neuroendocrine tumors, there is a note to code also any associated multiple endocrine neoplasia (MEN) syndrome (E31.2-). Another note instructs the coder to use an additional code to identify any associated endocrine syndrome, such as carcinoid syndrome (E34.0).

Determination of the Primary Site

The **primary site** is defined as the origin of the tumor. Physicians usually identify the origin of the tumor in the diagnostic statement. In some cases, however, the physician cannot identify the primary site. For these situations, ICD-10-CM provides an entry in the Table of Neoplasms titled "unknown site or unspecified" assigned to code C80.1 for malignant (primary) neoplasm, unspecified or C79.9 for secondary malignant neoplasm of unspecified site.

Category C76

Category C76, Malignant neoplasms of other and ill-defined sites, is available for use only when a more specific site cannot be identified. This category includes malignant neoplasms of contiguous sites, not elsewhere classified, whose point of origin cannot be determined.

> **EXAMPLE:** Carcinoma of the neck
>
> C76.0, Malignant neoplasm of head, face, and neck

Primary Malignant Neoplasm of Contiguous Sites or Overlapping Lesion

A tumor may develop at the junction of two parts of an organ or two organs next to each other. A primary malignant neoplasm that overlaps two or more sites may be called a contiguous neoplasm or an **overlapping lesion**. When the neoplasm is identified as located at an overlapping site, it will be classified to the subcategory code .8. A number of anatomic sites include an entry for an overlapping lesion with a code for the primary malignant site as the only entry on the row in the Table of Neoplasms.

For multiple neoplasms of the same site that are not contiguous, codes for each site should be assigned. For example, tumors of the upper outer quadrant and lower inner quadrant of the right breast would each be assigned a separate code.

EXAMPLE: A primary malignant lesion of the jejunum and ileum

Table of Neoplasms, Intestine, small, overlapping lesion C17.8

C17.8, Malignant neoplasm of overlapping sites of small intestine

Check Your Understanding 5.4

Using the Alphabetic Index and Tabular List, assign codes to the following.

1. Atypical chronic myeloid, BCR/ABL-negative leukemia
2. Basal cell carcinoma of lower and upper back
3. Adenocarcinoma of head of pancreas
4. Paget's disease with infiltrating duct carcinoma of right female breast involving central portion, nipple, and areola
5. Carcinoma *in situ* of the tongue, dorsal surface
6. Hemangioma of skin on the right lower leg
7. Papilloma of the cervix
8. Skin cancer (Squamous cell carcinoma) of the left leg
9. Hodgkin's lymphoma of intra-abdominal lymph nodes and spleen
10. Malignant neoplasm of face

Classification of Secondary Sites

The patient's health record is the best source of information for differentiating between a primary and a secondary site. A **secondary site** may be referred to as a metastatic site in the record documentation. The following subsection describes some of the principal terms used in diagnostic statements that refer to secondary malignant neoplasms.

Figure 5.2 depicts metastasis. The drawing shows how a primary cancer tumor has spread from the colon to the lung and brain, two metastatic sites. The inset shows how the cancer cells spread. The cells spread through the blood system and through lymph nodes to another part of the body and form a metastatic tumor. In metastasis, the original cancer cells move away from the primary site where it developed to another site in the body to form a second malignant neoplasm. The metastatic site or secondary neoplasm is always the same type of cancer as the primary tumor. For this reason, physicians are able to identify the source of the secondary neoplasm, that is, identify the primary site (NCI 2019b).

Metastatic Cancer

Metastatic cancer is a cancer that has spread from its original site, or what organ it first appeared, to another place in the body. A metastatic tumor is always caused by the cancer cells from another part of the body. Practically all cancers can form metastatic tumors. A metastatic tumor is one formed by metastatic cancer cells and is called a metastasis. The traveling of a cancer from one site to another site is also called metastasis. Metastatic cancer has the same name or cell type as the original or primary cancer. Microscopically, metastatic cancer cells look the same as the cells of the original cancer and have the same molecular features. For this reason, when a cancer spreads, the physician often continues to describe the cancer by its original site. For example, when a breast cancer spreads to the lungs and forms a metastatic tumor, the physician is likely to document the tumor as metastatic breast cancer, not lung cancer. In this example, the primary site is the breast, the secondary or metastatic site is the lung. This is an important concept for the coder to understand. Metastatic breast cancer is not likely to be a secondary cancer in the breast but instead a primary malignant neoplasm of the breast that has spread to another location (NCI 2018).

Figure 5.2.   **Metastasis**

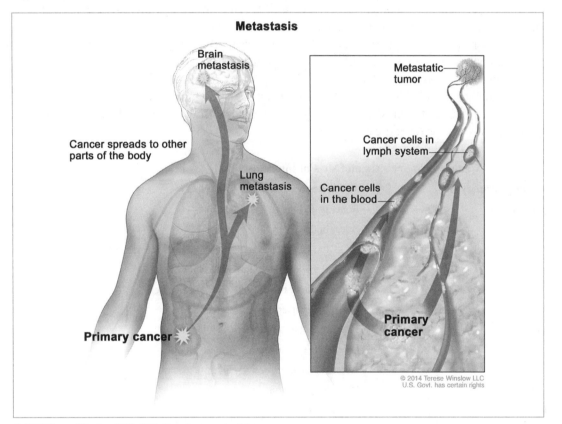

© 2014 Terese Winslow LLC, U.S. Govt. has certain rights

The sites of cancer metastasis are most commonly occurring in the bone, liver, and lung. Most cancers can spread to different parts of the body, but a particular primary site tumor usually spreads to one site more often than other sites in the body. Unfortunately, metastatic cancer cells can lie dormant and not grow at another body location for years before they grow into a tumor, if at all. Symptoms of metastatic cancer depend on the size and location of the metastasis. For example, cancer that spreads to the bone is likely to cause pain and can cause pathologic fractures. Cancer spreading to other sites can cause different symptoms, for example, cancer spread to the lungs causes shortness of breath. Abdominal swelling, pain, and jaundice can indicate that cancer has spread to the liver. There are circumstances when a patient's original cancer is discovered only after the metastatic tumor has spread to another site and caused symptoms. For example, a man with prostate cancer may not know it exists until the prostate cancer spreads to the bones in his pelvis that causes lower back pain.

It is also possible for a patient who was previously diagnosed with cancer to have cancer diagnosed a second time. Often this cancer is what physician's call a "new primary," for example, a patient with colon carcinoma is later diagnosed with breast cancer. The surgeon and pathologist can see that the cancer cells in the breast cancer did not come from the previous colon cancer. Other patients can have a "recurrence" or recurrent cancer, that is, the cancer occurs a second time in the same organ. If the cancer recurs in the same organ, it is usually call a "recurrence."

It is also possible to have a patient with a metastatic tumor, but the primary tumor cannot be found. The primary site may have been too small or it might have completely degenerated. However, when the secondary site is biopsied, the pathologist knows the secondary site is metastasis because the cells of the tumor do not resemble the cells of the organ where it was found. The physician may document this as a cancer of an unknown primary origin (CUP). In this situation with a CUP, the coder will assign a code for the secondary malignancy site for the site of the metastasis and a code for primary malignant of an unknown site. A patient may also develop a metastatic site after the primary site malignant tumor has been treated and is no longer under therapy. A patient with a history of a primary malignancy would be coded as a personal history of malignant neoplasm by site. Whenever a patient has a diagnosis of a metastatic cancer, two codes are required: one for the primary malignant site or personal history of primary malignant neoplasm and one for the secondary malignant site.

See table 5.2 for the most common sites of metastasis from a primary location, excluding the lymph nodes, for several cancer types:

Table 5.2. **Cancer primary sites and sites of metastasis**

Cancer primary site	Main sites of metastasis
Bladder	Bone, liver, lung*
Breast	Bone, brain†, liver, lung
Colorectal	Liver, lung, peritoneum
Kidney	Adrenal gland, bone, brain, liver, lung
Lung	Adrenal gland, bone, brain, liver, other lung
Melanoma	Bone, brain, liver, lung, skin/muscle
Ovary	Liver, lung, peritoneum
Pancreas	Liver, lung, peritoneum
Prostate	Adrenal gland, bone, liver, lung
Stomach	Liver, lung, peritoneum
Thyroid	Bone, liver, lung

*Lung includes the main part of the lung (parenchyma) as well as the pleura.
†Brain includes neural tissue or parenchyma and the meninges that surround the brain and the spinal cord.

Source: NCI 2018

Metastatic to and Direct Extension to

 The terms "metastatic to" and "direct extension to" are both used in classifying secondary malignant neoplasms in ICD-10-CM. For example, cancer described as "metastatic to" a specific site is interpreted as a secondary neoplasm of that site. Invasion through the entire wall of an organ into surrounding organs or adjacent tissues is referred to as "direct extension" or "contiguous spread" (NCI 2019b).

EXAMPLE: Metastatic carcinoma of the colon to the lung

C18.9, Malignant neoplasm of colon, unspecified

C78.00, Secondary malignant neoplasm of lung

The colon (C18.9) is the primary site, and the lung (C78.00) is the secondary site.

Spread to and Extension to

When expressed in terms of malignant neoplasm with "spread to" or "extension to," diagnoses should be coded as primary sites with metastases.

EXAMPLE: Adenocarcinoma of the stomach with spread to the peritoneum

C16.9, Malignant neoplasm of stomach, unspecified

C78.6, Secondary malignant neoplasm of retroperitoneum and peritoneum

The stomach (C16.9) is the primary site, and the peritoneum (C78.6) is the secondary site.

Malignant Neoplasm of Lymphatic and Hematopoietic Tissue

Chapter 2 includes the classification of malignant conditions of lymphatic and hematopoietic tissue. These conditions include lymphomas that arise out of lymph tissue, multiple myeloma that originates in bone marrow, and leukemia that forms in the blood with proliferation of abnormal leukocytes. These conditions are systemic and not isolated to a particular location, and the concept of metastatic coding discussed previously does not apply to these neoplasms. Lymphomas are classified according to their type and the specific lymph nodes involved when the diagnosis was made. Multiple myeloma is classified as to whether it is stated to be in remission, in relapse, or not having achieved remission. Leukemias are classified according to their type, such as lymphoid, myeloid, or monocytic, and how the condition currently exists (not having achieved remission, condition is in remission, or condition is in relapse). Remission occurs when the disease lessens in severity or the symptoms decrease and treatment may be discontinued. Relapse is the return of manifestations of the disease after an interval of improvement. Relapse may be considered a recurrence of the leukemia.

Check Your Understanding 5.5

Using the Alphabetic Index and Tabular List, assign codes to the following.

1. Burkitt's lymphoma in multiple lymph nodes and spleen

2. Recurrence of papillary carcinoma of the lateral wall of the bladder

3. Metastatic carcinoma of intrathoracic lymph nodes from small cell carcinoma of the right lower lobe of lung

4. Adenocarcinoma of sigmoid colon with extension to peritoneum

(Continued)

(Continued)

5. Adenocarcinoma of prostate with metastasis to spine

6. Metastatic carcinoma of bile duct to local (common duct) lymph nodes

7. Metastatic liver carcinoma with unknown primary site

8. Metastatic breast carcinoma

9. Glioblastoma of parietal and occipital lobes

10. B-cell lymphoma of multiple sites

Neoplasm-Related Pain

A patient with primary or secondary malignant neoplasms may seek medical care because of neoplasm-related pain. Code G89.3, neoplasm-related pain (acute)(chronic) is assigned to pain documented as being related, associated, or due to a primary or secondary malignant neoplasm. This code may be assigned for acute or chronic pain. The code may be assigned as a principal diagnosis or a first-listed diagnosis code when the stated reason for the admission or outpatient encounter is documented as pain control or pain management. The underlying neoplasm should also be reported as an additional diagnosis. When the reason for admission or outpatient care is the management of the neoplasm and the pain associated with the malignancy is also documented, code G89.3 can be assigned as an additional diagnosis code. It is not necessary to assign an additional code for the site of the pain.

Other Conditions Described as Malignant

The medical term "malignant" has two meanings: (1) tending to become worse and to cause death and (2) describing a cancer—anaplastic, invasive, metastatic (Mosby 2017, 805). In another context, it means resistant to treatment, occurring in severe form and frequently fatal, tending to become worse, and leading to an ingravescent (increasing in severity) course. In reference to a neoplasm, malignant means having the property of locally invasive and destructive growth and metastasis.

Effusion is the escape of fluid from blood vessels or lymphatics into the tissues or a cavity. This fluid can accumulate abnormally in the pleural cavity, pericardium, or peritoneum. Pleural effusions due to tumors may or may not contain malignant cells. When the condition is symptomatic, thoracentesis or chest tube drainage is required. Symptomatic pericardial effusion is treated by creating a pericardial window. Fluid in the peritoneum or ascites is usually treated with repeated paracentesis of small volumes of fluid.

A code for malignant ascites exists as R18.0 with a code first malignancy, such as malignant neoplasm of ovary (C56.-), or secondary malignant neoplasm of retroperitoneum and peritoneum (C78.6). Another condition described as malignant is malignant pleural effusion (J91.0). Beneath this code is a note to code first underlying neoplasm.

ICD-10-PCS Coding for Procedures Related to Neoplasms

ICD-10-PCS codes are found in the Index based on the general type of procedure. Based on the first three values of the code found in the Index, the corresponding table is located. The upper portion of each table contains a description of the first three characters of the procedure code listed in the Index, that is, the name of the section, the body system, and the root operation performed. The lower portion of the tables specifies all the valid combinations of character 4 through character 7. The four columns of the table represent the last four characters of the code. The four columns are labeled body part, approach, device, and qualifier in the Medical and Surgical section. The coder constructs the code selecting characters 4 through 7 based on the facts of the procedure documented in the operative or procedure report written by the physician.

Surgical procedures performed to treat neoplasms can occur in many body systems, such as central nervous system, respiratory system, gastrointestinal system, skin and breast, as well as other body systems. Tumors can develop in all parts of the body and multiple organ systems. Coders use ICD-10-PCS procedure codes from multiple parts of the Medical and Surgical Section of ICD-10-PCS as well as other sections of the coding system, such as administration and radiation therapy.

Neoplasms are often treated with removal of tumors via surgical procedures. There are three root operations that take out some or all of a body part with three root operations that are most likely related to removing a tumor: Excision, Resection, and Destruction.

Excision Procedures Related to Neoplasms

The root operation Excision is used for cutting out or off without replacement a part of the site identified by the body part values in the table. An Excision procedure may be done for the purpose of performing a biopsy of a tumor or lesion. A **biopsy** is the removal and examination, usually microscopic, of tissue from the body, performed to establish a precise diagnosis. The qualifier of X is used to indicate the excision is a diagnostic procedure, that is, the physician is submitting a specimen to pathology to determine if disease and what type is present in the specimen. Other therapeutic procedures would be the excision of body parts that contain malignant neoplasms, and the qualifier of Z would be used to indicate it was not a diagnostic procedure. A therapeutic procedure that involves an excision will always have the specimen submitted to pathology for a report describing the extent and type of disease present. When performing a therapeutic excision of a body part, the surgeon knows the disease is present and has made a decision on how to treat it. For example, a partial mastectomy or lumpectomy may be performed to remove a breast sparing procedure that removed the malignant lesion of the breast as the definitive treatment and leaves most of the breast in place. Refer to PCS Guideline B3.4b, biopsy followed by more definitive treatment. When a diagnostic biopsy procedure is followed by a more definitive procedure at the same procedure site, both the biopsy and the more definitive treatment are coded.

Resection Procedures Related to Neoplasms

The root operation **Resection** is used for the cutting out or off without replacement of all of a body part, as identified as one of the values of the body parts for various body systems. For example, a lumpectomy to treat carcinoma of the breast is coded with the root operation Excision. But if a total mastectomy, the complete removal of the breast, was performed, the root operation Resection would be used. This example can be applied to many organs that are removed in part or in total to treat a malignancy. However, the coder must apply the ICD-10-PCS definitions to the procedures described by physicians and not assume the physician's terminology is consistent with the PCS definitions. For example, the physician may identify the procedure performed as a transurethral resection of prostate or TURP. In the operative report, the coder notes the physician removed the posterior lobe of the prostate. In this example, the root operation of Resection would not be applied. Table 0VT for Resection within male reproductive system includes the body part "prostate" but does not include individual body parts for lobes of the prostate. Therefore, when only the posterior lobe of the prostate is removed, it does not qualify as a Resection as the entire prostate is not removed. The correct root operation would be Excision when a part or a lobe of the prostate is removed, with a code selected from the ICD-10-PCS table 0VB (see table 5.3). When the physician identifies the procedure as a retropubic prostatectomy or perineal prostatectomy, the operative report will describe the removal of the entire prostate. This procedure meets the definition of Resection in ICD-10-PCS and should be coded using the ICD-10-PCS table of 0VT (see table 5.4).

Table 5.3. ICD-10-PCS Table 0VB

Section	0	Medical and Surgical
Body System	V	Male Reproductive System
Operation	B	Excision: Cutting out or off, without replacement, a portion of a body part

Body Part	Approach	Device	Qualifier
0 Prostate	0 Open 3 Percutaneous 4 Percutaneous Endoscopic 7 Via Natural or Artificial Opening 8 Via Natural or Artificial Opening Endoscopic	Z No Device	X Diagnostic Z No Qualifier
1 Seminal Vesicle, Right 2 Seminal Vesicle, Left 3 Seminal Vesicles, Bilateral 6 Tunica Vaginalis, Right 7 Tunica Vaginalis, Left 9 Testis, Right B Testis, Left C Testes, Bilateral	0 Open 3 Percutaneous 4 Percutaneous Endoscopic	Z No Device	X Diagnostic Z No Qualifier
5 Scrotum S Penis T Prepuce	0 Open 3 Percutaneous 4 Percutaneous Endoscopic X External	Z No Device	X Diagnostic Z No Qualifier
F Spermatic Cord, Right G Spermatic Cord, Left H Spermatic Cords, Bilateral J Epididymis, Right K Epididymis, Left L Epididymis, Bilateral N Vas Deferens, Right P Vas Deferens, Left Q Vas Deferens, Bilateral	0 Open 3 Percutaneous 4 Percutaneous Endoscopic 8 Via Natural or Artificial Opening Endoscopic	Z No Device	X Diagnostic Z No Qualifier

Source: CMS 2019

Table 5.4.   **ICD-10-PCS Table 0VT**

Section	0	Medical and Surgical
Body System	V	Male Reproductive System
Operation	T	Resection: Cutting out or off, without replacement, all of a body part

Body Part	Approach	Device	Qualifier
0 Prostate	0 Open 4 Percutaneous Endoscopic 7 Via Natural or Artificial Opening 8 Via Natural or Artificial Opening Endoscopic	Z No Device	Z No Qualifier
1 Seminal Vesicle, Right 2 Seminal Vesicle, Left 3 Seminal Vesicles, Bilateral 6 Tunica Vaginalis, Right 7 Tunica Vaginalis, Left 9 Testis, Right B Testis, Left C Testes, Bilateral F Spermatic Cord, Right G Spermatic Cord, Left H Spermatic Cords, Bilateral J Epididymis, Right K Epididymis, Left L Epididymis, Bilateral N Vas Deferens, Right P Vas Deferens, Left Q Vas Deferens, Bilateral	0 Open 4 Percutaneous Endoscopic	Z No Device	Z No Qualifier
5 Scrotum S Penis T Prepuce	0 Open 4 Percutaneous Endoscopic X External	Z No Device	Z No Qualifier

Source: CMS 2019

Destruction Procedures Related to Neoplasms

The root operation Destruction is defined as the physical eradication of all or a portion of a body part by the direct use of energy, force, or a destructive agent. Destruction of a tumor or lesion may be performed using heat, cold, laser, or chemicals. There is usually no tissue to submit to pathology for examination after a destruction procedure as there is no tissue remaining from the site. Certain less invasive skin cancers are treated with cryotherapy or cryosurgery where lesions are destroyed by freezing the area with liquid nitrogen to destroy the cancer cells. Cryosurgery does not involve cutting, and the treated lesion becomes scabbed over and falls off the skin in a short period of time. Cryosurgery is a method of treatment that meets the definition of destruction.

Antineoplastic Chemotherapy

Antineoplastic chemotherapy is an infusion procedure coded with a procedure from the Administration section of ICD-10-PCS. The root operation Introduction is used to code chemotherapy. The main term is "Introduction of substance in or on." The subterm identifies where the infusion is introduced, which would be either a central vein or a peripheral vein. The approach is usually Percutaneous as the needle is introduced in the vein through the skin. The sixth character is the substance infused with value 0 for antineoplastic. Depending on the chemical infused, there may be an appropriate qualifier assigned as the seventh character for other antineoplastic or monoclonal antibody. When performed on a hospitalized inpatient, the coder would review the medication administration record or the chemotherapy infusion record to identify the substance infused and the location of introduction, that is, whether it was infused through a peripheral vein, a central line vein, or an implantable infusion port using a central vein.

ICD-10-CM and ICD-10-PCS Review Exercises: Chapter 5

Assign the correct ICD-10-CM diagnosis codes or ICD-10-PCS procedure codes for the following exercises.

1. Small cell carcinoma of the left lower lobe of the lung with metastasis to the intrathoracic lymph nodes, brain, and right rib

2. Benign carcinoid tumor of the jejunum

3. Subacute monocytic leukemia in remission

4. Malignant melanoma of the left shoulder area

5. The patient is seen in the pain clinic for chronic neoplasm-related pain that was known to be caused by the metastatic bone carcinoma of the vertebra that has spread from the left main bronchus of the lung.

6. The patient was diagnosed with carcinoma of the descending colon five years ago with surgical excision of the descending colon. The patient had completed chemotherapy for the primary malignancy and had no cancer treatment over the past three years. The patient's colostomy is functioning well. During a follow-up examination recently, a CT scan of the liver showed a suspicious lesion that was later biopsied and found to be a secondary malignant neoplasm that originated in the colon. The patient visited the oncologist today in Oncology Clinic to review possible treatment options.

7. The reason for the encounter is to receive chemotherapy following the recent diagnosis of malignant neoplasm of the upper lobe of the left lung. A partial lobectomy was performed two months ago, and the patient has been receiving chemotherapy.

8. The reason for the encounter is to receive radiation therapy following the recent diagnosis of carcinoma of the prostate to shrink the tumor prior to planned surgery to explore the tumor site in the next month.

ICD-10-CM and ICD-10-PCS Review Exercises: Chapter 5 (continued)

9. The patient was treated for carcinoma of the right kidney five years ago and was treated with chemotherapy and radiation therapy at that time. During this visit, the patient is being evaluated for the metastatic carcinoma of the right lung that was diagnosed recently. He will begin receiving radiation therapy again in the near future.

_____

10. The patient was diagnosed with an advanced malignant carcinoid tumor of the ascending colon with carcinoid syndrome. Medications are being prescribed to relieve the carcinoid syndrome symptoms.

_____

11. PROCEDURE: Transurethral endoscopic laser ablation of the prostate due to BPH

_____

12. PROCEDURE: Right breast lumpectomy with open sentinel lymph node biopsy, right axilla

_____

13. PROCEDURE: Open resection and removal of the right lobe of the liver due to metastasis from colon carcinoma

_____

14. PROCEDURE: Tube thoracostomy—chest tube insertion by incision—for drainage of malignant pleural effusion from right pleural cavity

_____

15. PROCEDURE: Rigid bronchoscopy with YAG laser photoresection for the destruction of tumor in the right main bronchus

_____

References

Centers for Disease Control and Prevention (CDC), National Center for Health Statistics (NCHS). 2019. *ICD-10-CM Official Guidelines for Coding and Reporting*, 2020. https://www.cdc.gov/nchs/data/icd/10cmguidelines_fy2020_final.pdf.

Centers for Medicare and Medicaid Services (CMS). 2019. 2020 ICD-10. https://www.cms.gov/medicare/Coding/ICD10/index.html.

Mosby. 2017. *Mosby's Pocket Dictionary of Medicine, Nursing, and Health Professions*, 8th ed. St. Louis: Mosby, Inc.

National Cancer Institute (NCI). 2019a. NCI Visuals Online. https://visualsonline.cancer.gov/.

National Cancer Institute (NCI). 2019b. SEER Training Modules: Regionalized. http://training.seer.cancer.gov/staging/systems/summary/regionalized.html.

National Cancer Institute (NCI). 2018. Metastatic Cancer. http://www.cancer.gov/types/metastatic-cancer.

U.S. National Library of Medicine, MedLinePlus (NLM). 2019. Cancer. https://www.nlm.nih.gov/medlineplus/cancer.html.

Chapter 6

Diseases of the Blood and Blood-Forming Organs and Certain Disorders Involving the Immune Mechanism (D50–D89)

Learning Objectives

At the conclusion of this chapter, you should be able to do the following:

- Describe the organization of the conditions and codes included in Chapter 3 of ICD-10-CM, Diseases of the Blood and Blood-forming Organs and Certain Disorders Involving the Immune Mechanism (D50–D89)

- Identify the causes of the specific types of anemia—deficiency, hemolytic, and aplastic

- Give specific examples of coagulation defects and briefly describe their treatments

- Describe primary and secondary thrombocytopenia and briefly describe their treatments

- Identify diseases of the white blood cells and give examples of these conditions

- Assign ICD-10-CM codes for conditions categorized in ICD-10-CM Chapter 3

- Assign ICD-10-PCS codes for procedures related to diseases of the blood and blood-forming organs

Key Terms

Acute posthemorrhagic anemia
Acquired hemolytic anemia
Anemia
Aplastic anemia
Aspiration
Bandemia
Biopsy
Coagulation defects
Hemolytic anemia

Heparin-induced thrombocytopenia
Hereditary hemolytic anemia
Neutropenia
Pernicious anemia
Sickle cell disorder
Thalassemia
Thrombocytopenia
Transplantation
von Willebrand's disease (vWD)

Overview of ICD-10-CM Chapter 3: Diseases of the Blood and Blood-Forming Organs and Certain Disorders Involving the Immune Mechanism (D50–D89)

Chapter 3 includes categories D50–D89 arranged in the following blocks:

D50–D53	Nutritional anemias
D55–D59	Hemolytic anemias
D60–D64	Aplastic and other anemias and other bone marrow failure syndromes
D65–D69	Coagulation defects, purpura and other hemorrhagic conditions
D70–D77	Other disorders of blood and blood-forming organs
D78	Intraoperative and postprocedural complications of the spleen
D80–D89	Certain disorders involving the immune mechanism

Diseases and disorders are grouped into subchapters or blocks making it easy to identify the type of conditions classified to ICD-10-CM Chapter 3. In Chapter 3, there is an increased level of specificity in the codes. This is intended to better identify specific disease types. The terminology used in the chapter is consistent with current clinical terminology.

Coding Guidelines and Instructional Notes for ICD-10-CM Chapter 3

At the time of this publication, there are no ICD-10-CM official coding guidelines for Chapter 3: Diseases of the Blood and Blood-Forming Organs and Certain Disorders involving the immune mechanism. An Excludes2 note is located under the Chapter 3 heading and includes several ICD-10-CM chapter codes. It is important for the coder to review this list.

Instructional Notes

 In ICD-10-CM Chapter 3, there are several codes with a note that states to "Use additional code for adverse effects, if applicable, to identify drug (T36–T50 with fifth or sixth character 5)."

EXAMPLES: D52.1, Drug-induced folate deficiency anemia
Use additional code for adverse effect, if applicable, to identify drug (T36–T50 with fifth or sixth character 5)

D59.0, Drug-induced autoimmune hemolytic anemia
Use additional code for adverse effect, if applicable, to identify drug (T36–T50 with fifth or sixth character 5)

D61.1, Drug-induced aplastic anemia
Use additional code for adverse effect, if applicable, to identify drug (T36–T50 with fifth or sixth character 5)

Another instructional note found in this chapter is "Code first, if applicable, toxic effects of substances chiefly nonmedicinal as to source (T51–T65)."

EXAMPLE: D61.2, Aplastic anemia due to other external agents
Code first, if applicable, toxic effects of substances chiefly nonmedicinal as to source (T51–T65)

Similarly, two instructional notes appear with the type of anemia as produced by either a poisoning or an adverse effect of a drug. The following type of anemia is produced by either a poisoning or an adverse effect of a drug.

EXAMPLE: D64.2, Secondary sideroblastic anemia due to drugs and toxins
Code first poisoning due to drug or toxin, if applicable (T36–T65 with fifth or sixth character 1–4, or 6)

Use additional code for adverse effect, if applicable, to identify drug (T36–T50 with fifth or sixth character 5)

Other instructional notes apply to the entire category of codes or an individual code to use additional codes for associated conditions.

EXAMPLES: D56.0, Alpha thalassemia
Use additional code, if applicable, for hydrops fetalis due to alpha thalassemia (P56.99)

D57, Sickle cell disorders
Use additional code for any associated fever (R50.81)

D59.3, Hemolytic-uremic syndromes
Use additional code to identify associated:
    E. coli infection (B96.2-)
    Pneumococcal pneumonia (J13)
    Shigella dysenteriae (A03.9)

D70, Neutropenia
Use additional code for any associated:
    Fever (R50.81)
    Mucositis (J34.81, K12.3-, K92.81, N76.81)

Instructions to "Code first" or "Code also" the underlying disease are also included in Chapter 3.

EXAMPLES: D61.82, Myelophthisis
Code also the underlying disorder, such as:
    Malignant neoplasm of breast (C50.-)
    Tuberculosis (A15.-)

D63.0, Anemia in neoplastic disease
Code first neoplasm (C00–D49)
D63.1, Anemia in chronic kidney disease
Code first underlying chronic kidney disease (CKD) (N18.-)

Another instruction recognizes external causes can produce a blood disorder.

EXAMPLE: D59.6, Hemoglobinuria due to hemolysis from other external causes
Use additional code (Chapter 20) to identify external cause

Certain blood disorders and disorders involving the immune mechanism are related to underlying diseases as well as influences of drugs and toxins. In addition, a blood disorder can produce other conditions or manifestations.

EXAMPLES: D70.1, Agranulocytosis secondary to cancer chemotherapy
Code also underlying neoplasm
Use additional code for adverse effect, if applicable, to identify drug (T45.1X5)

D89.81, Graft-versus-host disease
Code first underlying cause, such as:
    Complications of transplanted organs and tissue (T86.-)
    Complications of blood transfusion (T80.89)

Use additional codes to identify associated manifestations, such as:
    Desquamative dermatitis (L30.8)
    Diarrhea (R19.7)
    Elevated bilirubin (R17)
    Hair loss (L65.9)

Certain blood disorders in Chapter 3 of ICD-10-CM have at least three instructional notes, such as the following example.

EXAMPLE: D75.81, Myelofibrosis
Code first the underlying disorder, such as:
    Malignant neoplasm of breast (C50.-)
Use additional code, if applicable, for associated therapy-related myelodysplastic syndrome (D46.-)
Use additional code for adverse effect, if applicable, to identify drug (T45.1X5)

Coding Guidelines

There are no separate chapter-specific coding guidelines for Chapter 3 of ICD-10-CM. However, there are coding guidelines found in ICD-10-CM for Chapter 2 that apply to conditions coded in Chapter 3. Coding guideline, I.C.2.c.1, Neoplasms for anemia associated with malignancy states: "When the admission or encounter is for management of an anemia associated with the malignancy, and the treatment is only for anemia, the appropriate code for the *malignancy* is sequenced as the principal or first listed diagnosis followed by the appropriate code for the anemia (such as code D63.0, Anemia in neoplastic disease")) (CMS 2019).

There are directions provided in the guidelines for anemia associated with chemotherapy, immunotherapy, and radiation therapy. For example, when the patient is seen for management of anemia associated with an adverse effect of the administration of chemotherapy or immunotherapy and the only treatment is for the anemia, the following should be coded:

1.   The type of anemia treated and sequenced first

2.   The neoplasm being treated with chemo- or immunotherapy

3.   The adverse effect (T45.1X5) of antineoplastic and immunosuppressive drugs

Another example is when the patient is seen for management of anemia associated with an adverse effect of radiation, the following should be coded:

1. The type of anemia treated and sequenced first

2. The neoplasm being treated with radiation therapy

3. Y84.2, Radiological procedure and radiotherapy as the cause of abnormal reaction of the patient, or of later complication, without mention of misadventure at the time of the procedure

Coding Diseases of the Blood and Blood-Forming Organs and Certain Disorders Involving the Immune Mechanism in ICD-10-CM Chapter 3

As the reader begins to study the coding of blood disorders, it is important to understand the composition of blood. Blood contains three main types of cells: white blood cells, red blood cells, and platelets. White blood cells are also called monocytes, lymphocytes, neutrophils, eosinophils, basophils, and macrophages. Red blood cells are called erythrocytes. The third type are platelets. Figure 6.1 shows the different types of white blood cells, red blood cell, and platelets (NCI 2019).

Figure 6.1. **Blood cells**

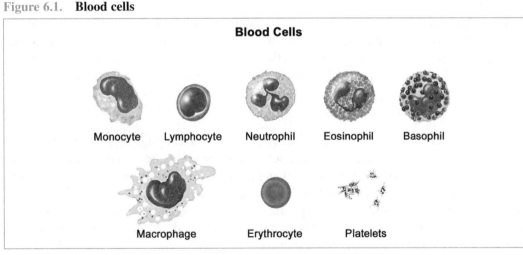

© 2007 Terese Winslow, U.S. Govt. has certain rights

Diseases of the blood include anemias, coagulation defects, purpura, and other hemorrhagic disorders as well as a variety of other disorders of blood-forming organs.

Anemias

Anemia is defined as a decrease in the number of erythrocytes (red blood cells), the quantity of hemoglobin, or the volume of packed red cells in the blood (Mosby 2017, 74).

Laboratory data reflect a decrease in red blood cells (RBCs), hemoglobin (Hgb), or hematocrit (Hct). Anemia is manifested by pallor of skin and mucous membranes, shortness of breath, palpitations of the heart, soft systolic murmurs, lethargy, and fatigability.

Nutritional Anemias (D50–D53)

Categories D50–D53 include codes for nutritional anemias. The most common type of anemia, iron deficiency anemia (category D50), is caused by an inadequate absorption of or excessive loss of iron. Iron deficiency anemia due to (chronic) blood loss is reported with code D50.0. The underlying cause of the bleeding should be coded when documented in the health record. Without further specification, iron deficiency anemia is reported with code D50.9. Other forms of nutritional anemias are vitamin B12 anemias caused by various factors and folate deficiency anemias related to dietary intake or drug-induced folate deficiencies. Another common nutritional anemia is due to protein deficiencies in people's diets.

Vitamin B12 Deficiency Anemia (D51)

Specific codes exist for vitamin B12 deficiencies due to intrinsic factor deficiency, B12 malabsorption, transcobalamin II, and other dietary vitamin B12 deficiency anemia, also known as vegan anemia.

Vitamin B12 and folate are important elements to enable the body to produce RBCs. The body's building blocks for its genetic code, DNA, also uses vitamin B12 in its production. The body stores vitamin B12 in the liver from various food sources, including seafood, meat, poultry, eggs, and dairy products. When the body does not have enough vitamin B12, a vitamin B12 deficiency anemia is produced and usually treated with replacement vitamin B12 orally or by injection.

Pernicious anemia is a form of vitamin B12 deficiency because of the body's inability to absorb vitamin B12 and make a sufficient number of RBCs. Other conditions can also produce pernicious anemia, for example, problems in the small intestine that prevent absorption of vitamin B12 from food. In addition, a vitamin B12 deficiency may occur with a folate deficiency.

Folate Deficiency Anemia (D52)

Specific codes exist for dietary folate deficiency and for drug-induced folate deficiency anemia as well as an unspecified folic acid deficiency anemia. Folic acid or folate aids in the production of RBCs. People get folate from eating green leafy vegetables, but the body does not store folate, so a consistent diet of these nutrients is essential in maintaining folate levels. Other causes of folate deficiency are long-term alcoholism and certain medications. However, the leading cause is a poor diet, especially in the elderly and people who do not eat fresh fruits and vegetables. Folic acid is also essential in pregnant women as it helps the fetus grow properly. Too little folic acid is suspected of causing birth defects in babies (NLM 2019a). A use additional code note appears under code D52.1, Drug-induced folate deficiency anemia, to use additional code for adverse effect, if applicable, to identify the drug (T36–T50 with fifth or sixth character 5).

Other Nutritional Anemia (D53)

Specific codes exist for protein deficiency anemia (D53.0), megaloblastic anemia NOS (D53.1), and simple chronic anemia, which is considered an unspecified form of nutritional anemia in ICD-10-CM (D53.9).

Hemolytic Anemias (D55–D59)

Hemolytic anemias are blood disorders that occur when RBCs are destroyed in a process called hemolysis. Hemolysis occurs before the normal time period in which the body normally destroys them, usually about 120 days after an RBC is created. The bone marrow that produces RBCs cannot keep up with the rapid destruction, even though it will try to speed up RBC production. With hemolysis, the body has a lower number of normal levels of RBCs. **Hemolytic anemia** is a condition in which the bone marrow cannot make enough new RBCs to replace the RBCs that are destroyed too early, before the RBCs can be replaced. There are many types and causes of hemolytic anemia. Hemolytic anemia can be acquired or inherited, but the cause may not be known (NHLBI 2019a).

In **acquired hemolytic anemia**, the body senses that something is wrong with the RBCs even though they are normal. For example, antibodies or proteins made by the immune system may signal to the body's immune system that the RBCs do not belong. In response, the body destroys the RBCs before their usual life span is up. The destruction of RBCs commonly occurs in the spleen but can also occur in the bloodstream. Causes of acquired hemolytic anemia include

- Autoimmune responses

- Physical damage to RBCs from certain conditions and factors

- Exposure to certain infectious organisms and toxins

- Reactions to certain medicines

Hereditary hemolytic anemia is related to problems with the genes that control how the RBCs are made in the body. This causes defects in the outer membranes of the RBCs, enzyme deficiencies inside RBCs, or hemoglobin disorders. The abnormal RBCs are fragile and may break down as they move through the bloodstream. If this happens, the spleen may remove the faulty RBCs from the blood. Types of hereditary hemolytic anemias include

- Glucose-6 phosphate dehydrogenase (G6PD) deficiency

- Pyruvate kinase deficiency

- Thalassemia

- Sickle cell

- Hereditary spherocytosis

- Hereditary elliptocytosis

ICD-10-CM classifies hereditary hemolytic anemias to the following categories or codes.

Glucose-6-Phosphate Dehydrogenase (G6PD) Deficiency (D55.0)

In Glucose-6-Phosphate Dehydrogenase (G6PD) Deficiency, the RBCs are missing an enzyme called G6PD. These enzymes are proteins that drive chemical reactions in the body. The missing enzyme makes the RBCs fragile and more likely to break down. If the RBCs come in contact with certain substances in the bloodstream, they rupture and die. Many factors, including those in certain medicines, foods (like fava beans), and infections, can trigger the breakdown of the RBCs. G6PD deficiency mostly affects men of African or Mediterranean descent. Some states require G6PD deficiency screening for newborns (NHLBI 2019a). Glucose-6-phosphate dehydrogenase (G6PD) without anemia is coded to D75.A.

Anemia Due to Disorders of Glycolytic Enzymes (Hemolytic Nonspherocytic Anemia, Hexokinase Deficiency Anemia, Pyruvate Kinase Deficiency Anemia, Triose-phosphate Isomerase Deficiency Anemia) (D55.2)

In Pyruvate Kinase (PK) Deficiency Anemia, the RBCs are missing an enzyme called pyruvate kinase. Not having enough of the PK enzyme causes RBCs to break down easily. Pyruvate kinase deficiency is more common among the Amish (NHLBI 2019a).

Thalassemia (D56)

Specific forms of thalassemia such as alpha, beta, delta-beta, as well as thalassemia minor and other thalassemias have individual codes. **Thalassemias** are inherited blood disorders, meaning that the disorder is passed from parents to children through genes. Thalassemias cause the body to make fewer healthy RBCs and less hemoglobin than normal, which can cause anemia. Hemoglobin is an iron-rich protein in RBCs. It carries oxygen to all parts of the body. Hemoglobin also carries carbon dioxide from the body to the lungs, where it is exhaled. People who have thalassemias can have mild or severe anemia. Thalassemias often affect people of Southeast Asian, Indian, Chinese, Filipino, Mediterranean, or African descent. The treatment for thalassemias are blood transfusions to replace destroyed RBCs, and blood and marrow stem cell transplants (NHLBI 2019a).

Sickle Cell Disorders (D57)

Different forms of sickle cell disorders are included in category D57. For example, specific codes exist for Hb-SS disease with crisis, including acute chest syndrome and splenic sequestration, each in a single code. Codes for other forms of sickle cell disorders including Hb-C, sickle-cell trait, sickle-cell thalassemia, Hb-SD, and Hb-SE disease are included in this category. In **sickle cell disorder**, the body makes abnormal hemoglobin that causes RBCs to have a sickle, or "C," shape. These sickle cells are sticky and do not travel easily through the blood vessels. Sickle cells live only about 10 to 20 days, and the bone marrow cannot make new RBCs fast enough to replace the dying ones. In the United States, sickle cell anemia mainly affects people of African descent (NHLBI 2019a). Some states require sickle cell anemia screening for newborn babies. The treatments for sickle cell anemia include folic acid supplements made from the synthetic form of folate, antibiotics to prevent infection, medicine to reduce the number of faulty RBCs in the blood, and a medicine called hydroxyurea, which may help the body make more healthy hemoglobin and reduce the amount of faulty hemoglobin that leads to sickle cells.

Other Hereditary Hemolytic Anemias (D58)

Other hereditary hemolytic anemias that are classified to category D58 include some less common hemolytic anemias such as spherocytosis, elliptocytosis, and other hemoglobinemias, including Hb-C disease and Hb-D disease.

Hereditary Spherocytosis (D58.0)

Hereditary spherocytosis is caused by a defect in the RBCs' outer membranes that causes them to have a spherical or ball-like shape. The ball-shaped RBCs have a shorter than normal life span. Hereditary spherocytosis is the most common cause of hemolytic anemia among people of Northern European descent (NHLBI 2019a).

Hereditary Elliptocytosis (D58.1)

Hereditary elliptocytosis is caused by a defect in the RBCs' outer membranes that makes them oval shaped and less flexible than normal. The RBCs have a shorter than normal life span. Disorders of the RBC outer membrane, both hereditary spherocytosis and hereditary elliptocytosis, are treated with folic acid supplements, blood transfusions, and, rarely, removal of the spleen (NHLBI 2019a).

Acquired Hemolytic Anemia (D59)

Typically, **acquired hemolytic anemias** are caused by extrinsic factors such as drugs or toxins, systemic diseases, liver or renal disease, or abnormal immune responses. Treatments for acquired hemolytic anemia are dependent on the type of anemia. Examples of some treatments are as follows:

- Corticosteroids and other medicines to suppress the immune system

- Intravenous gammaglobulin, a medication that can increase the life span of RBCs and possibly reduce the amount of antibodies produced

- Iron and folic acid supplements

- Eculizumab, an antibody that blocks the destruction of RBCs in this form of anemia

- Plasmapheresis, or a procedure to remove antibodies from the blood

- Blood transfusion

- Removal of the spleen

- Avoidance of cold temperatures

ICD-10-CM classifies acquired hemolytic anemia to category D59, with the fourth character describing the specific type or cause of disorder; for example:

D59.0, Drug-induced autoimmune hemolytic anemia with the instructional note "use additional code for adverse effect, if applicable, to identify drug (T36–T50 with fifth or sixth character 5)"

D59.1, Other autoimmune hemolytic anemia, which may be described as cold agglutinin disease or cold or warm type hemolytic anemia

D59.3, Hemolytic–uremic syndrome with the instructional note "use additional code to identify associated *E. coli* infection, pneumococcal pneumonia, or *Shigella dysenteriae*" (NHLBI 2019a)

Aplastic and Other Anemias and Other Bone Marrow Failure Syndromes (D60–D64)

Aplastic anemia is a condition in which the bone marrow is damaged. As a result, the stem cells are destroyed or develop abnormally. In this situation, the body cannot make enough RBCs, WBCs, or platelets. This type of anemia is rare, but it can be fatal. Aplastic anemia can be acquired or inherited. Many times, the cause of the aplastic anemia or the condition that triggers it is unknown. There are known causes of acquired aplastic anemia that include the following:

- High-dose radiation or chemotherapy: These cancer treatments kill cancer cells, but they also may damage other cells, such as stem cells. When stem cells are damaged, healthy RBCs, WBCs, and platelets cannot develop. Aplastic anemia may resolve after these cancer treatments are stopped.

- Environmental toxins: Substances such as pesticides, arsenic, and benzene can damage bone marrow, causing aplastic anemia.

- Certain medicines: Certain medications used to treat rheumatoid arthritis and some antibiotics, such as chloramphenicol (which is rarely used in the United States), can damage the bone marrow and cause aplastic anemia.

- Viral infections: Hepatitis, Epstein-Barr virus, parvovirus B-19, human immunodeficiency virus (HIV), mononucleosis, and cytomegalovirus can damage the bone marrow and lead to aplastic anemia.

- Autoimmune diseases: These diseases, such as lupus and rheumatoid arthritis, may cause the immune system to attack its own cells. This can damage bone marrow cells and prevent them from making healthy new blood cells.

- Other hereditary conditions can damage your stem cells, leading to aplastic anemia. These conditions include Fanconi anemia, Shwachman-Diamond syndrome, dyskeratosis congenita, Diamond-Blackfan anemia, and a megakaryocytic thrombocytopenia. Some women may develop mild aplastic anemia during pregnancy. This anemia tends to go away after childbirth.

- In some cases, aplastic anemia is associated with another blood disorder called paroxysmal nocturnal hemoglobinuria (PNH). A genetic mutation causes PNH. The disorder develops when abnormal stem cells in the bone marrow make blood cells with a faulty outer membrane (outside layer). This destroys RBCs and prevents the body from making enough WBCs and platelets. Aplastic anemia may only last a short time if it is due to a short-term condition, illness, or other factor. However, aplastic anemia can be a long-term condition if its cause is unknown or if an inherited condition, long-term illness, or other factor causes it (NHLBI 2019b).

ICD-10-CM classifies aplastic anemias to categories D60–D64, with the fourth, fifth, and sixth characters indicating the specific type as shown in the following categories.

Other Aplastic Anemias and Other Bone Marrow Failure Syndromes (D61)

Within category D61 are codes for constitutional anemias such as Blackfan-Diamond syndrome (D61.01), Fanconi's anemia (D61.09), drug-induced aplastic anemia (D61.1), aplastic anemia due to other external agents (D61.2), and idiopathic aplastic anemia (D61.3). The codes for pancytopenia are included in category D61. Specific codes exist for antineoplastic chemotherapy-induced pancytopenia (D61.810) and other drug-induced pancytopenia.

Acute Posthemorrhagic Anemia (D62)

Acute posthemorrhagic anemia or anemia due to acute blood loss is reported with code D62. Acute posthemorrhagic anemia is a normocytic, normochromic anemia developing as a result of rapid loss of large quantities of RBCs during bleeding (Encyclopedia Britannica 2019). It may occur as a result of a massive hemorrhage that may be due to spontaneous or traumatic rupture of a large blood vessel, rupture of an aneurysm, arterial erosion from a peptic ulcer or neoplastic process, or complications of surgery from excessive blood loss. Coders should not assume that anemia following a procedure, or postoperative anemia, is acute blood loss anemia. Coding postoperative anemia as a diagnosis needs more information than this phrase. Postoperative anemia must be specified as due to (acute) blood loss (D62) or due to chronic blood loss (D50.). If the physician specifies the postoperative anemia further, it is assigned to D64.9, anemia, unspecified.

Anemia in Chronic Diseases Classified Elsewhere (D63)

Conditions classified to code D63 develop in patients with chronic diseases.

> **EXAMPLE:** Anemia in neoplastic disease (D63.0)
> This code includes an instructional note to "code first neoplasm (C00–D49)."
>
> Anemia in chronic kidney disease (CKD) (D63.1)
> This condition is also known as erythropoietin-resistant anemia (EPO-resistant anemia). The code includes an instructional note to "code first underlying chronic kidney disease (CKD) (N18.-)."
>
> Anemia in other chronic disease classified elsewhere (D63.8)
> The "code first underlying disease, such as:" instruction note is included here. Examples of the underlying diseases that may be coded here are hypothyroidism, malaria, symptomatic late syphilis, and tuberculosis.

Check Your Understanding 6.1

Assign diagnosis codes to the following conditions.

1. Sickle cell disease with crisis and acute chest syndrome

2. Hereditary megaloblastic anemia

3. Orotaciduric anemia

4. Pyruvate kinase (PK) deficiency anemia

5. Acute chest syndrome in sickle-cell thalassemia

6. Chronic acquired pure red cell aplasia

7. Sideroblastic anemia due to rheumatoid arthritis

8. Nutritional megaloblastic anemia

9. Antineoplastic chemotherapy-induced pancytopenia

10. Beta thalassemia minor

Coagulation Defects, Purpura, and Other Hemorrhagic Conditions (D65–D69)

Coagulation defects are disorders of the platelets that result in serious bleeding due to a deficiency of one or more clotting factors. ICD-10-CM classifies coagulation defects to categories D65–D68 (NLM 2019b).

Coagulation defects include

- Disseminated intravascular coagulation [defibrination syndrome], D65

- Hereditary factor VIII deficiency, D66

  - This category includes classical hemophilia or hemophilia A.

- Hereditary factor IX deficiency, D67

  - Factor IX deficiency disorder includes Christmas disease or hemophilia B.

- Other coagulation defects, D68

Subcategory D68.0 classifies **von Willebrand's disease (vWD)**. This is a bleeding disorder that affects the blood's ability to clot. If the blood does not clot, the person will have heavy, difficult to control hemorrhage after an injury. The bleeding can damage the internal organs and can be life threatening. In vWD, there is either one of two low levels of a certain protein in the blood, or the protein itself does not function well. The protein is called von Willebrand's factor, and it helps to make the blood clot. Small blood cell fragments called platelets clump together to plug the hole in the blood vessel and stop the bleeding. von Willebrand's factor acts like glue to help the platelets stick together and form a blood clot. von Willebrand's factor also carries clotting factor VIII (8), another important protein that helps the blood clot. Factor VIII is the protein that is missing or nonfunctioning in people who have hemophilia, another bleeding disorder. vWD is more common and usually milder than hemophilia. In fact, vWD is the most common inherited bleeding disorder. vWD affects both males and females, while hemophilia mainly affects males (NLM 2019c).

Category D69 includes codes that describe purpura, thrombocytopenia, and other hemorrhagic disorders. **Thrombocytopenia** is diagnosed when the platelets fall below 100,000/mm. Two types of thrombocytopenia are recognized: primary, or idiopathic, and secondary. Idiopathic, or immune thrombocytopenic purpura (ITP), is an autoimmune disorder with development of antibodies to one's own platelets. In children, the condition often resolves without treatment. In adults, medications such as corticosteroids or thrombopoietins are given. In severe cases, the spleen may be removed to eliminate the platelet destruction by phagocytosis. Primary thrombocytopenia may also be congenital or hereditary. Primary thrombocytopenia is classified in ICD-10-CM to D69.4- subcategory depending on the type.

Secondary thrombocytopenia is a complication of another disease. The treatment of the secondary form of this condition centers on treating the underlying disease or changing medication. ICD-10-CM classifies secondary thrombocytopenia to code D69.59. Post-transfusion purpura (PTP) is coded to D69.51. This condition is characterized by a sudden and severe thrombocytopenia (a platelet count of less than 10,000), usually occurring 5 to 10 days following transfusions of whole blood, plasma, platelets, or red blood cells. PTP is a reaction associated with the presence of antibodies directed against the Human Platelet Antigen (HPA) system.

Assign diagnosis codes to the following conditions.

1. Owren's disease
2. Primary hypercoagulable state
3. Post-transfusion purpura
4. Splenic torsion
5. Christmas disease, factor IX deficiency

Other Disorders of Blood and Blood-Forming Organs

ICD-10-CM classifies neutropenia to category D70 with fourth-character codes for the various specific forms of neutropenia. **Neutropenia** is a decrease in the number of neutrophils, a type of white blood cell. Codes in the range of D70.0–D70.9 describe congenital agranulocytosis, agranulocytosis secondary to cancer chemotherapy, other drug-induced agranulocytosis, neutropenia due to infection, and cyclic neutropenia as well as other and unspecified forms of neutropenia.

Bandemia is defined as the presence of an excess number of immature WBCs or band cells, while the total WBC count is normal (Taber's Cyclopedic Medical Dictionary 2018). Bandemia is frequently present in patients with bacterial infections. However, bandemia may be identified when a diagnosis of infection has not been established. Pediatricians frequently use this diagnosis in children when the source of an infection is unknown. ICD-10-CM specifically identifies bandemia with code D72.825. Category D72, other disorders of white blood cells, also includes codes for eosinophilia and leukopenia.

Diseases of the spleen, a blood-forming organ, are included in category D73. Specific codes exist for hyposplenism, hypersplenism, chronic congestive splenomegaly, abscess, cyst, and infarction of spleen.

Methemoglobinemia, both congenital and acquired forms, are classified to codes within category D74. Other and unspecified diseases of blood and blood-forming organs are included in category D75. It includes myelofibrosis, a chronic progressive disease in which fibrous tissue replaces normal bone marrow. A progressive anemia results even though the spleen attempts to replace the lost blood production and splenomegaly can occur. Secondary polycythemia occurs as a result of tissue hypoxia and is associated with chronic obstructive pulmonary disease, congenital heart disease, and prolonged exposures to high altitudes (higher than 10,000 feet). ICD-10-CM classifies secondary polycythemia to code D75.1. Myelofibrosis can be a primary hematologic disease or a secondary process. Code D47.1, Chronic myeloproliferative disease, is the primary form of the disease. Code D75.81 is used to code the unspecified form or the secondary form of myelofibrosis.

Heparin-induced thrombocytopenia (HIT) is a life-threatening clinical event that can occur in 3 to 5 percent of all patients receiving unfractionated heparin for at least five days or in about 0.5 percent of patients receiving low molecular-weight heparin (NLM 2019d). HIT is a hypercoagulable state, not a hemorrhagic condition. The diagnosis is first suspected based on a fall in the platelet count by 50 percent or more occurring 5 to 12 days after beginning heparin therapy. Treatment involves the initiation of an alternative anticoagulant or direct thrombin inhibitor drugs. Code D75.82 is included in ICD-10-CM for HIT.

Intraoperative and Postprocedural Complications of the Spleen

Category D78, Intraoperative and postprocedural complications of the spleen, includes codes for intraoperative hemorrhage and hematoma of the spleen, accidental puncture and laceration of the spleen, and postprocedural hemorrhage and hematoma of the spleen. These combination codes identify the specific complication and whether the complication occurred during a procedure on the spleen or the complication occurred during another surgical procedure. Two codes, D78.81 and D78.89, are available to identify another specified type of complication of the spleen beyond the codes in the range of D78.01–D78.22. An additional code is used to further identify what the complication was.

Check Your Understanding 6.3

Assign diagnosis codes to the following conditions.

1. Congenital neutropenia with fever
2. Postoperative hematoma of spleen following surgery on liver
3. Post spleen procedure seroma (of spleen)
4. Eosinophilic leukopenia
5. Selective deficiency of immunoglobulin A (IgA disease)

ICD-10-PCS Coding for Procedures Related to Blood Disorders

The types of procedures that are most closely related to the treatment of blood disorders are administration of transfusions, aspiration, biopsy, and transplant.

Administration

Transfusion of blood and blood components is a treatment for various types of blood disorders. Transfusions are coded with ICD-10-PCS codes from the Administration section. There are seven characters to the administration codes:

Character 1: Section

Character 2: Physiological System and Anatomical Region

Character 3: Root Operation

Character 4: Body System/Region

Character 5: Approach

Character 6: Substance

Character 7: Qualifier

Administration codes represent procedures for putting in or on a therapeutic, prophylactic, protective, diagnostic, nutritional, or physiological substance. This section includes codes for transfusions, infusions, and injections as well as similar procedures such as irrigations.

Section

Character 1, which represents the section, uses the value 3 for Administration.

Body System

Character 2 for the body part contains only three values: Indwelling Device (value C), Physiological Systems and Anatomical Regions (value E), or Circulatory System (value 0).

Root Operation

Character 3 is for the root operation. There are only three root operations in the Administration section:

- Introduction (value 0): Putting in or on a therapeutic, diagnostic, nutritional, physiological, or prophylactic substance except blood or blood products

- Irrigation (value 1): Putting in or on a cleansing substance

- Transfusion (value 2): Putting in blood or blood products

Body/System Region

Character 4 specifies the body system/region. This character identifies the site where the substance is administered, not the site where the substance administered takes effect.

Sites include Skin and Mucous Membrane, Subcutaneous Tissue, and Muscle. Other sites include Eye, Respiratory Tract, Peritoneal Cavity, and Epidural Space. The body systems/regions for arteries and veins are Peripheral Artery, Central Artery, Peripheral Vein, and Central Vein.

Approach

Character 5 specifies the approach. The Percutaneous approach is for intradermal, subcutaneous, and intramuscular introductions or injections. Other approaches are Open, Via Natural or Artificial Opening, External, and Via Natural or Artificial Opening Endoscopic, as defined in the Medical and Surgical section.

Substance

Character 6 specifies the substance being administered or introduced. Broad categories of substances are defined, for example, anesthetic, antineoplastic, contrast, dialysate, and blood products.

Qualifier

Character 7 is the qualifier. A qualifier for autologous and nonautologous specifies the type of substance. Other qualifiers further specify a substance.

When accessing the Index to identify a code for a transfusion, the main term is Transfusion followed by subterms for artery, products of conception, and vein for further indentations. Under artery, the coder must know if it is a central or peripheral artery. Under the type of artery, the coder must identify the substance being administered, such as antihemophilic factors, blood, bone marrow, and such. The same factors are found under the subterm vein, that is, is it a central vein or a peripheral vein, where the administration is the site where the substance is to be administered. For transfusions, under both artery and vein, the type of blood products must be known: platelets, red cells, frozen red cells, white cells, or whole blood.

Aspiration, Biopsy, and Transplant

Biopsies are common procedures that are used to diagnose blood disorders and disorders of blood-forming organs. In the ICD-10-PCS Index, the entry for Biopsy states, "see Drainage with qualifier Diagnostic" and "see Excision with qualifier Diagnostic." A **biopsy** or another procedure may also be described as an aspiration biopsy or simply an aspiration. The Index entry for Aspiration tells the coder to see Drainage. **Aspiration**, or drainage, is defined as taking or letting out fluids or gases from a body part.

Two common sites for biopsies for these conditions in blood and blood-forming organs are bone marrow and lymph nodes. A bone marrow aspiration is found in the Index under the main term Drainage, bone marrow with a four-character code of 079T. An aspiration is taking out fluids from the bone marrow through a needle. The coder must identify the approach for this procedure as Open, Percutaneous, or Percutaneous Endoscopic. There is no choice for the device. The seventh character for an aspiration that is a diagnostic procedure would be value X.

When the coder accesses the Index for a bone marrow biopsy under the main term Excision, there is no entry for bone marrow. This is not a mistake. A bone marrow biopsy does not meet the definition of an Excision as there is no cutting out or off of a body part. A bone marrow "biopsy" is, by definition, an Extraction, meaning the bone marrow is pulled or stripped out or off all or a portion of a body part by the use of force. Under the main term Extraction, bone marrow, the coder must know the location of the extraction, that is, iliac, sternum, or vertebral. All three entries lead to the three-character code of 07D. The fourth character is value Q for Sternum, R for Iliac, or S for Vertebral. The approach is either Open or Percutaneous, which is the typical approach. There is no value for device except for Z for no device. The qualifier is either X for diagnostic or Z for no qualifier.

A bone marrow transplant is coded as a Transfusion in ICD-10-PCS because it meets the definition of the root operation of "putting in blood or blood products." **Transplantation** is defined as putting in or on all or a portion of a living body part taken from another individual or animal to physically take the place or function of all or a portion of a similar body part. A bone marrow transplant is a procedure to replace damaged or destroyed bone marrow with healthy bone marrow stem cells. Bone marrow is the soft, fatty tissue inside your bones. Stem cells are immature cells in the bone marrow that give rise to all of your blood cells. Stem cell transplants are also coded with the root operation Transfusion.

Coding of a lymph node biopsy is coded to the root operation Excision or Aspiration, depending on how the specimen is removed. Usually a lymph node biopsy is performed by cutting or excision. The main term Excision is located in the ICD-10-PCS Index. The body part needs to be identified as the location of the lymphatic structure, for example, Axillary, Inguinal, Neck, and such. The three-character code given is 07B. The approach options are Open, Percutaneous, or Percutaneous Endoscopic. There is no option for device other than Z for no device. A biopsy would have the qualifier of X for diagnostic.

Table 6.1.   **ICD-10-PCS Table 07D**

Section	0	Medical and Surgical
Body System	7	Lymphatic and Hemic Systems
Operation	D	Extraction: Pulling or stripping out or off all or a portion of a body part by the use of force

Body Part	Approach	Device	Qualifier
0 Lymphatic, Head 1 Lymphatic, Right Neck 2 Lymphatic, Left Neck 3 Lymphatic, Right Upper Extremity 4 Lymphatic, Left Upper Extremity 5 Lymphatic, Right Axillary 6 Lymphatic, Left Axillary 7 Lymphatic, Thorax 8 Lymphatic, Internal Mammary, Right 9 Lymphatic, Internal Mammary, Left B Lymphatic, Mesenteric C Lymphatic, Pelvis D Lymphatic, Aortic F Lymphatic, Right Lower Extremity G Lymphatic, Left Lower Extremity H Lymphatic, Right Inguinal J Lymphatic, Left Inguinal K Thoracic Duct L Cisterna Chyli	3 Percutaneous 4 Percutaneous Endoscopic 8 Via Natural or Artificial Opening Endoscopic	Z No Device	X Diagnostic
M Thymus P Spleen	3 Percutaneous 4 Percutaneous Endoscopic	Z No Device	X Diagnostic
Q Bone Marrow, Sternum R Bone Marrow, Iliac S Bone Marrow, Vertebral	0 Open 3 Percutaneous	Z No Device	X Diagnostic Z No Qualifier

Source: CMS 2019

ICD-10-CM and ICD-10-PCS Review Exercises: Chapter 6

Assign the correct ICD-10-CM diagnosis codes and ICD-10-PCS procedure codes for the following exercises.

1.   Chronic posthemorrhagic anemia

2.   von Willebrand's disease

3.   Chronic congestive splenomegaly

4.   Hereditary type II nonspherocytic hemolytic anemia

5.   Idiopathic thrombocytopenic purpura

(Continued on next page)

ICD-10-CM and ICD-10-PCS Review Exercises: Chapter 6 *(continued)*

6. Anemia due to malignant neoplasm of the pylorus

7. Disseminated intravascular coagulation

8. Idiopathic aplastic anemia

9. Hemoglobin H disease

10. Polycythemia secondary to living in high-altitude region

11. Glucose-6-phosphate dehydrogenase (G6PD) without anemia

12. Heparin-induced thrombocytopenia (HIT)

13. Sickle cell thalassemia with crisis

14. Anemia in end-stage renal disease (ESRD)

15. Severe combined immunodeficiency caused by adenosine deaminase.

16. PROCEDURE: Donor-fresh frozen plasma (FFP) transfusion through a central venous line

17. PROCEDURE: Therapeutic plasmapheresis, single session

18. PROCEDURE: Bone marrow needle extraction biopsy, iliac

19. PROCEDURE: Laparoscopic total splenectomy

20. PROCEDURE: Lymph node open biopsy by excision, right axilla

References

Centers for Medicare and Medicaid Services (CMS). 2019. *ICD-10-CM Official Guidelines for Coding and Reporting*, 2020. https://www.cms.gov/medicare/coding/icd10/index.html.

Encyclopedia Britannica. 2019. Blood disease: Normocytic normochromic anemias. https://www.britannica.com/science/blood-disease/Normocytic-normochromic-anemias.

Mosby. 2017. *Mosby's Pocket Dictionary of Medicine, Nursing, and Health Professions*, 8th ed. St. Louis: Mosby, Inc.

National Cancer Institute (NCI). 2019. NCI Visuals Online. https://visualsonline.cancer.gov/.

National Heart, Lung and Blood Institute (NHLBI). 2019a. What is Hemolytic Anemia? http://www.nhlbi.nih.gov/health/health-topics/topics/ha.

National Heart, Lung and Blood Institute (NHLBI). 2019b. What is Aplastic Anemia? http://www.nhlbi.nih.gov/health/health-topics/topics/aplastic.

Taber's Cyclopedic Medical Dictionary. 2018 Philadelphia: F. A. Davis & Company. https://www.tabers.com/tabersonline/view/Tabers-Dictionary/737751/0/bandemia?q=Bandemia.

U.S. National Library of Medicine, MedLinePlus (NLM). 2019a. Folate-Deficiency Anemia. https://medlineplus.gov/ency/article/000551.htm.

U.S. National Library of Medicine, MedLinePlus (NLM). 2019b. Bleeding Disorders. https://www.nlm.nih.gov/medlineplus/bleedingdisorders.html.

U.S. National Library of Medicine, MedLinePlus (NLM). 2019c. What Is von Willebrand's Disease. http://www.nhlbi.nih.gov/health/health-topics/topics/vwd.

U.S. National Library of Medicine, MedlLinePlus (NLM). 2019d. Thrombocytopenia.https://www.nhlbi.nih.gov/health-topics/thrombocytopenia

Chapter 7

Endocrine, Nutritional and Metabolic Diseases (E00–E89)

Learning Objectives

At the conclusion of this chapter, you should be able to do the following:

- Describe the organization of the conditions and codes included in Chapter 4 of ICD-10-CM, Endocrine, Nutritional and Metabolic Diseases (E00–E89)

- Describe the different types of diabetes and how the type of diabetes impacts code selection in ICD-10-CM

- Identify the codes included in Chapter 4 of ICD-10-CM that describe nutritional and metabolic disorders

- Assign ICD-10-CM diagnosis codes for endocrine, nutritional, and metabolic diseases

- Assign ICD-10-PCS procedure codes for procedures related to endocrine, nutritional, and metabolic diseases

Key Terms

Cystic fibrosis
Dehydration
Diabetes mellitus
Type 1 diabetes
Type 2 diabetes
Endocrine glands
Excision

Hypoglycemia
Hypovolemia
Kwashiorkor
Malnutrition
Marasmus
Resection
Stereotactic radiosurgery (SRS)

Overview of ICD-10-CM Chapter 4: Endocrine, Nutritional and Metabolic Diseases

Chapter 4 includes categories E00–E89 arranged in the following blocks:

E00–E07	Disorders of thyroid gland
E08–E13	Diabetes mellitus
E15–E16	Other disorders of glucose regulation and pancreatic internal secretion
E20–E35	Disorders of other endocrine glands
E36	Intraoperative complications of endocrine system
E40–E46	Malnutrition
E50–E64	Other nutritional deficiencies
E65–E68	Overweight, obesity and other hyperalimentation
E70–E88	Metabolic disorders
E89	Postprocedural endocrine and metabolic complications and disorders, not elsewhere classified

Diabetes mellitus and malnutrition have their own subchapter codes in this chapter. Additional codes can be found for other diseases of other endocrine glands and nutritional deficiencies.

All neoplasms, whether functionally active or not, are classified in Chapter 2 of ICD-10-CM (Neoplasms). Appropriate codes in Chapter 4 of ICD-10-CM (namely, E05.8-, E07.0, E16–E31, and E34.-) may be used as additional codes to indicate either functional activity by neoplasms and ectopic endocrine tissue or hyperfunction and hypofunction of endocrine glands associated with neoplasms and other conditions classified elsewhere.

Coding Guidelines and Instructional Notes for ICD-10-CM Chapter 4

The National Center for Health Statistics (NCHS) has published chapter-specific guidelines for Chapter 4 in the *ICD-10-CM Official Guidelines for Coding and Reporting*. The coding student should review all of the coding guidelines for Chapter 4 of ICD-10-CM, which appear in an ICD-10-CM code book or at the CDC website (CDC 2019) or in appendix F.

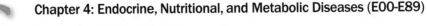

CG

Chapter 4: Endocrine, Nutritional, and Metabolic Diseases (E00-E89)

Guideline I.C.4.a. Diabetes mellitus

The diabetes mellitus codes are combination codes that include the type of diabetes mellitus, the body system affected, and the complications affecting that body system. As many codes within a particular category as are necessary to describe all of the complications of the disease may be used. They should be sequenced based on the reason for a particular encounter. Assign as many codes from categories E08–E13 as needed to identify all of the associated conditions that the patient has.

1. Type of diabetes

   The age of a patient is not the sole determining factor, though most type 1 diabetics develop the condition before reaching puberty. For this reason type 1 diabetes mellitus is also referred to as juvenile diabetes.

2. Type of diabetes mellitus not documented

   If the type of diabetes mellitus is not documented in the medical record the default is E11.-, Type 2 diabetes mellitus.

3. Diabetes mellitus and the use of insulin and oral hypoglycemics

   If the documentation in a medical record does not indicate the type of diabetes but does indicate that the patient uses insulin, code E11-, Type 2 diabetes mellitus, should be assigned. An additional code should be assigned from category Z79 to identify the long-term (current) use of insulin or oral hypoglycemic drugs. If the patient is treated with both oral medications and insulin, only the code for long-term (current) use of insulin should be assigned. Code Z79.4 should not be assigned if insulin is given temporarily to bring a type 2 patient's blood sugar under control during an encounter.

4. Diabetes mellitus in pregnancy and gestational diabetes

   See Section I.C.15. Diabetes mellitus in pregnancy. See Section I.C.15. Gestational (pregnancy induced) diabetes

5. Complications due to insulin pump malfunction

   a. Underdose of insulin due to insulin pump failure

      An underdose of insulin due to an insulin pump failure should be assigned to a code from subcategory T85.6, Mechanical complication of other specified internal and external prosthetic devices, implants and grafts, that specifies the type of pump malfunction, as the principal or first-listed code, followed by code T38.3x6-, Underdosing of insulin and oral hypoglycemic [antidiabetic] drugs. Additional codes for the type of diabetes mellitus and any associated complications due to the underdosing should also be assigned.

   b. Overdose of insulin due to insulin pump failure

      The principal or first-listed code for an encounter due to an insulin pump malfunction resulting in an overdose of insulin, should also be T85.6-, Mechanical complication of other specified internal

(Continued)

185

(Continued)

and external prosthetic devices, implants and grafts, followed by code T38.3x1-, Poisoning by insulin and oral hypoglycemic [antidiabetic] drugs, accidental (unintentional).

6. Secondary diabetes mellitus

    Codes under categories E08, Diabetes mellitus due to underlying condition, and E09, Drug or chemical induced diabetes mellitus, and E13, Other specified diabetes mellitus, identify complications/manifestations associated with secondary diabetes mellitus. Secondary diabetes is always caused by another condition or event (e.g., cystic fibrosis, malignant neoplasm of pancreas, pancreatectomy, adverse effect of drug, or poisoning).

    a. Secondary diabetes mellitus and the use of insulin or oral hypoglycemic drugs

        For patients with secondary diabetes mellitus who routinely use insulin or oral hypoglycemic drugs, an additional code from category Z79 should be assigned to identify long-term (current) use of insulin or oral hypoglycemic drugs. If the patient is treated with both oral medications and insulin, only the code for long-term (current) use of insulin should be assigned. Code Z79.4 should not be assigned if insulin is given temporarily to bring a type 2 secondary diabetic patient's blood sugar under control during an encounter.

    b. Assigning and sequencing secondary diabetes codes and its causes

        The sequencing of the secondary diabetes codes in relationship to codes for the cause of the diabetes is based on the Tabular List instructions for categories E08, E09, and E13.

        i. Secondary diabetes mellitus due to pancreatectomy

            For postpancreatectomy diabetes mellitus (lack of insulin due to the surgical removal of all or part of the pancreas), assign code E89.1, Postprocedural hypoinsulinemia. Assign a code from category E13 and a code from subcategory Z90.41, Acquired absence of pancreas, as additional codes.

        ii. Secondary diabetes due to drugs

            Secondary diabetes may be caused by an adverse effect of correctly administered medications, poisoning or sequela of poisoning. *See section I.C.19.e for coding of adverse effects and poisoning, and section I.C.20 for external cause code reporting.*

Coding Endocrine, Nutritional and Metabolic Diseases in ICD-10-CM Chapter 4

Chapter 4 of ICD-10-CM, Endocrine, Nutritional and Metabolic Diseases (E00–E89) contains many frequently coded conditions such as disorders of the thyroid gland, obesity, dehydration, and diabetes mellitus. There is an Excludes1 note at the beginning of ICD-10-CM, Chapter 4 for transitory endocrine and metabolic disorders specific to the newborn (P70–P74). An illustration of the organs of the endocrine system is shown in figure 7.1.

Figure 7.1. Endocrine system

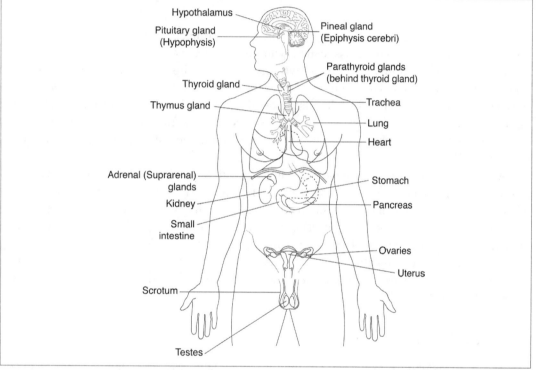

Hypothalamus
Pituitary gland (Hypophysis)
Pineal gland (Epiphysis cerebri)
Parathyroid glands (behind thyroid gland)
Thyroid gland
Thymus gland
Trachea
Lung
Heart
Adrenal (Suprarenal) glands
Stomach
Kidney
Pancreas
Small intestine
Ovaries
Uterus
Scrotum
Testes

©AHIMA

Disorders of Thyroid Gland (E00–E07)

The category Disorders of Thyroid Gland contains the frequently coded conditions of hypothyroidism, nontoxic goiter, thyrotoxicosis or hyperthyroidism, and thyroiditis. For the thyroid conditions that are related to drugs such as hypothyroidism or thyroiditis, there are notes to "code first" poisoning due to drug or toxin and use additional code for adverse effect. For acute thyroiditis, another note reminds the coder to use additional code (B95–B97) to identify the infectious agent.

The thyroid gland is located in the neck in front of the trachea. It consists of two lobes that are connected by an isthmus or space. The thyroid gland produces two hormones, thyroxine (T4) and triiodothyronine (T3), that regulate metabolic functions in the body including growth and development, body temperature, how fast the heart beats, and how the body burns calories. Four parathyroid glands are located to the dorsal area of the thyroid lobes. The parathyroid hormone helps to maintain blood calcium, normal neuromuscular function, blood clotting, and cell membrane permeability (NLM 2019a; Mosby 2017, 1000–1001).

Hypothyroidism

Hypothyroidism is the condition caused by decreased production of the thyroid hormones. This can be an acquired condition caused by surgical removal of part or all of the thyroid, or hypothyroidism can be caused by medications to treat hyperthyroidism or various other congenital or autoimmune factors. Examples of these conditions are described with code E03.0, congenital hypothyroidism with diffuse goiter, and E03.2, hypothyroidism due to medicaments and other exogenous substances. There is a "code first" note and a "use additional code" note following E03.2 to remind the coder to identify the drug that is involved with producing the hypothyroidism (NLM 2019b; Mosby 2017, 659).

Goiter

A goiter is an enlargement of the thyroid gland that produces a prominent swelling in the neck. The enlargement may be associated with normal levels of thyroid hormones or may be present with hyperthyroidism and hypothyroidism. The condition is called a diffuse nontoxic goiter or a simple goiter. The gland may be cystic or fibrous with single or multiple nodules present. Treatment is usually the administration of antithyroid or thyroid hormones depending on the patient's thyroid function. Surgery is rarely done for diffuse nontoxic or simple goiters except when there is evidence of tracheal compression or obstruction of the thoracic outlet (Mosby 2017, 576).

A toxic goiter is an enlargement of the thyroid with numerous nodules and excessive thyroid hormone production. It occurs most frequently in elderly individuals and produces signs of thyrotoxicosis such as nervousness, tremor, weakness, irritability, fatigue, and weight loss, as anorexia is common. Heart failure and cardiac arrhythmia are produced by a toxic goiter or thyrotoxicosis. Management of this condition may be difficult, but treatment is usually antithyroid drugs in combination with beta-blocker heart medications to normalize the thyroid function. After the diagnosis is confirmed, treatment with radioactive iodine may be required (Mosby 2017, 1363).

Thyrotoxicosis

Thyrotoxicosis is defined as the state of thyroid hormone excess and is not the same as hyperthyroidism, that is, the result of excessive thyroid function. Hyperthyroidism is usually caused by Graves' disease, toxic multinodular goiter, and toxic adenomas. In hyperthyroidism, the gland is excreting greater than normal amounts of thyroid hormone. This produces accelerated metabolic processes in the body. Symptoms include nervousness, fatigue, heat intolerance, palpitations, constant hunger with weight loss, tremors, and exophthalmos. Treatment usually prescribed is antithyroid drugs with radioactive iodine for certain scenarios. Untreated hyperthyroidism can lead to serious heart failure. Surgical removal of part or all of the thyroid gland may be necessary (Mosby 2017, 1351).

Thyroiditis

Thyroiditis is an inflammation of the thyroid that may be caused by viral or bacterial infections, certain medications, genetics, or autoimmune disease, such as type 1 diabetes and rheumatoid arthritis. Two of the more common types of thyroiditis are Hashimoto's disease and postpartum thyroiditis. Inflammation of the thyroid after giving birth, postpartum thyroiditis, is often underdiagnosed because the symptoms may be considered the "baby blues" that may follow a delivery. Postpartum women may feel very tired and moody. Within a month of delivery, the patient may have signs and symptoms of hyperthyroidism with excess thyroid hormones in the bloodstream, but several months later, symptoms of hypothyroidism are exhibited when the hormones decrease and the thyroid begins to recover. The condition is more likely to occur in women who have a personal or family history of thyroid disorders or have chronic viral hepatitis. Treatment depends on the patient's symptoms and the stage of the disease.

Hashimoto's disease is also known as autoimmune thyroiditis or Hashimoto's thyroiditis. In this condition, the immune system produces antibodies that interfere with the thyroid's ability to make thyroid hormone. This causes the thyroid levels to be too low, and hypothyroidism is produced. An underactive thyroid causes the body's metabolic functions to slow down, including maintaining heart rate and producing energy from food. Hashimoto's disease (named after a Japanese surgeon) is closely related to Graves' disease, another autoimmune disease of the thyroid. Symptoms of Hashimoto's disease are usually a goiter and a feeling of fullness in the throat making it difficult to swallow. The patient also has fatigue, weight gain, pale coloring in the face with fullness, slower heart rate, and various other symptoms that could be attributed to many other disorders. Replacement therapy with thyroid hormone is the usual treatment (Mosby 2017, 598, 1350).

Diabetes Mellitus (E08–E13)

Diabetes mellitus is a metabolic disease in which the pancreas does not produce insulin normally. The cause of diabetes mellitus can be attributed to both hereditary and nonhereditary factors, such as obesity, surgical removal of the pancreas, or the action of certain drugs. When the pancreas fails to produce insulin, glucose (sugar) is not broken down to be used and stored by the body's cells. As a result, too much sugar accumulates in the blood, causing hyperglycemia and resulting in spillover into the urine, causing glycosuria. Saturating the blood and urine with glucose draws water out of the body, causing dehydration and thirst. Other symptoms include excessive hunger, marked weakness, and weight loss. Treatment may consist of insulin regulation by either insulin injection or oral antidiabetic agents, along with physical activity and a healthy diet. Over time, high blood glucose can lead to serious problems in the heart, eyes, kidneys, nerves, gums, and teeth. According to the American Diabetes Association (ADA), 29.1 million Americans, or 9.3 percent of the population, have diabetes according to statistics collected in 2015. Approximately 1.25 million American children have type 1 diabetes, as the incidence of type 2 diabetes is much greater. Americans aged 65 years and older have a high prevalence of diabetes, with 25.9 percent, or 11.8 million, of seniors diagnosed and undiagnosed (ADA 2019a).

Type 1 diabetes is usually diagnosed in children and young adults and was previously known as juvenile diabetes but can appear at any age. In type 1 diabetes, the body does not produce insulin. According to the American Diabetes Association, only 5 percent of people with diabetes have this form of the disease. Symptoms of type 1 diabetes include frequent urination, unusual thirst, extreme hunger, unusual weight loss, and extreme fatigue and irritability (ADA 2019b).

The most common type of diabetes is **type 2 diabetes**. The body does not produce enough insulin or the cells ignore the insulin or do not use insulin well. A patient who is older, is obese, has a family history of diabetes, and does not exercise is at higher risk of type 2 diabetes. The symptoms of type 2 diabetes appear slowly. Symptoms include the same symptoms type 1 diabetic patients experience in addition to frequent infections, blurred vision, cuts and bruises that are slow to heal, and tingling and numbness in the hands and feet. However, some people do not notice symptoms at all (ADA 2019c).

There are five categories for diabetes mellitus in ICD-10-CM. The diabetes mellitus codes reflect manifestations and complications of the disease by using the fourth or fifth characters. ICD-10-CM classifies inadequately controlled, out of control, and poorly controlled diabetes mellitus by reporting diabetes mellitus, by type, with hyperglycemia.

The diabetes mellitus codes are combination codes that include the

- type of diabetes (type 1, type 2, due to underlying condition or due to drug or chemical)

- body system affected

- complications affecting that body system

For type 1 and type 2 diabetes, the diabetes code contains the details about the type of diabetes and most of the associated complications. A few of the diabetes codes require the use of an additional code, for example, to identify the stage of the chronic kidney disease caused by the diabetes. For other types of diabetes, the underlying condition is listed first, followed by the diabetes code that includes any associated complication.

Each type of diabetes has a particular category of codes, some examples include:

- E08, Diabetes mellitus due to underlying condition

  ○ Code first the underlying condition, such as forms of Cushing's syndrome (category E24.-)

- E09, Drug or chemical-induced diabetes mellitus

  ○ Code first poisoning due to drug or toxin, if applicable, (T36–T65 with fifth or sixth character 1–4 or 6)

  ○ Use additional code for adverse effect, if applicable, to identify drug (T36–T50 with fifth or sixth character 5)

  ○ Use additional code to identify control using insulin (Z79.4), oral antidiabetic drugs (Z79.85), oral hypoglycemic drugs (Z79.84)

- E10, Type 1 diabetes mellitus

  ○ Includes brittle diabetes (mellitus), diabetes (mellitus) due to autoimmune process, diabetes (mellitus) due to immune-mediated pancreatic islet beta-cell destruction, idiopathic diabetes (mellitus), juvenile-onset diabetes (mellitus), and ketosis-prone diabetes (mellitus)

- E11, Type 2 diabetes mellitus

  ○ Includes diabetes (mellitus) due to insulin secretory defect, diabetes NOS, insulin-resistant diabetes (mellitus)

  ○ Use additional code to identify control using: insulin (Z79.4), oral antidiabetic drugs (Z79.84), oral hypoglycemic drugs (Z79.84)

- E13, Other specified diabetes mellitus

  ○ Includes diabetes mellitus due to genetic defects of beta-cell function, diabetes mellitus due to genetic defects in insulin action, postpancreatectomy diabetes mellitus, postprocedural diabetes mellitus, secondary diabetes mellitus NEC

  ○ Use additional code to control using: insulin (Z79.4), oral antidiabetic drugs (Z79.84), oral hypoglycemic drugs (Z79.84)

Other forms of diabetes are coded elsewhere in ICD-10-CM:

- Gestational diabetes (O24.4-)

- Neonatal diabetes mellitus (P70.2)

In addition to identifying the type of diabetes, the ICD-10-CM code includes one or more of the complications or manifestations that exists in a particular body system. For example,

- E08.21, Diabetes mellitus due to underlying condition with diabetic nephropathy

- E09.610, Drug or chemical-induced diabetes mellitus with diabetic neuropathic arthropathy

- E10.321, Type 1 diabetes mellitus with mild nonproliferative diabetic retinopathy with macular edema. Use seventh character to designate laterality.

- E11.51, Type 2 diabetes mellitus with diabetic peripheral angiopathy without gangrene. Use seventh character to designate laterality.

- E13.620, Other specified diabetes mellitus with diabetic dermatitis. Use seventh character to designate laterality.

The coder may assign as many codes from categories E08–E13 as needed to identify all the associated conditions that a patient may have had treated. An additional code of Z79.4 is used to identify patients who routinely use insulin for the management of their type 2 or other forms of diabetes, except for type 1 diabetes. Type 1 diabetes mellitus is typically treated with insulin, and therefore, the additional code Z79.4 would not be used. Other forms of diabetes may or may not use insulin as part of the treatment. When insulin is used with other types of diabetes, for example, with type 2 diabetes, the additional code of Z79.4 provides more information about the patient's disease and what is required to treat it.

Check Your Understanding 7.1

Assign diagnosis codes to the following conditions.

1. Hyperthyroidism with nodular goiter without crisis

2. Mild proliferative diabetic retinopathy, type 2 diabetes with macular edema, on daily insulin injections and oral hypoglycemic drugs with diabetic cataract in right eye

3. Type 1 diabetic with diabetic chronic kidney disease, stage 4, being seen for regulation of insulin dosage. Patient also has abscessed right molar

4. Secondary diabetes due to acute idiopathic pancreatitis with diabetic hyperglycemia; long-term insulin use

5. Steroid-induced diabetes mellitus due to the prolonged use of corticosteroids, which have been discontinued at a previous visit. The patient's diabetes is managed with insulin. This is a follow-up visit for the diabetes.

6. Type 1 diabetes with severe chronic diabetic left foot ulcer with diabetic peripheral angiopathy. Foot ulcer is under treatment and currently has breakdown of skin only. Patient also has stage 2 chronic kidney disease.

7. Secondary diabetes mellitus, poorly controlled, due to postpancreatectomy

8. Graves' disease with thyrotoxic crisis or strom

9. Nonsuppurative thyroiditis

10. Type 2 diabetes with polyneuropathy

Other Disorders of Glucose Regulation and Pancreatic Internal Secretion (E15–E16)

Codes for nondiabetic hypoglycemic coma, other hypoglycemic conditions, and Zollinger-Ellison syndrome are included in this block of codes. Code E16.0, Drug-induced hypoglycemia without coma, has a "use additional code" note to add a code for adverse effect, if applicable, to identify a drug (T36–T50 with fifth or sixth character 5).

Codes for specified forms of hypoglycemia or the unspecified diagnosis of hypoglycemia are included in category E16, other disorders of pancreatic internal secretion. The body needs glucose, a form of sugar, to have enough energy. After a meal, the person's blood absorbs glucose. If the person eats more sugar than needed, muscles and the liver store the extra. When the blood sugar declines, a hormone causes the liver to release glucose. Usually, this raises blood sugar. If it does not elevate the blood sugar level, the person has a condition called **hypoglycemia**. In some situations, the blood sugar can be dangerously low. Physical signs and symptoms of hypoglycemia include hunger, confusion, shakiness, dizziness, weakness, anxiety, and sometimes difficulty speaking (NLM 2019c).

Hypoglycemia is usually a side effect of diabetes medicine. However, a person can also have hypoglycemia without having diabetes. In order to find the cause of hypoglycemia, certain laboratory tests will be performed to measure blood glucose, insulin, and other chemicals that play a part in the body's use of energy. The code for unspecified hypoglycemia in the category E16 will likely be used for the patient's reason for theses diagnostic studies.

Zollinger-Ellison syndrome is not a common condition but is a serious one when it occurs in early childhood and in adults between the second and fifth decades of life. Figure 7.2 shows the

Figure 7.2. **Organs affected by Zollinger-Ellison syndrome**

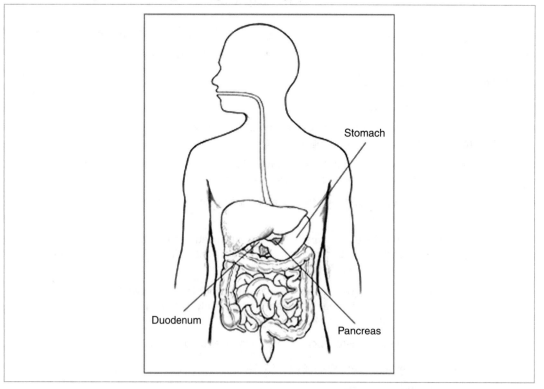

Source: National Institute of Diabetes and Digestive and Kidney Diseases (NIDDK) 2013

organs that are affected by Zollinger-Ellison syndrome, specifically the stomach, duodenum, and pancreas. One or more gastrinomas develop in the pancreas and duodenum and release abnormally large amounts of the gastrin hormone that causes the stomach to produce excessive amounts of acid. This produces severe peptic ulcerations in the duodenum and other parts of the upper intestine, such as the stomach. Sometimes the tumors are cancerous and may spread to other parts of the body. A total gastrectomy may be needed if medications to control the gastric hypersecretion are unsuccessful and the peptic ulcers do not heal (Mosby 2017, 1467; NIH 2013).

Disorders of Other Endocrine Glands (E20–E35)

The endocrine system is made up of the endocrine glands that secrete hormones. There are eight major **endocrine glands**: pituitary, pineal, thyroid, thymus, adrenal, pancreas, testes in males, and ovaries in females. These glands are scattered throughout the body but are considered one body system because of their similar functions and mechanisms of influence as well as important interrelationships.

Codes for disorders of the parathyroid gland, pituitary gland, adrenal gland, thymus gland, as well as testicular and ovarian dysfunction are included here. Some of the commonly coded conditions in this block of codes are Cushing's syndrome, Addison's disease, polycystic ovarian syndrome, premature menopause, multiple endocrine neoplasia (MEN) syndromes, and carcinoid syndrome. For conditions related to the use of medications, notes are included to "use additional code" for adverse effect to identify the drug or drugs that are responsible for the gland's dysfunction.

Cushing's syndrome is a metabolic disorder resulting from the excessive production of or exposure to the hormone cortisol. Cortisol is produced by the adrenal gland, also known as adrenocorticotropic hormone (ACTH). The most common cause of Cushing's syndrome is a pituitary tumor. Other causes include taking a synthetic hormone drug that is used to treat an inflammatory disease elsewhere in the body. Fortunately, Cushing's syndrome is rare. The treatment depends on the cause of the excessive hormone. Medications may be prescribed to lower the cortisol levels or surgery may be required to remove the pituitary gland that is increasing the secretion of ACTH (Mosby 2017, 352; NLM 2019d; NLM 2019e).

Addison's disease, also known as primary adrenocortical insufficiency, is a serious metabolic condition caused by complete or partial failure of the adrenocortical function in the body. The adrenal glands, located above the kidneys, simply do not make enough of the hormone cortisol and androgens. The causes may be an autoimmune process where the body's immune system attacks its own tissue, damaging the adrenal glands or causing tubercular or fungal infection or a hemorrhage in the adrenal gland. If left untreated, the condition can be life threatening. Treatment includes replacement therapy with glucocorticoid and mineral corticoid drugs and careful regulation of fluids and diet intake (NLM 2019f; Mosby 2017, 29; NLM 2019g).

Polycystic ovarian syndrome or polycystic ovary disease is an endocrine disorder characterized by anovulation, amenorrhea, hirsutism, and infertility. The cause of the disease is unknown but suspected to be the result of various factors working together, including insulin resistance, increased levels of the hormone androgen, and irregular menstrual cycles. Androgens are steroid hormones produced by the adrenal glands or the ovaries. Women with polycystic ovary disease also tend to have endometrial hyperplasia where the lining of the uterus becomes too thick. This condition is a risk factor for endometrial cancer. Treatment depends on the woman's symptoms, whether she wants to become pregnant, and other health conditions that coexist. Women who do not desire a pregnancy may be treated with a combined hormonal birth control pill with estrogen and progestin that regulates the menstrual cycle and decreases androgen levels to reduce hirsutism and acne. Insulin-sensitizing drugs will help the body respond to insulin as well as reduce the androgen levels in the blood (ACOG 2017; Mosby 2017, 1065; NLM 2019h).

Malnutrition (E40–E46)

Malnutrition is the condition that occurs when the body does not get enough nutrients. There are a number of causes of malnutrition. It may result from inadequate or unbalanced diet, problems with digestion or absorption, and certain medical conditions. Malnutrition can occur if a person does not eat enough food. Starvation is a form of malnutrition. A person may develop malnutrition if there is a lack of a single vitamin in the diet. In some cases, malnutrition is very mild and causes no symptoms. However, sometimes it can be so severe that the damage done to the body is permanent (NLM 2019e, 2019g).

ICD-10-CM contains a code for **kwashiorkor**, a severe malnutrition with nutritional edema with dyspigmentation of the skin and hair. This condition is most common in areas where there is famine, limited food supply, and low levels of education of how to eat a proper diet. This disease is more common in very poor countries. It often occurs during a drought or other natural disaster, or during political unrest. These conditions are responsible for a lack of food, which leads to malnutrition. Kwashiorkor is very rare in children in the United States. When kwashiorkor does occur in the United States, it is usually a sign of child abuse and severe neglect (NLM 2019h).

Marasmus is a severe deficiency of calories and protein. It tends to develop in infants and very young children. It typically results in weight loss and dehydration. Breast-feeding usually protects against marasmus (Mosby 2017, 810).

ICD-10-CM contains a limited number of malnutrition codes in this chapter. Codes are included for severe malnutrition, moderate and mild degree protein–calorie malnutrition, and malnutrition unspecified. The documentation required to best describe the type of malnutrition would include the degree of malnutrition (first, mild, moderate, second, severe, third) or the type of protein–calorie or protein–energy malnutrition (mild, moderate, or severe).

Other Nutritional Deficiencies (E50–E64)

Codes in this section classify a variety of vitamin and other nutrient deficiencies. For example, the conditions included here are vitamin A, thiamine, B group, and D and K deficiencies. Other conditions include dietary deficiencies of calcium, zinc, iron, magnesium, and other specified nutrient elements. Also in this block of codes is category E64, Sequelae of malnutrition and other nutritional deficiencies. This category is used to indicate conditions in categories E43, E44, E46, and E50–63 as the cause of sequelae, which are themselves classified elsewhere. These are the late effects of diseases classifiable to the above categories if the disease itself is no longer present. A "code first" note to code the condition resulting from (sequela) of malnutrition and other nutritional deficiencies is included here.

Check Your Understanding 7.2

Assign diagnosis codes to the following conditions.

1. Zollinger-Ellison syndrome

2. Moderate protein–calorie malnutrition due to AIDS

(Continued)

(*Continued*)

3. Hypoglycemic coma in a nondiabetic patient

4. Bartter's syndrome

5. Symptomatic premature menopause

6. Alcoholic pellagra

7. Vitamin B6 deficiency

8. Thymus hypertrophy

9. Polycystic ovarian syndrome

10. Vitamin A deficiency with corneal xerosis

Overweight, Obesity, and Other Hyperalimentation (E65–E68)

Both overweight and obesity mean a person's weight is greater than what is considered healthy for his or her height. A person described as obese means the person has too much body fat. A person described as overweight means the person weighs too much. Both terms means the person's weight is greater than what is considered healthy for his or her height. Obesity occurs when a person eats more calories than the person burns in activities or exercise. Each person has a balance their body needs for calories in and calories out. Factors that also affect weight include a person's genetic composition, overeating, eating high-fat foods, and not being physically active. Obesity increases the person's risk for diabetes, heart disease, stroke, arthritis, and some cancers (NLM 2019i). The title of this section of codes includes "hyperalimentation," which means overfeeding or the ingestion of an amount of nutrients that exceeds the demands of the appetite (Mosby 2017, 645).

Body mass index (BMI) is used as a screening tool for overweight or obesity. BMI is a person's weight in kilograms divided by the square of height in meters. The BMI measurement is a screening tool but is not a diagnostic indicator of body fatness or health of an individual. Appropriate health assessments are necessary to evaluate an individual's status and risks. According to the Centers for Disease Control and Prevention (2016), the following BMI ranges indicate underweight, normal weight, overweight, and obese status:

- If the BMI is less than 18.5, it indicates the person is within the underweight range.

- If the BMI is 18.5 to 24.9, it indicates the person is within the normal or healthy weight range.

- If the BMI is 25.0 to 29.9, it indicates the person is within the overweight range.

- If the BMI is 30.0 or higher, it indicates the person is within the obese range.

With category E66, overweight and obesity, two instructional notes are included. A "code first" note appears here to code obesity complicating pregnancy, childbirth, and the puerperium if applicable; that is, if the patient is pregnant or in the postpartum period. Another note states "use additional code to identify body mass index (BMI) if known (Z68.1-)" for all the codes in category E66. Coding guideline 1.B.14 addresses documentation for BMI and pressure ulcer stages, coma scale, and NIH stroke scale codes. The BMI level can be coded based on clinicians' documentation other than the physician if the BMI meets the requirements for a reportable additional diagnosis.

Metabolic Disorders (E70–E88)

The category Metabolic Disorders is a mixture of both common and uncommon diseases. The commonly coded conditions here are hypercholesterolemia, hyperlipidemia, cystic fibrosis, dehydration, hyper- and hypokalemia, electrolyte imbalance, and metabolic syndrome. Less commonly occurring conditions coded here are a variety of metabolism disorders including fatty acid, amino acid, purine, and porphyrin metabolism.

Volume depletion may refer to depletion of total body water (dehydration) or depletion of the blood volume (hypovolemia). **Dehydration**, a lack of adequate water in the body, can be a medical emergency. This condition is classified to E86.0. Common in infants and elderly people, severe dehydration can occur with vomiting, excessive heat and sweating, diarrhea, or lack of food or fluid intake. Blood volume may be maintained despite dehydration, with fluid being pulled from other tissues. Conversely, hypovolemia may occur without dehydration when "third spacing" of fluids occurs, for example, with significant edema or ascites. **Hypovolemia** is an abnormally low circulating blood volume and is classified to E86.1. Blood loss may be due to internal bleeding from the intestine or stomach, external bleeding from an injury, or loss of blood volume and body fluid associated with diarrhea, vomiting, dehydration, or burns. If hypovolemia is severe, hypovolemic shock can occur with symptoms such as rapid or weak pulse, feeling faint, pale skin, cool or moist skin, rapid breathing, anxiety, overall weakness, and low blood pressure. Emergency medical attention must be sought. Given that the nature of these two conditions and their respective treatments are different, coding of hypovolemia is different from dehydration (NLM 2019j).

> **EXAMPLE:** Patient admitted with severe dehydration and gastroenteritis
> Treatment was directed toward resolving the dehydration
> E86.0, Dehydration
> K52.9, Gastroenteritis

Cystic fibrosis is an inherited disease of the exocrine glands that affects the gastrointestinal and respiratory systems. Category codes for cystic fibrosis (CF) (category E84) describe the complications that occur with CF in the respiratory system, digestive system, and other manifestations that often occur. Cystic fibrosis is characterized by chronic obstructive pulmonary disease, pancreatic insufficiency, and abnormally high sweat electrolytes. The degree of pulmonary involvement usually determines the course of the disease. The patient's demise is often the result of respiratory failure and cor pulmonale. A note to "use additional code to identify any infectious organism present, such as: Pseudomonas (B96.5)" appears under code E84.0 for cystic fibrosis with pulmonary manifestations (NLM 2019k).

Postprocedural Endocrine and Metabolic Complications and Disorders, Not Elsewhere Classified (E89)

A limited number of postprocedural, postsurgical, or postirradiation complications and disorders are coded in Chapter 4 of ICD-10-CM. Such conditions include postprocedural hypothyroidism, hypoinsulinemia, hypoparathyroidism, hypopituitarism, and postprocedural ovarian failure. As in other chapters, postprocedural hemorrhage and hematoma of an endocrine system organ are included at the end of the block of codes.

Check Your Understanding 7.3

Assign diagnosis codes to the following conditions.

1. Morbid obesity with a BMI of 40 in an adult

2. Overweight 10-year-old male child, height 56 inches, weight 102 pounds, BMI 22.9, 85th percentile for BMI

3. Alkaptonuria

4. Zellweger-like syndrome

5. Salmonella gastroenteritis complicated by dehydration (child was admitted primarily for dehydration treatment but both conditions treated)

6. Familial hypercholesterolemia

7. Fredrickson's hyperlipoproteinemia, Type IIb

8. Transfusion-associated circulatory overload (TACO)

9. Localized amyloidosis

10. Metabolic syndrome with obesity

ICD-10-PCS Procedure Codes for Procedures Related to Chapter 4: Endocrine, Nutritional and Metabolic Disorders

The procedures performed on organs in the endocrine system appear in the ICD-10-PCS code book in tables that start with the two characters 0 and G followed by five characters representing the root operation, body part, approach, device, and qualifier:

Character 1 is Value 0—Medical and Surgical

Character 2 is Value G—Endocrine System

Root Operation

Character 3 of the ICD-10-PCS codes is the root operation. The root operations that represent the objectives of procedures for surgical treatment of the diseases of the Endocrine system are shown in table 7.1.

Table 7.1. **Root operations, values, and definitions for procedures on body parts within the Endocrine system**

Change (2): Taking out or off a device from a body part and putting back an identical or similar device in or on the same body part without cutting or puncturing the skin or a mucous membrane
Destruction (5): Physical eradication of all or a portion of a body part by the direct use of energy, force, or a destructive agent
Division (8): Cutting into a body part, without draining fluids and/or gases from the body part, in order to separate or transect a body part

(Continued)

Drainage (9): Taking or letting out fluids and/or gases from a body part
Excision (B): Cutting out or off, without replacement, a portion of a body part
Extirpation (C): Taking or cutting out solid matter from a body part
Insertion (H): Putting in a nonbiological appliance that monitors, assists, performs, or prevents a physiological function but does not physically take the place of the body part
Inspection (J): Visually and/or manually exploring a body part
Reattachment (M): Putting back in or on all or a portion of a separated body part to its normal location or other suitable location
Release (N): Freeing a body part from an abnormal physical constraint by cutting or by the use of force
Removal (P): Taking out or off a device from a body part
Repair (Q): Restoring, to the extent possible, a body part to its normal anatomic structure and function
Reposition (S): Moving to its normal location, or other suitable location, all or a portion of a body part
Resection (T): Cutting out or off, without replacement, all of a body part
Revision (W): Correcting, to the extent possible, a portion of a malfunctioning device or the position of a displaced device

Source: CMS 2019

Body Part

Character 4 identifies the body part involved in the procedure. The body parts in ICD-10-PCS have individual values that include laterality when a pair of glands exists, for example, as shown in table 7.2.

Table 7.2. **Body parts and values included in the ICD-10-PCS codes for the Endocrine system**

0—Pituitary Gland
1—Pineal Body
2—Adrenal Gland, left
3—Adrenal Gland, right
4—Adrenal Gland, bilateral
5—Adrenal Gland
6—Carotid Body, left
7—Carotid Body, right
8—Carotid Bodies, bilateral
9—Para-aortic Body
B—Coccygeal Glomus
C—Glomus Jugulare
D—Aortic Body
F—Paraganglion Extremity
G—Thyroid Gland Lobe, left
H—Thyroid Gland Lobe, right
J—Thyroid Gland Isthmus
K—Thyroid Gland
L—Superior Parathyroid Gland, right

| M—Superior Parathyroid Gland, left |
| N—Inferior Parathyroid Gland, right |
| P—Inferior Superior Parathyroid Gland, left |
| Q—Parathyroid Glands, multiple |
| R—Parathyroid Gland |
| S—Endocrine Gland |

Source: CMS 2019

Approach

Character 5 identifies the approach used in the procedure. The approach for procedures performed on organs within the Endocrine system are limited to three options and are shown in table 7.3. The qualifier value of X for diagnostic procedure is available for the root operations of Drainage and Excision.

Table 7.3.   **Approaches, definitions, and values included in the ICD-10-PCS codes for the Endocrine system**

| **Open** (0): Cutting through the skin or mucous membrane and any other body layers necessary to expose the site of the procedure |
| **Percutaneous** (3): Entry, by puncture or minor incision, of instrumentation through the skin or mucous membrane and any other body layers necessary to reach the site of the procedure |
| **Percutaneous endoscopic** (4): Entry, by puncture or minor incision, of instrumentation through the skin or mucous membrane and any other body layers necessary to reach and visualize the site of the procedure |
| **External** (X): Performed directly on the skin or mucous membrane and procedures performed indirectly by the application of external force through the skin or mucous membrane |

Source: CMS 2019

Device

Character 6 identifies if a device remains in the patient's body after the procedure is concluded. The devices used to code procedures performed on organs within the Endocrine system are limited to a few devices, as shown in table 7.4.

Table 7.4.   **Devices and values included in the ICD-10-PCS codes for the Endocrine system**

| 0—Drainage Device |
| 2—Monitoring Device |
| 3—Infusion Device |
| Y—Other Device |
| Z—No Device |

Source: CMS 2019

Qualifier

Character 7 is a qualifier that specifies an additional attribute of the procedure, if applicable. The qualifier characters used to code procedures performed on organs within the Endocrine system are limited to two values, as shown in table 7.5.

Table 7.5.   **Qualifiers used to code procedures within the Endocrine system**

X—Diagnostic
Z—No Qualifier

Source: CMS 2019

Resection, Excision, and Destruction of Endocrine Glands

The more common procedures on the endocrine glands are Excision, Resection, and Destruction. The surgical removal of all of a body part (**Resection**), part of a body part (**Excision**), or the physical eradication (**Destruction**) of all or a portion of the endocrine glands are coded based on the body part involved. Biopsy procedures are performed on endocrine glands by excision or by fine needle aspiration that could be either an excision of tissue or drainage of fluid or gases.

Laterality is used to identify the body parts within the endocrine system, for example, left, right, and bilateral adrenal glands as well as left and right inferior and superior parathyroid glands. Of particular importance in coding thyroid procedures, the coder must note that the lobes of the thyroid gland are individual body parts. If the physician describes the procedure as a thyroidectomy of the left lobe, the procedure is coded as a Resection of the thyroid gland lobe, left, as PCS identifies this site as a body part. Coding the thyroidectomy of the left lobe as an Excision would be incorrect as an Excision is cutting out or off a portion of a body part.

The coder should review the following ICD-10-PCS guidelines for a complete description of coding biopsy, excision, and resection procedures.

CG

B3.4a Biopsy Procedures

Biopsy procedures are coded using the root operations Excision, Extraction, or Drainage and the qualifier Diagnostic. Examples: Fine needle aspiration biopsy of lung is coded to the root operation Drainage with the qualifier Diagnostic. Biopsy of bone marrow is coded to the root operation Extraction with the qualifier Diagnostic. Lymph node sampling for biopsy is coded to the root operation Excision with the qualifier Diagnostic.

B3.4b Biopsy followed by more definitive treatment

If a diagnostic Excision, Extraction, or Drainage procedure (biopsy) is followed by a more definitive procedure, such as Destruction, Excision, or Resection at the same procedure site, both the biopsy and the more definitive treatment is coded. Example: Biopsy of breast followed by partial mastectomy at the same procedure site, both the biopsy and the partial mastectomy procedure are coded.

B3.8 Excision vs. Resection

PCS contains specific body parts for anatomical subdivisions of a body part, such as lobes of the lungs or liver and regions of the intestine. Resection of the specific body part is coded whenever all of the body part is cut out and off, rather than coding Excision of a less specific body part. Example: Left upper lung lobectomy is coded to Resection of Upper Lung Lobe, Left rather than Excision of Lung, Left.

B4.1a General Guidelines for Body Part

If a procedure is performed on a portion of a body part that does not have a separate body part value, code the body part value corresponding to the whole body part. Example: A procedure performed on the alveolar process of the mandible is coded to the mandible body part (CMS 2019).

Stereotactic radiosurgery using a gamma beam, particulate type, or other photon radiosurgery is available to destroy lesions on endocrine glands such as the adrenal, parathyroid, pineal body, pituitary, and thyroid glands. Stereotactic radiosurgery is classified in the Radiation Therapy section of ICD-10-PCS. The main term to use in the Index to locate these procedures is "Stereotactic radiosurgery" with subterms of gamma beam, other photon, and particulate with additional entries of the body part involved. **Stereotactic radiosurgery (SRS)** is a form of radiation therapy that focuses high-powered x-rays on a small area of the body. For example, SRS is used to treat tumors within the pituitary gland located beneath the brain in the pituitary fossa of the sphenoid bone. SRS requires placing the patient in a rigid head frame attached to the skull to aim a single large dose of radiation directly to a tumor. This causes less damage to healthy tissue that is near the tumor. Other types of radiation therapy can affect nearby healthy tissue; SRS better targets the abnormal area. Despite its name, radiosurgery is a treatment, not a surgical procedure (NCI 2019).

For SRS on the endocrine glands, that is, pituitary gland, pineal body, adrenal glands, parathyroid glands, and thyroid, the ICD-10-PCS DG2 table in the Radiation Therapy section is used for coding the procedures:

Table 7.6. **ICD-10-PCS Table DG2**

D Radiation Therapy
G Endocrine System
2 Stereotactic Radiosurgery

Treatment Site (4th)	Modality Qualifier (5th)	Isotope (6th)	Qualifier (7th)
0 Pituitary Gland 1 Pineal Body 2 Adrenal Glands 4 Parathyroid Glands 5 Thyroid	D Stereotactic Other Photon radiosurgery H Stereotactic Particulate radiosurgery J Stereotactic Gamma Bean radiosurgery	Z None	Z None

Source: CMS 2019

ICD-10-CM and ICD-10-PCS Review Exercises: Chapter 7

Assign the correct ICD-10-CM diagnosis codes and ICD-10-PCS procedure codes for the following exercises.

1. Type 2 diabetic with stage 1 diabetic chronic kidney disease

(Continued on next page)

ICD-10-CM and ICD-10-PCS Review Exercises: Chapter 7 (continued)

2. Toxic diffuse goiter with thyrotoxic storm

3. Type 2 diabetic due to Cushing's syndrome

4. Hypokalemia

5. Cystic fibrosis with pulmonary manifestations due to Pseudomonas

6. Uncontrolled (hyperglycemia) type 2 diabetes mellitus; mild degree malnutrition

7. Panhypopituitarism

8. Lower extremity ulcer on skin of left heel secondary to brittle diabetes mellitus, type 1, uncontrolled

9. Diabetic proliferative retinopathy in a patient with controlled type 1 diabetes

10. Overweight adult with a body mass index (BMI) of 26.5

11. Syndrome of inappropriate secretion of antidiuretic hormone (SIADH)

12. Hypoglycemia in type 1 diabetes with coma

13. Postsurgical hypothyroidism

14. Folic acid deficiency

15. Partial androgen insensitivity syndrome

16. PROCEDURE: Open total left lobe thyroidectomy

ICD-10-CM and ICD-10-PCS Review Exercises: Chapter 7 (continued)

17. PROCEDURE: Partial right lobectomy, thyroid gland, open

_____

18. PROCEDURE: Right carotid body biopsy, open, by excision

_____

19. PROCEDURE: Laparoscopic partial left hypophysectomy

_____

20. PROCEDURE: Stereotactic gamma beam radiosurgery, parathyroid gland tumor

_____

References

The American College of Obstetricians and Gynecologists (ACOG). 2017. Polycystic Ovary Syndrome (PCOS). http://www.acog.org/~/media/For%20Patients/faq121.pdf.

American Diabetes Association (ADA). 2019a. Statistics About Diabetes. http://www.diabetes.org/diabetes-basics/statistics/.

American Diabetes Association (ADA). 2019b. Type 1. http://www.diabetes.org/diabetes-basics/type-1/.

American Diabetes Association (ADA). 2019c. Type 2. http://www.diabetes.org/diabetes-basics/type-2/.

Centers for Disease Control and Prevention (CDC), National Center for Health Statistics (NCHS). 2019. *ICD-10-CM Official Guidelines for Coding and Reporting*, 2020. https://www.cdc.gov/nchs/data/icd/10cmguidelines_fy2019_final.pdf.

Centers for Medicare and Medicaid Services (CMS). 2019. *ICD-10-PCS Official Guidelines for Coding and Reporting*, 2020. http://www.cms.gov/Medicare/Coding/ICD10/.

Mosby. 2017. *Mosby's Pocket Dictionary of Medicine, Nursing, and Health Professions*, 8th ed. St. Louis: Mosby, Inc.

National Cancer Institute (NCI). 2019. Pituitary Tumors Treatment (PDQ®): Treatment Option Overview. http://www.cancer.gov/types/pituitary/patient/pituitary-treatment-pdq#section/_53.

National Institute of Diabetes and Digestive and Kidney Diseases (NIDDK), National Institute of Health (NIH). 2013. Zollinger-Ellison Syndrome. http://www.niddk.nih.gov/health-information/health-topics/digestive-diseases/zollinger-ellison-syndrome/Pages/facts.aspx.

U.S. National Library of Medicine, MedLinePlus (NLM). 2019a. Thyroid Diseases. https://www.nlm.nih.gov/medlineplus/thyroiddiseases.html.

U.S. National Library of Medicine, MedLinePlus (NLM). 2019b. Hypothyroidism. https://www.nlm.nih.gov/medlineplus/hypothyroidism.html.

U.S. National Library of Medicine, MedLinePlus (NLM). 2019c. Hypoglycemia. https://medlineplus.gov/hypoglycemia.html.

U.S. National Library of Medicine, MedLinePlus (NLM). 2019d. Cushing's Syndrome. https://www.nlm.nih.gov/medlineplus/cushingssyndrome.html.

U.S. National Library of Medicine, MedLinePlus (NLM). 2019e. Malnutrition. https://www.nlm.nih.gov/medlineplus/malnutrition.html.

U.S. National Library of Medicine, MedLinePlus (NLM). 2019f. Addison Disease. https://www.nlm.nih.gov/medlineplus/addisondisease.html.

U.S. National Library of Medicine, MedLinePlus (NLM). 2019g. Malnutrition. https://www.nlm.nih.gov/medlineplus/ency/article/000404.htm.

U.S. National Library of Medicine, MedLinePlus (NLM). 2019h. Kwashiorkor. https://www.nlm.nih.gov/medlineplus/ency/article/001604.htm.

U.S. National Library of Medicine, MedLinePlus (NLM). 2019i. Obesity. https://www.nlm.nih.gov/medlineplus/obesity.html.

U.S. National Library of Medicine, MedLinePlus (NLM). 2019j. Dehydration. https://www.nlm.nih.gov/medlineplus/dehydration.html.

U.S. National Library of Medicine, MedLinePlus (NLM). 2019k. Cystic Fibrosis. https://www.nlm.nih.gov/medlineplus/cysticfibrosis.html.

Chapter 8

Mental, Behavioral and Neurodevelopmental Disorders (F01–F99)

Learning Objectives

At the conclusion of this chapter, you should be able to do the following:

- Describe the organization of the conditions and codes included in Chapter 5 of ICD-10-CM, Mental, Behavioral and Neurodevelopmental Disorders (F01–F99)

- Describe the DSM-5 and explain its purpose

- Apply the multiple coding rules related to the coding of mental disorders

- Apply the inclusion and exclusion notes for the classification of mental disorders

- Describe the ICD-10-CM coding guidelines for the selection of principal diagnosis for patients admitted for alcohol or drug dependence treatment

- Assign ICD-10-CM codes for mental and behavioral disorders

- Assign ICD-10-PCS codes for mental disorder- and behavioral-disorder–related procedures

Key Terms

Alcohol use disorder
Bipolar disorder
Borderline personality disorder
Diagnostic and Statistical Manual of Mental Disorders, Fifth Edition (DSM-5)

Drug dependence
Eating disorder
Generalized anxiety disorder (GAD)
Intellectual disabilities
Schizophrenia

Overview of ICD-10-CM Chapter 5: Mental, Behavioral and Neurodevelopmental Disorders (F01–F99)

Chapter 5 organizes mental and behavioral disorders in the following blocks:

F01–F09	Mental disorders due to known physiological conditions
F10–F19	Mental and behavioral disorders due to psychoactive substance use
F20–F29	Schizophrenia, schizotypal, delusional, and other non-mood psychotic disorders
F30–F39	Mood [affective] disorders
F40–F48	Anxiety, dissociative, stress-related, somatoform and other nonpsychotic mental disorders
F50–F59	Behavioral syndromes associated with physiological disturbances and physical factors
F60–F69	Disorders of adult personality and behavior
F70–F79	Intellectual Disabilities
F80–F89	Pervasive and specific developmental disorders
F90–F98	Behavioral and emotional disorders with onset usually occurring in childhood and adolescence
F99	Unspecified mental disorder

Chapter 5, Mental, Behavioral, and Neurodevelopmental Disorders (F01–F99), allows for more specific coding of these conditions consistent with the language of behavioral health and substance abuse services as documented in health and client records today. For example, mental and behavioral disorders due to psychoactive substance use (F10–F19) include an extensive number of codes that link the substance involved (alcohol or specific drug) with the specific disorder caused by it. For instance, code F14.280 identifies cocaine dependence with cocaine-induced anxiety disorder. The Index to Diseases and Injuries provides access to these codes under the main term "dependence," with the substance and subterms beneath it to identify the behavioral disturbance associated with the substance.

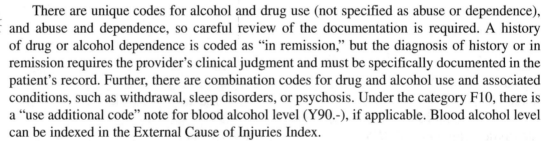

There are unique codes for alcohol and drug use (not specified as abuse or dependence), and abuse and dependence, so careful review of the documentation is required. A history of drug or alcohol dependence is coded as "in remission," but the diagnosis of history or in remission requires the provider's clinical judgment and must be specifically documented in the patient's record. Further, there are combination codes for drug and alcohol use and associated conditions, such as withdrawal, sleep disorders, or psychosis. Under the category F10, there is a "use additional code" note for blood alcohol level (Y90.-), if applicable. Blood alcohol level can be indexed in the External Cause of Injuries Index.

Other categories in this chapter, including schizophrenia, mood disorders, anxiety, dissociative, or other nonpsychotic disorders, allow for more specific reporting of the current episode of illness. Chapter 5 also includes codes for eating disorders, sleep disorders not due to a substance or known physiological condition, impulse disorders, and gender identity disorders, as well as specific developmental disorders.

DSM-5

The Diagnostic and Statistical Manual of Mental Disorders, Fifth Edition (**DSM-5**) is a nomenclature developed by the American Psychiatric Association (APA) to standardize the diagnostic process for patients with psychiatric disorders (APA 2017) and incorporates the Chapter 5 ICD-10-CM codes. Because the DSM-5 diagnostic codes are limited to codes in the ICD system, new DSM-5 disorders are assigned to the best available ICD codes. DMS-5 and ICD-9-CM previously used the same codes. Some DSM-5 disorders are assigned to the same ICD code, which is unavoidable because the selection of diagnostic codes in DSM-5 is limited to those already included in ICD-9-CM. It was expected that DSM-5 and ICD-10-CM would be available at the same time in May 2013 when DSM-5 was published. Since ICD-10-CM was delayed until October 2015, DSM-5 used ICD-9-CM codes. The ICD-10-CM codes are now shown in parentheses in the DSM-5 book with the ICD-9-CM following the DSM-5 disorder. The names connected with the ICD-10-CM codes sometimes do not match the DSM-5 name. For example, the diagnosis of persistent depressive disorder in DSM-5 is classified to 300.4 in ICD-9-CM and F34.1 in ICD-10-CM as Dysthymic Disorder. The APA continues to work with the National Center for Health Statistics (NCHS) and the Centers for Medicare and Medicaid Services to include the new DSM-5 terms in ICD-10-CM. The APA and DSM-5 websites provide resources about the DSM-5 classification for mental disorders (APA 2019; APA 2018).

The purpose of DSM-5 is to provide clear descriptions of diagnostic categories that allow clinicians and investigators to diagnose, communicate about, study, and treat people with various mental disorders. Keep in mind that coders must assign diagnosis codes based on health record documentation by a provider who is legally qualified to render a medical diagnosis. DSM-5 uses the codes within ICD-9-CM and ICD-10-CM for all mental disorders, including personality disorders and intellectual disabilities, but the ICD system does not contain the detailed descriptions of how to diagnose these conditions as used by the psychiatrists and mental health practitioners. The GP v-5 book contains dual codes for every psychiatric diagnosis to account for the ICD-10-CM diagnosis codes. The inclusion of ICD-10-CM codes in the DSM-5 code book allows the physician or practitioner to assign valid ICD-10-CM codes for services after October 1, 2015 for the purposes of proper billing and insurance claims (APA 2017).

Coding Guidelines and Instructional Notes for ICD-10-CM Chapter 5

The NCHS has published chapter-specific guidelines for Chapter 5 in the *ICD-10-CM Official Guidelines for Coding and Reporting*. The coding student should review all of the coding guidelines for Chapter 5 of ICD-10-CM, which appear in an ICD-10-CM code book, at the CDC website (CDC 2019), or in appendix F.

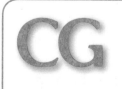

Chapter 5: Mental, Behavioral and Neurodevelopmental disorders (F01-F99)

Guideline I.C.5.a. Pain disorders related to psychological factors

Assign code F45.41 for pain that is exclusively related to psychological disorders. As indicated in the Excludes1 note under category G89, a code from category G89 should not be assigned with code F45.41.

Code F45.42, Pain disorders with related psychological factors, should be used with a code from category G89, Pain, not

(Continued)

(Continued)

elsewhere classified, if there is documentation of a psychological component for a patient with acute or chronic pain.

See Section I.C.6 Pain

Guideline I.C.5.b. Mental and behavioral disorders due to psychoactive substance use

1. In Remission

    Selection of codes for "in remission" for categories F10–F19, mental and behavioral disorders due to psychoactive substance use (categories F10–F19 with -11, -.21) requires the provider's clinical judgment. The appropriate codes for "in remission" are assigned only on the basis of provider documentation (as defined in the Official Guidelines for Coding and Reporting), unless otherwise instructed by the classification.

    Mild substance use disorders early or sustained remission are classified to the appropriate codes for substance abuse in remission, and moderate or severe substance use disorders in early or sustained remission are classified to appropriate codes for substance dependence in remission.

2. Psychoactive Substance Use, Abuse, and Dependence

    When the provider documentation refers to use, abuse and dependence of the same substance (that is, alcohol, opioid, cannabis, etc.), only one code should be assigned to identify the pattern of use based on the following hierarchy:

    - If both use and abuse are documented, assign only the code for abuse

    - If both abuse and dependence are documented, assign only the code for dependence

    - If use, abuse, and dependence are all documented, assign only the code for dependence

    - If both use and dependence are documented, assign only the code for dependence.

3. Psychoactive Substance Use, Unspecified

    As with all other unspecified diagnoses, the codes for unspecified psychoactive substance use (F10.9-, F11.9-, F12.9-, F13.9-, F14.9-, F15.9-, F16.9-, F18.9, F19.9) should only be assigned based on provider documentation and when they meet the definition of a reportable diagnosis (see Section III, Reporting Additional Diagnoses). These codes are to be used only when the psychoactive substance use is associated with

(Continued)

a physical, mental or behavioral disorder, and such a relationship is documented by the provider.

Guideline I.C.5.c. Factitious Disorder

Factitious disorder imposed on self or Munchausen's syndrome is a disorder in which a person falsely reports or causes his or her own physical or psychological signs or symptoms. For patients with documented factitious disorder on self or Munchausen's syndrome, assign the appropriate code from subcategory F68.1-, Factitious disorder imposed on self.

Munchausen's syndrome by proxy (MSBP) is a disorder in which a caregiver (perpetrator) falsely reports or causes an illness or injury in another person (victim) under his or her care, such as a child, an elderly adult, or a person who has a disability. The condition is also referred to as "factitious disorder imposed on another" or "factitious disorder by proxy." The perpetrator, not the victim, receives this diagnosis. Assign code F68.A, Factitious disorder imposed on another, to the perpetrator's record. For the victim of a patient suffering from MSBP, assign the appropriate code from categories T74, Adult and child abuse, neglect and other maltreatment, confirmed, or T76, Adult and child abuse, neglect and other maltreatment, suspected.

See Section I.C.19.f. Adult and child abuse, neglect and other maltreatment

Coding Mental, Behavioral and Neurodevelopmental Disorders in ICD-10-CM Chapter 5

The codes in this chapter include mental, behavioral, and neurodevelopmental disorders, including disorders of psychological development, but exclude symptoms, signs, and abnormal clinical laboratory findings (R00–R99). Chapter 5 of ICD-10-CM does not contain symptoms and signs that might be attributed to a mental or behavioral disorder. For example, category R25, Abnormal involuntary movements, contains symptoms of abnormal head movements, twitching, or tremors. However, when these symptoms are caused by conditions such as stereotyped movement disorders or tic disorders, the conditions are coded in categories F95 and F98 in Chapter 5 of ICD-10-CM.

Within Chapter 5 of ICD-10-CM, the behavioral health conditions are organized into related sections. Each section has specific Index entries with Includes, Excludes1, and Excludes2 notes, along with directional notes to further explain the coding of the conditions. The terminology used by the physicians must be carefully followed in the Index and Tabular List to code accurately.

The diagnosis codes must be used and reported to the highest level of specificity provided by the physician. In this chapter, many of the codes have been expanded to include related conditions and manifestations. An understanding of the diseases and updated clinical terminology in the behavioral health setting is crucial to accurately code the conditions treated. Coders should make no assumptions about the meaning of physician diagnostic statements; when in doubt, the physician should be asked for clarification.

Direction notes are included in the chapter to direct the coder how to use the codes appropriately. A note appears to explain what conditions are included in a section. For example, under the block of codes for mental disorders due to known physiological conditions (F01–F09), a note explains these codes include a group of mental disorders that have a common etiology in cerebral disease, brain injury, or other disorder leading to cerebral dysfunction. Other instructional notes appear to direct the coder when multiple coding is required to describe the coexistence of physical and psychological conditions.

Multiple Coding

When coding mental disorders, instructional notations to assign additional codes to fully describe the patient's condition are frequently encountered. Examples of such instructional notations follow:

- Instructional note to assign an additional code to identify any associated behavioral disorder

> **EXAMPLE:**   F01.51, Vascular dementia with behavioral disturbance
>
> Use additional code, if applicable, to identify wandering in vascular dementia (Z91.83)

- Instructional note to code first the underlying physiological condition

> **EXAMPLE:**   F07.0, Personality change due to known physiological condition
>
> Code first the underlying physiological condition

- Instructional note to code first the associated physical disorder

> **EXAMPLE:**   F54, Psychological and behavioral factors associated with disorders or disease classified elsewhere
>
> Code first the associated physical disorder, such as:
>
> Asthma (J45.-)
>
> Dermatitis (L23–L25)
>
> Gastric ulcer (K25.-)
>
> Mucous colitis (K58.-)
>
> Ulcerative colitis (K51.-)
>
> Urticaria (L50.-)

- Instructional note to use additional code to identify other conditions

  EXAMPLE: F84, Pervasive developmental disorders

  Use additional code to identify any associated medical condition and intellectual disabilities

Inclusion and Exclusion Notes

Chapter 5 of ICD-10-CM contains many special inclusion notes, such as those in the following two examples:

Inclusion note says that ecstasy, PCP, and phencyclidine are included in hallucinogen-related disorders, as these are hallucinogen drugs.

EXAMPLE: F16, Hallucinogen-related disorders
   Includes: ecstasy
        PCP
        phencyclidine

Inclusion note that serves to advise that conditions described as conversion hysteria, conversion reaction, hysteria, and hysteria psychosis are coded to category F44.

EXAMPLE: F44, Dissociative and conversion disorders
   Includes: conversion hysteria
        conversion reaction
        hysteria
        hysterical psychosis

Exclusion notes also are used frequently in Chapter 5 to warn that specified forms of a condition are classified elsewhere, such as

- The Excludes1 note advises that the codes for alcohol dependence and alcohol use cannot be used with code F10.1- for alcohol abuse as these terms are mutually exclusive. Patients will have only one of these conditions: abuse, dependence, or use.

  EXAMPLE: F10.1, Alcohol abuse
       Excludes1: Alcohol dependence (F10.2-)
            Alcohol use, unspecified (F10.9-)

- The Excludes2 note indicates that a code for cocaine-related disorders (F14.-) can be used with a code from other stimulant-related disorders (F15.-) because a patient can have both a stimulant-related disorder and a cocaine-related disorder. An Excludes2 note indicates that both conditions can be coded when a patient is treated for both conditions.

  EXAMPLE: F15, Other stimulant-related disorders
       Excludes2: cocaine-related disorders (F14.-)

Check Your Understanding 8.1

Answer the following questions about Chapter 5 of ICD-10-CM and the coding guidelines.

1. What is the purpose of DSM-5?

2. Can you find the detailed descriptions of how to diagnose conditions within chapter 5 of ICD-10-CM? If not, where are they located? What is included in chapter 5 of ICD-10-CM?

3. When a provider documents both use and dependence of a psychoactive substance in a patient's health record, what code(s) should be assigned by the coder?

4. Assign the appropriate code(s) for the following condition: Organic brain syndrome due to poorly controlled grand mal seizures

5. Assign the appropriate code(s) for the following condition: Major neurocognitive disorder with combative behavior and wandering

---

Alcohol-Related Disorders

ICD-10-CM Category F10, Alcohol-related disorders, with intoxication, withdrawal, and alcohol-induced related disorders, is further subdivided into three disorders:

- F10.1—Alcohol abuse

- F10.2—Alcohol dependence

- F10.9—Alcohol use, unspecified

According to DSM-5 criteria, **alcohol use disorder** describes a problematic pattern of alcohol use leading to clinically significant impairment or distress. DSM-5 removed the separate diagnoses of substance "dependence" and substance "abuse" and replaced them with a single diagnosis, "substance use disorder." A minimum of two to three criteria must be met in the patient's presentation to establish the diagnosis. For example, two to three criteria must be met for a mild substance use disorder diagnosis, while four to five is moderate, and six to seven is severe (APA 2019).

A criteria threshold is in place to establish a substance use disorder. As stated above, in DSM-5, it is a minimum of meeting two to three of the criteria to establish the diagnosis. Past abuse was one or more with three or more for dependence. Criteria are provided for a "substance use disorder" with severity judged on the number of criteria met. Also included are criteria for intoxication, withdrawal, substance-induced disorders, and unspecified substance-related disorders.

What might be documented by some physicians as alcoholism but is more appropriately diagnosed as alcohol dependence is classified to subcategory F10.2-, Alcohol dependence. The fifth character identifies the following:

- alcohol dependence, uncomplicated (F10.20)

- alcohol dependence, in remission (F10.21)

- alcohol dependence with intoxication (F10.22-) with a sixth character to identify alcohol dependence with intoxication, uncomplicated, with delirium, or unspecified as to the type

- alcohol dependence with withdrawal (F10.23-) with a sixth character to identify alcohol dependence with withdrawal uncomplicated, with delirium, with perceptional disturbance or unspecified as to the type

- alcohol dependence with alcohol-induced mood disorder (F10.24)

- alcohol dependence with alcohol-induced psychotic disorder (F10.25-) with a sixth character to identify alcohol dependence with delusions, hallucinations, or unspecified as to the type

- alcohol dependence with alcohol-induced persisting amnestic disorder (F10.26)

- alcohol dependence with alcohol-induced persisting dementia (F10.27)

- alcohol dependence with other alcohol-induced disorders (F10.28-) with a sixth character to identify alcohol dependence with anxiety disorder, sexual dysfunction, sleep disorder, and other alcohol-induced disorder

- alcohol dependence with unspecified alcohol-induced disorder (F10.29)

Other codes exist in ICD-10-CM for alcohol abuse (F10.1-) with fifth and sixth characters to classify alcohol abuse with intoxication, alcohol-induced mood disorder, alcohol-induced psychotic disorder, and other alcohol-induced disorders. When the terminology of "alcohol use" is used by a healthcare provider without further specification as to whether the disorder is a dependence or an abuse type, there are ICD-10-CM codes with five and six characters for alcohol use, unspecified, with other alcohol-induced disorders, such as anxiety disorder, sexual dysfunction, sleep disorder, and other alcohol-induced disorder (F10.9-).

Substance Use Disorders

DSM-5 does not use the terminology of substance abuse and substance dependence. Instead, the conditions are referred to substance use disorders, which are defined as mild, moderate, or severe to indicate the level of severity, which is determined by the number of diagnostic criteria met by the individual as outlined in the DSM-5 criteria. Substance use disorders are diagnosed when the recurrent use of drugs causes clinically and functionally significant impairment, such as health problems, disability, and failure to meet the responsibilities at work, school, or home. Substance abuse professionals use the criteria published in DSM-5 to make the diagnosis of substance use disorder in an individual based on evidence of impaired control, social impairment, risky use, and pharmacological criteria (SAMHSA 2019).

ICD-10-CM includes a series of three-character categories for drug-related disorders including abuse, dependence and use with intoxication, withdrawal, and other substance-related disorders.

- F11, Opioid-related disorders

- F12, Cannabis-related disorders

- F13, Sedative, hypnotic or anxiolytic-related disorders

- F14, Cocaine-related disorders

- F15, Other stimulant-related disorders

- F16, Hallucinogen-related disorders

- F17, Nicotine dependence

- F18, Inhalant-related disorders

- F19, Other psychoactive substance–related disorders

All of the categories have a similar outline: four-character codes for drug abuse, drug dependence, and drug use, unspecified. The codes are further divided into drug abuse, drug dependence, and drug use that exist with intoxication, mood disorder, psychotic disorder, and other drug-induced disorders. For example, opioid-related disorder category F11 includes codes for

- F11.120, Opioid abuse with intoxication, uncomplicated

- F11.24, Opioid dependence with opioid-induced mood disorder

- F11.251, Opioid dependence with opioid-induced psychotic disorder with hallucinations

- F11.982, Opioid use, unspecified, with opioid-induced sleep disorder

Nicotine Dependence

Codes exist in Chapter 5: Mental, Behavioral and Neurodevelopmental Disorders as well as other chapters of ICD-10-CM to describe the current or past use of nicotine or tobacco. Category F17, Nicotine dependence, is included in Chapter 5 of ICD-10-CM. Only nicotine dependence is included here as the terminology of nicotine abuse or use is not used. The provider documentation about the patient's tobacco use determines the code assigned:

- If the provider describes the patient as a "smoker" and the coder uses that term in the ICD-10-CM Alphabetic Index to Diseases, the coder is directed to see Dependence, drug, nicotine and assign a code from that category F17.

- If the provider simply documents tobacco use as a diagnosis for the patient, another code in Chapter 21 provides a description of the patient's status, that is, tobacco use, Z72.0.

- If a patient is no longer smoking or using tobacco products, a personal history of nicotine dependence, Z87.891, is present in Chapter 21: The Factors Influencing Health Status and Contact with Health Services.

- If a pregnant woman uses tobacco during her pregnancy, a code in Chapter 15: Pregnancy, Childbirth and the Puerperium, is available to describe smoking or tobacco use complicating the pregnancy (O99.33-), with a sixth character to identify the trimester of pregnancy of the woman. An additional code appears under this code to use additional code from F17 to identify the type of tobacco used.

The coder must consider the guidelines, I.C.5.b. Mental and behavioral disorders due to psychoactive substance use.

The coder cannot decide when to use the terminology of alcohol or drug use in remission as the codes must be based on the provider's documentation as described in the following guideline:

EXAMPLE: I.C.5.b.1. In Remission

Selection of codes for "in remission" for categories F10–F19, mental and behavioral disorders due to psychoactive substance use (categories F10–F19 with -11, -.21) requires the provider's clinical judgment. The appropriate codes for "in remission" are assigned only on the basis of provider documentation (as defined in the *Official*

Guidelines for Coding and Reporting), unless otherwise instructed by the classification. Mild substance use disorders in early or sustained remission are classified to the appropriate codes for substance abuse in remission, and moderate or severe substance use disorders in early or sustained remission are classified to the appropriate codes for substance dependence in remission.

It is common for different providers to describe the patient's use, abuse, or dependence on the same substance within the same record for the same encounter. The documentation of the attending physician should be the clinical information used to code. Only one code should be assigned, even when the physician describes the patient's disorder as use, abuse, and dependence according to the hierarchy provided in the following guideline:

EXAMPLE: I.C.5.b.2. Psychoactive Substance Use, Abuse, and Dependence

When the provider documentation refers to use, abuse and dependence of the same substance (that is, alcohol, opioid, cannabis, etc.), only one code should be assigned to identify the pattern of use based on the following hierarchy:

If both use and abuse are documented, assign only the code for abuse.

If both abuse and dependence are documented, assign only the code for dependence.

If use, abuse, and dependence are all documented, assign only the code for dependence.

If both use and dependence are documented, assign only the code for dependence.

As the following guideline states, the coders should assign codes for psychoactive substance use only when the condition meets the definition of a reportable diagnosis, usually as an additional diagnosis. A reportable diagnosis is a condition that affects patient care in terms of requiring either clinical evaluation or therapeutic treatment or diagnostic procedures or extended length of hospital stay or increased nursing care or monitoring.

EXAMPLE: I.C.5.b.3. Psychoactive Substance Use, Unspecified

As with all other unspecified diagnoses, the codes for unspecified psychoactive substance use (F10.9-, F11.9-, F12.9-, F13.9-, F14.9-, F15.9-, F16.9-, F18.9-, F19.9-) should only be assigned based on provider documentation and when they meet the definition of a reportable diagnosis (see Section III, Reporting Additional Diagnoses). The codes are to be used only when the psychoactive substance use is associated with a physical, mental or behavioral disorder, and such a relationship is documented by the provider.

Other Mental, Behavioral, and Neurodevelopmental Disorders (F20–F29)

Categories F20–F29 contain blocks of codes that classify schizophrenia, schizotypal, delusional, and other nonmood psychotic disorders. Specific forms of schizophrenia are contained in category F20, Schizophrenia, such as paranoid, disorganized, catatonic, undifferentiated, residual, and other forms of schizophrenia. **Schizophrenia** is a chronic mental health condition that can be a severe and disabling disorder in some patients while other individuals with the condition can cope with the symptoms and lead normal lives. Some individuals with schizophrenia hear voices, may not make sense when they talk, and believe other people are controlling their thoughts or intending to harm them. While some patients can be independent while taking their medications, other patients have difficulty holding a job or caring for themselves so they rely on family and others for assistance with their day-to-day lives (NLM 2019a).

Mood (affective) disorders are classified with the codes in the block of codes from F30 to F39. A **bipolar disorder** is also known as manic-depressive illness. Various forms of this illness are classified with category F31 to the fifth character level for the specific forms of the illness. Bipolar disorder or manic-depressive illness, psychosis, or reaction is a mental health disorder that produces unusual mood swings in a patient as well as varying levels of functioning, for example, in handling the everyday activities of daily life. The bipolar disorder usually develops when a person is in his or her late teen or early adult years. Patients with bipolar disorder experience intense emotional episodes that can be overly excited, which are called manic episodes. ICD-10-CM contains codes in the range from F31.0 to F31.2 for manic episodes. The patient can experience a sad and hopeless state that is called a depressive episode. ICD-10-CM contains codes in the range from F31.30 to F31.5 for depressive episodes. Physicians may also describe a patient as having a mixed state, which includes symptoms of both mania and depression. A patient with a mixed type of bipolar disorder is classified to the range of codes from F31.60 to F31.64. A patient with bipolar disorder may be very irritable and explosive during a mood episode. People with bipolar disorder may also abuse alcohol or other substances, have difficulty maintaining positive personal relationships, and perform poorly in school or on the job. Often, these problems are not recognized as a sign of this major mental illness. Bipolar disease is a long-term illness, and patients need long-term treatment to maintain control of their symptoms. There are effective treatments using medications and psychotherapy for reducing the severity of a patient's symptoms and preventing a relapse (NLM 2019b).

Code F41.1 classifies **generalized anxiety disorder (GAD)**. This condition is usually diagnosed in patients who are excessively worried about many things even when there is little to no reason to worry about them. The patients are very anxious about activities of daily life. They expect things will go poorly for them, and this keeps them from doing normal everyday tasks. GAD may be an inherited condition. It may develop slowly, often starting during the teen years or early adult life. Symptoms get better and worse over time and are often severe during times of stress. Better treatments have been developed as researchers learn more about fear and anxiety as it is produced in the brain. The condition is first suspected in a patient who complains about headaches, stomach and muscle aches, unexplained pain, and difficulty sleeping with feeling tired all the time. It is hard to diagnose as it develops slowly and may take time to be diagnosed while other causes are ruled out. Patients worry about everyday things, have trouble controlling their constant worries, have a hard time concentrating in school and on the job, and are not able to relax. GAD is usually treated with psychotherapy, medication, or both. Cognitive behavior therapy is often useful for the patient by teaching the patient different ways to think, behave, and react to situations that they worry about. Two types of medications that may be beneficial include antianxiety medications and antidepressants (NLM 2019c).

An **eating disorder** is an illness that causes disturbances in eating, such as consuming very small amounts of food or consuming excessive amounts of food. A person with an eating disorder usually has severe concerns about his or her body weight or appearance. Eating disorders frequently begin during teen and young adult years but may also start in childhood or later in life. Common eating disorders are anorexia nervosa, bulimia nervosa, and binge eating disorder. These conditions are treatable medical and mental illnesses. Frequently, the conditions coexist with other mental illnesses such as depression, anxiety disorders, and substance abuse. If a patient does not seek or receive treatment, the conditions can be life threatening. Some patients who do not continue their treatment are frequently hospitalized. Patients with anorexia nervosa require hospital care because of severe metabolic disorder and nutritional deficiencies that result from the condition that make the individual very ill. ICD-10-CM classifies the various forms of eating disorders that exist. Code F50.01, Anorexia nervosa restricting type, and code F50.02, anorexia nervosa binge eating/purging type are available to classify the patient. Other codes exist for bulimia nervosa (F50.2), other eating disorders (F50.3), and unspecified types of eating disorders (F50.9) in ICD-10-CM (NLM 2019d).

ICD-10-CM provides a block of codes for disorders of adult personality and behavior (F60–F69). One example of a condition classified with a code from this section is **borderline personality disorder**, code F60.3. This is a serious mental illness marked by unstable moods with difficulty in controlling behavior and maintaining positive interpersonal relationships. Most people who suffer from borderline personality disorder have problems regulating their emotions and thoughts and exhibit impulsive and reckless behavior. As a result, the patients have unstable relationships with other people including multiple marriages and alienating friends. Patients with this disorder also have other mental health illnesses such as depression, anxiety, substance abuse, and eating disorders. The condition is difficult to identify and often underdiagnosed or misdiagnosed. Borderline personality disorder can be treated with different types of psycho-therapy, such as cognitive behavioral therapy, dialectical behavior therapy, and schema-focused therapy. It is important for the therapy to be effective, so the patient must get along with and trust the therapist; otherwise the patient often abandons the treatment. Unfortunately, there are no medications recognized as effective to treat the condition. However, some patients benefit from medications to treat their symptoms of anxiety, depression, and aggression (NIH 2017).

Intellectual disabilities (F70–F79) is another description for mental retardation. The phrase intellectual disabilities is used to describe a person's ability to learn and function at an expected level for his or her age in the activities of daily life. The level of intellectual disability can vary for both children and adults with this condition. Some individuals have very minor problems, while others are severely disabled by the lack of ability to function at a normal level. The intellectual disabilities can be coded according to the severity of the disability as described by the physician as mild (F70), moderate (F71), profound (F72), severe (F73), or if the patient has other intellectual disability (F78) or if simply stated the patient has an intellectual disability that is coded to an unspecified code (F79). An Excludes1 note appears under section F70–F79, Intellectual Disabilities that states "borderline intellectual functioning, IQ above 70 to 84, is to be coded to a symptom code of R41.83" (CDC n.d.).

There is an instructional note that follows the section heading to code first any associated physical or developmental disorder. In ICD-10-CM, the associated physical or developmental disorder is listed first, followed by the appropriate code from F70 to F79.

Factitious Disorder

Factitious disorder imposed on self (Munchausen's syndrome) is a disorder in which a person falsely reports or causes his or her own physical or psychological signs or symptoms. For patients with documented factitious disorder on self (Munchausen's syndrome), assign the appropriate code from subcategory F68.1-, Factitious disorder imposed on self.

Munchausen's syndrome by proxy (MSBP) is a disorder in which a caregiver (perpetrator) falsely reports or causes an illness or injury in another person (victim) under his or her care, such as a child, an elderly adult, or a person who has a disability. The condition is also referred to as "factitious disorder imposed on another" or "factitious disorder by proxy." The perpetrator, not the victim, receives this diagnosis. Assign code F68.A, Factitious disorder imposed on another, to the perpetrator's record. For the victim of a patient suffering from MSBP, assign the appropriate code from categories T74, Adult and child abuse, neglect and other maltreatment, confirmed, or T76, Adult and child abuse, neglect and other maltreatment, suspected.

Check Your Understanding 8.2

Assign diagnosis codes to the following conditions.

1. Bipolar disorder, partial remission with most recent episode as mixed
2. Hoarding disorder
3. Attention deficit hyperactivity disorder, predominantly inattentive presentation
4. Pathological gambling
5. Factitious disorder on self including physical signs
6. Prolonged grief with anxiety and depressed mood
7. Body dysmorphic disorder
8. Neurotic hypochondria
9. Social anxiety disorder of childhood
10. Panic attack

ICD-10-PCS Coding for Procedures Related to Mental Health and Substance Abuse Services

Therapies for patients that include behavior health procedures have ICD-10-PCS procedures in the Mental Health (GZ1–GZJ) and Substance Abuse (HZ2–HZ9) sections. Within the Mental Health section, the procedures available to be coded include psychological tests, crisis intervention, individual psychotherapy, and counseling. Within the Substance Abuse section, the services available to be coded include detoxification, counseling, and psychotherapy.

ICD-10-PCS Index Entries for Mental Health and Substance Abuse

In ICD-10-PCS, there are Index entries for mental health and substance abuse treatment procedures under "substance abuse treatment" and under the titles of the various procedures for both mental health and substance abuse therapy. For example, under substance abuse treatment are entries for counseling, detoxification services, medication management, pharmacotherapy, and psychotherapy. These same procedure titles are listed under separate entries in the Index as well. Currently, there are no specific coding guidelines published for coding mental health and substance abuse treatment procedures.

Mental Health Section GZ1–GZJ

Services provided to patients with mental, behavioral, and neurodevelopment disorders are included in the Mental Health section GZ1–GZJ in ICD-10-PCS and are built using the following characters:

Character 1: Section
Character 2: Body System

Character 3: Root Type
Character 4: Qualifier
Character 5: Qualifier
Character 6: Qualifier
Character 7: Qualifier

Section

Character 1, which represents the Mental Health section, uses the value G.

Body System

The body system is not specified for mental health. The placeholder character value of Z is reported in the second character position.

Root Type

Character 3 is for the root type that is applicable to the Medical Health section. There are 12 root types; the value and the definition are as follows:

- Psychological Tests (value 1)—The administration and interpretation of standardized psychological tests and measurement instruments for the assessment of psychological function

- Crisis Intervention (value 2)—Treatment of a traumatized, acutely disturbed, or distressed individual for the purpose of short-term stabilization

- Medication Management (value 3)—Monitoring and adjusting the use of medications for the treatment of a mental health disorder

- Individual Psychotherapy (value 5)—Treatment of an individual with a mental health disorder by behavioral, cognitive, psychoanalytic, psychodynamic, or psychophysiological means to improve functioning or well-being

- Counseling (value 6)—The application of psychological methods to treat and individual with normal developmental issues and psychological problems in order to increase function, improve well-being, alleviate distress or maladjustment, or resolve crisis

- Family Psychotherapy (value 7)—Treatment that includes one or more family members of an individual with a mental health disorder by behavioral, cognitive, psychoanalytic, psychodynamic, or psychophysiological means to improve functioning or well-being

- Electroconvulsive Therapy (value B)—The application of controlled electrical voltages to treat a mental health disorder

- Biofeedback (value C)—Provision of information from the monitoring and regulating of physiological processes in conjunction with cognitive-behavioral techniques to improve patient functioning or well-being

- Hypnosis (value F)—Induction of a state of heightened suggestibility by auditory, visual, and tactile techniques to elicit an emotional or behavioral response

- Narcosynthesis (value G)—Administration of intravenous barbiturates in order to release suppressed or repressed thoughts

- Group Psychotherapy (value H)—Treatment of two or more individuals with a mental health disorder by behavioral, cognitive, psychoanalytic, psychodynamic, or psycho-physiological means to improve functioning or well-being

- Light Therapy (value J)—Application of specialized light treatments to improve functioning or well-being

Qualifier Character 4

Character 4 further specifies the root type procedure:

Psychological Tests
    0—Developmental
    1—Personality and Behavioral
    2—Intellectual and Psychoeducational
    3—Neuropsychological
    4—Neurobehavioral and Cognitive Status

Individual Psychotherapy
    0—Interactive
    1—Behavioral
    2—Cognitive
    3—Interpersonal
    4—Psychoanalysis
    5—Psychodynamic
    6—Supportive
    8—Cognitive-Behavioral
    9—Psychophysiological

Counseling
    0—Educational
    1—Vocational
    3—Other counseling

Family Psychotherapy
    2—Other Family Psychotherapy

Electroconvulsive Therapy
    0—Unilateral–Single Seizure
    1—Unilateral–Multiple Seizure
    2—Bilateral–Single Seizure
    3—Bilateral–Multiple Seizure
    4—Other Electroconvulsive therapy

Biofeedback
    9—Other biofeedback

All other root types: Crisis Intervention, Medication Management, Hypnosis, Narcosynthesis, Group Psychotherapy, and Light Therapy

    Z—None

Qualifier Character 5

This qualifier represents an additional attribute for the procedure when applicable. Currently, there are no qualifiers in the Mental Health section. Therefore, the placeholder character value of Z is reported for character 5.

Qualifier Character 6

This qualifier represents an additional attribute for the procedure when applicable. Currently, there are no qualifiers in the Mental Health section. Therefore, the placeholder character value of Z is reported for character 6.

Qualifier Character 7

This qualifier represents an additional attribute for the procedure when applicable. Currently, there are no qualifiers in the Mental Health section. Therefore, the placeholder character value of Z is reported for character 7.

Substance Abuse Section HZ2–HZ9

Services provided to patients with substance abuse disorders are included in the Substance Abuse section HZ2–HZ9 in ICD-10-PCS and are built using the following characters:

Character 1: Section
Character 2: Body System
Character 3: Root Type
Character 4: Qualifier
Character 5: Qualifier
Character 6: Qualifier
Character 7: Qualifier

Section

Character 1, which represents the Substance Abuse section, uses the value H.

Body System

The body system is not specified for substance. The placeholder character value of Z is reported in the second character position.

Root Type

Character 3 is for the root type that applicable to the Substance Abuse section. There are seven root types; the value and the definition are as follows:

- Detoxification Services (value 2)—Detoxification from alcohol or drugs

- Individual Counseling (value 3)—The application of psychological methods to treat an individual with addictive behavior

- Group Counseling (value 4)—The application of psychological methods to treat two or more individuals with addictive behavior

- Individual Psychotherapy (value 5)—Treatment of an individual with addictive behavior by behavioral, cognitive, psychoanalytic, psychodynamic, or psychophysiological means

- Family Counseling (value 6)—The application of psychological methods that includes one or more family members to treat an individual with addictive behavior

- Medication Management (value 8)—Monitoring and adjusting the use of replacement medications for the treatment of addiction

- Pharmacotherapy (value 9)—The use of replacement medications for the treatment of addiction

Qualifier Character 4

Character 4 further specifies the root type procedure:

Detoxification
    Z—None

Individual Counseling
    0—Cognitive
    1—Behavioral
    2—Cognitive-Behavioral
    3—12-step
    4—Interpersonal
    5—Vocational
    6—Psychoeducation
    7—Motivational Enhancement
    8—Confrontational
    9—Continuing Care
    B—Spiritual
    C—Pre-/Post-Test Infectious Disease

Group Counseling
    0—Cognitive
    1—Behavioral
    2—Cognitive-Behavioral
    3—12-step
    4—Interpersonal
    5—Vocational
    6—Psychoeducation
    7—Motivational Enhancement
    8—Confrontational
    9—Continuing Care
    B—Spiritual
    C—Pre-/Post-Test Infectious Disease

Individual Psychotherapy
    0—Cognitive
    1—Behavioral
    2—Cognitive-Behavioral
    3—12-step
    4—Interpersonal

5—Interactive
6—Psychoeducation
7—Motivational Enhancement
8—Confrontational
9—Supportive
B—Psychoanalysis
C—Psychodynamic
D—Psychophysiological

Family Counseling
3—Other Family Counseling

Medication Management
0—Nicotine Replacement
1—Methadone Maintenance
2—Levo-alpha-acetylmethadol (LAAM)
3—Antabuse
4—Naltrexone
5—Naloxone
6—Clonidine
7—Bupropion
8—Psychiatric Medication
9—Other Replacement Medication

Pharmacotherapy
0—Nicotine Replacement
1—Methadone Maintenance
2—Levo-alpha-acetylmethadol (LAAM)
3—Antabuse
4—Naltrexone
5—Naloxone
6—Clonidine
7—Bupropion
8—Psychiatric Medication
9—Other Replacement Medication

Qualifier Character 5

This qualifier represents an additional attribute for the procedure when applicable. Currently, there are no qualifiers in the Substance Abuse section. Therefore, the placeholder character value of Z is reported for character 5.

Qualifier Character 6

This qualifier represents an additional attribute for the procedure when applicable. Currently, there are no qualifiers in the Substance Abuse section. Therefore, the placeholder character value of Z is reported for character 6.

Qualifier Character 7

This qualifier represents an additional attribute for the procedure when applicable. Currently, there are no qualifiers in the Substance Abuse section. Therefore, the placeholder character value of Z is reported for character 7.

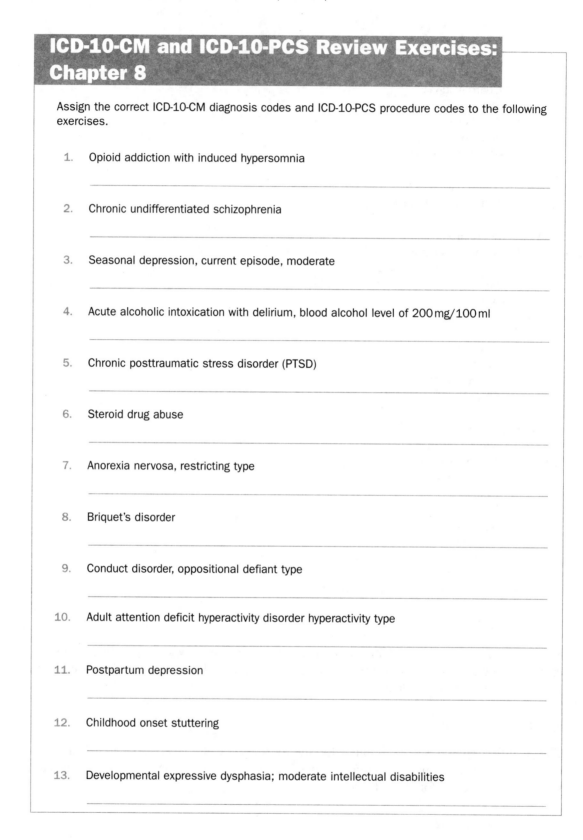

ICD-10-CM and ICD-10-PCS Review Exercises: Chapter 8

Assign the correct ICD-10-CM diagnosis codes and ICD-10-PCS procedure codes to the following exercises.

1. Opioid addiction with induced hypersomnia

2. Chronic undifferentiated schizophrenia

3. Seasonal depression, current episode, moderate

4. Acute alcoholic intoxication with delirium, blood alcohol level of 200 mg/100 ml

5. Chronic posttraumatic stress disorder (PTSD)

6. Steroid drug abuse

7. Anorexia nervosa, restricting type

8. Briquet's disorder

9. Conduct disorder, oppositional defiant type

10. Adult attention deficit hyperactivity disorder hyperactivity type

11. Postpartum depression

12. Childhood onset stuttering

13. Developmental expressive dysphasia; moderate intellectual disabilities

ICD-10-CM and ICD-10-PCS Review Exercises: Chapter 8 (continued)

14. Cigarette dependence smoker (listed as a diagnosis by physician as part of the final diagnoses in the discharge summary)

   _____

15. Cocaine abuse with cocaine-induced sleep disorder

   _____

16. PROCEDURE: Individual psychophysiological psychotherapy for mental health treatment

   _____

17. PROCEDURE: Electroconvulsive therapy, bilateral, single seizure

   _____

18. PROCEDURE: Intellectual and psychoeducational psychological test

   _____

19. PROCEDURE: Family counseling for substance abuse treatment

   _____

20. PROCEDURE: Drug detoxification treatment for substance abuse

   _____

References

American Psychiatric Association (APA). 2019a. https://www.psychiatry.org/.

American Psychiatric Association (APA). 2019b. Substance Related and Addictive Disorders. https://www.psychiatry.org/psychiatrists/practice/dsm/educational-resources/dsm-5-fact-sheets.

American Psychiatric Association (APA). 2018. Diagnostic and Statistical Manual of Mental Disorders (DSM–5). https://www.psychiatry.org/psychiatrists/practice/dsm.

American Psychiatric Association (APA). 2017. Guide to Using DSM-5 In the Transition to ICD-10. http://psychnews.psychiatryonline.org/doi/full/10.1176/appi.pn.2015.8b15.

Centers for Medicare and Medicaid Services (CMS). 2019. *ICD-10-PCS Official Guidelines for Coding and Reporting*, 2020. http://www.cms.gov/Medicare/Coding/ICD10/.

Centers for Disease Control and Prevention (CDC). n.d. Facts About Intellectual Disability. http://www.cdc.gov/ncbddd/actearly/pdf/parents_pdfs/IntellectualDisability.pdf.

National Institute of Health (NIH). 2017. Borderline Personality Disorder. http://www.nimh.nih.gov/health/topics/borderline-personality-disorder/index.shtml.

Substance Abuse and Mental Health Services Administration (SAMHSA). 2019. Substance Abuse Disorders. http://www.samhsa.gov/disorders/substance-use.

U.S. National Library of Medicine, MedLinePlus (NLM). 2019a. Schizophrenia. https://www.nlm.nih.gov/medlineplus/schizophrenia.html.

U.S. National Library of Medicine, MedLinePlus (NLM). 2019b. Bipolar Disorder. https://www.nlm.nih.gov/medlineplus/bipolardisorder.html.

U.S. National Library of Medicine, MedLinePlus (NLM). 2019c. Generalized Anxiety Disorder. https://www.nlm.nih.gov/medlineplus/ency/article/000917.htm.

U.S. National Library of Medicine, MedLinePlus (NLM). 2019d. Eating Disorders. https://www.nlm.nih.gov/medlineplus/eatingdisorders.html.

Chapter 9

Diseases of the Nervous System (G00–G99)

Learning Objectives

At the conclusion of this chapter, you should be able to do the following:

- Describe the organization of the conditions and codes included in Chapter 6 of ICD-10-CM, Diseases of the Nervous System (G00–G99)

- Differentiate the coding of hemiplegia and hemiparesis and other paralytic conditions

- Distinguish the coding of epilepsy, seizures, and convulsions

- Describe different types of headaches coded with ICD-10-CM

- Assign ICD-10-CM codes for diseases of the nervous system

- Assign ICD-10-PCS code for procedures related to diseases of the nervous system

Key Terms

Bypass
Central pain syndrome
Cerebral palsy
Dementia
Epilepsy
Hemiplegia
Meningitis
Migraine

Mild cognitive impairment
Neoplasm-related pain
Release
Repair
Reposition
Seizure
Transfer

Overview of ICD-10-CM Chapter 6: Diseases of the Nervous System

Chapter 6 of ICD-10-CM includes categories G00–G99 arranged in the following blocks:

G00–G09	Inflammatory diseases of the central nervous system
G10–G14	Systemic atrophies primarily affecting the central nervous system
G20–G26	Extrapyramidal and movement disorders
G30–G32	Other degenerative diseases of the nervous system
G35–G37	Demyelinating diseases of the central nervous system
G40–G47	Episodic and paroxysmal disorders
G50–G59	Nerve, nerve root and plexus disorders
G60–G65	Polyneuropathies and other disorders of the peripheral nervous system
G70–G73	Diseases of myoneural junction and muscle
G80–G83	Cerebral palsy and other paralytic syndromes
G89–G99	Other disorders of the nervous system

Chapter 6 of ICD-10-CM contains diseases of the nervous system. Figure 9.1 illustrates the anatomical structure of the brain. Figure 9.2 illustrates the peripheral nervous system. Conditions within the central nervous system, including the brain and spinal cord, as well as disorders of the peripheral nervous system are included in this chapter in ICD-10-CM.

Figure 9.1. **Anatomy of the brain**

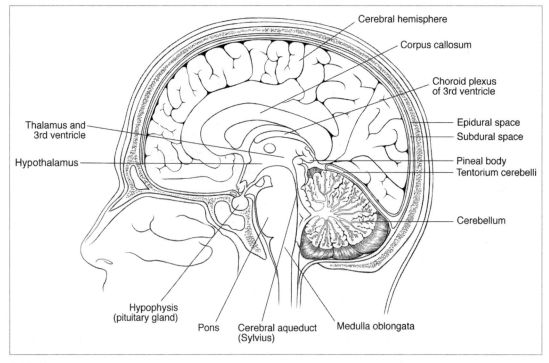

© AHIMA

Figure 9.2. **Peripheral nervous system**

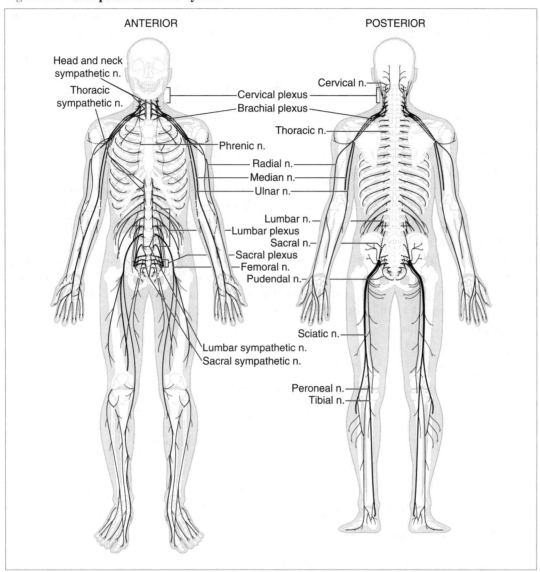

ANTERIOR   POSTERIOR

Head and neck sympathetic n.

Thoracic sympathetic n.

Cervical n.

Cervical plexus

Brachial plexus

Thoracic n.

Phrenic n.

Radial n.

Median n.

Ulnar n.

Lumbar n.

Lumbar plexus

Sacral n.

Sacral plexus

Femoral n.

Pudendal n.

Sciatic n.

Lumbar sympathetic n.

Sacral sympathetic n.

Peroneal n.

Tibial n.

© AHIMA

A number of codes include a combination of conditions, such as persistent migraine aura with cerebral infarction, intractable (G43.61-). Additionally, a number of codes for diseases of the nervous system include facts concerning the onset of the disease. For example, G30.0, Alzheimer's disease with early onset, and G30.1, Alzheimer's disease with late onset, are available in ICD-10-CM. ICD-10-CM has codes for the nervous system diseases that exist with and without associated symptoms. For example, there are two codes for phantom limb syndrome, differentiating whether pain is present or not (G54.6–G54.7).

Classification of sleep disorders is included in Chapter 6 instead of in the signs and symptoms chapter. Sleep apnea has its own subcategory with fifth-character specificity identifying the type.

Epilepsy and recurrent seizures are classified to category G40 in ICD-10-CM. The Alphabetic Index also refers the coder to category G40 for the diagnosis of "seizure disorder."

In contrast, the diagnoses of "seizure(s)" or "convulsion(s)" or "convulsive seizure" are classified to a symptom code, R56.9 in category R56, Convulsions, not elsewhere classified. Coders must follow the Alphabetic Index entries cautiously to distinguish these diagnoses when coding.

Coding Guidelines and Instructional Notes for ICD-10-CM Chapter 6

At the start of Chapter 6 in ICD-10-CM, a series of excluded conditions are listed that are applicable to all conditions classifiable to Chapter 6. For example, at the start of Chapter 6 of ICD-10-CM, there is an Excludes2 note that states conditions from other chapters can be used in addition to the codes for diseases of the nervous system. For example, if the patient also has certain conditions originating in the perinatal period, codes from categories P04–P96 may be assigned with the nervous system condition.

Throughout the chapter, there are instructional notes to "use additional code to identify organism," "code first underlying disease," "use additional code for adverse effect, if applicable, to identify drug," and "code also any associated condition" (CDC 2019). Multiple coding is frequently required to fully describe diseases of the nervous system. Examples of these instructional notes include

- G00.2, Streptococcal meningitis

    ◦ Use additional code to further identify organism (B95.0–B95.5)

- G53, Cranial nerve disorders in diseases classified elsewhere

    ◦ Code first underlying disease, such as neoplasm (C00–D49)

- G90.4, Autonomic dysreflexia

    ◦ Use additional code to identify the cause, such as fecal impaction (K56.41), pressure ulcer (pressure area) (L89.-), or urinary tract infection (N39.0)

- G47.3, Sleep Apnea

    ◦ Code also any associated underlying condition

Another instructional note appears in ICD-10-CM beneath category G89, Pain, not elsewhere classified, stating, "Code also related psychological factors associated with pain (F45.42)."

> An Excludes1 note here at code G89, Pain, not elsewhere classified, reminds the coders what is not coded with codes from category G89, specifically generalized pain (R52), pain disorders exclusively related to psychological factors (F45.41), or pain unspecified (R52) (CDC 2019). In addition, there is an Excludes2 note that reminds the coder what other pain codes can be assigned with a code from category G89, Pain, not elsewhere classified. The category G89 codes describe acute pain, chronic pain, and neoplasm-related pain. Included in the Excludes2 codes under category G89 are codes for the site of the pain, such as abdominal or back, with other terms such as myalgia or pain from prosthetic devices, implants, and grafts (CDC 2019).

The NCHS has published chapter-specific guidelines for Chapter 6 in the *ICD-10-CM Official Guidelines for Coding and Reporting*. The coding student should review all of the coding guidelines for Chapter 6 of ICD-10-CM, which appears in an ICD-10-CM code book or at the CDC website (CDC 2019) or in appendix F.

CG

Chapter 6 : Diseases of the Nervous System (G00-G99)

Guideline I.C.6.a. Dominant/nondominant side: Codes from category G81, hemiplegia and hemiparesis, and subcategories G83.1–G83.3, Monoplegia of lower limb, upper limb or unspecified, identify whether the dominant or non-dominant side is affected. Should the affected side be documented, but not specified as dominant or non-dominant, and the classification does not indicate a default, code selection is as follows:

- For ambidextrous patients, the default should be dominant

- If the left side is affected, the default is non-dominant

- If the right side is affected, the default is dominant

Guidelines I.C.6.b. Pain—Category G89

1. General coding information

   Codes in category G89, Pain, not elsewhere classified, may be used in conjunction with codes from other categories and chapters to provide more detail about acute or chronic pain and neoplasm-related pain, unless otherwise indicated below.

   If the pain is not specified as acute or chronic, post-thoracotomy, postprocedural, or neoplasm-related, do not assign codes from category G89.

   A code from category G89 should not be assigned if the underlying (definitive) diagnosis is known, unless the reason for the encounter is pain control/management and not management of the underlying condition

   When an admission or encounter is for a procedure aimed at treating the underlying condition (e.g., spinal fusion, kyphoplasty), a code for the underlying condition (e.g., vertebral fracture, spinal stenosis) should be assigned as the principal diagnosis. No code from category G89 should be assigned.

   a. Category G89 Codes as Principal or First-listed Diagnosis

   Category G89 codes are acceptable as principal diagnosis or the first-listed code:

   - When pain control or pain management is the reason for the admission/encounter (e.g., a patient with displaced intervertebral disc, nerve impingement and severe back pain presents for injection of steroid into

   (Continued)

(Continued)

the spinal canal). The underlying cause of the pain should be reported as an additional diagnosis, if known.

- When a patient is admitted for the insertion of a neurostimulator for pain control, assign the appropriate pain code as the principal or first-listed diagnosis. When an admission or encounter is for a procedure aimed at treating the underlying condition and a neurostimulator is inserted for pain control during the same admission/encounter, a code for the underlying condition should be assigned as the principal diagnosis and the appropriate pain code should be assigned as a secondary diagnosis

b. Use of Category G89 Codes in Conjunction with Site Specific Pain Codes

i. Assigning Category G89 and Site-Specific Pain Codes

Codes from category G89 may be used in conjunction with codes that identify the site of pain (including codes from chapter 18) if the category G89≈code provides additional information. For example, if the code describes the site of the pain, but does not fully describe whether the pain is acute or chronic, then both codes should be assigned.

ii. Sequencing of Category G89 Codes with Site-Specific Pain Codes

The sequencing of category G89 codes with site-specific pain codes (including chapter 18 codes), is dependent on the circumstances of the encounter/admission as follows:

- If the encounter is for pain control or pain management, assign the code from category G89 followed by the code identifying the specific site of pain (e.g., encounter for pain management for acute neck pain from trauma is assigned code G89.11, Acute pain due to trauma, followed by code M54.2, Cervicalgia, to identify the site of pain).

- If the encounter is for any other reason except pain control or pain management, and a related definitive diagnosis has not been established (confirmed) by the provider, assign the code for the specific site of pain first, followed by the appropriate code from category G89.

2. Pain due to devices, implants and grafts

   See Section I.C.19. Pain due to medical devices

3. Postoperative Pain

   The provider's documentation should be used to guide the coding of postoperative pain, as well as *Section III. Reporting Additional Diagnoses and Section IV. Diagnostic Coding and Reporting in the Outpatient Setting.*

   The default for post-thoracotomy and other postoperative pain not specified as acute or chronic is the code for the acute form.

   Routine or expected postoperative pain immediately after surgery should not be coded.

   a. Postoperative pain not associated with specific postoperative complication

      Postoperative pain not associated with a specific postoperative complication is assigned to the appropriate postoperative pain code in category G89.

   b. Postoperative pain associated with specific postoperative complication

      Postoperative pain associated with a specific postoperative complication (such as painful wire sutures) is assigned to the appropriate code(s) found in Chapter 19, Injury, poisoning, and certain other consequences of external causes. If appropriate, use additional code(s) from category G89 to identify acute or chronic pain (G89.18 or G89.28).

4. Chronic pain

   Chronic pain is classified to subcategory G89.2. There is no time frame defining when pain becomes chronic pain. The provider's documentation should be used to guide use of these codes.

5. Neoplasm Related Pain

   Code G89.3 is assigned to pain documented as being related, associated or due to cancer, primary or secondary malignancy, or tumor. This code is assigned regardless of whether the pain is acute or chronic.

   This code may be assigned as the principal or first-listed code when the stated reason for the admission/encounter is documented as pain control/pain management. The underlying neoplasm should be reported as an additional diagnosis.

(Continued)

(Continued)

When the reason for the admission/encounter is management of the neoplasm and the pain associated with the neoplasm is also documented, code G89.3 may be assigned as an additional diagnosis. It is not necessary to assign an additional code for the site of the pain.

See Section I.C.2 for instructions on the sequencing of neoplasms for all other stated reasons for the admission/ encounter (except for pain control/pain management).

6. Chronic pain syndrome

Central pain syndrome (G89.0) and chronic pain syndrome (G89.4) are different than the term "chronic pain," and therefore codes should only be used when the provider has specifically documented this condition.

See Section I.C.5. Pain disorders related to psychological factors

Coding Diseases of the Nervous System for ICD-10-CM Chapter 6

Chapter 6: Diseases of the Nervous System (G00–G99) includes diseases of the central and peripheral nervous systems as well as epilepsy, migraine, and other headache syndromes. Laterality is included in the nerve root and plexus disorders to identify whether the mononeuropathy occurs on the right or left side. Codes from category G81, Hemiplegia and hemiparesis, and subcategories G83.1-, G83.2-, G83.3-, Monoplegias, identify whether the right or left dominant or nondominant side is affected.

Meningitis

Meningitis is the inflammation of the meninges, which cover the brain and the spinal cord. Figure 9.3 illustrates the layers of the cerebral meninges. The three layers of the meninges are the dura mater, pia mater, and arachnoid membrane. The most common type of meningitis is viral meningitis. Bacterial meningitis occurs less frequently than does viral meningitis and can be life threatening. The pia mater and the arachnoid membrane can be inflamed by bacterial meningitis (Mosby 2017, 831). Both conditions can start with a cold-like infection. The infection can damage blood vessels in the brain and lead to a stroke and cause other organ damage. Pneumococcal and meningococcal infections can cause bacterial meningitis. Symptoms of meningitis include a sudden fever, stiff neck, and headache. Meningitis can progress rapidly but can be treated to prevent serious complications including death. Since meningitis frequently occurs in adolescents and young adults living in dorms or in close contact in schools, many physicians recommend vaccinations to prevent some of the bacterial infections that can cause meningitis (NLM 2019a). As a variety of microorganisms or viruses can cause meningitis, they are classified to either ICD-10-CM in Chapter 6: Diseases of the Nervous System, or Chapter 1:

Certain Infectious and Parasitic Diseases. The instructions provided in the Alphabetic Index to Diseases must be followed to ensure accurate code assignment. For example, the following entry in the ICD-10-CM Index to Diseases and Injuries includes types of meningitis, such as:

EXAMPLE: Meningitis G03.9
abacterial G03.0
actinomycotic A42.81
adenoviral A87.1
arbovirus A87.8
aseptic (acute) G03.0
bacterial G00.9

Figure 9.3. **Cerebral meninges**

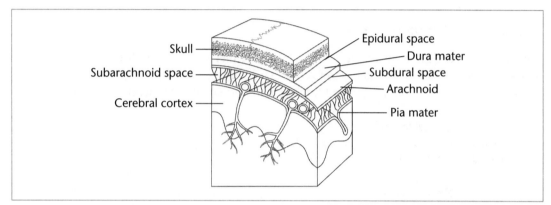

© AHIMA

Organic Sleep Disorders (G47)

The category G47, Sleep disorders, includes fourth and fifth digit codes to classify various types of sleep disorder and the range of ICD-10-CM codes, such as:

- Insomnia, G47.00–G47.09

- Hypersomnia, G47.10–G47.19

- Circadian rhythm sleep disorders, G47.20–G47.29

- Sleep apnea, G47.30–G47.39

- Narcolepsy and cataplexy, G47.411–G47.429

- Parasomnia, G47.50–G47.59

- Sleep-related movement disorders, G47.61–G47.69

- Other sleep disorders, G47.8

- Sleep disorder, unspecified, G47.9

Several of the subclassification codes contain the direction "Code first underlying condition" and "Code also associated medical condition" (CDC 2019). Additional codes for sleep disorders not due to a substance or known physiological condition (F51) and due to substance-related conditions are included in Chapter 5: Mental, Behavioral and

Neurodevelopmental Disorders. For example, a patient with a cocaine dependence may experience cocaine-induced insomnia that is assigned two codes:

G47.01, Insomnia due to medical condition
F14.282, Cocaine dependence with cocaine-induced sleep disorder

Other Degenerative Diseases of the Nervous System (G30–G32)

Categories G30–G32 describe hereditary and degenerative diseases of the central nervous system that range in severity from mild to severe (see figure 9.1 for an illustration of right hemisphere of the brain or central nervous system and the anatomical structures within it).

Alzheimer's Disease (G30)

Four character codes are available to classify Alzheimer's disease with early onset (G30.0) and Alzheimer's disease with late onset (G30.1), as well as other and unspecified Alzheimer's disease. An important note is included to use an additional code to identify

Delirium, if applicable (F05)
Dementia with behavioral disturbance (F02.81)
Dementia without behavioral disturbance (F02.80)

There is an Excludes1 note at the start of category G30, Alzheimer's disease, that reminds the coder of three conditions: senile degeneration of brain NEC; senile dementia, unspecified; and senility, unspecified. These three conditions are not coded with the specific Alzheimer disease codes G30.0–G30.9.

A patient with **dementia** can experience a variety of symptoms that are attributed to a neurological disorder with behavioral features. The patient's relatives may first notice a loss of the patient's memory of recent events. Memory loss by itself does not establish the diagnosis of dementia. However, if a patient has other symptoms such as language difficulties and the ability to carry out normal everyday functions, the diagnosis of dementia is more likely to be made. Patients with dementia can have difficulty handling their financial responsibilities, such as writing checks, or taking care of their home, such as cooking, cleaning, washing dishes, and laundry. As the disease progresses, the patients may lose their problem-solving thought processes and may have personality changes. Patients with dementia may become agitated and experience visual delusions, such as seeing objects that are not present. Another symptom is memory loss that progresses from mild to severe. Patients with dementia may not recognize loved ones as their disease progresses and lose their ability to express themselves or to even speak (NLM 2019b).

Other Degenerative Diseases of the Nervous System, Not Elsewhere Classified (G31)

Category G31, Other degenerative diseases of the nervous system, not elsewhere classified, also has the instruction to use an additional code to identify dementia with and without behavioral disturbance. ICD-10-CM code F02.81 identifies behavioral disturbance examples as aggressive, combative, violent behavior. Another note states to use an additional code to identify wandering in dementia that is also considered a behavioral disturbance (CDC 2019).

Acute and chronic forms of cerebral degenerative disease are included in this category, such as Pick's disease, G31.01; Degeneration of nervous system due to alcohol, G31.2; and Dementia with Lewy bodies, G31.83.

Code G31.84 identifies the condition described by physicians as **mild cognitive impairment**. This disease entity is defined as impairment in memory (or any other cognitive domain) that is beyond what is normal for age, with relatively intact function in the other cognitive domains. The patient will first have a memory complaint that is corroborated by other individuals and, for this reason, seek medical evaluation. The diagnosis is used by physicians as the reason for diagnostic testing services, for example, for brain imaging to rule out other conditions that could be causing the symptoms (NIH 2017).

Other Degenerative Disorders of the Nervous System in Diseases Classified Elsewhere (G32)

Included in category G32, Other degenerative disorders of the nervous system in diseases classified elsewhere, are italicized codes to identify degenerative disorders that are the consequence of other diseases. "Code first underlying disease" directions remind the coder that entries such as vitamin B12 deficiency, amyloidosis, and cerebellar ataxia in neoplastic disease should be coded first when these conditions are the known causes of the degenerative disorder.

- For example, if the patient has vitamin B12 deficiency that is causing subacute combined degeneration of the spinal cord, two codes are assigned:

    ○ Vitamin B12 deficiency, E53.8

    ○ Subacute combined degeneration of spinal cord in diseases classified elsewhere, G32.0

Check Your Understanding 9.1

Assign diagnosis codes for the following conditions.

1. Streptococcus meningitis, due to group A strep
2. Tardive dyskinesia
3. Huntington's chorea
4. Restless legs syndrome
5. Primary lateral sclerosis

Pain, Not Elsewhere Classified (G89)

The Pain, Not Elsewhere Classified category in ICD-10-CM has unique codes for encounters for pain management. A "use additional code" note appears at the top of this category to direct the coder to assign a code for pain associated with psychological factors, as documented by the physician (CDC 2019). Excludes notes under this category state that generalized pain is coded to the ICD-10-CM symptoms chapter (R52), and localized pain should be coded to pain by the site identified. The excludes note also states that a pain disorder exclusively attributed to psychological factors should not be coded with category G89, but instead with code F45.41.

Code G89.0, **central pain syndrome**, describes the condition that can be caused by damage to the central nervous system by trauma- or brain-related disease (for example, cardiovascular accident [CVA], multiple sclerosis, tumors, epilepsy, or Parkinson's disease). The condition may also be described as "thalamic pain syndrome."

Other codes exist for acute pain (G89.11–G89.19) and chronic pain (G89.21–G89.29) due to trauma or surgery. There is no time frame defining when pain becomes chronic. The physician's documentation should be used to guide the use of chronic pain codes.

Neoplasm-related pain may be described with code G89.3 for pain due to the primary or secondary malignancy or tumor. This code is assigned regardless of whether the pain is described as acute or chronic. Code G89.4 can be used as a principal diagnosis or first-listed diagnosis if the reason for the admission or outpatient visit is for pain control or pain management. The underlying neoplasm should be reported as an additional diagnosis code. The neoplasm-related pain code can be reported as an additional diagnosis when the reason for the admission or outpatient visit is management of the neoplasm, and the pain associated with the neoplasm is also documented.

Finally, a single code, G89.4, is provided for the diagnostic statement "chronic pain syndrome," often stated as the reason for ongoing pain management services. The code for chronic pain syndrome should only be used when the physician has specifically documented this condition.

Category G89 codes are acceptable as the principal or first-listed diagnosis codes. Codes from category G89 can be reported with codes that identify the site of the pain, including symptom codes from the ICD-10-CM body system or symptoms chapters, if the category G89 code provides additional information. For example, if a code from the body system or symptoms chapters identifies the site of the pain but does not describe the pain as acute or chronic, both codes should be assigned.

The sequencing of category G89 codes with site-specific pain codes depends on the circumstances of the admission or outpatient visit. For example, if the patient is being seen in the Pain Clinic to treat his neoplasm-related pain in the lumbar region of his back due to the bone metastatic carcinoma from his prostate carcinoma, the first-listed code would be the code G89.3, neoplasm-related pain, followed by codes for lumbar region pain, M54.5; carcinoma of prostate, C61; and secondary carcinoma of bone, C79.51. If the patient was in the Oncology Clinic for the management of his carcinoma of the prostate and also complains of the lumbar back pain that is attributed to the bone metastasis in the lumbar vertebrae, code C61 for the carcinoma of the prostate would be listed as the first diagnosis with the other diagnoses listed as additional diagnosis codes.

If the encounter is for pain control or pain management, the code from category G89 is sequenced first, followed by the code for the specific site of the pain or the underlying cause of the pain, if known. For example, assume a patient with known displacement of lumbar intervertebral disc is seen in the Pain Clinic for management of his chronic low back pain secondary to displacement of the lumbar intervertebral disc. For this encounter, the chronic pain, G89.29, would be listed first with an additional code, M51.26, for the underlying condition of the displacement of the lumbar intervertebral disc.

When an admission or encounter is for a procedure aimed at treating the underlying condition, a code for the underlying condition should be assigned as the principal or first-listed diagnosis. No code from category G89 should be assigned. For example, assume a patient with known displacement of lumbar intervertebral disc and chronic back pain due to the displaced disc is admitted for a laminectomy with excision of the herniated intervertebral disc. This patient's principal diagnosis is the displacement of the lumbar intervertebral disc, M51.26.

When an admission or encounter is for any other reason except pain control or pain management, and a related definitive diagnosis has not been established or confirmed by the provider, the coder should assign the code for the specific site of pain first, followed by the appropriate code from category G89. For example, assume a patient comes to the physician's office complaining of left hip pain that has been present for several months. The physician orders x-rays to be performed and concludes the patient has chronic hip pain of unknown etiology. For this encounter, the code for the left hip pain, M25.552, is listed as the first code with an additional code for the chronic pain, G89.2-.

Codes for postoperative or postthoracotomy pain are classified to the subcategories of G89.1 or G89.2 depending on whether the pain is acute or chronic. If the postoperative pain is not specified as acute or chronic, G89.18 is the default code for the acute form. Postoperative pain may be a principal or first-listed diagnosis when the reason for the admission or outpatient visit is documented as postoperative pain control or management. Postoperative pain can be reported as a secondary diagnosis code when a patient has outpatient surgery and develops an unusual amount of postoperative pain. Routine or expected postoperative pain immediately after surgery is not coded.

Check Your Understanding 9.2

Assign diagnosis codes to the following conditions.

1. Patient was admitted for treatment of acute abdominal pain due to acute appendicitis with peritonitis

2. Acute knee pain, left, due to accident

3. Chronic pain syndrome

4. Chronic back pain, lumbosacral region

5. Cancer-associated severe back pain related to secondary (metastatic) cancer in bone

---

Cerebral Palsy and Other Paralytic Syndromes (G80–G83)

The following subsections discuss the categories of other disorders of the nervous system, including paralytic conditions and epilepsy.

Cerebral Palsy, Category G80

Cerebral palsy is one of a group of neurological disorders that appear in infancy or early childhood. The condition permanently affects body movement and muscle coordination but usually does not worsen as the person ages. It is thought to be caused by abnormalities in parts of the brain that control muscle movements. The most common signs are a lack of muscle coordination when trying to walk, stiff muscles, dragging one leg or foot when walking, and exaggerated reflexes or spasticity. Other suspected causes of cerebral palsy are brain damage that occurs in the first few months of life, for example, from a fall, motor vehicle accident, or child abuse. Bacterial or viral meningitis in a young child may also be a cause of cerebral palsy. Cerebral palsy produces varying degrees of disability. One patient may be unable to walk and require lifelong care. Another person may have difficulty walking but does not require special assistance and leads a normal life. Fourth-digit subcategories identify the different forms of infantile cerebral palsy, such as spastic quadriplegic, spastic diplegic, spastic hemiplegic, athetoid, ataxic, or other forms of cerebral palsy (NINDS 2019).

Hemiplegia and Hemiparesis, Category G81

The terms **hemiplegia** and **hemiparesis** both refer to the paralysis of either the left side or the right side of the body. Paralysis is the loss of muscle function. Hemiplegia can be complete on one side of the body that affects both arm and leg or partial when only the arm or leg affected on one side of the body. Most hemiplegia is the result of a stroke or an injury such as a spinal cord injury (NLM 2019d).

Category G81 has fourth- and fifth-digit subcategories that differentiate between flaccid and spastic hemiplegia. Flaccid refers to the loss of muscle tone in the paralyzed parts with the absence of tendon reflexes, whereas spastic refers to the spasticity of the paralyzed parts with increased tendon reflexes. The G81 codes often are assigned when the health record provides no further information, when the cause of the hemiplegia and hemiparesis is unknown, or as an additional code when the condition results from a specified cause.

A note on how to use the codes in the categories G81 (Hemiplegia and hemiparesis), G82 (Paraplegia and quadriplegia), and G83 (Other paralytic syndromes) is provided: the categories are to be used only when the listed conditions are reported without further specification or are stated to be old or long-standing but of unspecified cause. The category is also for use in multiple coding to identify these conditions resulting from any cause. Paralytic sequelae of cerebral infarct/stroke are in ICD-10-CM Chapter 9: Diseases of the Circulatory System. An example of the use of the hemiplegia codes with another condition is when a patient has a cerebral infarction that produces dominant right-sided flaccid hemiplegia:

> **EXAMPLE:**   Cerebral infarction, unspecified, I63.9
> Flaccid hemiplegia affecting right dominant side, G81.01

A fifth-digit subclassification is included in category G81–G83 to identify whether the dominant or nondominant side of the body is affected. This type of specificity may not be available in the health record; if the information is not available, assign the fifth digit 0. However, if the affected side is documented but not specified as the dominant or nondominant side for the patient, and the classification does not provide a default code, the code is based on I.C.6.a. Diseases of the Nervous System, Dominant/Nondominant side.

Codes from category G81, Hemiplegia and hemiparesis, and subcategories G83.1, Monoplegia of upper limb, and G83.3, Monoplegia, unspecified, identify whether the dominant or nondominant side is affected. Should the affected side be documented, but not specified as dominant or nondominant, and the classification system does not indicate a default, code selection is as follows:

- For ambidextrous patients, the default should be the dominant side.

- If the left side is affected, the default is nondominant.

- If the right side is affected, the default is dominant (CMS 2019).

> **EXAMPLE:**   The patient had a cerebral infarction due to a thrombosis of right middle cerebral artery with monoplegia of the upper limb on the left side. The physician does not document whether the patient is right-hand or left-hand dominant. There would be two codes assigned: one code for the type of cerebral infarction that occurred and a second code for the monoplegia that was the current result of cerebral infarction:
>
> Cerebral infarction due to thrombosis of right middle cerebral artery, I63.311
> Monoplegia, upper, limb left side, G83.14

Epilepsy and Recurrent Seizures, Category G40

An instructional note appears under the category heading G40, Epilepsy and recurrent seizures; it explains that terminology that is the same as "intractable" may be documented as pharmacoresistant, pharmacologically resistant, treatment resistant, refractory, medically refractory, and poorly controlled. If the physician uses any of these terms, the coder can assign the ICD-10-CM diagnosis code for the intractable form of the disease (CDC 2019).

The term **epilepsy** denotes any disorder characterized by recurrent seizures. A **seizure** is a transient disturbance of cerebral function caused by an abnormal paroxysmal neuronal discharge in the brain.

Physicians often document "recurrent seizure" or "seizure disorder" as well as epilepsy in a health record. Recurrent seizures or seizure disorders are classified in the same category as epilepsy because the terminology is synonymous in medicine. Localization-related epilepsy is the terminology used today for an older term, partial epilepsy.

Other terms used to describe convulsions are not classified to category G40. Such phrases as convulsion or convulsive disorder, convulsive seizures, fits, or recurrent convulsions are not accepted as equivalent to epilepsy or recurrent seizures. Instead the codes for the convulsive conditions are included in category R56 within ICD-10-CM Chapter 18 for symptoms. The term seizure and the plural term seizures are also coded to the symptom code R56.9 by following the Alphabetic Index carefully. Coders must not use the terms seizures and convulsions interchangeably. By using the physician's description of the patient's condition and following the Alphabetic Index precisely, different terminology will produce different ICD-10-CM diagnosis codes. Conditions documented as convulsions, posttraumatic seizures, seizures, and convulsive seizures are not coded to category G40, Epilepsy and recurrent seizures. Instead, these conditions are coded to category R56, Convulsions, not elsewhere classified. Recurrent seizures, epileptic convulsions or seizures, and seizure disorders are assigned to category G40, Epilepsy and recurrent seizures.

The ICD-10-CM Index to Diseases provides the following entries under the main term of seizure. The following conditions are classified to category R56, Convulsions, not elsewhere classified:

Seizure, convulsive—see Convulsions, R56.9
Seizure, febrile, R56.00
Seizure, posttraumatic, R56.1

The following conditions are classified to category G40, Epilepsy and recurrent seizures

Seizure, disorder, G40.909
Seizure, epileptic—see Epilepsy, G40.909
Seizure, grand mal, G40.409
Seizure, petit mal, G40.409
Seizure, recurrent, G40.909

Migraine, Category G43

A note with G43, Migraine provides the following terms to be considered equivalent to intractable: pharmacoresistant (pharmacologically resistant), treatment resistant, refractory (medically), and poorly controlled.

Migraine headaches are recurrent headaches that produce moderate to severe head pain for the patient. The pain may be pulsing or throbbing and may appear on only one side of the head. In addition to pain, the patient often experiences nausea and vomiting. The patient prefers to rest in a darkened, quiet room as light and sound exacerbate the patient's symptoms. Some patients experience what is called an "aura," that is, a warning to the patient that he or she is about to have a migraine headache. The aura may be flashing lights or zigzag lines that the patient sees in the patient's visual field. Some patients have momentary loss of vision during their aura stage. Some research has suggested that migraines may be linked to the alternating dilation and narrowing of blood vessels in the brain. Migraines may be an inherited condition and have a genetic component that affects the activity of brain cells. Some medications have helped to prevent the severity of migraine attacks, while other medications relieve the symptoms that patients with migraines experience. Some patients experience migraines for most of their adult life, while other patients report fewer migraines as the person ages (NLM 2019c).

The classification of migraine headaches is reported with category codes G43, Migraine. Many types of migraine headaches can be identified with specific codes in subcategories for migraine with aura, migraine without aura, hemiplegic migraine, persistent migraine aura with and without cerebral infarction, chronic migraine, and other forms of migraine. Category G43 codes include a sixth digit to identify the manifestation of the migraine in several of the individual codes. For example, migraine, not intractable with status migrainous, and migraine, intractable, without status migrainous, are both options for the sixth character.

An additional code to identify the cerebral infarction (codes from I63.-) is required with subcategory codes from G43.6, Persistent migraine aura with cerebral infarction. The definition of "chronic" in primary episodic headache disorders is a headache that occurs on more days than not for more than three months.

ICD-10-CM provides codes for other types of headaches. Chapter 6: Diseases of the Nervous System, also includes category G44, other headache syndromes. This includes headaches described with terminology other than migraine headache. Headaches without a known cause are included in ICD-10-CM Chapter 18: Signs, Symptoms, and Ill-Defined Conditions.

Examples of headaches that are classified to category G43, Migraine include the following:

- Migraine without aura and migraine with aura

- Hemiplegic migraine

- Persistent migraine without cerebral infarction and with cerebral infarction

- Chronic migraine without aura

- Cyclical vomiting

- Ophthalmoplegic migraine

- Periodic headache syndromes in child or adult

- Abdominal migraine

- Other specified migraines such as menstrual migraine

Examples of headaches that are classified to category G44, Other headache syndrome include the following:

- Cluster headache

- Vascular headache

- Tension-type headache

- Posttraumatic headache

- Drug-induced headache

- Complicated and other specified headache syndromes

A diagnosis of "headache" or "facial pain" is coded to category R51, Headache, that is included in Chapter 18: Symptoms, Signs, and Abnormal Clinical and Laboratory Findings, not elsewhere classified.

Intraoperative and Postprocedural Complications, Category G97

Also in this chapter are the intraoperative and postprocedural complication codes. Intraoperative complications include such conditions as:

- Intraoperative hemorrhage and hematoma of a nervous system organ or structure complicating a nervous system procedure or complicating other body system procedure

- Accidental puncture or laceration of dura during a procedure

- Accidental puncture and laceration of other nervous system organ or structure during a nervous system procedure or during other procedure

Postprocedural complications include such conditions as:

- Cerebrospinal fluid leak from spinal puncture

- Intracranial hypotension following ventricular shunting

- Postprocedural hemorrhage, hematoma, and seroma of a nervous system organ or structure following a nervous system procedure or following other procedure.

Coders must be aware that the documentation of complications of care must be clearly indicated. *ICD-10-CM Official Guidelines for Coding and Reporting*, I.B.16, Documentation of complications of care provides the following direction: Code assignment is based on the provider's documentation of the relationship between the condition and the care or procedure. The guideline extends to any complication of care, regardless of the chapter the code is located in. It is important to note that not all conditions that occur during or following medical care or surgery are classified as complications. There must be a cause-and-effect relationship between the care provided and the condition, and an indication in the documentation that it is a complication. Query the provider for clarification, if the complication is not clearly documented (CDC 2019).

Check Your Understanding 9.3

Assign diagnosis codes to the following conditions.

1. Absence epileptic syndrome, not stated as intractable

2. Recurrent seizures

3. Intractable chronic cluster headaches

4. Retinal migraine

5. Narcolepsy with cataplexy

(Continued)

(*Continued*)

6. Stroke with current resulting left dominant-sided hemiplegia

7. Cerebral infarction, due to thrombosis, cerebral artery with resulting monoplegia of right arm, dominant side

8. Guillain-Barré syndrome

9. Facial (Bell's) Palsy

10. Headache following lumbar puncture procedure

ICD-10-PCS Coding for Procedures Related to Nervous System

There are two sections of ICD-10-PCS related to procedures performed on the nervous system:

Central Nervous System tables 001–00X
Peripheral Nervous System tables 012–01X

Central Nervous System

The procedures performed on organs in the central nervous system appear in the ICD-10-PCS code book in tables that start with the two characters 0 and 0 followed by five characters representing root operation, body part, approach, device, and qualifier:

Character 1 is Value 0—Medical and Surgical
Character 2 is Value 0—Central Nervous System

Root Operation

Character 3 of the ICD-10-PCS codes is the root operation. The root operations that represent the objectives of procedures for surgical treatment of the diseases of the Central Nervous system are shown in table 9.1.

Table 9.1.   **Root operations for procedures on body parts within the Central Nervous system**

Bypass: Altering the route of passage of the contents of a tubular body part
Change: Taking out or off a device from a body part and putting back an identical or similar device in or on the same body part without cutting or puncturing the skin or a mucous membrane.
Destruction: Physical eradication of all or a portion of a body part by the direct use of energy, force, or a destructive agent
Dilation: Expanding an orifice or the lumen of a tubular body part
Division: Cutting into a body part, without draining fluids and/or gases from the body part, in order to separate or transect a body part
Drainage: Taking or letting out fluids and/or gases from a body part
Excision: Cutting out or off, without replacement, a portion of a body part
Extirpation: Taking or cutting out solid matter from a body part
Extraction: Pulling or stripping out or off all or a portion of a body part by the use of force
Fragmentation: Breaking solid matter in a body part into pieces

Insertion: Putting in a nonbiological appliance that monitors, assists, performs, or prevents a physiological function but does not physically take the place of the body part
Inspection: Visually and/or manually exploring a body part
Map: Locating the route of passage of electrical impulses and/or locating functional area in a body part
Release: Freeing a body part from an abnormal physical constraint by cutting or by the use of force
Removal: Taking out or off a device from a body part
Repair: Restoring, to the extent possible, a body part to its normal anatomic structure and function
Reposition: Moving to its normal location, or other suitable location, all or a portion of a body part
Resection: Cutting out or off, without replacement, all of a body part
Supplement: Putting in or on biologic or synthetic material that physically reinforces and/or augments the function of a portion of a body part
Revision: Correcting, to the extent possible, a portion of a malfunctioning device or the position of a displaced device
Transfer: Moving, without taking out, all or a portion of a body part to another location to take over the function of all or a portion of a body part

Source: CMS 2019

Body Part

Character 4 identifies the body part involved in the procedure. The body part and the values for the Central Nervous system procedures are in table 9.2.

Table 9.2. **Body parts and values included in the ICD-10-PCS codes for the Central Nervous system**

0—Brain
1—Cerebral meninges
2—Dura Mater
3—Epidural Space, Intracranial
4—Subdural Space, Intracranial
5—Subarachnoid Space, Intracranial
6—Cerebral Ventricle
7—Cerebral Hemisphere
8—Basal Ganglia
9—Thalamus
A—Hypothalamus
B—Pons
C—Cerebellum
D—Medulla Oblongata
E—Cranial Nerve
F—Olfactory Nerve
G—Optic Nerve
H—Oculomotor Nerve
J—Trochlear Nerve
K—Trigeminal Nerve
L—Abducens Nerve
M—Facial Nerve

(Continued)

N—Acoustic Nerve
P—Glossopharyngeal Nerve
Q—Vagus Nerve
R—Accessory Nerve
S—Hypoglossal Nerve
T—Spinal Meninges
U—Spinal Canal
V—Spinal Cord
W—Cervical Spinal Cord
X—Thoracic Spinal Cord
Y—Lumbar Spinal Cord

Source: CMS 2019

Approach

Character 5 identifies the approach, value, and definition used in the procedure. The approaches for procedures performed on organs within the Central Nervous system are shown in table 9.3.

Table 9.3. **Approaches included in the ICD-10-PCS codes for the Central Nervous system**

Open (0): Cutting through the skin or mucous membrane and any other body layers necessary to expose the site of the procedure
Percutaneous (3): Entry, by puncture or minor incision, of instrumentation through the skin or mucous membrane and any other body layers necessary to reach the site of the procedure
Percutaneous endoscopic (4): Entry, by puncture or minor incision, of instrumentation through the skin or mucous membrane and any other body layers necessary to reach and visualize the site of the procedure.
External (X): Procedure performed directly on the skin or mucous membrane or procedures performed indirectly by the application of external force through the skin or mucous membrane.

Source: CMS 2019

Device

Character 6 identifies if a device remains in the patient's body after the procedure is concluded. The devices used to code procedures performed on organs within the Central Nervous system are limited to the devices as shown in table 9.4.

Table 9.4. **Devices included in the ICD-10-PCS codes for the Central Nervous system**

0—Drainage Device
2—Monitoring Device
3—Infusion Device
4—Radioactive Element, Cesium-131 Collagen Implant
7—Autologous Tissue Substitute
J—Synthetic Substitute
K—Nonautologous Tissue Substitute
M—Neurostimulator Lead
Y—Other Device
Z—No Device

Source: CMS 2019

Qualifier

Character 7 is a qualifier that specifies an additional attribute of the procedure, if applicable. The qualifier characters used to code procedures performed on organs within the Central Nervous system are limited to two values, as shown in table 9.5.

Table 9.5. Qualifiers used to code procedures within the Central Nervous system

X—Diagnostic
Z—No Qualifier

Source: CMS 2019

Peripheral Nervous System

The procedures performed on organs in the peripheral nervous system appear in the ICD-10-PCS code book in tables that start with the two characters 0 and 1 followed by five characters representing root operation, body part, approach, device, and qualifier:

Character 1 is Value 0—Medical and Surgical
Character 2 is Value 1—Peripheral Nervous System

Root Operation

Character 3 of the ICD-10-PCS codes is the root operation. The root operations that represent the objectives of procedures for surgical treatment of the diseases of the Peripheral Nervous system are shown in table 9.6.

Table 9.6. Root operations for procedures on body parts within the Peripheral Nervous system

Change: Taking out or off a device from a body part and putting back an identical or similar device in or on the same body part without cutting or puncturing the skin or a mucous membrane.
Destruction: Physical eradication of all or a portion of a body part by the direct use of energy, force, or a destructive agent
Division: Cutting into a body part, without draining fluids and/or gases from the body part, in order to separate or transect a body part
Drainage: Taking or letting out fluids and/or gases from a body part
Excision: Cutting out or off, without replacement, a portion of a body part
Extirpation: Taking or cutting out solid matter from a body part
Extraction: Pulling or stripping out or off all or a portion of a body part by the use of force
Insertion: Putting in a nonbiological appliance that monitors, assists, performs, or prevents a physiological function but does not physically take the place of the body part
Inspection: Visually and/or manually exploring a body part
Release: Freeing a body part from an abnormal physical constraint by cutting or by the use of force
Removal: Taking out or off a device from a body part
Repair: Restoring, to the extent possible, a body part to its normal anatomic structure and function
Replacement: Putting in or on biological or synthetic material that physically takes the place and/or function of all or a portion of a body part
Reposition: Moving to its normal location, or other suitable location, all or a portion of a body part

(Continued)

Supplement: Putting in or on biologic or synthetic material that physically reinforces and/or augments the function of a portion of a body part
Revision: Correcting, to the extent possible, a portion of a malfunctioning device or the position of a displaced device
Transfer: Moving, without taking out, all or a portion of a body part to another location to take over the function of all or a portion of a body part

Source: CMS 2019

Body Part

Character 4 identifies the body part involved in the procedure. Table 9.7 identifies the body parts and values for the Peripheral Nervous system.

Table 9.7. **Body parts and values included in the ICD-10-PCS codes for the Peripheral Nervous system**

0—Cervical Plexus
1—Cervical Nerve
2—Phrenic Nerve
3—Brachial Plexus
4—Ulnar Nerve
5—Median Nerve
6—Radial Nerve
8—Thoracic Nerve
9—Lumbar Plexus
A—Lumbosacral Plexus
B—Lumbar Nerve
C—Pudendal Nerve
D—Femoral Nerve
F—Sciatic Nerve
G—Tibial Nerve
H—Peroneal Nerve
K—Head and Neck Sympathetic Nerve
L—Thoracic Sympathetic Nerve
M—Abdominal Sympathetic Nerve
N—Lumbar Sympathetic Nerve
P—Sacral Sympathetic Nerve
Q—Sacral Plexus
R—Sacral Nerve
Y—Peripheral Nerve

Source: CMS 2019

Approach

Character 5 identifies the approach, value, and definition used in the procedure. The approach for procedures performed on organs within the Peripheral Nervous system are shown in table 9.8.

Table 9.8. **Approaches, values, and definitions included in the ICD-10-PCS codes for the Peripheral Nervous system**

Open (0): Cutting through the skin or mucous membrane and any other body layers necessary to expose the site of the procedure
Percutaneous (3): Entry, by puncture or minor incision, of instrumentation through the skin or mucous membrane and any other body layers necessary to reach the site of the procedure
Percutaneous endoscopic (4): Entry, by puncture or minor incision, of instrumentation through the skin or mucous membrane and any other body layers necessary to reach and visualize the site of the procedure.
External (X): Procedure performed directly on the skin or mucous membrane or procedures performed indirectly by the application of external force through the skin or mucous membrane.

Source: CMS 2019

Device

Character 6 identifies if a device remains in the patient's body after the procedure is concluded. The devices used to code procedures performed on organs within the Peripheral Nervous system are limited to a few devices as shown in table 9.9.

Table 9.9. **Devices and values included in the ICD-10-PCS codes for the Peripheral Nervous system**

0—Drainage Device
2—Monitoring Device
7—Autologous Tissue Substitute
J—Synthetic Substitute
K—Nonautologous Tissue Substitute
M—Neurostimulator Lead
Y—Other Device
Z—No Device

Source: CMS 2019

Qualifier

Character 7 is a qualifier that specifies an additional attribute of the procedure, if applicable. The qualifier characters used to code procedures performed on organs within the Peripheral Nervous system are limited to two values as shown in table 9.10.

Table 9.10. **Qualifier used to code procedures within the Peripheral Nervous system**

X—Diagnostic
Z—No Qualifier

Source: CMS 2019

One frequently performed procedure in the central nervous system is the creation of a shunt to drain fluid from one site to another cavity. For example, shunting from the cerebral ventricle to a peritoneal location is coded as a **Bypass** in ICD-10-PCS. Guideline B3.6a includes the instruction that a bypass procedure is coded using the body part that is the origin of the shunt in the fourth character code of the code and the destination of the shunt in the seventh character (qualifier). Bypass procedures therefore are coded as from a body part to another body part.

Procedures frequently performed on the peripheral nervous system include Release, Repair, Reposition, and Transfer procedures. The Index entries for **Release** include a subterm of "nerve" with the peripheral nerves as well as other nerves listed beneath it. A Release procedure involves freeing a nerve from a body part from an abnormal physical constraint. The three-digit code for release of a peripheral nerve is 01N. The fourth character identifies the nerve released, such as ulnar, median, radial, and such. The approach choices are Open, Percutaneous, or Percutaneous Endoscopic. There is no device or qualifier option in this table, as neither will apply to this type of procedure.

A **Repair** of a nerve involves restoring the nerve to the extent position or restoring the nerve to its normal anatomic structure and function. The broad terms of neuroplasty or neurorrhaphy refer the coder to the root operations of Repair and Supplement. The suture repair of a nerve is coded as a Repair. Root Operation Supplement of a nerve would involve an autologous tissue substitute to reinforce the nerve structure.

Other procedures performed on nerves may be described as a transposition. Transposition is not a root operation in ICD-10-PCS. Instead, the Index refers the coder to the root operations of Reposition or Transfer for a transposition of a nerve. A **Reposition** of a nerve involves moving it to its normal location or other suitable location all of a portion of the nerve. Under the main term Reposition in the Index, the coder will find a subterm of nerve with specific nerves listed beneath it. Table 01S for Reposition of a peripheral nerve includes the identified nerve as the fourth body part character. The approach for a Reposition is Open, Percutaneous, or Percutaneous Endoscopic. There is no applicable value for the sixth or seventh characters of device or qualifier.

A nerve transfer is coded to the root operation **Transfer**. In ICD-10-PCS, a nerve transfer is the moving, without taking it out, all of a portion of the nerve to another location to take over the function of all or a portion of the nerve. Transfer is a main term in the Index with nerve as a subterm and the specific nerves listed with the three-digit code table 01X. Again, the "from" and "to" concept is used for transfers with the body part used for the nerve transferred from and the qualifier as the nerve transferred to. There are two choices for the approach used, that is, Open and Percutaneous Endoscopic, and there is no choice for a device as it does not apply.

ICD-10-CM and ICD-10-PCS Review Exercises: Chapter 9

Assign the correct ICD-10-CM diagnosis codes and ICD-10-PCS procedure codes to the following exercises.

1. A patient had been noted to have dementia and forgetfulness. He has been leaving his home and forgetting where he is or where he is going. The diagnosis of dementia due to early-onset Alzheimer's was established.

2. Juvenile myoclonic epilepsy with intractable seizures, status epilepticus

3. Chronic cluster headaches

4. Chronic Migraine without aura, not intractable with status migrainous

5. Autonomic dysreflexia due to urinary tract infections

ICD-10-CM and ICD-10-PCS Review Exercises: Chapter 9 *(continued)*

6. Obstructive hydrocephalus

7. The patient, a type 2 diabetic with neuropathy, developed weakness of the left arm and leg. The patient was brought to the emergency room where he could speak but was unable to use his left arm and leg. The patient was able to ambulate with no neurological deficits within 24 hours. Due to the complete recovery, it was determined that the patient had experienced a TIA. During this encounter, the patient also was treated for an intractable classical migraine.

8. Myasthenia gravis in crisis

9. Alcoholic encephalopathy

10. Complex regional pain syndrome I, bilateral lower legs

11. Intracranial subdural abscess due to methicillin–resistant *Staphylococcus aureus*

12. Carpal tunnel syndrome and tarsal tunnel syndrome, both on left side

13. Spastic diplegic cerebral palsy

14. Dementia with Lewy body disease and violent behavior

15. Postpolio syndrome

16. PROCEDURE: Diagnostic lumbar spinal puncture

17. PROCEDURE: Transposition/reposition radial nerve, open, right arm

18. PROCEDURE: Ulnar nerve release by fasciotomy, left arm

19. PROCEDURE: Cerebral ventricular-peritoneal shunt using synthetic shunt material for shunt creation via open technique

20. PROCEDURE: Open neurorrhaphy, Femoral nerve

References

Centers for Disease Control and Prevention (CDC), National Center for Health Statistics (NCHS). 2019. *ICD-10-CM Official Guidelines for Coding and Reporting*, 2020. https://www.cdc.gov/nchs/data/icd/10cmguidelines_fy2019_final.pdf.

Centers for Medicare and Medicaid Services (CMS). 2019. *ICD-10-PCS Official Guidelines for Coding and Reporting*, 2020. http://www.cms.gov/Medicare/Coding/ICD10/.

Mosby. 2017 *Mosby's Pocket Dictionary of Medicine, Nursing, and Health Professions*, 8th ed. St. Louis: Mosby, Inc.

National Institute of Health (NIH). 2017. About Alzheimer's Disease: Mild Cognitive Impairment. https://www.nia.nih.gov/alzheimers/topics/mild-cognitive-impairment.

National Institute of Neurological Disorders and Stroke (NINDS). 2019. NINDS Cerebral Palsy Information Page. http://www.ninds.nih.gov/disorders/cerebral_palsy/cerebral_palsy.htm.

U.S. National Library of Medicine, MedLinePlus (NLM). 2019a. Meningitis. https://www.nlm.nih.gov/medlineplus/meningitis.html.

U.S. National Library of Medicine, MedLinePlus (NLM). 2019b. Dementia. https://www.nlm.nih.gov/medlineplus/dementia.html.

U.S. National Library of Medicine, MedLinePlus (NLM). 2019c. Migraine. https://www.nlm.nih.gov/medlineplus/migraine.html.

U.S. National Library of Medicine, MedLinePlus (NLM). 2019d. Paralysis. https://www.nlm.nih.gov/medlineplus/paralysis.html.

Chapter 10

Diseases of the Eye and Adnexa (H00–H59)

Learning Objectives

At the conclusion of this chapter, you should be able to do the following:

- Describe the organization of the conditions and codes included in Chapter 7 of ICD-10-CM, Diseases of the Eye and Adnexa (H00–H59)

- Identify and describe the various types of eye disorders, including retinopathy, glaucoma, and cataract

- Explain how the glaucoma stage relates to the coding of glaucoma

- Assign ICD-10-CM codes for diseases of the eyes and adnexa

- Assign ICD-10-PCS codes for procedures related to diseases of the eyes and adnexa

Key Terms

Bullous keratopathy

Cataract

Chemical conjunctivitis

Cortical cataract

Cystoid macular edema (CME)

Glaucoma

Glaucoma suspect

Infantile and juvenile cataract

Morgagnian type cataract

Nuclear cataracts

Retained lens fragment

Retinal detachment

Retinopathy of prematurity (ROP)

Rhegmatogenous (retinal) detachment

Subcapsular cataract

Traction (retinal) detachment

Overview of ICD-10-CM Chapter 7: Diseases of the Eye and Adnexa

Chapter 7 of ICD-10-CM includes categories H00–H59 arranged in the following blocks:

H00–H05	Disorders of eyelid, lacrimal system and orbit
H10–H11	Disorders of conjunctiva
H15–H22	Disorders of sclera, cornea, iris and ciliary body
H25–H28	Disorders of lens
H30–H36	Disorders of choroid and retina
H40–H42	Glaucoma
H43–H44	Disorders of vitreous body and globe
H46–H47	Disorders of optic nerve and visual pathways
H49–H52	Disorders of ocular muscles, binocular movement, accommodation and refraction
H53–H54	Visual disturbances and blindness
H55–H57	Other disorders of eye and adnexa
H59	Intraoperative and postprocedural complications and disorders of eye and adnexa, not elsewhere classified

The structure of the codes for diseases of the eye and adnexa is by site. The terminology for some of the categories in Chapter 7 has been updated to reflect current terminology. For example, senile cataract terminology has been updated to age-related cataract. There has been an expansion of the number of characters in the codes for eye and adnexa diseases to describe right side, left side, and in some cases bilateral conditions. There is also a code for "unspecified" side to use when the health record documentation does not specify the laterality of the condition.

Coding Guidelines and Instructional Notes for ICD-10-CM Chapter 7, Diseases of the Eye and Adnexa

At the start of Chapter 7 in ICD-10-CM, a "use an external cause code" appears following the code for the eye condition to identify the cause of the eye condition, if applicable (CDC 2019).

A series of Excludes2 conditions are listed that are applicable to all conditions classifiable to Chapter 7. The conditions described in the Excludes2 note are diseases that can be coded in addition to the Chapter 7 codes for eye conditions.

The NCHS has published chapter-specific guidelines for Chapter 7 in the *ICD-10-CM Official Guidelines for Coding and Reporting*. The coding student should review all of the coding guidelines for Chapter 7 of ICD-10-CM, which appear in an ICD-10-CM code book or at the CDC website (CDC 2019) or in appendix F.

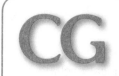

Chapter 7 : Diseases of the Eye and Adnexa (H00-H59)

Guideline I.C.7.a Glaucoma

1. Assigning Glaucoma Codes

   Assign as many codes from category H40, Glaucoma, as needed to identify the type of glaucoma, the affected eye, and the glaucoma stage.

2. Bilateral glaucoma with same type and stage

   When a patient has bilateral glaucoma and both eyes are documented as being the same type and stage, and there is a code for bilateral glaucoma, report only the code for the type of glaucoma, bilateral, with the seventh character for the stage.

   When a patient has bilateral glaucoma and both eyes are documented as being the same type and stage, and the classification does not provide a code for bilateral glaucoma (i.e. subcategories H40.10, H40.11 and H40.20) report only one code for the type of glaucoma with the appropriate seventh character for the stage.

3. Bilateral glaucoma stage with different types or stages

   When a patient has bilateral glaucoma and each eye is documented as having a different type or stage, and the classification distinguishes laterality, assign the appropriate code for each eye rather than the code for bilateral glaucoma.

   When a patient has bilateral glaucoma and each eye is documented as having a different type, and the classification does not distinguish laterality (i.e. subcategories H40.10, H40.11 and H40.20), assign one code for each type of glaucoma with the appropriate seventh character for the stage.

   When a patient has bilateral glaucoma and each eye is documented as having the same type, but different stage, and the classification does not distinguish laterality (i.e. subcategories H40.10, H40.11 and H40.20), assign a code for the type of glaucoma for each eye with the seventh character for the specific glaucoma stage documented for each eye.

4. Patient admitted with glaucoma and stage evolves during the admission

   If a patient is admitted with glaucoma and the stage progresses during the admission, assign the code for highest stage documented.

   (Continued)

(Continued)

5. Indeterminate stage glaucoma

    Assignment of the seventh character "4" for "indeterminate stage" should be based on the clinical documentation. The seventh character "4" is used for glaucomas whose stage cannot be clinically determined. This seventh character should not be confused with the seventh character "0", unspecified, which should be assigned when there is no documentation regarding the stage of the glaucoma.

Guideline I.C.7.b Blindness

If "blindness" or "low vision" of both eyes is documented but the visual impairment category is not documented, assign code H54.3, Unqualified visual loss, both eyes. If "blindness" or "low vision" in one eye is documented but the visual impairment category is not documented, assign a code from H54.6-, Unqualified visual loss, one eye. If "blindness" or "visual loss" is documented without any information about whether one or both eyes are affected, assign code H54.7, Unspecified visual loss.

Coding Diseases of the Eye and Adnexa in ICD-10-CM Chapter 7

Chapter 7 of ICD-10-CM contains specific codes for diseases of the eye that include infections, inflammations, lesions, deformities, and visual impairments among the many afflictions that a person can experience in the eye and the supporting structures. As stated in the Excludes2 note, diseases of the eye can be coded with conditions classified in other chapters. Diseases of the eye and adnexa coexist with infectious and parasitic diseases, diabetes, eye injuries, and other conditions. Coding diseases of the eye requires the coder's attention to detail including the specific forms of the disease and whether the condition occurs on the right side, left side, or is present in both eyes. A diagram of the eye and its structures is shown in figure 10.1.

Disorders of the Eyelid, Lacrimal System and Orbit (H00–H05)

ICD-10-CM codes in the range of H00–H05 describe disorders of the eyelid, lacrimal system, and orbit. The lacrimal system, as seen in figure 10.2, is a collection of structures that produce tears and drain the tears from the surface of the eyeball (Mosby 2017, 747). The orbits are a pair of bony cavities in the skull that house the eyeballs and associated eye muscles, nerves, and blood vessels (Mosby 2017, 960). Examples of conditions coded to the range of codes H00–H05 include hordeolum, chalazion, entropion, ectropion, blepharochalasis, inflammations, deformities of the lacrimal system and orbit, and other conditions. The codes include specific codes for the right eye, right upper and lower eyelid, left eye, left upper and lower eyelid,

Figure 10.1. **Diagram of the eye**

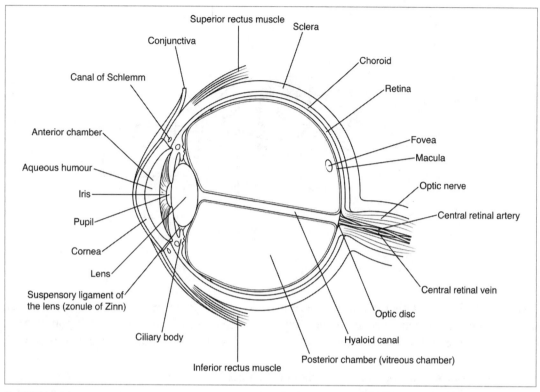

© AHIMA

and bilateral eyes, and a code for those conditions that do not have the laterality documented, for example:

H00.11, Chalazion right upper eyelid
H00.12, Chalazion right lower eyelid
H00.13, Chalazion right eye, unspecified eyelid
H00.14, Chalazion left upper eyelid
H00.15, Chalazion left lower eyelid
H00.16, Chalazion left eye, unspecified eyelid
H00.19, Chalazion unspecified eye, unspecified eyelid

H05.221, Edema of right orbit
H05.222, Edema of left orbit
H05.223, Edema of bilateral orbit
H05.229, Edema of unspecified orbit

Disorders of Conjunctiva (H10–H11)

Disorders of the conjunctiva are classified in the range of H10–H11. The conjunctiva is the mucous membrane lining of the inner surface of the eyelids and anterior part of the sclera (Mosby 2017, 320). Included in this range of codes are acute and chronic conjunctivitis and blepharoconjunctivitis that are bacterial or viral inflammations of the conjunctiva and eyelids

Figure 10.2.   **The lacrimal system**

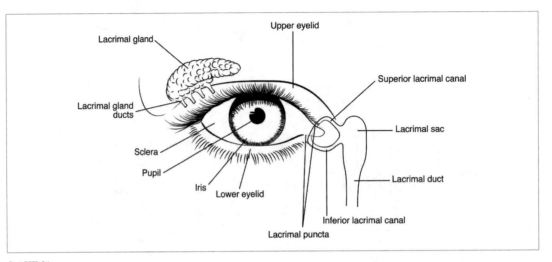

© AHIMA

(Mosby 2017, 320). Other conditions here include specific disorders of the conjunctiva such as pterygium, conjunctival scars, hemorrhages, cysts, and other disorders of the conjunctiva. Right eye, left eye, bilateral eyes, and unspecified sides of these conditions are classified with individual codes.

A note follows the code for acute chemical conjunctivitis (H10.21-) to direct the coder to "code first" T51–T65 to identify the chemical and intent of the toxic chemical that caused the damage to the eye. The toxic chemicals could be alcohol, organic solvents, corrosive substances, soaps, and detergents, as well as pesticides and other substances. **Chemical conjunctivitis** occurs when a person develops an inflammation of the conjunctiva after a substance gets in the eye. This event is an injury, and that is the reason the T51–T65 code is used first. As a result of the exposure to the chemical, the patient suffers eye pain, redness, and swelling. Often this is an occupational injury with workers in the construction, manufacturing, and agriculture industry injured when working with chemicals. The treatment usually occurs in an Emergency Department or Urgent Care Center with prolonged eye washing, antibiotic eyedrops, and artificial tears prescribed.

EXAMPLE: The patient was exposed to an accidental release of chlorine gas in the manufacturing plant where he worked and developed acute bilateral eye pain. The patient was diagnosed with acute bilateral chemical conjunctivitis due to chlorine gas and coded as follows:

T59.4X1A, Toxic effect of chlorine gas, accidental, initial encounter
H10.213, Acute toxic conjunctivitis, bilateral

Disorders of Sclera, Cornea, Iris and Ciliary Body (H15–H22)

The block of codes H15–H22 describes disorders of the sclera, cornea, iris, and ciliary body as shown in the figures 10.1 and 10.2 within the diagrams of the eye and the lacrimal system. Conditions classified with these codes include many inflammations of these sites such as episcleritis, keratitis, keratoconjunctivitis, and iridocyclitis. Other corneal conditions such as bullous keratopathy, corneal edema, keratoconus, and other corneal deformities are also included. Diseases of the iris and ciliary body such as hyphema and cysts of the iris as well as anterior and posterior synechiae complete the block of codes. Right eye, left eye, bilateral, and unspecified laterality are included for the conditions in these codes, for example:

H18.10, Bullous keratopathy, unspecified eye
H18.11, Bullous keratopathy, right eye
H18.12, Bullous keratopathy, left eye
H18.13, Bullous keratopathy, bilateral

Disorders of Lens (H25–H28)

Disorders of the lens (H25–H28) includes commonly coded conditions of the eye. These conditions are age-related cataract, infantile and juvenile cataract, traumatic cataract, cataract secondary to ocular disorders, drug-induced cataract, and other disorders of the lens including aphakia and dislocation of the lens. Codes also exist for laterality and bilateral conditions.

Age-Related Cataract (Category H25)

A **cataract** is the opacity of the crystalline lens of the eye, or its capsule, which results in a loss of vision (NEI 2015a). ICD-10-CM identifies different types of age-related or senile cataracts. A common age-related cataract in the elderly is a **cortical cataract** (H25.0-), which creates an opacity and swelling of the entire lens in a mature cataract. The cataract is white wedge-like opacities that look like spokes around the periphery of the cortex of the lens that is part of the lens surrounding the central nucleus. Other common cataracts produce an opacity at the anterior subcapsular (anterior pole cataract, H25.03-) or the posterior subcapsular (posterior pole cataract, H25.04-) pole of the lens. **Subcapsular cataracts** develop in the back of the eye and are more common in patients with diabetes or patients taking high doses of steroid medications. Other age-related cataracts are **nuclear cataracts**, or an opacity in the central nucleus of the eye (H25.1-), or **morgagnian type cataracts** (H25.2-), which are a mature cataract in which the cortex has liquefied and the nucleus moves freely in the lens. Examples of cataracts are coded as follows:

H25.011, Cortical age-related cataract, right eye
H25.12, Age-related nuclear cataract, left eye
H25.21, Age-related cataract, morgagnian type, right eye

Infantile and Juvenile Cataract (H26.0-)

Infantile and juvenile cataracts are congenital cataracts that are present at birth but may not be identified until the child is older (MedicineNet 2019). Cataracts that require treatment include lamellar, polar, total, or nuclear types. Congenital cataracts may occur as part of other birth defects such as congenital rubella, Down syndrome, familial congenital cataract, and trisomy 13 (NLM 2019). The cataracts in category H26.0- are coded according to the type: cortical, lamellar, zonular, nuclear, or polar as follows:

H26.011, Infantile and juvenile cortical, lamellar, or zonular cataract, right eye
H26.032, Infantile and juvenile nuclear cataract, left eye
H26.041, Anterior subcapsular polar infantile and juvenile cataract, right eye

Check Your Understanding 10.1

Assign ICD-10-CM diagnosis codes to the following conditions.

1. Acute mucopurulent follicular conjunctivitis, left eye
2. Bilateral marginal corneal ulcer
3. Stable keratoconus, right eye
4. Cortical age-related cataract, bilateral
5. Juvenile nuclear cataract

Disorders of Choroid and Retina (H30–H36)

Codes in the range of H30–H36 are describing disorders of choroid and retina including the laterality. The more frequently coded conditions in this section are retinal detachments, retinopathy due to hypertension, vasculitis, prematurity, and macular degeneration of various types.

Retinal Detachments and Breaks (H33)

A **retinal detachment** is the separation of the inner layers of the retina from the underlying retinal pigment epithelium that is attached to the choroid (NEI 2009). The choroid is a vascular membrane containing large branched pigment cells sandwiched between the retina and sclera. Separation of the sensory retina from the underlying epithelium occurs in different ways. A hole, tear, or break occurs when fluid from the vitreous cavity seeps in between the retina and the retinal pigment epithelium, the cell layer that nourishes the retina. This type is called a **rhegmatogenous detachment** or a retinal detachment with a retinal break (H33.0-). This is the most common type of detachment. Rhegma means a break. Vitreous fluid enters the break and separates the sensory retina from the epithelium resulting in the "detachment" (NEI 2009).

The second type is a **traction detachment** of the retina (H33.4-), which is caused by traction from inflammatory or vascular fibrous membranes on the surface of the retina, which attaches to the vitreous. The most common causes of tractional retinal detachment are proliferative diabetic retinopathy, sickle cell disease, advanced retinopathy of prematurity, and penetrating trauma. Vitreoretinal traction increases with age, as the vitreous gel shrinks and collapses over time, frequently causing posterior vitreous detachments in approximately two-thirds of persons older than 70 years (NEI 2009).

Symptoms of a retinal detachment are what may be described as vitreous "floaters," which is a floating spot or oval in the patient's vision. Another symptom a patient may describe is tiny black flecks appearing suddenly. Later as the condition progresses, the patients describe cobwebs in their vision. Other common symptoms described by patients are flashing lights or prisms with floaters in their vision (NEI 2009). Examples of retinal detachments and breaks are as follows:

H33.011, Retinal detachment with single break, right eye
H33.052, Total retinal detachment, left eye
H33.311, Horseshoe tear of retina without detachment, right eye

Retinopathy of Prematurity (H35.1-)

Retinopathy of prematurity (ROP) is a serious vasoproliferative disorder involving the developing retina in premature infants (NEI 2014). ROP primarily affects premature infants weighing about 2¾ pounds or less and born before 31 weeks of gestation. The disorder usually develops in both eyes and is one of the most common causes of visual loss in childhood and can produce lifelong vision impairment. Mild forms usually cause little or no vision loss. Severe forms lead to vision loss due to retinal scarring and damage. Even with optimal treatment, many preterm infants will develop some level of ROP, especially the smallest and most premature infants. Retrolental fibroplasia is an older medical term used to describe the condition in which the retina is actually scarred. Codes in the range of H35.10- through H35.17- identify the specific stages of ROP as well as retrolental fibroplasia. Codes for retinopathy of prematurity identify the stage of the disorder and the right eye, left eye, or bilateral status of the disease. For example:

H35.111, Retinopathy of prematurity, stage 0, right eye
H35.143, Retinopathy of prematurity, stage 3, bilateral
H35.172, Retrolental fibroplasia, left eye

Check Your Understanding 10.2

Assign ICD-10-CM diagnosis codes to the following conditions.

1. Posterior cyclitis, right eye

2. Traction detachment of retina, left eye

3. Operculum of retina without detachment, left eye

4. Retinitis pimentosa

5. Macula scars of posterior pole, right eye

Glaucoma (H40–H42)

Detailed glaucoma coding guidelines appear in the *Official Guidelines for Coding and Reporting*. Part I.C.7a1–a5 must be reviewed prior to coding these conditions. Included in the guidelines are five directions:

- I.C.7.a.1 Assign as many codes from category H40, Glaucoma, as needed to identify the type of glaucoma, the affected eye, and the glaucoma stage.

- I.C.7.a.2 When a patient has bilateral glaucoma and both eyes are documented as being the same type and stage, and there is a code for bilateral glaucoma, report only the code for the type of glaucoma, bilateral, with the seventh character for the stage.

- I.C.7.a.3 When a patient has bilateral glaucoma and each eye is documented as having a different type or stage, and the classification distinguishes laterality, assign the appropriate code for each eye rather than a code for bilateral glaucoma.

When a patient has bilateral glaucoma and each eye is documented as having a different type, and the classification does not distinguish laterality, assign one code for each type of glaucoma with appropriate seventh character for the stage.

When a patient has bilateral glaucoma and each eye is documented as having the same type but different stage, and the classification does not distinguish laterality, assign a code for the type of glaucoma for each eye with the seventh character for the specific glaucoma stage documented for each eye.

- I.C.7.a.4 If a patient is admitted with glaucoma and the stage progresses during the admission, assign the code for the highest stage documented.

- I.C.7.a.5 Assign the seventh character "4" for "indeterminate stage" when the glaucoma's stage cannot be clinically determined. The seventh character of "0" is for unspecified when no documentation is available for the stage of glaucoma (CDC 2019).

Specific forms of glaucoma are coded with ICD-10-CM codes in the block of codes from H40 and H42. The official coding guidelines describe the requirement to assign as many codes from category H40, Glaucoma, as needed to identify the type of glaucoma, the affected eye, and the glaucoma stage. The stage of glaucoma is specified with a seventh character:

0—stage unspecified
1—mild stage
2—moderate stage
3—severe stage
4—indeterminate stage

The assignment of the seventh character 4 for "indeterminate stage" of glaucoma should be based on the clinical documentation. The seventh character 4 is used for glaucomas in which the stage cannot be clinically determined. The seventh character 4 should not be confused with seventh character 0 for unspecified stage. Unspecified stage should be assigned when there is no documentation regarding the stage of the glaucoma.

Glaucoma is a group of diseases that damage the eye's optic nerve and can result in vision loss and blindness. The space in the front of the eye is the anterior chamber. The anterior chamber is filled with fluid known as aqueous humor that is produced continually and protects the tissues of the eye. In a normal eye, the aqueous humor flows in and out of the anterior chamber maintaining a constant pressure. In a diseased eye, the fluid does not drain out of the eye as it should, and pressure builds up in the anterior chamber. This pressure over time damages the optic nerve. Damage to the optic nerve impairs vision and is irreversible. If the high pressure is not treated, the damage to the optic nerve can lead to blindness. Ocular hypertension is another term that describes the high intraocular pressure in the eye that has not damaged the optic nerve at a point in time (NEI 2015b).

Category H40 is subdivided to identify the various types of glaucoma. Subcategory codes exist for glaucoma suspect (H40.0-), open-angle glaucoma (H40.1-), and primary angle-closure glaucoma (H40.2-). Other forms of glaucoma are the result of eye trauma (H40.3-), eye inflammation (H40.4-), secondary to other eye diseases (H40.5-), or due to the adverse effects of prescription drugs (H40.6-).

Glaucoma suspect (H40.0-) is a condition identified in a patient who has risk factors that may cause glaucoma in the future. When described as having glaucoma suspect, the patient does not have damage to the optic nerve as the result of the increased pressure in the anterior chamber, but there is an abnormal appearance of the optic nerve upon examination. The patients are monitored over time to begin treatment if glaucoma is found. Glaucoma suspect is the name of this condition and should not be considered the equivalent of a diagnosis stated as "suspected" glaucoma. Examples of this type of glaucoma are as follows:

H40.003, Preglaucoma, unspecified, bilateral
H40.011, Open angle with borderline findings, low risk, right eye
H40.062, Primary angle closure without glaucoma damage, left eye

Open-angle glaucoma (H40.1-) is a chronic form of glaucoma that gets its name from the fact that the angle between the iris and the cornea remains open and looks normal upon examination of the eye. However, for an unknown reason, the draining system in the eye fails to function correctly. This causes pressure to build up in the eye slowly and gradually damages the optic nerve. The patient has no visual symptoms, has no pain in the eye, and only experiences vision problems as the nerve damage progresses. Physicians may describe this form of glaucoma as simple chronic glaucoma or low-tension glaucoma, and it usually affects both eyes. Examples of open-angle glaucoma are as follows:

H40.11X1, Primary open-angle glaucoma, mild stage
H40.1223, Low-tension glaucoma, left eye, severe stage
H40.151, Residual stage of open-angle glaucoma, right eye

Primary angle-closure glaucoma (H40.2-) is an acute form of the disease. This form occurs suddenly with significant eye pain and visual defects. The disease is called angle-closure because the angle between the iris and the cornea closes and prevents the aqueous humor from draining, raising pressure in the anterior chamber. Usually this "attack" of glaucoma affects one eye. The occurrence of primary angle-closure glaucoma is a medical emergency and if left untreated will result in permanent damage to the patient's vision in less than two days. The emergency is usually treated with surgery to open the blockage and allow normal flow of aqueous humor. Physicians may describe this form of glaucoma as acute angle-closure glaucoma, acute glaucoma, or a glaucoma attack or crisis. It may also be described as narrow-angle glaucoma. A chronic and intermittent form of angle-closure glaucoma also exists when the normal flow of drainage cannot be sustained. Examples of primary angle-closure glaucoma are as follows:

H40.211, Acute angle-closure glaucoma, right eye
H40.2223, Chronic angle-closure glaucoma, left eye, severe stage
H40.233, Intermittent angle-closure glaucoma, bilateral

There are also secondary forms of glaucoma that develop as a complication of other diseases. Secondary glaucoma can be the result of eye trauma and eye inflammations such as uveitis, as well as a complication of eye surgery or a complication of advanced cataracts left untreated. Secondary forms of glaucoma are coded in ICD-10-CM as glaucoma secondary to eye trauma (H40.3-), secondary to eye inflammation (H40.4-), secondary to other eye disorders (H40.5-), and glaucoma secondary to drugs (H40.6-). Patients developing glaucoma as a result of corticosteroid therapy are classified to subcategory H40.6. A "use additional code" note appears beneath subcategory H40.6 to code the drug that is causing the adverse effect of glaucoma that would be in the range of T36–T50 with the fifth or sixth character 5. Examples of the secondary forms of glaucoma are as follows:

H40.31X1, Glaucoma secondary to eye trauma, right eye, mild stage
H40.42X2, Glaucoma secondary to eye inflammation, left eye, moderate stage

H40.53X2, Glaucoma secondary to other eye disorders, bilateral, moderate stage

H40.63X3, Glaucoma secondary to drugs, bilateral, severe stage

T38.0X5A, Adverse effect of glucocorticoids and synthetic analogues, initial encounter (the seventh character depends on the episode of care)

Subcategory H40.83- includes codes for aqueous misdirection, also known as malignant glaucoma. It is not "malignant" as in the sense of a cancerous condition. The term "malignant" is used in medicine to identify any condition that is severe and becomes progressively worse over time. Aqueous misdirection is usually a complication of eye surgery and requires additional surgical treatment. It is neither angle-closure nor open-angle glaucoma. In this form of glaucoma, the aqueous flows into the vitreous or posteriorly instead of flowing into the anterior chamber. Finally, if documentation in the health record states glaucoma only, code H40.9, Unspecified glaucoma, should be assigned. Examples of these conditions are as follows:

H40.833, Aqueous misdirection, bilateral

H40.89, Other specified glaucoma

H40.9, Unspecified glaucoma

Blindness and Low Vision (H54–H54.8)

A new guideline appears in the *Official Guidelines for Coding and Reporting* Part I.C.7b that must be reviewed prior to coding for blindness and low vision. Included in the guidelines are the following directions: If "blindness" or "low vision" of both eyes is documented but the visual impairment category is not documented, assign code H54.3, Unqualified visual loss, both eyes. If "blindness" or "low vision" in one eye is documented but the visual impairment category is not documented, assign a code from H54.6-, Unqualified visual loss, one eye. If "blindness" or "visual loss" is documented without any information about whether one or both eyes are affected, assign code H54.7, Unspecified visual loss.

Intraoperative and Postprocedural Complications and Disorders of Eye and Adnexa, Not Elsewhere Classified

The final category in this chapter is H59, for intraoperative and postprocedural complications and disorders of the eye and adnexa, not elsewhere classified. These include disorders of the eye following cataract surgery as well as eye conditions that are complications of ophthalmic and other procedures. Codes in this section also identify if the right eye, left eye, or both eyes (bilateral) are affected by the complication.

There are three specific disorders of the eye that occur following cataract surgery: keratopathy (bullous aphakic), cataract (lens) fragments in the eye, and cystoid macular edema. Codes in the range of H59.0- to H59.09- identify these conditions. **Bullous keratopathy** (H59.01-) is a condition of the cornea with excess accumulation of fluid in the cornea. It occurs occasionally after cataract extraction from the loss of corneal endothelium as the result of surgery. The patients report that their vision is not as clear as it was immediately after surgery. Any type of intraocular surgery, especially cataract surgery, may damage endothelial cells and hasten the decline in endothelial cell count. Various treatments exist for this condition from simple observing to see if the condition resolves after the surgery to the most intensive therapy being a corneal transplant (Roat 2018).

An infrequent but well-known complication of cataract surgery is some form of **retained lens fragments**, particularly posterior dislocation of lens fragments. This is coded as H59.02-, Cataract (lens) fragments in eye following cataract surgery. Depending on the severity of the case, associated side effects range from uncomfortable inflammation and elevated intraocular pressure to cystoid macular edema and retinal detachment. With timely and appropriate management, the final visual outcome for the majority of patients with retained lens material is positive. Removing the retained lens fragments is usually a straightforward task for the ophthalmologist with a pars plana vitrectomy, effective for removing retained lens fragments, lowering the intraocular pressure, and reducing inflammation (Vision and Eye Health 2019).

Cystoid macular edema (CME) (H59.03-) is a complication that occurs during the first year after cataract surgery in a very small number of patients who have had a lens extraction procedure. It is a disease of the macula or the central retina. It is painless with multiple cyst-like areas of fluid that causes retinal swelling. The symptoms of the edema include blurred, decreased central vision and a painless swelling of the eye. The retinal inflammation is treated with anti-inflammatory medications that can be administered as eyedrops, by injection, or as medications taken orally. Sometime diuretics help reduce the swelling. If necessary, a vitrectomy is done to relieve the pressure of the vitreous pulling on the macular (Comer 2019). Examples of this complication following cataract surgery are as follows:

H59.031, Cystoid macular edema following cataract surgery, right eye
H59.032, Cystoid macular edema following cataract surgery, left eye
H59.033, Cystoid macular edema following cataract surgery, bilateral
H59.039, Cystoid macular edema following cataract surgery, unspecified eye

The other intraoperative and postprocedural complications include the following:

- Intraoperative hemorrhage and hematoma of eye and adnexa complicating a ophthalmic procedure (H59.11-)

- Intraoperative hemorrhage and hematoma of eye and adnexa complicating other procedure (H59.12-)

- Accidental puncture and laceration of eye and adnexa during an ophthalmic procedure (H59.21-)

- Accidental puncture and laceration of eye and adnexa during other procedure (H59.22-)

- Postprocedural hemorrhage, hematoma, and seroma of eye and adnexa following an ophthalmic procedure (H59.31-)

- Postprocedural hemorrhage, hematoma, and seroma of eye and adnexa following other procedure (H59.32)

- Inflammation (infections) of postprocedural bleb (H59.4-)

- Chorioretinal scars after surgery for detachment (H59.81-)

Check Your Understanding 10.3

Assign ICD-10-CM diagnosis codes to the following conditions.

1. Ocular hypertension of the left eye
2. Chronic angle-closure glaucoma, left eye, moderate stage
3. Residual stage of primary open-angle glaucoma, right eye
4. Bilateral low vision
5. Postprocedural hemorrhage of right eye following eye surgery

ICD-10-PCS Coding for Procedures Related to the Eye and Adnexa

The procedures performed on the eye appear in the ICD-10-PCS code book in tables that start with the two characters 0 and 8, followed by five characters representing root operation, body part, approach, device, and qualifier:

Character 1 is Value 0—Medical and Surgical
Character 2 is Value 8—Eye

Root Operation

Character 3 of the ICD-10-PCS codes in the Medical Surgical section is the root operation. The root operations that represent the objectives of procedures for surgical treatment of the diseases of the eye and adnexa are shown in table 10.1.

Table 10.1. **Root operations for procedures on body parts within the eye and adnexa**

Alteration: Modifying the anatomic structure of a body part without affecting the function of the body part
Bypass: Altering the route of passage of the contents of a tubular body part
Change: Taking out or off a device from a body part and putting back an identical or similar device in or on the same body part without cutting or puncturing the skin or a mucous membrane.
Destruction: Physical eradication of all or a portion of a body part by the direct use of energy, force, or a destructive agent
Dilation: Expanding the orifice or lumen of a tubular body part
Drainage: Taking or letting out fluids and/or gases from a body part
Excision: Cutting out or off, without replacement, a portion of a body part
Extirpation: Taking or cutting out solid matter from a body part
Extraction: Pulling or stripping out or off all or a portion of a body part by the use of force
Fragmentation: Breaking solid matter in a body part into pieces

Insertion: Putting in a nonbiological appliance that monitors, assists, performs, or prevents a physiological function but does not physically take the place of the body part
Inspection: Visually and/or manually exploring a body part
Occlusion: Completely closing an orifice or the lumen of a tubular body part
Reattachment: Putting back in or on all or a portion of a separated body part to its normal location or other suitable location
Release: Freeing a body part from an abnormal physical constraint by cutting or by the use of force
Removal: Taking out or off a device from a body part
Repair: Restoring, to the extent possible, a body part to its normal anatomic structure and function
Replacement: Putting in or on biological or synthetic material that physically takes the place and/or function of all or a portion of a body part
Reposition: Moving to its normal location, or other suitable location, all or a portion of a body part
Resection: Cutting out or off, without replacement, all of a body part
Supplement: Putting in or on biological or synthetic material that physically reinforces and/or augments the function of a portion of a body part
Restriction: Partially closing an orifice or the lumen of a tubular body part
Revision: Correcting, to the extent possible, a portion of a malfunctioning device or the position of a displaced device
Transfer: Moving, without taking out, all or a portion of a body part to another location to take over the function of all or a portion of a body part

Source: CMS 2019

Body Part

Character 4 identifies the body part involved in the procedure. The body parts in ICD-10-PCS have individual values that include laterality, as shown in table 10.2.

Table 10.2. **Body parts and values included in the ICD-10-PCS codes for the eye and adnexa**

0—Eye, right
1—Eye, left
2—Anterior Chamber, right
3—Anterior Chamber, left
4—Vitreous, right
5—Vitreous, left
6—Sclera, right
7—Sclera, left
8—Cornea, right

(*Continued*)

9—Cornea, left
A—Choroid, right
B—Choroid, left
C—Iris, right
D—Iris, left
E—Retina, right
F—Retina, left
G—Retinal Vessel, right
H—Retinal Vessel, left
J—Lens, right
K—Lens, left
L—Extraocular Muscle, right
M—Extraocular Muscle, left
N—Upper Eyelid, right
P—Upper Eyelid, left
Q—Lower Eyelid, right
R—Lower Eyelid, left
S—Conjunctiva, right
T—Conjunctive, left
V—Lacrimal Gland, right
W—Lacrimal Gland, left
X—Lacrimal Duct, right
Y—Lacrimal Duct, left

Source: CMS 2019

Approach

Character 5 identifies the approach used in the procedure. The approach for procedures performed on organs within the eye and adnexa as shown in table 10.3.

Table 10.3.   **Approaches, definitions, and values included in the ICD-10-PCS codes for the eye and adnexa**

Open (0): Cutting through the skin or mucous membrane and any other body layers necessary to expose the site of the procedure
Percutaneous (3): Entry, by puncture or minor incision, of instrumentation through the skin or mucous membrane and any other body layers necessary to reach the site of the procedure
Via Natural or Artificial Opening (7): Entry of instrumentation through a natural or artificial external opening to reach the site of the procedure

Via Natural or Artificial Opening Endoscopic (8): Entry of instrumentation through a natural or artificial external opening to reach and visualize the site of the procedure
External (X): Procedures performed directly on the skin or mucous membrane and procedures performed indirectly by the application of external force through the skin or mucous membrane

Source: CMS 2019

Device

Character 6 identifies if a device remains in the patient's body after the procedure is concluded. The devices used to code procedures performed on organs within the eye and adnexa are limited to the devices as shown in table 10.4.

Table 10.4.   **Devices and values included in the ICD-10-PCS codes for the eye**

0—Drainage Device
0—Synthetic Substitute, Intraocular Telescope
1—Radioactive Element
3—Infusion Device
5—Epiretinal Visual Prosthesis
7—Autologous Tissue Substitute
C—Extraluminal Device
D—Intraluminal Device
J—Synthetic Substitute
K—Nonautologous Tissue Substitute
Y—Other Device
Z—No Device

Source: CMS 2019

Qualifier

Character 7 is a qualifier that specifies an additional attribute of the procedure, if applicable. The qualifier characters used to code procedures performed on organs within the eye and adnexa are four values as shown in table 10.5. The qualifier value of X for diagnostic procedure is available for the root operations of Drainage and Excision.

Table 10.5.   **Qualifiers used to code procedures within the eye**

4—Sclera
3—Nasal Cavity
X—Diagnostic
Z—No Qualifier

Source: CMS 2019

Procedures performed on the eye are included in the tables from 080–08X with the root operations Alteration, Bypass, Change, Destruction, Dilation, Drainage, Excision, Extirpation, Extraction, Fragmentation, Insertion, Inspection, Occlusion, Reattachment, Release, Removal, Repair, Replacement, Reposition, Resection, Supplement, Restriction, Revision, and Transfer. Like procedures in other body systems, in order to code eye procedures, the coder needs to know the definition of root operations and the anatomy of the eye to identify the body parts.

Using strictly the titles of operations of eye procedures is not sufficient to code in ICD-10-PCS. A term used by a physician may be the equivalent of multiple possible root operations that the coder has to analyze by reading the operative report to determine the primary objective of the procedure (what the procedure accomplished). For example, consider the following eye procedure terminology and the possible root operations that may be used based on what was performed:

Keratoplasty:
– Repair (LASIK to correct refractive error)
– Replacement (Corneal transplant)
– Supplement (Lamellar keratoplasty)

Phacoemulsification:
– Replacement (if an intraocular lens (IOL) is inserted)
– Extraction (if there is no IOL inserted)

ICD-10-PCS procedures are produced by building a code using the values provided for each root operation performed on a particular body system and body part. A keratoplasty is surgery on the cornea that may also be called corneal transplant or corneal grafting. A penetrating keratoplasty is the removal of the full thickness of the cornea and replacing it with donor corneal tissue. Usually this is called a corneal transplant. A lamellar keratoplasty is a partial-thickness graft of the cornea. In this procedure, only the epithelium and superficial stroma of the cornea are removed and are replaced with donor tissue that supplements the remaining corneal tissue that was not removed from the eye. Based on the type of keratoplasty performed, the root operation may be Repair as the procedure is restoring, to the extent possible, a body part to its normal anatomic structure and function. A Replacement is defined as putting in or on biological or synthetic material that physically takes the place or function of all or a portion of a body part. The Supplement root operation, defined as putting in or on biological or synthetic material that physically reinforces or augments the function of a portion of a body part, is used for the lamellar keratoplasty as the donor tissue reinforces the existing cornea in the patient's eye (Dorland 2012).

For cataract surgery, the root operation may be Replacement or Extraction depending on whether the intraocular lens is placed in the eye at the same procedure. Replacement is used when the artificial lens is placed in the eye to replace the lens that was removed with the cataract. Extraction, defined as pulling or stripping out or off all or a portion of a body part by the use of force, is the root operation when the cataract or the diseased lens in the eye is removed without replacement by an artificial lens during the same procedure.

Other examples of eye procedures and the possible root operations used to code them include:

• Blepharoplasty: Alteration, Repair, Replacement, Reposition, or Supplement

• Dacryocystostomy or sclerotomy: Drainage

- Enucleation or evisceration: Replacement or Resection

- Photocoagulation: Destruction or Repair

- Probing lacrimal duct: Inspection or Dilation

- Removal of foreign body: Extirpation

- Scleral buckling: Supplement

- Strabismus: Reposition

- Trabeculectomy: Drainage

- Vitrectomy: Excision or Resection

ICD-10-CM and ICD-10-PCS Review Exercises: Chapter 10

Assign the correct ICD-10-CM diagnosis codes or ICD-10-PCS procedure codes to the following exercises.

1. Macular drusen, right eye

   _____

2. Irregular astigmatism, both eyes

   _____

3. Presenile cortical cataract, left eye

   _____

4. Retained metal foreign body fragments, right upper eyelid

   _____

5. Low-tension glaucoma, severe stage unilateral

   _____

6. Floppy iris syndrome, right eye, due to the patient's prescription Flomax taken as prescribed, follow-up visit

   _____

7. Single break retinal detachment, left eye

   _____

8. Acute atopic conjunctivitis, right eye

   _____

9. Bilateral retinopathy of prematurity, stage 2

   _____

(Continued on next page)

ICD-10-CM and ICD-10-PCS Review Exercises: Chapter 10 (continued)

10. Monocular exotropia with V pattern, left eye

11. Right eye blindness category 3 and left eye low vision category 1

12. Bullous keratopathy, left eye, due to cataract surgery

13. Chronic iridocyclitis and cataract with neovascularization, right eye

14. Chronic lacrimal dacryocystitis, right eye

15. Essential hypertension with hypertensive retinopathy

16. PROCEDURE: Removal of foreign body (glass) from right eye

17. PROCEDURE: Transnasal endoscopy for dilation and stent placement in left lacrimal duct

18. PROCEDURE: Penetrating keratoplasty of right cornea with donor matched cornea for transplant, percutaneous approach

19. PROCEDURE: Cataract extraction by phacoemulsification, left eye, with prosthetic lens immediate insertion

20. PROCEDURE: Lamellar keratoplasty, onlay supplement type, right cornea, using autograft

References

Centers for Disease Control and Prevention (CDC), National Center for Health Statistics. 2019. *ICD-10-CM Official Guidelines for Coding and Reporting*, 2020. http://www.cdc.gov/nchs/icd/icd10cm.htm.

Comer, G. M. 2019. Cystoid Macular Edema (CME). University of Michigan Kellogg Eye Center. http://www.kellogg.umich.edu/patientcare/conditions/cystoid.macular.edema.html.

Dorland. 2012. *Dorland's Illustrated Medical Dictionary*, 32nd ed. Philadelphia: Elsevier.

MedicineNet. 2019. Cataracts in Infants. http://www.medicinenet.com/cataracts_in_infants/views.htm.

Mosby. 2017. *Mosby's Pocket Dictionary of Medicine, Nursing, and Health Professions*, 8th ed. St. Louis: Mosby, Inc.

National Eye Institute (NEI). 2015a. Facts About Cataract. https://nei.nih.gov/health/cataract/cataract_facts.

National Eye Institute (NEI). 2015b. Facts About Glaucoma. https://nei.nih.gov/health/glaucoma/glaucoma_facts.

National Eye Institute (NEI). 2014. Facts About Retinopathy of Prematurity (ROP). https://nei.nih.gov/health/rop/rop.

National Eye Institute (NEI). 2009. Facts About Retinal Detachment. https://nei.nih.gov/health/retinaldetach/retinaldetach.

Roat, M. I. 2018. Bullous Keratopathy. Merck Manual-Consumer Version. http://www.merckmanuals.com/home/eye-disorders/corneal-disorders/bullous-keratopathy.

U.S. National Library of Medicine, MedLinePlus (NLM). 2019. Congenital Cataract. https://www.nlm.nih.gov/medlineplus/ency/article/001615.htm.

Vision and Eye Health. 2019. Cataract Surgery: Complications During Surgery. http://www.vision-and-eye-health.com/cataractsurgery-intraopcomplications.html.

Chapter 11

Diseases of the Ear and Mastoid Process (H60–H95)

Learning Objectives

At the conclusion of this chapter, you should be able to do the following:

- Describe the organization of the conditions and codes included in Chapter 8 of ICD-10-CM, Diseases of the Ear and Mastoid Process (H60–H95)

- Identify and describe the various types of ear infections, including otitis externa and otitis media

- Identify and describe the various types of hearing loss

- Assign ICD-10-CM codes for diseases of the ear and mastoid process

- Assign ICD-10-PCS codes for procedures related to the ear and mastoid process

Key Terms

Conductive hearing loss
Deaf nonspeaking
Dizziness
Mastoiditis
Ménière's disease
Otitis externa

Otitis media (OM)
Otosclerosis
Salpingitis
Sensorineural hearing loss
Vertigo

Overview of ICD-10-CM Chapter 8: Diseases of the Ear and Mastoid Process (H60–H95)

Chapter 8 of ICD-10-CM includes categories H60–H95 arranged in the following blocks:

H60–H62	Diseases of external ear
H65–H75	Diseases of middle ear and mastoid
H80–H83	Diseases of inner ear
H90–H94	Other disorders of ear
H95	Intraoperative and postprocedural complications and disorders of ear and mastoid process, not elsewhere classified

Chapter 8 in ICD-10-CM classifies the Diseases of the Ear and Mastoid Process. Blocks of codes have been created to identify the types of conditions that would occur in the external ear, middle ear and mastoid, and inner ear. Like many chapters, the intraoperative and postprocedural complications are grouped at the end of the chapter rather than included in different categories. The codes include greater specificity at the fourth-, fifth-, and sixth-character levels, for example, acute otitis media (AOM) with and without spontaneous rupture of the ear drum with specific codes for the type of perforation. Also included are codes for laterality for the right, left, bilateral, and unspecified sides of the body for the sites and more "code first underlying disease" notes.

EXAMPLES: H65, Nonsuppurative otitis media
H71, Cholesteatoma of middle ear
H81, Disorders of vestibular function

Coding Guidelines and Instructional Notes for ICD-10-CM Chapter 8, Diseases of the Ear and Mastoid Process (H60–H95)

At the time of this publication, the NCHS has not published chapter-specific guidelines for Chapter 8 in the *ICD-10-CM Official Guidelines for Coding and Reporting*. The coding student should review all of the coding guidelines for ICD-10-CM, which appear in an ICD-10-CM code book, at the CDC website (CDC 2019) or in appendix F.

There are instructional notes throughout Chapter 8 to direct the coder for correct and complete coding. At the start of Chapter 8 in ICD-10-CM, there is a note to use an external cause code following the code for the ear condition, if applicable, to identify the cause of the ear condition. An Excludes2 note includes a series of excluded conditions that are applicable to all conditions classifiable to Chapter 8. For example, certain conditions originating in the perinatal period of the first 28 days of life are coded to Chapter 16 of ICD-10-CM, and certain infectious and parasitic diseases are coded to Chapter 1 instead of to the chapter for diseases of the ear and mastoid process (CDC 2019).

An example of an instructional note appears at category H72, Perforation of tympanic membrane, to recognize the importance of coding first the associated otitis media with the diagnosis of perforation of the tympanic membrane. The Excludes1 note that follows explains other conditions that are not to be coded to category H72 as these excluded conditions cannot occur together.

> **EXAMPLE:** H72, Perforation of tympanic membrane
> Code first any associated otitis media (H65.-, H66.1-, H66.2-, H66.3-, H66.4-, H66.9-, H67.-)
>
> Excludes1:
> acute suppurative otitis media with rupture of the tympanic membrane (H66.01-)
> traumatic rupture of ear drum (S09.2-)

There is an instructional note in categories H65, H66, and H67 to use an additional code for any associated perforated tympanic membrane (H72.-). This is a reminder to the coder that two codes are required when a patient has both otitis media and perforated tympanic membrane.

Another instructional note is found under the category for suppurative and unspecified otitis media (H66). The note instructs coding professionals to use an additional code to identify the following:

- Z77.22, Exposure to environmental tobacco smoke

- P96.81, Exposure to tobacco smoke in the perinatal period

- Z87.891, History of tobacco dependence

- Z57.31, Occupational exposure to environmental tobacco smoke

- F17.-, Tobacco dependence

- Z72.0, Tobacco use

Coding Diseases of the Ear and Mastoid Process in ICD-10-CM Chapter 8

The chapter is organized into five blocks of codes:

- Diseases of the External Ear, H60–H62

- Diseases of the Middle Ear and Mastoid, H65–H75

- Diseases of the Inner Ear, H80–H83

- Other Disorders of the Ear, H90–H94

- Intraoperative and Postprocedural Complications and Disorders of Ear and Mastoid Process, Not Elsewhere Classified, H95

A diagram of the ear is shown in figure 11.1 that illustrates the structures within the outer or external ear, within the middle ear, and within the internal ear.

Figure 11.1.   **Diagram of the ear**

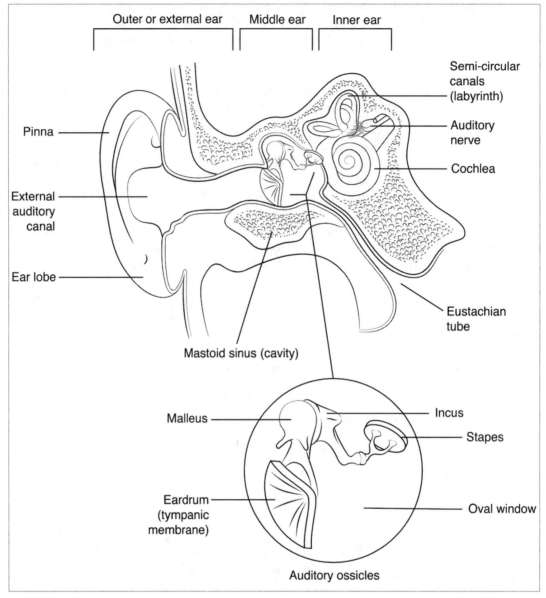

© AHIMA

Diseases of External Ear (H60–H62)

The external ear is the outer part of the ear consisting of the auricle and the external acoustic meatus that is the auditory canal, or the passage leading to the ear drum (Mosby 2017, 492). It may also be called the outer ear. **Otitis externa** (external otitis, swimmer's ear) is an infection of the external auditory canal that may be classified as acute or chronic. Acute otitis externa is characterized by moderate to severe pain, fever, regional cellulitis, and partial hearing loss. Instead of pain, chronic otitis externa is characterized by pruritus, which leads to scaling and a thickening of the skin.

ICD-10-CM classifies otitis externa to category H60, Otitis externa. Subcategories H60.0 for abscess of external ear, H60.1 for cellulitis of external ear, and H60.2 for malignant otitis externa include codes for unspecified, right, left, and bilateral ears. Similarly, subcategory

H60.3 includes fifth and sixth character codes for diffuse otitis externa, hemorrhagic otitis externa, swimmer's ear, and other infective otitis media with specific codes for unspecified, right, left, and bilateral ears.

Subcategories H62.4 and H62.8 classify otitis externa and other disorders of the external ear in diseases classified elsewhere. These codes require the reporting of the underlying disease that has caused the external ear condition. A "code first underlying disease" note appears under each subcategory, such as coding erysipelas, impetigo, or gout as the underlying disease.

EXAMPLE: Otitis externa, right ear, due to erysipelas
A46, Erysipelas
H62.41, Otitis externa in other diseases classified elsewhere, right ear

Diseases of Middle Ear and Mastoid (H65–H75)

Diseases of the middle ear and mastoid is a series of codes from H65–H75. A note to use additional code for any associated perforated tympanic membrane is included with the otitis media codes at the H65 and H66 category level. Other notes to use additional codes for exposure to smoke from environment and personal use of tobacco products are also included with the codes for otitis media or middle ear infections.

Otitis Media

Otitis media (OM) is an inflammation of the middle ear (Mosby 2017, 973) that may be further specified in ICD-10-CM codes as suppurative or secretory, and acute or chronic. These variations and their symptoms are as follows:

- Acute suppurative OM is characterized by severe, deep, throbbing pain; sneezing and coughing; mild to high fever; hearing loss; dizziness; nausea; and vomiting. Suppurative infections involve the formation of pus.

- Acute secretory or serous OM results in severe conductive hearing loss and, in some cases, a sensation of fullness in the ear with popping, crackling, or clicking sounds on swallowing or with jaw movement. Secretory infections produce a secretion or serous exudate.

- Chronic OM has its origin in the childhood years but usually persists into adulthood. Cumulative effects of chronic OM include thickening and scarring of the tympanic membrane, decreased or absent tympanic mobility, cholesteatoma, and painless purulent discharge (NIDCD 2017a).

Acute, chronic, and unspecified types of otitis media can be coded with laterality identified for right, left, bilateral, or unspecified ears. ICD-10-CM classifies OM to categories H65, Nonsuppurative otitis media, and H66, Suppurative and unspecified otitis media. Both of these categories are subdivided to identify acute and chronic forms of OM and other specific types of OM.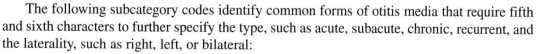

The following subcategory codes identify common forms of otitis media that require fifth and sixth characters to further specify the type, such as acute, subacute, chronic, recurrent, and the laterality, such as right, left, or bilateral:

H65.0	Acute serous otitis media
H65.1	Other acute nonsuppurative otitis media
H65.4	Other chronic nonsuppurative otitis media
H66.0	Acute suppurative otitis media
H66.3	Other chronic suppurative otitis media

There are instructional notes with categories H65, H66, and H67 to use an additional code for any associated perforated tympanic membrane. Another instructional note is found under the categories H65 and H66 to use an additional code to identify use of or exposure to tobacco products.

Eustachian Salpingitis and Obstruction (H68)

Acute and chronic infections of the eustachian tube as well as obstruction of the eustachian tube can be coded with category H68. The term "salpingitis" is included in the codes. **Salpingitis** is the inflammation of a tubular site, such as a fallopian tube in the female reproductive tract as well as the eustachian tube in the middle ear. Examples of eustachian salpingitis and obstruction are as follows:

> H68.011, Acute Eustachian Salpingitis, right ear
> H68.022, Chronic Eustachian Salpingitis, left ear
> H68.113, Osseous Obstruction of Eustachian Tube, bilateral

Mastoiditis and Related Conditions (H70)

Category H70, Mastoiditis and related conditions, includes four-, five-, and six-character codes to identify acute mastoiditis, chronic mastoiditis, petrositis, and other related conditions. Laterality is included in this category to identify if the patient's right, left, or bilateral ears are involved. Codes for an unspecified ear are also included.

The definition of **mastoiditis** is an infection of one of the mastoid bones; usually, it is an extension of a middle ear infection (Mosby 2017, 814) that includes all inflammatory processes of the mastoid bone air cells of the temporal bone. As the mastoid bone is an extension of the middle ear cleft, many children or adults with AOM or chronic middle ear inflammatory disease will have mastoiditis. In most cases, middle ear symptoms are more obvious in the patients (that is, fever, pain, conductive hearing loss), and the disease within the mastoid is not considered a separate disease when it occurs together.

Acute mastoiditis is present with AOM. In some patients, the infection spreads, and patients develop osteitis or periosteitis of the mastoid process. These patients have acute surgical mastoiditis (ASM), a complication of otitis media.

Chronic mastoiditis most commonly occurs with chronic suppurative otitis media and with cholesteatoma formation. Cholesteatomas are growths in the lining of the middle ear that invade and change the normal structure and function of surrounding soft tissue and bone. It is a destructive process accelerated in the presence of active infection.

With AOM as the underlying disease, the most common organism causing surgical mastoiditis is *Streptococcus pneumoniae*, followed by *Haemophilus influenzae* and group A *Streptococcus pyogenes*. Gram-negative organisms and *Staphylococcus aureus* are the organisms that develop more frequently in patients with chronic mastoiditis.

Most of the children admitted with acute mastoiditis have no history of recurrent AOM. In those children, *S. pneumoniae* has been the leading pathogen, while *Pseudomonas aeruginosa* causes the disease in children with recurrent AOM. Persistent otorrhea that persists more than three weeks is the most consistent sign that a process involving the mastoid has evolved.

A patient with acute mastoiditis may have a high and unrelenting fever. Some of this symptomatology may be related to the associated AOM. However, if a patient has a persistent fever, particularly when the patient is receiving adequate and appropriate antimicrobial agents, this is the indication the patient has ASM.

The patient feels pain deep in and behind the ear with mastoiditis, and it is typically worse at night when the patient is lying down and trying to sleep. This persistent pain is a warning sign of mastoid disease. Hearing loss is common with all infectious processes that involve the middle ear (Devan 2017).

Examples of coding mastoiditis and related conditions are as follows:

H70.002, Acute mastoiditis without complications, left ear

H70.011, Subperiosteal abscess of mastoid, right ear

H70.12, Chronic mastoiditis, left ear

H70.211, Acute petrositis, right ear

Perforation of Tympanic Membrane (H72)

The most common use of the codes in category H72 is to classify the condition of a "ruptured" tympanic membrane that can occur at the same time as acute and chronic middle ear infections. The tympanic membrane is a thin covering in the middle ear that transmits sound vibrations to the internal ear by means of the auditory ossicles. As the result of infection or inflammation, the membrane swells and then can break or rupture (Mosby 2017, 1392). However, the includes note under category H72 states that persistent posttraumatic perforation of the ear drum and postinflammatory perforation of the ear drum are included in this category (CDC 2019). There is a note to code first any associated otitis media with the codes from category H72 when the two conditions occur together. The code first note acknowledges that the otitis media is the cause of the perforation in many patients.

> **EXAMPLE:** Central perforation of the tympanic membrane of the right ear due to acute otitis media of right ear
> H66.91, Otitis media (includes acute otitis media NOS)
> H72.01, Central perforation of the tympanic membrane, right ear

---

Check Your Understanding 11.1

Assign ICD-10-CM diagnosis codes to the following conditions.

1. Keratosis obturans of left ear canal

2. Impacted cerumen, bilateral ears

3. Acute allergic serous otitis media, recurrent, bilateral

4. Otitis media with effusion, right and left ears

5. Acute myringitis, left ear

Diseases of the Inner Ear (H80–H83)

Diseases of the inner ear include such conditions as otosclerosis, disorders of vestibular function, such as Ménière's disease, and different types of vertigo. Vertiginous syndromes in diseases classified elsewhere as well as other diseases of the inner ear may be coded with laterality.

Otosclerosis (H80)

Otosclerosis is the growth of spongy bone in the inner ear where it causes obstruction. It causes slowly progressive conductive hearing loss. Otosclerosis affects 10 percent of the Caucasian population and is more likely to occur in middle-aged women (NIDCD 2018a). Frequency is thought to be decreasing because more people now are receiving the measles vaccination. Often the patient with otosclerosis has a family history of the disease. Pregnancy and estrogen therapy is suspected to increase the progression of otosclerosis. Symptom onset usually occurs by age 40 but can also occur later in life. The most common symptom is slowly progressive bilateral hearing loss. Vertigo is uncommon, but tinnitus or ringing in the ears may be present. These symptoms often resolve after successful surgical treatment. On physical examination, patients with conductive hearing loss often speak softly but do not realize it because they hear their voices as louder because of the enhanced bone conduction of sound (NIDCD 2018a).

> **EXAMPLE:** The patient has obliterative otosclerosis of the oval window within the left ear
> H80.12, Otosclerosis involving oval window, obliterative, left ear

Ménière's Disease (H81.0-)

Ménière's disease is a disorder of the inner ear that causes severe dizziness (vertigo), ringing in the ears (tinnitus), hearing loss, and a feeling of fullness or congestion in the ear. Ménière's disease usually affects only one ear (NIDCD 2017b). It may be documented as idiopathic endolymphatic or labyrinthine hydrops. Endolymphatic hydrops is increased pressure within the inner ear lymphatic system. Excess pressure accumulation causes symptoms of fluctuating hearing loss, occasional episodic vertigo, tinnitus, and pressure or fullness sensation in the ears. The terms of Ménière's disease, Ménière's syndrome, and endolymphatic hydrops may be used as synonymous terms. However, Ménière's disease has an unknown cause, but Ménière's syndrome is due to endocrine abnormalities, trauma, electrolyte imbalance, autoimmune dysfunction, medications, parasitic infections, or hyperlipidemia. Finding the cause and treatment can be a difficult medical task. The cause may be a simple condition like dehydration or a serious disease such as a brain tumor. Medical therapy can be directed toward treatment of the actual symptoms of the acute attack or directed toward prophylactic prevention of the attacks. If Ménière's syndrome is the final diagnosis, treatment is directed as the primary disease (that is, thyroid disease). In ICD-10-CM, Ménière's disease, labyrinthine hydrops, Ménière's syndrome, or vertigo is coded to one subcategory, H81.0-, with fifth characters for right ear, left ear, bilateral ears, or unspecified ear.

EXAMPLES: H81.01, Ménière's disease, right ear
H81.02, Ménière's disease, left ear
H81.03, Ménière's disease, bilateral
H81.09, Ménière's disease, unspecified ear

Benign Paroxysmal Vertigo (H81.1-)

A common type of vertigo is benign paroxysmal positional vertigo (BPPV). The subcategory of codes H81.10–H81.13 identify laterality for right, left, bilateral, and unspecified ears. Patients describe their **vertigo** as a feeling that their surroundings seem to whirl around them. Dizziness is not the same as vertigo. **Dizziness** is a sensation of unsteadiness accompanied by a feeling of movement within the head. Many patients who present to their physician's office complaining of the vertigo sensation are diagnosed with BPPV. In addition, BPPV can occur at the same time with other inner ear diseases, for example, with Ménière's disease (NIDCD 2017c).

Classic BPPV is usually triggered by sitting up quickly from a supine position. Patients describe the feeling of the room spinning around them. The onset is typically sudden. Patients state that they are more likely to experience the condition in the morning while trying to sit up when they are getting out of bed. The symptoms resolve quickly. However, the sensation can occur again when the person moves to a sitting position while getting out of bed. This sensation can occur for a period of days to weeks. Sometimes the symptoms periodically resolve but later recur. Patients report that if they get up slowly and pause while sitting on the edge of the bed before standing they do not have the same vertigo sensations. People who have BPPV may not feel dizzy but can experience severe dizziness triggered by head movements. Many patients have few or no symptoms between the episodes of vertigo. However, some patients complain of a continual "foggy or cloudy" sensation after their vertigo starts. The cause of the vertigo may never be found. Patients who are at risk for vertigo are people who have been inactive, such as patients recovering from surgery and illnesses and spending a lot of time lying down in bed. It is also common in patients with central nervous system diseases and ear diseases, but the connection has not been established. Vertigo is also common in patients with acute alcoholism. Treatment of the condition may be vertigo-suppressant medications that relieve some of the symptoms. However, many patients simply experience a resolution of the problem on its own but continue to observe the pattern of rising slowly from bed or from a reclining position to prevent a recurrence (NLM 2019). The codes for benign paroxysmal vertigo in ICD-10-CM are as follows:

H81.10, Benign paroxysmal vertigo, unspecified ear
H81.11, Benign paroxysmal vertigo, right ear
H81.12, Benign paroxysmal vertigo, left ear
H81.12, Benign paroxysmal vertigo, bilateral

Check Your Understanding 11.2

Assign diagnosis codes to the following conditions.

1. Cochlear otosclerosis, right ear
2. Vestibular neuronitis, bilateral
3. Ménière's disease, right ear
4. Cochlear otosclerosis, left ear
5. Central positional nystagmus, left ear

Other Disorders of Ear (H90–H94)

The block of codes H90–H94 includes specific codes with laterality for many different types of hearing loss. Other conditions such as otalgia, tinnitus, and disorders of acoustic or the eighth cranial nerve can be coded with laterality.

Conductive and Sensorineural Hearing Loss, Other and Unspecified Hearing Loss (H90–H91)

ICD-10-CM category codes H90 and H91 contain several subcategory codes that describe various forms of hearing loss or deafness. **Conductive hearing loss** or impairment is hearing loss caused by dysfunction of the outer or middle ear (NIDCD 2018b). It is the decreased ability to hear sounds because of a defect of the sound-conducting apparatus of the ear. Conductive hearing loss in one ear (unilateral) is classified with codes H90.11–H90.12 when the patient has unrestricted hearing on the contralateral, or opposite, site. Conductive hearing loss that occurs bilaterally is classified with code H90.0. There is also the option for unspecified conductive hearing loss with code H90.2.

Sensorineural hearing loss is the decreased ability to hear sounds due to a defect in the sensory mechanisms within the ear or the nerves within the ear (NIDCD 2018b). Sensorineural hearing loss may be described as sensory, neural, or central hearing loss. Sensorineural hearing loss with unrestricted hearing in the opposite ear is classified with codes H90.41–H90.42. The code for bilateral conductive hearing loss is H90.3. Again, there is a code H90.5 for unspecified sensorineural hearing loss.

Specific codes exist for unilateral mixed conductive and sensorineural hearing loss (H90.7-) and bilateral mixed hearing loss (H90.6), as well as code H90.8 for use when the condition is not specified as unilateral or bilateral. Another condition described as **deaf nonspeaking** or "deafmutism" is classified with code H91.3 to identify the condition when a patient has the absence of both hearing and the faculties of speech.

Examples of ICD-10-CM codes for hearing loss include the following:

H90.0, Conductive hearing loss, bilateral
H90.441, Sensorineural hearing loss, unilateral, right ear, with unrestricted hearing on the contralateral side
H90.6, Mixed conductive and sensorineural hearing loss, bilateral

Intraoperative and Postprocedural Complications and Disorders of Ear and Mastoid Process, Not Elsewhere Classified (H95)

Finally, intraoperative and postprocedural complications and disorders of ear and mastoid process, not elsewhere classified, are the block of codes at the end of the chapter. These codes identify conditions such as the following:

- Recurrent cholesteatoma of postmastoidectomy cavity (H95.0-)

    EXAMPLE: H95.01, Recurrent cholesteatoma of postmastoidectomy cavity, right ear

- Other disorders of ear and mastoid process following mastoidectomy (H95.1-)

    EXAMPLE: H95.132, Mucosal cyst of postmastoidectomy cavity, left ear

- Intraoperative hemorrhage and hematoma of ear and mastoid procedure complicating a procedure on the ear and mastoid process (H95.2-)

    EXAMPLE: H95.21, Intraoperative hemorrhage and hematoma of ear and mastoid process complicating a procedure on the ear and mastoid process

- Accidental puncture and laceration of ear and mastoid process during a procedure on the ear and mastoid process (H95.3-)

    EXAMPLE: H95.31, Accidental puncture and laceration of ear and mastoid process during a procedure on the ear and mastoid process

- Postprocedural hemorrhage of ear and mastoid process following a procedure on the ear and mastoid process (H95.4-)

    EXAMPLE: H95.41, Postprocedural hemorrhage of ear and mastoid process following a procedure on the ear and mastoid process

- Postprocedural stenosis of external ear canal (H95.81-)

    EXAMPLE: H95.812, Postprocedural stenosis of left external ear canal

Check Your Understanding 11.3

Assign diagnosis codes to the following conditions.

1. Conductive hearing loss, right side, with normal hearing in left ear

2. Mixed conductive and sensorineural hearing loss in left ear with normal hearing in right ear

3. Pulsatile tinnitus in right ear

4. Recurrent cholesteatoma of postmastoidectomy cavity, left ear

5. Otorrhea and otorrhagia, right ear

ICD-10-PCS Coding for Procedures Related to Ear and Mastoid Process

 The procedures performed on the ear and mastoid process appear in the ICD-10-PCS code book in tables that start with the two characters 0 and 9, followed by five characters representing root operation, body part, approach, device, and qualifier:

Character 1 is Value 0—Medical and Surgical
Character 2 is Value 9—Ear, Nose, and Sinus

Root Operation

Character 3 of the Medical and Surgical section ICD-10-PCS codes is the root operation. The root operations that represent the objectives of procedures for surgical treatment of the diseases of the ear are shown in table 11.1.

Table 11.1. **Root operations for procedures on body parts within the ear**

Alteration: Modifying the anatomic structure of a body part without affecting the function of the body part
Bypass: Altering the route of passage of the contents of a tubular body part
Change: Taking out or off a device from a body part and putting back an identical or similar device in or on the same body part without cutting or puncturing the skin or a mucous membrane
Destruction: Physical eradication of all or a portion of a body part by the direct use of energy, force, or a destructive agent
Dilation: Expanding the orifice or lumen of a tubular body part
Division: Cutting into a body part, without draining fluid and/or gases from the body part, in order to separate or transect a body part
Drainage: Taking or letting out fluids and/or gases from a body part
Excision: Cutting out or off, without replacement, a portion of a body part
Extirpation: Taking or cutting out solid matter from a body part
Extraction: Pulling or stripping out or off all or a portion of a body part by the use of force
Insertion: Putting in a nonbiological appliance that monitors, assists, performs, or prevents a physiological function but does not physically take the place of the body part
Inspection: Visually and/or manually exploring a body part
Reattachment: Putting back in or on all or a portion of a separated body part to its normal location or other suitable location
Release: Freeing a body part from an abnormal physical constraint by cutting or by the use of force
Removal: Taking out or off a device from a body part
Repair: Restoring, to the extent possible, a body part to its normal anatomic structure and function

Replacement: Putting in or on biological or synthetic material that physically takes the place and/or function of all or a portion of a body part
Reposition: Moving to its normal location, or other suitable location, all or a portion of a body part
Resection: Cutting out or off, without replacement, all of a body part
Supplement: Putting in or on biological or synthetic material that physically reinforces and/or augments the function of a portion of a body part
Revision: Correcting, to the extent possible, a portion of a malfunctioning device or the position of a displaced device

Source: CMS 2019

Body Part

Character 4 identifies the body part involved in the procedure. The body parts in ICD-10-PCS have individual values that include laterality, as shown in table 11.2.

Table 11.2. Body parts and values included in the ICD-10-PCS codes for the ear and mastoid process

0—External Ear, right
1—External Ear, left
2—External Ear, bilateral
3—External Auditory Canal, right
4—External Auditory Canal, left
5—Middle Ear, right
6—Middle Ear, left
7—Tympanic Membrane, right
8—Tympanic Membrane, left
9—Auditory Ossicle, right
A—Auditory Ossicle, left
B—Mastoid Sinus, right
C—Mastoid Sinus, left
D—Inner Ear, right
E—Inner Ear, left
F—Eustachian Tube, right
G—Eustachian Tube, left
H—Ear, right
J—Ear, left
K—Nasal Mucosa and Soft Tissue

(Continued)

L—Nasal Turbinate
M—Nasal Septum
N—Nasopharynx
P—Accessory Sinus
Q—Maxillary Sinus, right
R—Maxillary Sinus, left
S—Frontal Sinus, right
T—Frontal Sinus, left
U—Ethmoid Sinus, right
V—Ethmoid Sinus, left
W—Sphenoid Sinus, right
X—Sphenoid Sinus, left
Y—Sinus

Source: CMS 2019

Approach

Character 5 identifies the approach used in the procedure. The approach for procedures performed on organs within the ear and mastoid process are shown in table 11.3.

Table 11.3. **Approaches, definitions, and values included in the ICD-10-PCS codes for the ear**

Open (0): Cutting through the skin or mucous membrane and any other body layers necessary to expose the site of the procedure
Percutaneous (3): Entry, by puncture or minor incision, of instrumentation through the skin or mucous membrane and any other body layers necessary to reach the site of the procedure
Percutaneous Endoscopic (4): Entry, by puncture of minor incision, of instrumentation through the skin or mucous membrane and any other body layers necessary to reach and visualize the site of the procedure
Via Natural or Artificial Opening (7): Entry of instrumentation through a natural or artificial external opening to reach the site of the procedure
Via Natural or Artificial Opening Endoscopic (8): Entry of instrumentation through a natural or artificial external opening to reach and visualize the site of the procedure
External (X): Procedures performed directly on the skin or mucous membrane and procedures performed indirectly by the application of external force through the skin or mucous membrane

Source: CMS 2019

Device

Character 6 identifies if a device remains in the patient's body after the procedure is concluded. The devices used to code procedures performed on organs within the ear and mastoid process are limited to a few devices as shown in table 11.4.

Table 11.4.   Devices and values included in the ICD-10-PCS codes for the ear and mastoid process

0—Drainage Device
4—Hearing Device, Bone Conduction
5—Hearing Device, Single Channel Cochlear Prosthesis
6—Hearing Device, Multiple Channel Cochlear Prosthesis
7—Autologous Tissue Substitute
B—Intraluminal Device, Airway
D—Intraluminal Device
J—Synthetic Substitute
K—Nonautologous Tissue Substitute
S—Hearing Device
Y—Other Device
Z—No Device

Source: CMS 2019

Qualifier

Character 7 is a qualifier that specifies an additional attribute of the procedure, if applicable. The qualifier characters used to code procedures performed on organs within the ear and mastoid process are limited to three values as shown in table 11.5. The qualifier value of X for diagnostic procedure is available for the root operations of Drainage and Excision.

Table 11.5.   Qualifiers used to code procedures within the ear and mastoid process

0—Endolymphatic
X—Diagnostic
Z—No Qualifier

Source: CMS 2019

Procedures performed on the ear, nose, and sinus are included in the tables from 090–09W with root operations Alteration, Bypass, Change, Destruction, Dilation, Division, Drainage, Excision, Extirpation, Extraction, Insertion, Inspection, Reattachment, Release, Removal, Repair, Replacement, Reposition, Resection, Supplement, and Revision. Like procedures in other body systems, in order to code ear, nose, and sinus procedures, the coder needs to know the definition of root operations and the anatomy to identify the body parts.

Using strictly the titles of operations of ear procedures is not sufficient to code in ICD-10-PCS. A term used by a physician may be the equivalent of multiple possible root operations that the coder has to analyze by reading the operative report to determine the primary objective of the procedure—what did the procedure accomplish? Different types of devices are inserted into the body for hearing assistance, for example, bone conduction hearing implants and cochlear devices. Numerous other surgical and diagnostic procedures are performed in the ear, nose, and sinuses. For example, consider the following ear, nose, and sinus procedure terminology and the possible root operations that may be used based on what was performed:

Rhinoplasty may be performed for a variety of objectives as described by these root operations:

- Alteration: cosmetic repair for improved appearance

- Repair: restoring, to the extent possible, the body part to its normal anatomic structure and function

- Replacement: putting in or on biological or synthetic material that physically takes the place or function of all or a portion of a body part

- Supplement: putting in or on biological or synthetic material that physically reinforces or augments the function of a portion of a body part

Ethmoidectomy, myringectomy, sinusotomy, stapedectomy, and turbinectomy procedures all involve the removal of these body parts as described by these root operations:

- Excision: cutting out or off, without replacement, a portion of a body part

- Resection: cutting out or off, without replacement, all of a body part

Otoplasty, septoplasty, and turbinoplasty are procedures that correct a condition at the body part as described by these root operations:

- Repair: restoring, to the extent possible, the body part to its normal anatomic structure and function

- Replacement: putting in or on biological or synthetic material that physically takes the place or function of all or a portion of a body part

- Reposition: moving to its normal location or other suitable location all or a portion of a body part

- Supplement: putting in or on biological or synthetic material that physically reinforces or augments the function of a portion of a body part

Otoscopy, rhinoscopy, and sinusoscopy may be performed without an accompanying surgical procedure through the scope. When the procedure is strictly an examination, it is coded with the following root operation:

- Inspection: visually or manually exploring a body part

Myringotomy or turbinotomy are procedures performed to drain or destroy a lesion in the body part and are described by one of the following operations:

- Drainage: taking or letting out fluids or gases from a body part

- Destruction: physical eradication of all or a portion of a body part by the direct use of energy, force, or a destructive agent

Removal of foreign body is a common procedure performed on the ear. The root operation is:

- Extirpation: taking or cutting out solid matter from a body part

ICD-10-CM and ICD-10-PCS Review Exercises: Chapter 11

Assign the correct ICD-10-CM diagnosis codes or ICD-10-PCS procedures codes to the following exercises.

1. Chronic serous otitis media, bilateral

   _____

2. Acute subperiosteal abscess of mastoid, right ear

   _____

3. Left acute serous otitis media with a total perforated tympanic membrane of the right ear

   _____

4. Left acute eustachian salpingitis

   _____

5. Bilateral conductive hearing loss due to nonobliterative otosclerosis of the stapes at the oval window. The patient is unable to hear with hearing aids and has decided to undergo left stapedectomy. During the surgery, an inadvertent laceration was made to the tympanic metal flap, which was repaired. Assign the diagnosis codes only.

   _____

6. Pulsatile Tinnitus, bilateral

   _____

7. Right-sided otitis externa in erysipelas

   _____

8. Acoustic trauma both ears

   _____

9. Acute eczematoid otitis externa, right ear

   _____

10. Acute suppurative otitis media with rupture of the right ear drum

    _____

11. Right tubotympanic suppurative otitis media, chronic. Patient has history of tobacco dependence.

    _____

12. Suppurative otitis media with central perforation of tympanic membrane, left ear

    _____

13. (1) Tinnitus, right ear; (2) otalgia, left ear

    _____

14. Left acute myringitis

    _____

(Continued on next page)

ICD-10-CM and ICD-10-PCS Review Exercises: Chapter 11 *(continued)*

15. Chronic postmastoidectomy cavity inflammation, left ear

16. PROCEDURE: Stapedectomy (removal of entire stapes), left ear

17. PROCEDURE: Removal of impacted foreign body (bead) left external auditory canal via ear canal

18. PROCEDURE: Insertion of a multiple channel cochlear prosthesis into right inner ear, open approach

19. PROCEDURE: Bilateral myringotomy and placement of tubes behind the tympanic membrane

20. PROCEDURE: Excision of cholesteatoma, left middle ear, open approach

References

Centers for Disease Control and Prevention (CDC), National Center for Health Statistics. 2019. *ICD-10-CM Official Guidelines for Coding and Reporting*, 2020. http://www.cdc.gov/nchs/icd/icd10cm.htm.

Centers for Medicare and Medicaid Services (CMS). 2019. *ICD-10-PCS Official Guidelines for Coding and Reporting*, 2020. http://www.cms.gov/Medicare/Coding/ICD10/.

Devan, P. P. 2018. Mastoiditis. Medscape. http://emedicine.medscape.com/article/2056657-overview.

Mosby. 2017. *Mosby's Pocket Dictionary of Medicine, Nursing, and Health Professions*, 8th ed. St. Louis: Mosby, Inc.

National Institute on Deafness and Other Communication Disorders (NIDCD). 2017a. Ear Infections in Children. http://www.nidcd.nih.gov/health/hearing/pages/earinfections.aspx.

National Institute on Deafness and Other Communication Disorders (NIDCD). 2017b. Ménière's Disease. http://www.nidcd.nih.gov/health/balance/pages/meniere.aspx.

National Institute on Deafness and Other Communication Disorders (NIDCD). 2017c. Balance Disorders. http://www.nidcd.nih.gov/health/balance/pages/balance_disorders.aspx.

National Institute on Deafness and Other Communication Disorders (NIDCD). 2018a. Otosclerosis. http://www.nidcd.nih.gov/health/hearing/Pages/otosclerosis.aspx.

National Institute on Deafness and Other Communication Disorders (NIDCD). 2018b. Glossary. http://www.nidcd.nih.gov/health/glossary/Pages/glossary.aspx.

U.S. National Library of Medicine, MedlinePlus, (NLM). 2019. Benign Positional Vertigo. https://www.nlm.nih.gov/medlineplus/ency/article/001420.htm.

Chapter 12

Diseases of the Circulatory System (I00–I99)

Learning Objectives

At the conclusion of this chapter, you should be able to do the following:

- Describe the organization of the conditions and codes included in Chapter 9 of ICD-10-CM, Diseases of the Circulatory System (I00–I99)

- Apply the ICD-10-CM coding guidelines for the correct coding of circulatory diagnoses

- Explain the circulatory system diseases of rheumatic fever, chronic rheumatic heart disease, hypertension, hypertensive disease, angina, acute myocardial infarction, chronic ischemic heart disease, heart failure, cardiac arrhythmias, cardiac arrest, cerebrovascular disease, and sequelae of cerebrovascular disease

- Assign ICD-10-CM codes for ICD-10-CM Chapter 9, Diseases of the Circulatory System

- Assign ICD-10-PCS codes for procedures related to diseases of the circulatory system

Key Terms

Abdominal-coronary artery bypass
Acute myocardial infarction (AMI)
Angina pectoris
Aortocoronary bypass
Atherosclerosis
Arteriosclerotic heart disease
Atherosclerotic heart disease
Atrial fibrillation
Atrial flutter
Automatic implantable cardioverter-defibrillator (AICD)
Benign hypertension
Cardiac arrhythmia

Cardiac catheterization
Cerebral infarction
Cerebrovascular accident (CVA)
Cerebrovascular disease
Congestive heart failure
Coronary angiography
Coronary arteriography
Deep vein thrombosis (DVT)
Electrode
Heart block: First-, Second-, and Third-degree
Heart failure
Hypertensive chronic kidney disease
Hypertensive heart disease

Hypertensive heart and chronic kidney disease
Internal mammary-coronary artery bypass
Intravenous tissue plasminogen activator (tPA)
Left-sided heart failure
Malignant hypertension
Non-ST elevation myocardial infarction (NSTEMI)
Normal blood pressure (BP)
Pacing lead
Paroxysmal tachycardia
Percutaneous transluminal coronary angioplasty (PTCA)
Pulse generator

Rheumatic chorea
Rheumatic fever
Rheumatic heart disease
Right-sided heart failure
Secondary hypertension
Sick sinus syndrome (SSS)
ST elevation myocardial infarction (STEMI)
Supraventricular tachycardia
Unstable angina
Venous thromboembolism (VTE)
Ventricular fibrillation
Ventriculography
Wolff-Parkinson-White (WPW) syndrome

Overview of ICD-10-CM Chapter 9: Diseases of the Circulatory System

Chapter 9 of ICD-10-CM includes categories I00–I99 arranged in the following blocks:

I00–I02	Acute rheumatic fever
I05–I09	Chronic rheumatic heart diseases
I10–I16	Hypertensive diseases
I20–I25	Ischemic heart disease
I26–I28	Pulmonary heart disease and diseases of pulmonary circulation
I30–I52	Other forms of heart disease
I60–I69	Cerebrovascular disease
I70–I79	Diseases of arteries, arterioles and capillaries
I80–I89	Diseases of veins, lymphatic vessels and lymph node, not elsewhere classified
I95–I99	Other and unspecified disorders of the circulatory system

The terminology used to describe several cardiovascular conditions has been revised to reflect more current medical practice. For example, acute myocardial infarction (AMI) is identified as **ST elevation myocardial infarction (STEMI)**, or Type 1 ST elevation myocardial infarction, and **non-ST myocardial infarction elevation (NSTEMI)**, or Type 1 non-ST myocardial infarction. A STEMI is a myocardial infarction in which the ST segment is elevated in one lead or several leads. The ST segment on an electrocardiogram is the interval from the end of the ventricular depolarization to the onset of the T wave and is usually isoelectric in normal patients (Dorland 2012, 935, 1687). An NSTEMI may also be referred to as a non-Q-wave myocardial infarction, subendocardial myocardial infarction, or a nontransmural myocardial infarction. This is a type of myocardial infarction that involves less than the full thickness of the myocardial wall (Dorland 2012, 935). Type 2 through Type 5 myocardial infarctions are included in category I21.A, other type myocardial infarction. Intermediate coronary syndrome is identified in ICD-10-CM as unstable angina (CDC 2019). Acute coronary occlusion without myocardial infarction is better classified in ICD-10-CM as acute coronary thrombosis not resulting in myocardial infarction. Hypertension codes do not identify the type of hypertension such as benign, malignant, or unspecified. There is only one code for essential hypertension (I10.-). Hypertensive crisis, also known as hypertensive urgency or emergency, is identified with category code I16.

The terminology used to describe several cardiovascular conditions has been revised to reflect more current medical practice.

> **EXAMPLES:** I21, ST elevation (STEMI) and non-ST elevation (NSTEMI) myocardial infarction
> I20.0, Unstable angina
> I24.0, Acute coronary thrombosis not resulting in myocardial infarction

The category for late effects of cerebrovascular disease is titled "Sequelae of cerebrovascular disease." The codes in the category include the type of stroke, such as hemorrhage or infarction, and the specific sequela, such as cognitive or speech deficits, monoplegia or hemiplegia, and aphasia or dysphagia. In addition, the laterality of the affliction and whether the dominant or nondominant side is affected is included in the codes' descriptions.

Coding Guidelines and Instructional Notes for ICD-10-CM Chapter 9

At the beginning of Chapter 9, a series of excluded conditions are listed that are applicable to all conditions classifiable to Chapter 9. For example, the Excludes2 note includes conditions that can be coded with codes from Chapter 9. Such conditions include but are not limited to certain conditions originating in the perinatal period, certain infectious and parasitic diseases, and complications of pregnancy, childbirth, and the puerperium.

Under several blocks of codes including hypertensive disease (I10–I16) and ischemic heart disease (I20–I25), there are "use additional code to identify" notes to code exposure to environmental tobacco smoke, history of tobacco use, occupational exposure to environmental tobacco smoke, tobacco dependence, and tobacco use.

Other codes, including cardiomyopathy in diseases classified elsewhere (I43) and paroxysmal tachycardia (I47), include "code first" notes, such as underlying diseases of amyloidosis; glycogen storage disease; gout and thyrotoxicosis; or abortion, ectopic, or molar pregnancy, and obstetric surgery and procedures.

The NCHS has published chapter-specific guidelines for Chapter 9 in the *ICD-10-CM Official Guidelines for Coding and Reporting*. The coding student should review all of the coding guidelines for Chapter 9 of ICD-10-CM, which appear in an ICD-10-CM code book, on the CDC website (CDC 2019) or in appendix F.

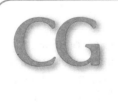

Chapter 9: Diseases of the Circulatory System (I00-I99)

Guideline I.C.9.a Hypertension: The classification presumes a causal relationship between hypertension and heart involvement and between hypertension and kidney involvement, as the two conditions are linked by the term "with" in the Alphabetic

(Continued)

(Continued)

Index. These conditions should be coded as related even in the absence of provider documentation explicitly linking them, unless the documentation clearly states the conditions are unrelated.

For hypertension and conditions not specifically linked by relational terms such as "with," "associated with" or "due to" in the classification, provider documentation must link the conditions in order to code them as related.

Guideline I.C.9.a.1. Hypertensive with Heart Disease: Hypertension with heart conditions classified to I50.- or I51.4–I51.7, I51.89, I51.9 are assigned to a code from category I11, Hypertensive heart disease. Use an additional code from category I50, Heart failure, to identify the type(s) of heart failure in those patients with heart failure.

The same heart conditions (I50.-, I51.4–I51.7, I51.89, I51.9) with hypertension are coded separately if the provider has documented they are unrelated to the hypertension. Sequence according to the circumstances of the admission/encounter.

Guideline I.C.9.a.2. Hypertensive Chronic Kidney Disease: Assign codes from category I12, Hypertensive chronic kidney disease, when both hypertension and a condition classifiable to category N18, Chronic kidney disease (CKD), are present. CKD should not be coded as hypertensive if the provider indicates the CKD is not related to the hypertension.

The appropriate code from category N18 should be used as a secondary code with a code from category I12 to identify the stage of chronic kidney disease.

See Section I.C.14.a. Chronic kidney disease.

If a patient has hypertensive chronic kidney disease and acute renal failure, an additional code for the acute renal failure is required.

Guideline I.C.9.a.3. Hypertensive Heart and Chronic Kidney Disease: Assign codes from combination category I13, Hypertensive heart and chronic kidney disease, when there is hypertension with both heart and kidney involvement. If heart failure is present, assign an additional code from category I50 to identify the type of heart failure.

The appropriate code from category N18, Chronic kidney disease, should be used as a secondary code from category I13 to identify the stage of chronic kidney disease.

See Section I.C.14. Chronic kidney disease.

The codes in category I13, Hypertensive heart and chronic kidney disease, are combination codes that include hypertension, heart disease and chronic kidney disease. The Includes note at I13 specifies that the condition included in I11 and I12 are included together in I13. If a patient has hypertension, heart disease and chronic kidney disease then a code from I13 should be used, not individual codes for hypertension, heart disease and chronic kidney disease, or codes from I11 or I12.

For patients with both acute renal failure and chronic kidney diseases an additional code for acute renal failure is required.

Guideline I.C.9.a.4. Hypertensive Cerebrovascular Disease: For hypertensive cerebrovascular disease, first assign the appropriate code from categories I60–I69, followed by the appropriate hypertension code.

Guideline I.C.9.a.5. Hypertensive Retinopathy: Subcategory I35.0, Background retinopathy and retinal vascular changes, should be used with a code from category I10-I15, Hypertensive disease to include the systemic hypertension. The sequencing is based on the reason for the encounter.

Guideline I.C.9.a.6. Hypertension, Secondary: Secondary hypertension is due to an underlying condition. Two codes are required: one to identify the underlying etiology and one from category I15 to identify the hypertension. Sequencing of codes is determined by the reason for admission/encounter.

Guideline I.C.9.a.7. Hypertension, Transient: Assign code R03.0, Elevated blood pressure reading without diagnosis of hypertension, unless patient has an established diagnosis of hypertension. Assign code O13.-, Gestational [pregnancy-induced] hypertension without significant proteinuria, or O14, Pre-eclampsia, for transient hypertension of pregnancy.

Guideline I.C.9.a.8. Hypertension, Controlled: This diagnosis statement usually refers to an existing state of hypertension under control by therapy. Assign the appropriate code from categories I10–I15, Hypertensive diseases.

Guideline I.C.9.a.9. Hypertension, Uncontrolled: Uncontrolled hypertension may refer to untreated hypertension or hypertension not responding to current therapeutic regimen. In either case, assign the appropriate code from categories I10–I15, Hypertensive diseases.

Guideline I.C.9.a.10 Hypertensive Crisis Assign a code from category I16, Hypertensive crisis, for documented hypertensive urgency, hypertensive emergency or unspecified hypertensive crisis. Code also any identified hypertensive disease (I10-I15). The sequencing is based on the reason for the encounter.

Guideline I.C.9.a.11 Pulmonary Hypertension Pulmonary hypertension is classified to category I27, Other pulmonary heart disease. For secondary pulmonary hypertension (I27.1, I27.2-), code also any associated conditions or adverse effects of drugs or toxins. The

(Continued)

(Continued)

sequencing is based on the reason for the encounter except for adverse effects of drugs (See Section I.C.19.e).

Guideline I.C.9.b. Atherosclerotic Coronary Artery Disease and Angina: ICD-10-CM has combination codes for atherosclerotic heart disease with angina pectoris. The subcategories for these codes are I25.11, Atherosclerotic heart disease of native coronary artery with angina pectoris and I25.7, Atherosclerosis of coronary artery bypass graft(s) and coronary artery of transplanted heart with angina pectoris.

When using one of these combination codes it is not necessary to use an additional code for angina pectoris. A causal relationship can be assumed in a patient with both atherosclerosis and angina pectoris, unless the documentation indicates the angina is due to something other than atherosclerosis.

If a patient with coronary artery disease is admitted due to an acute myocardial infarction (AMI), the AMI should be sequenced before the coronary artery disease.

See Section I.C.9. Acute myocardial infarction (AMI).

Guideline I.C.9.c Intraoperative and Postprocedural Cerebrovascular Accident: Medical record documentation should clearly specify the cause-and-effect relationship between the medical intervention and the cerebrovascular accident in order to assign a code for intraoperative or postprocedural cerebrovascular accident.

Proper code assignment depends on whether it was an infarction or hemorrhage and whether it occurred intraoperatively or postoperatively. If it was a cerebral hemorrhage, code assignment depends on the type of procedure performed.

Guideline I.C.10.d.1. Category I69, Sequelae of Cerebrovascular Disease: Category I69 is used to indicate conditions classifiable to categories I60–I67 as the causes of sequela (neurologic deficits), themselves classified elsewhere. These "late effects" include neurologic deficits that persist after initial onset of conditions classifiable to categories I60–I67. The neurologic deficits caused by cerebrovascular disease may be present from the onset or may arise at any time after the onset of the condition classifiable to categories I60–I67.

Codes from category I69, Sequelae of cerebrovascular disease, that specify hemiplegia, hemiparesis and monoplegia identify whether the dominant or nondominant side is affected. Should the affected side be documented, but not specified as dominant or nondominant, and the classification system does not indicate a default, code selection is as follows:

- For ambidextrous patients, the default should be dominant.
- If the left side is affected, the default is nondominant.
- If the right side is affected, the default is dominant.

Guideline I.C.10.d.2. Codes from category I69 with codes from I60–I67: Codes from category I69 may be assigned on a health care record with codes from I60–I67, if the patient has a current cerebrovascular disease and deficits from an old cerebrovascular disease.

Guideline I.C.10.d.3. Codes from category I69, Personal history of transient ischemic attack (TIA) and cerebral infarction (Z86.73): Codes from category I69 should not be assigned if the patient does not have neurologic deficits.

See Section I.C.21.c.4. History (of) for use of personal history codes

Guideline I.C.9.e.1. Type I Acute myocardial infarction (AMI) ST Elevation Myocardial Infarction (STEMI) and Non-ST Elevation Myocardial Infarction (NSTEMI): The ICD-10-CM codes for type 1 acute myocardial infarction (AMI) identify the site, such as anterolateral wall or true posterior wall. Subcategories I21.0–I21.2 and code I21.3 are used for type 1 ST elevation myocardial infarction (STEMI). Code I21.4, Non-ST elevation (NSTEMI) myocardial infarction, is used for type 1 non-ST elevation myocardial infarction (NSTEMI) and nontransmural MIs.

If a type 1 NSTEMI evolves to STEMI, assign the STEMI code. If a type 1 STEMI converts to NSTEMI due to thrombolytic therapy, it is still coded as a STEMI.

For encounters occurring while the myocardial infarction is equal to, or less than, four weeks old, including transfers to another acute setting or a postacute setting, and the myocardial infarction meets the definition for "other diagnoses" (see Section III, Reporting Additional Diagnoses), codes from category I21 may continue to be reported. For encounters after the 4 week time frame and the patient is still receiving care related to the myocardial infarction, the appropriate aftercare code should be assigned, rather than a code from category I21. For old or healed myocardial infarctions not requiring further care, code I25.2, Old myocardial infarction, may be assigned.

Guideline I.C.9.e.2. Acute myocardial infarction, unspecified: Code I21.9, Acute myocardial infarction, unspecified is the default for unspecified acute myocardial infarction or unspecified type. If only type 1 STEMI or transmural MI without the site is documented, assign code I21.3, ST elevation (STEMI) myocardial infarction of unspecified type.

(Continued)

(Continued)

Guideline I.C.9.e.3. AMI documented as nontransmural or subendocardial but site provided: If an AMI is documented as nontransmural or subendocardial, but the site is provided, it is still coded as subendocardial AMI.

See Section I.C.21.3 for information on coding status post administration of tPA in a different facility within the last 24 hours.

Guideline I.C.9.e.4. Subsequent acute myocardial infarction: A code from category I22, Subsequent ST elevation (STEMI) and non-ST elevation (NSTEMI) myocardial infarction is to be used when a patient who has suffered a type 1 or unspecified AMI has a new AMI within the 4 week time frame of the initial AMI. A code from category I22 must be used in conjunction with a code from category I21. The sequencing of I22 and I21 codes depends on the circumstances of the encounter.

Do not assign code I22 for subsequent myocardial infarctions other than type 1 or unspecified. For subsequent type 2 AMI assign only code I21.A1. For subsequent type 4 or type 5 AMI, assign code I21.A9.

If a subsequent myocardial infarction of one type occurs within 4 weeks of a myocardial infarction of a different type, assign the appropriate codes from category I21 to identify each type. Do not assign a code from I22. Codes from category I22 should only be assigned if both the initial and subsequent myocardial infarctions are type 1 or unspecified.

Guideline I.C.9.e.5. Other types of myocardial infarction: The ICD-10-CM provides codes for different types of myocardial infarction. Type 1 myocardial infarctions are assigned to codes I21.0-I21.4.

Type 2 myocardial infarction (myocardial infarction due to demand ischemia or secondary to ischemic imbalance) is assigned to code I21.A1, Myocardial infarction type 2 with a code for the underlying cause coded first. Do not assign code I24.8, Other forms of acute ischemic heart disease, for the demand ischemia. If a type 2 AMI or the underlying cause is dependent on the circumstances of admission. When a type 2 AMI is described as NSTEMI or STEMI, only assign code I21.A1. Codes I21.01-I21.4 should only be assigned for type 1 AMIs.

Acute myocardial infarctions type 3, 4a, 4b, 4c, and 5 are assigned to code I21.A9, Other myocardial infection type.

The "Code also" and "Code first" notes should be followed related to complications, and for coding of postprocedural myocardial infarctions during or following cardiac surgery.

Check Your Understanding 12.1

Answer the following questions about the Official Guidelines for Chapter 9 of ICD-10-CM diagnosis code.

1. What is coded in addition to category I12, Hypertensive chronic kidney disease when both hypertension and chronic kidney disease are present in a patient?

2. What other conditions may be coded for a patient with secondary pulmonary hypertension (I27.1, I27.2-)?

3. What assumption can be made by the coder when a physician describes a patient has having atherosclerotic coronary artery disease with angina?

4. When can a code from category I69 be used with a code from categories I60–I67?

5. When is it appropriate to use an I22 subsequent type 1 AMI code?

Coding Diseases of the Circulatory System in ICD-10-CM Chapter 9

Chapter 9 contains an expanded number of specific codes that describe coronary, cerebral, and vascular diseases. "Use additional code to identify" notes appear throughout the chapter to direct the coder to identify exposure to, history of, current use of, and dependence on tobacco. Codes also specify the laterality of vessels to identify the specific location of disease, for example, left middle cerebral artery.

Beneath categories I21, I22, and I23 for AMI are notes that state the specific category to be used to identify myocardial infarctions specified as acute or with a stated duration of four weeks (28 days) or less from onset.

The instructional notes and guidelines are very important for these three categories to indicate correct code usage. A code from category I22, Subsequent AMI, must be used in conjunction with a code from category I21, for type 1 STEMI and type 1 NSTEMI. Do not assign code I22 for subsequent myocardial infarctions other than type 1 or unspecified. For subsequent type 2 AMI assign only code I21.A1. For subsequent type 4 or type 5 AMI, assign code I21.A9. A code from category I23, Certain current complications following STEMI and NSTEMI, must be used in conjunction with a code from category I21 or I22.

Acute Rheumatic Fever and Rheumatic Heart Disease (I00–I09)

Acute and chronic diseases of rheumatic origin are classified in categories I00 through I09. This section also covers diseases of mitral and aortic valves. Rheumatic heart disease continues to be the most common cause for mitral stenosis that develops in people with an untreated streptococcal infection such as a strep throat (NLM 2019a).

Acute Rheumatic Fever (I00–I02)

Rheumatic fever occurs after a streptococcal sore throat (group A *Streptococcus hemolyticus*). The acute phase of the illness is marked by fever, malaise, sweating, palpitation, and polyarthritis, which varies from vague discomfort to severe pain felt chiefly in the large joints. Most patients have elevated titers of antistreptolysin antibodies and increased sedimentation rates (AACC 2019).

The importance of rheumatic fever derives entirely from its capacity to cause severe heart damage. Salicylates markedly reduce fever, relieve joint pain, and may reduce joint swelling, if present. Because rheumatic fever often recurs, prophylaxis with penicillin is recommended and has markedly reduced the incidence of rheumatic heart disease in the general population.

ICD-10-CM codes for acute rheumatic fever include categories for rheumatic fever without heart involvement (I00), rheumatic fever with heart involvement (I01), and rheumatic chorea (I02) for the following diseases:

I00,   Rheumatic fever without heart involvement
I01,   Rheumatic fever with heart involvement
     I01.0,   Acute rheumatic pericarditis
     I01.1,   Acute rheumatic endocarditis
     I01.2,   Acute rheumatic myocarditis
     I01.8,   Other acute rheumatic heart disease
     I01.9,   Acute rheumatic heart disease, unspecified
I02,   Rheumatic chorea
     I02.0,   Rheumatic chorea with heart involvement
     I02.9,   Rheumatic chorea without heart involvement

Rheumatic chorea is also known as Sydenham's chorea. The condition occurs more often in children but can also occur in adults. Chorea is the result of acute rheumatic fever but may not be evident for as long as six months after the original streptococcal infection. It can be present with or without rheumatic fever damage to the heart. A patient with rheumatic chorea will have a variety of symptoms including muscle weakness, difficulty in gripping objects, difficulty walking, and a slurred or garbled speech pattern. Psychological symptoms may be present with the physical signs. The patient may have emotional displays that are out of proportion with the events occurring around the patient. The patient may also have attention deficits, experience anxiety when separated from parents or caregivers, and have some obsessive-compulsive tendencies. In adult women, poststreptococcal chorea may complicate pregnancy, known as chorea gravidarum (NLM 2019b).

Using the ICD-10-CM Index to Diseases and Injuries, the entry for chorea is coded depending on whether heart involvement is present:

Chorea,
   with
      heart involvement I02.0
         acute or active (conditions in I01.-) I02.0
         rheumatic I02.9
            with valvular disease I02.0
      rheumatic heart disease (chronic)(inactive) (quiescent)—code to rheumatic heart condition involved

Sydenham's I02.9
     with heart involvement—see Chorea, with rheumatic heart disease
     nonrheumatic G25.5

Chronic Rheumatic Heart Disease (I05–I09)

Instructional notes that clarify code usage are also found under specific codes. Under code I05, Rheumatic mitral valve diseases, is a note that states this category includes conditions classifiable to both I05.0 and I05.2–I05.9, whether specified as rheumatic or not.

Rheumatic heart disease develops with an initial attack of rheumatic fever. It is thought that the degree of heart inflammation from rheumatic fever determines whether patients develop rheumatic heart disease. About 1 percent of people who had no heart inflammation with the initial rheumatic fever develop rheumatic heart disease. However, about 30 percent of patients who had mild heart inflammation and 70 percent of patients who had severe heart inflammation develop rheumatic heart disease (Weinberg 2019). The cardiac involvement may affect all three layers of the heart muscle, causing pericarditis, scarring and weakening of the myocardium, and endocardial involvement of heart valves. The latter condition occurs more often in children who have had rheumatic fever and, to a lesser extent, in adults with rheumatic fever. A murmur heard over the heart is symptomatic of a valvular lesion. Rheumatic fever causes inflammation of the valves, thus damaging the valve cusps so that the opening may become permanently narrowed (stenosis). The mitral valve is involved in the great majority of such cases; the aortic valve is involved to a lesser extent; and the tricuspid and pulmonary valves are involved in a small percentage of the patients (Weinberg 2019).

When stenosis affects the mitral valve, blood flow decreases from the left atrium into the left ventricle. As a result, blood is held back in the lungs, then in the right side of the heart, and, finally, in the veins of the body. Incompetence of a valve may also occur because the cusps will not retract. If the mitral valve cannot close, blood escapes from the mitral valve back into the left atrium. In the case of the aortic valve, blood escapes from the aorta into the left ventricle. In such cases, plastic and metal replacement valves that function as well as normal valves may be surgically inserted.

In coding diseases of the mitral valve and diseases affecting both the mitral and aortic valves, the Index to Diseases offers direction to codes from categories I05–I09. Remember to always trust the Index to Diseases and assign the code it indicates.

EXAMPLE: Insufficiency, insufficient.
    mitral (valve) I34.0
        with
            aortic (valve) disease I08.0
                with tricuspid (valve) disease I08.3
            obstruction or stenosis I05.2
                with aortic valve disease I08.0
            tricuspid (valve) disease 108.1
                with aortic (valve) disease 108.3
            congenital Q23.3
            rheumatic I05.1
                with
                    aortic valve disease I08.0
                        with tricuspid (valve) disease I08.3
                  obstruction or stenosis I05.22
                      with aortic valve disease I08.0
                          with tricuspid valve disease I08.3

Diseases of the mitral valve, aortic valve, tricuspid valve, and pulmonary valve that are identified by the physician as nonrheumatic are classified to categories I34–I37 as directed by the Index to Diseases and the Excludes1 notes under the chronic rheumatic heart disease subcategory codes.

Hypertensive Disease (I10–I16)

The Index to Diseases uses the main terms "Hypertension" and "Hypertensive" to list the disease of hypertension and the other conditions caused by hypertension. ICD-10-CM has one category for "Hypertension," I10, even though different forms of hypertension may be described by a physician for a patient. Hypertension is a treatable disease but is also a major risk factor for coronary heart disease, stroke, congestive heart failure, end-stage renal disease, and peripheral vascular disease.

Definition of Hypertension

Blood pressure (BP) readings, which are described in mm Hg, for adults aged 18 years or older are as follows:

- Normal: systolic lower than 120 mm Hg, diastolic lower than 80 mm Hg

- Prehypertension: systolic 120–139 mm Hg, diastolic 80–89 mm Hg

- Stage 1 hypertension: systolic 140–159 mm Hg, diastolic 90–99 mm Hg

- Stage 2 hypertension: systolic 160 mm Hg or greater, diastolic 100 mm Hg or greater

The definition above is based on the average of two or more readings taken at each of two or more visits after the initial measurement. **Normal blood pressure (BP)**, with respect to cardiovascular risk, is less than 120/80 mm Hg (Riaz 2014).

The prevalence of hypertension increases with age. About 90 to 95 percent of hypertension is primary (essential hypertension), and its cause is unknown. The remaining 2 to 10 percent is secondary hypertension (Madhur 2019). Both essential and secondary hypertension can be either benign or malignant. Complications of hypertension include left ventricular failure, arteriosclerotic heart disease, retinal hemorrhages, cerebrovascular insufficiency, and renal failure (Madhur 2019).

Benign Hypertension (I10)

In most cases, **benign hypertension** remains fairly stable over many years and is compatible with a long life. If untreated, however, it becomes an important risk factor in coronary heart disease and cerebrovascular disease. Benign hypertension is also asymptomatic until complications develop. Effective antihypertensive drug therapy is the treatment of choice. The ICD-10-CM Index to Diseases and Injuries provides the following entry for hypertension that includes the nonessential modifiers that have no influence on the code assignment of I10:

Hypertension, hypertensive (accelerated)(benign)(essential)(idiopathic)(malignant) (systemic) I10

Malignant Hypertension (I10)

Malignant hypertension is far less common, occurring in only a small percent of patients with elevated blood pressure. It is also known as accelerating hypertension. The malignant form is frequently of abrupt onset. It often ends with renal failure or cerebral hemorrhage. Usually a person with malignant hypertension will complain of headaches and difficulties with vision. Blood pressures of 180/120 are common, and an abnormal protrusion of the optic nerve (papilledema) occurs with microscopic hemorrhages and exudates seen in the retina. The initial event appears to be some form of vascular damage to the kidneys. This may result from long-standing benign hypertension with damage of the arteriolar walls, or it may derive from arteritis of some form. The chances for long-term survival depend on early treatment before significant renal insufficiency has developed (Bisognano 2017). As stated previously, there is no distinction in ICD-10-CM for different types of hypertension. The following conditions are all coded to ICD-10-CM code I10, Essential (primary) Hypertension:

I10,   High blood pressure
I10,   Arterial hypertension
I10,   Benign hypertension
I10,   Essential hypertension
I10,   Malignant hypertension
I10,   Primary hypertension
I10,   Systemic hypertension

Hypertensive Heart Disease (I11)

Hypertensive heart disease refers to the secondary effects on the heart of prolonged sustained systemic hypertension (Riaz 2014). The heart must work against greatly increased resistance in the form of high blood pressure. The primary effect is thickening of the left ventricle, finally resulting in heart failure. The symptoms are similar to those of heart failure from other causes. Many persons with controlled hypertension do not develop heart failure. However, when a patient has heart failure with hypertension, additional codes are required to be used with category I11 to specify the type of heart failure that exists, such as I50.1–I50.9, if known. The separate hypertensive heart disease codes are as follows:

I11.0,   Hypertensive heart disease with heart failure
    Hypertensive heart failure
    Use additional code to identify the type of heart failure (I50.-)

I11.9,   Hypertensive heart disease without heart failure
    Hypertensive heart disease NOS

Heart conditions such as heart failure and other forms of heart disease (I50.- or I51.4–I51.9) with hypertension are assigned to a code from category I11, Hypertensive heart disease.

Hypertensive Chronic Kidney Disease (I12)

Hypertensive chronic kidney disease is any chronic kidney disease (N18.-) or contracted kidney (N26.-) that is due to hypertension. A code from category I12, Hypertensive chronic kidney disease, is assigned when both the diagnosis of hypertension and chronic kidney disease are present and documented by the physician. ICD-10-CM presumes a cause-and-effect relationship and classifies chronic kidney disease with hypertension as hypertensive chronic kidney disease. An additional code from category N18 should be used with a code from category I12 to identify the stage of chronic kidney disease. If a patient has hypertensive chronic kidney disease and acute renal failure, an additional code for the acute renal failure is required. Separate codes exist for hypertension with different stages of chronic kidney disease:

I12.0,   Hypertensive chronic kidney disease with stage 5 chronic kidney disease or end-stage renal disease
    Use additional code to identify the stage of chronic kidney disease
    (N18.5, N18.6)

I12.9,   Hypertensive chronic kidney disease with stage 1 through stage 4 chronic kidney disease or unspecified chronic kidney disease
    Use additional code to identify the stage of chronic kidney disease (N18.1–N18.4, N18.9)

Hypertensive Heart and Chronic Kidney Disease (I13)

Hypertensive heart and chronic kidney disease is any heart disease due to hypertension (I11) with chronic kidney disease and hypertension (I12). Separate subcategory codes exist for hypertensive heart disease with chronic kidney disease, stage 1 through stage 4, and hypertensive heart disease with chronic kidney disease, stage 5 or end-stage renal disease:

I13.0,	Hypertensive heart and chronic kidney disease with heart failure and stage 1 through stage 4 chronic kidney disease or unspecified chronic kidney disease Use additional code to identify the type of heart failure (I50.-) Use additional code to identify the stage of chronic kidney disease (N18.1–N18.4, N18.9)
I13.10,	Hypertensive heart and chronic kidney disease without heart failure with stage 1 through stage 4 chronic kidney disease, or unspecified chronic kidney disease Use additional code to identify the stage of chronic kidney disease (N18.1–N18.4, N18.9)
I13.11,	Hypertensive heart and chronic kidney disease without heart failure with stage 5 or end-stage renal disease Use additional code to identify the stage of chronic kidney disease (N18.5, N18.6)
I13.2,	Hypertensive heart and chronic kidney disease with heart failure and with stage 5 or end-stage renal disease Use additional code to identify type of heart failure (I50.-) Use additional code to identify the stage of chronic kidney disease (N18.5, N18.6)

Secondary Hypertension (I15)

Secondary hypertension is due to another disease or underlying condition. Two codes are required: one to identify the underlying etiology and one from category I15 to identify the hypertension. Beneath category code I15 is an instructional note to "code also underlying condition." The sequencing of the two codes depends on the circumstances of the visit or admission, that is, what the primary focus of attention is. The codes in category I15 include a broad description of the underlying cause:

I15.0,	Renovascular hypertension
I15.1,	Hypertension secondary to other renal disorders
I15.2,	Hypertension secondary to endocrine disorders
I15.8,	Other secondary hypertension
I15.9,	Secondary hypertension, unspecified

Secondary hypertension identified as renovascular hypertension is hypertension usually due to renal artery or renal vascular disease. This is the opposite of the conditions in category I12.0 where the chronic kidney disease is due to hypertension, not the other way around as in secondary hypertension (I15.0).

Hypertensive Crisis (I16)

Category I16 classifies the conditions referred to as hypertensive crisis. Code I16.0 identifies hypertensive urgency. Code I16.1 describes hypertensive emergency. The unspecified condition of hypertensive crisis is classified with code I16.9. According to the *Official Guidelines for Coding and Reporting*, coder should assign a code from category I16 when the provider has identified the condition of hypertensive crisis, hypertensive urgency or hypertensive emergency. The I16 category code would be used with another code that identifies the type of hypertensive disease the patient has from categories I10–I15. Depending on the circumstances of the admission or visit, the I10–I15 code may be listed first or the I16 code may be listed first. For example, if the patient was admitted because of a hypertensive emergency due to the patient's essential hypertension, the principal diagnosis is likely to be I16.1 with a secondary diagnosis code of I10 (CDC 2019).

Check Your Understanding 12.2

Assign diagnosis codes to the following conditions.

1. Hypertension due to renovascular disease

2. Hypertensive heart disease with heart failure

3. Hypertensive cardiorenal disease with stage 5 chronic kidney disease (without heart failure)

4. Hypertensive emergency in a patient with essential hypertension

5. Hypertensive renal disease with chronic kidney disease, stage 4

Ischemic Heart Disease (I20–I25)

Combination codes in ICD-10-CM include **atherosclerotic heart disease** with angina and appear in category I25, Chronic ischemic heart disease. This placement eliminates the need to use an additional code for angina pectoris or unstable angina. The I25 category codes in ICD–10–CM contain details about the location of the coronary artery disease, such as native vessel or bypass graft, and the type of angina, such as unstable, with documented spasm, as well as other forms of angina pectoris. An illustration of the coronary arteries of the heart is shown in figure 12.1.

Angina Pectoris (I20)

There are two types of angina: unstable angina and angina pectoris.

Unstable Angina

Unstable angina, also known as crescendo and preinfarction angina, is defined as the development of prolonged episodes of anginal discomfort, usually occurring at rest and requiring hospitalization to rule out a myocardial infarction. ICD-10-CM classifies unstable angina with code I20.0. Code I20.0 is assigned when a patient is admitted to the hospital and treated for unstable angina without documentation of infarction, occlusion, or thrombosis (Tan 2019). Unstable angina may also be described as intermediate coronary syndrome (CDC 2019). The adjective of "unstable" is an indented subterm under the main term of Angina in the ICD-10-CM Index to Diseases and Injuries and coded differently than the diagnosis of angina.

> **EXAMPLE:** Angina (attack)(cardiac)(chest)(heart)(pectoris)(syndrome)(vasomotor) I20.9
>
> ...
>
> Unstable I20.0

Figure 12.1.   **Diagram of coronary arteries**

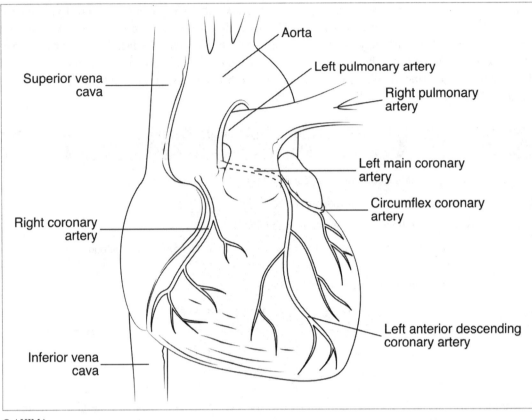

© AHIMA

Angina Pectoris

Angina pectoris refers to chest pain due to ischemia (loss of blood supply to a part) of the heart. The blood flow, with its supply of oxygen, is reduced because of atherosclerosis (hardening of arteries). Immediate causes of angina pectoris can be exertion, stress, cold weather, or digestion of a large meal. Pain is most commonly felt beneath the sternum, and a vague or a sharp pain sometimes radiates down the left arm. Blood pressure and heart rate are increased during an attack; however, angina lasts only a few minutes and is relieved by rest and/or sublingual nitroglycerin. Angina pectoris is a warning of more severe heart disease, such as myocardial infarction or congestive heart failure (Alaeddini 2018).

ICD-10-CM classifies angina pectoris to category I20. The fourth-digit subcategories identify specific types of angina pectoris, such as angina pectoris with documented spasm, which may also be described as Prinzmetal angina, variant angina, or spasm-induced angina (I20.1). The definition of Prinzmetal or variant angina is chest pain at rest secondary to myocardial ischemia. Other forms of angina pectoris are classified as I20.8 and may be described as stable angina, angina equivalent, or coronary slow flow syndrome. There is also a code I20.9 for angina pectoris NOS or angina NOS, which may also be described as ischemic chest pain.

ICD-10-CM has combination codes for atherosclerotic heart disease with angina pectoris. The subcategories for these codes are I25.11, Atherosclerotic heart disease of native coronary artery with angina pectoris, and I25.7, Atherosclerosis of coronary artery bypass graft(s) and coronary artery of transplanted heart with angina pectoris. When using one of these combination codes, it is not necessary to use an additional code for angina pectoris. A causal relationship can be assumed in a patient with both atherosclerosis and angina pectoris, unless the documentation indicates the angina is due to something other than atherosclerosis. If a patient with coronary artery disease is admitted due to an AMI, the AMI should be sequenced before the coronary artery disease as these are two separate clinical conditions. When angina is present with atherosclerotic heart disease, the ICD-10-CM Index to Diseases and Injuries provides the following direction to indicate that a combination code will be used to describe the angina with atherosclerotic heart disease:

> Angina (attack)(cardiac)(chest)(heart)(pectoris)(syndrome)(vasomotor) I20.9
> > With
> > > Atherosclerotic heart disease—see Arteriosclerosis, coronary artery

Angina and Coronary Disease

In ICD-10-CM, there are combination codes for patients with angina and coronary artery disease. Within the ICD-10-CM Index to Diseases and Injuries, there are repeated entries that link the two conditions of angina and arteriosclerosis. The coder must be diligent to find two entries in the Index to Diseases and Injuries for the specific two conditions that exist (the location of the coronary arteriosclerosis within the heart and the type of angina):

> Arteriosclerosis, arteriosclerotic
> > coronary
> > > bypass graft I25.810
> > > > with
> > > > > angina pectoris I25.709
> > > > > > with documented spasm I25.701
> > > > > > specified type NEC I25.708
> > > > > > unstable I25.700
>
> Arteriosclerosis, arteriosclerotic
> > coronary
> > > native vessel
> > > > with
> > > > > angina pectoris I25.119
> > > > > > with documented spasm I25.111
> > > > > > specified type NEC I25.118
> > > > > > unstable I25.110
> > > > > ischemic chest pain I25.769

EXAMPLE: A patient was admitted with angina. Diagnostic cardiac catheterizations determined that the angina was due to coronary arteriosclerosis of the native vessels. The patient was discharged on antianginal medications.

The combination code I25.119, Atherosclerotic heart disease of native coronary with unspecified angina pectoris, is listed as the principal diagnosis. There is no requirement to add an additional code for the angina.

EXAMPLE: A patient was admitted with symptomatic angina that evolved into an AMI.

The AMI is sequenced as the principal diagnosis, I21.3, ST elevation

(STEMI) of unspecified site. No additional code is assigned for angina as it is an inherent part of the condition.

EXAMPLE: A patient with unstable angina was admitted to the hospital for left heart cardiac catheterization. He was found to have significant four-vessel coronary atherosclerosis. He had four-native-vessel coronary artery bypass surgery performed during the same admission. The combination code I25.110, Atherosclerotic heart disease of native coronary artery with unstable angina, is the principal diagnosis. The diagnosis of unstable angina is not assigned as an additional diagnosis because it is included in code I25.110.

Acute and Subsequent STEMI and NSTEMI and Certain Complications (I21–I23)

Acute myocardial infarction (AMI) usually occurs as a result of a sudden inadequacy of coronary flow. The first symptom of AMI is the development of deep substernal pain described as aching or pressure, often with radiation to the back or left arm. The patient may be pale, diaphoretic (sweaty), and in severe pain; however, the symptoms may vary between men and women. Peripheral or carotid cyanosis may be present, as well as arrhythmias. Treatment is designed to relieve the patient's distress, reduce cardiac work, and prevent and treat complications. Major complications include tachycardia, frequent ventricular premature beats, heart block, and ventricular fibrillation. Heart failure often occurs. Physicians may refer to an AMI as a type 1 STEMI or type 1 NSTEMI (NHLBI 2019a).

Included under category I21, type 1 STEMI and type 1 NSTEMI myocardial infarction, is the terminology of cardiac infarction, coronary (artery) embolism, coronary (artery) occlusion, coronary (artery) rupture, coronary (artery) thrombosis, and infarction of heart, myocardium, or ventricle. This code is intended to represent a myocardial infarction specified as acute or with a stated duration of four weeks (28 days) or less from onset. Specific ICD-10-CM coding guidelines exist for the coding of current and subsequent type 1 AMIs with AMI complication codes and likely will challenge new ICD-10-CM coders as they begin to use the classification system. Also included in codes I21.A1-I21.A9 are other types of myocardial infarctions, such as myocardial infarction type 2 that is also known as myocardial infarction due to demand ischemia or ischemic imbalance. This occurs when a condition other than coronary artery disease results in an imbalance between myocardial oxygen supply and/or demand. A "code also" note appears under code I21.A1 to identify the underlying cause, if known and applicable. Other types of myocardial infarction are known as type 3, type 4 and type 5 that occur from presumed cardiac etiology or associated with revascularization procedures. A "code first" and "code also" note appear under code I21.A9 to identify a postprocedural myocardial infarction or a cardiac complication if known and applicable.

The note with category I22 says that a code from category I22 must be used in conjunction with a code from category I21 for type 1 or unspecified ST elevation and type 1 or unspecified non-ST elevation myocardial infarction. The I22 code should be sequenced first if it is the reason for encounter, or it should be sequenced after the I21 code if the subsequent MI occurs during the encounter for the initial MI. Also watch for notes to use additional codes to identify body mass index (BMI), if known, and tobacco use or exposure. Should a patient who is in the hospital due to a type 1 or unspecified AMI have a subsequent AMI while still in the hospital, code I21 would be sequenced first as the reason for admission, with code I22 sequenced as a secondary code. Should a patient have a subsequent AMI after discharge for care of an initial type 1 or unspecified AMI, and the reason for admission is the subsequent AMI, the I22 code should be sequenced first followed by the I21. An I21 code must accompany an I22 code to identify the site of the initial AMI and to indicate that the patient is still within the four-week time frame of healing from the initial AMI. Do not assign code I22 for subsequent myocardial infarctions other than type 1 or unspecified. For subsequent type 2 AMI assign only code I21.A1. For subsequent type 4 or type 5 AMI, assign code I21.A9.

Certain current complications following STEMI and NSTEMI myocardial infarctions are reported with category I23 codes when the condition occurs within four weeks after the infarction. Code I25.2, Old myocardial infarction, is assigned when the diagnostic statement mentions the presence of a healed MI presenting no symptoms during the current episode of care.

EXAMPLE: A patient was admitted on 1/1/20XX and diagnosed with a type 1 ST elevation anterior wall myocardial infarction. Three days after admission, the patient suffered a subsequent ST elevation inferior wall myocardial infarction. Two diagnosis codes would be assigned and sequenced in the following order:

I21.09, ST elevation myocardial infarction, anterior wall

I22.1, Subsequent ST elevation myocardial infarction, inferior wall

EXAMPLE: A patient was admitted on 2/1/20XX and diagnosed with a type 1 STEMI involving the diagonal artery of the anterior wall. The patient was discharged on 2/7/20XX to his home. On 2/17/20XX, the patient is readmitted to the hospital with a second STEMI also involving the coronary artery of the anterior wall. The two admissions would be coded and sequenced as follows:

Admission 2/1/20XX   I21.02, ST elevation myocardial infarction, diagonal coronary artery

Admission 2/17/20XX   I22.0, Subsequent ST elevation myocardial infarction, anterior wall

I21.02, ST elevation myocardial infarction, diagonal coronary artery

EXAMPLE: A patient was admitted on 3/1/20XX and diagnosed with a type 1 non-ST elevation myocardial infarction. The patient was admitted six months ago with an acute STEMI of the inferoposterior wall. The admission of 3/1/20XX would be coded and sequenced as follows:

I21.4, Non-ST elevation (NSTEMI) myocardial infarction

I25.2, Healed or old myocardial infarction (occurred six months ago)

Diagnostic Tools for AMI

The diagnosis of AMI depends on the patient's clinical history, the physical examination, interpretation of the electrocardiogram (EKG) and chest radiograph, and measurement of serum levels of cardiac enzymes, such as troponins or the MB isoenzyme of creatine kinase (CK-MB).

Diagnostic uncertainty frequently arises because of various factors. Many patients with acute AMI have atypical symptoms. Other people with typical physical symptoms do not have

AMI. EKGs may also be nondiagnostic. Laboratory tests known as biochemical or serum markers of cardiac injury are commonly relied upon to diagnose or exclude an AMI.

Creatine kinase and lactate dehydrogenase have been the "gold standard" for the diagnosis of AMI for many years. However, single values of these tests have limited sensitivity and specificity. Serum markers currently in use are troponin T and I, myoglobin, and CK-MB. These markers are used instead of, or along with, the standard markers.

EKGs also prove useful in diagnosing myocardial infarctions. The initial EKG may be diagnostic in acute transmural myocardial infarction, but serial EKGs may be necessary to confirm the diagnosis for other myocardial infarction sites.

A patient diagnosed with an acute myocardial infarction or an acute ischemic stroke may be given **intravenous tissue plasminogen activator (tPA)**, which is a thrombolytic agent also known as a "clot-busting drug." Studies have shown that tPA and other clot-dissolving agents can reduce the amount of damage to the heart muscle and save lives. In order to be effective, tPA must be given within the first three hours after the onset of symptoms. The fact that a patient has received tPA is important information. A patient may be seen in Hospital A and receive tPA intravenously and then be transferred to Hospital B for further management of the AMI. If the patient has received tPA within the 24 hours prior to admission to the current facility, then the coder at Hospital B should code Z92.82, Status post administration of tPA (rtPA) in a different facility within the last 24 hours prior to admission to the current facility. The condition requiring the tPA administration is coded first, such as acute MI or acute cerebral infarction. Hospital A does not use diagnosis code Z92.82.

Chronic Ischemic Heart Disease (I25)

ICD-10-CM classifies chronic ischemic heart disease to category I25. Chronic ischemic heart disease or **atherosclerotic** or **arteriosclerotic heart disease** refers to those cases in which ischemia has induced general myocardial atrophy and scattered areas of interstitial scarring. This heart disease results from slow, progressive narrowing of the coronary arteries. This course may be altered by episodes of sudden severe coronary insufficiency. The patient with chronic ischemic heart disease may develop angina or an AMI.

In order to code the diagnosis of chronic ischemic heart disease, the ICD-10-CM Index to Diseases and Injuries provides the following entries:

Disease, coronary (artery)—see Disease, heart, ischemic, atherosclerotic
Disease, heart, ischemic (chronic or with a stated duration of over four weeks) I25.9
Disease, heart, ischemic, atherosclerotic (of) I25.10

Atherosclerosis

Atherosclerosis is the formation of lesions on the inside of arterial walls from the accumulation of fat cells and platelets (Dorland 2012, 172). Another term for atherosclerosis is arteriosclerosis. The gradual enlargement of the lesion eventually weakens the arterial wall and narrows the lumen, or channel of the blood vessel, decreasing the volume of blood flow. The large arteries—the aorta and its main branches—are primarily affected, but smaller arteries such as the coronary and cerebral arteries can also be affected. In such a case, the patient experiences chest pain, shortness of breath, and sweating. Blood pressure is high; pulse is rapid and weak. An x-ray reveals cardiomegaly and narrowing, or occlusion, of the affected vessel wall. Blood tests may show hypercholesterolemia.

Atherosclerosis is the major cause of ischemia of the heart, brain, and extremities. Its complications include stroke, congestive heart failure, angina pectoris, myocardial infarction, and kidney failure. Treatment is directed toward the specific manifestation.

Subcategories of I25, Chronic Ischemic Heart Disease

ICD-10-CM classifies atherosclerotic heart disease and coronary artery disease to category I25, Chronic ischemic heart disease. The fourth-, fifth-, and sixth-digit subcategories describe specific types of ischemic heart diseases. The ICD-10-CM subcategories under I25 describe specific types of ischemic heart disease, such as

I25.1,   Atherosclerotic heart disease of native coronary artery, with and without types of angina pectoris

 I25.10, Atherosclerotic heart disease of native coronary artery without angina pectoris

 I25.110-I25.119, Atherosclerotic heart disease of native coronary artery with angina pectoris. Sixth characters are used to identify the atherosclerotic heart disease with unstable angina, angina pectoris with documented spasm, with other forms of angina pectoris and unspecified angina pectoris.

I25.2,   Old myocardial infarction

I25.3,   Aneurysm of the heart

I25.4,   Coronary artery aneurysm and dissection

 I25.41, Coronary artery aneurysm

 I25.42, Coronary artery dissection

I25.5,   Ischemic cardiomyopathy

I25.6,   Silent myocardial ischemia

I25.7,   Atherosclerosis of coronary artery bypass graft(s) and coronary artery of transplanted heart with angina pectoris, specifying the type of graft involved

 I25.70, Atherosclerosis of coronary artery bypass graft(s), unspecified, with angina pectoris

 I25.71, Atherosclerosis of autologous vein coronary artery bypass graft(s) with angina pectoris

 I25.72, Atherosclerosis of autologous artery coronary artery bypass graft(s) with angina pectoris

 I25.73, Atherosclerosis of nonautologous biological coronary artery bypass graft(s) with angina pectoris

 I25.75, Atherosclerosis of native coronary artery of transplanted heart with angina pectoris

 I25.76, Atherosclerosis of bypass graft of coronary artery of transplanted heart with angina pectoris

 I25.79, Atherosclerosis of other coronary artery bypass graft(s) with angina pectoris

 Sixth characters represent the atherosclerosis with unstable angina, angina pectoris with documented spasm, with other forms of angina pectoris and unspecified angina pectoris.

I25.8,   Other forms of chronic heart disease

    I25.81,   Atherosclerosis of other coronary vessels without angina pectoris

        Sixth characters represent the type of coronary artery such as bypass graft(s), native coronary artery of transplanted heart, bypass graft of coronary artery of transplanted heart.

    I25.82,   Chronic total occlusion of coronary artery

    I25.83,   Coronary atherosclerosis due to lipid-rich plaque

    I25.84,   Coronary atherosclerosis due to calcified coronary lesion

    I25.89,   Other forms of chronic ischemic heart disease

I25.9,   Chronic ischemic heart disease, unspecified

Important "use additional code" notes appear throughout category I25, Chronic ischemic heart disease. These notes remind the coder to add a code, depending on the particular subcategory code:

Chronic total occlusion of coronary artery, I25.82
Coronary atherosclerosis due to calcified coronary lesion, I25.84
Coronary atherosclerosis due to lipid-rich plaque, I25.83
Various codes for tobacco use and exposure to tobacco smoke

The instructional code of "use additional code" appears under codes I25.1-, I25.7-, I25.8- for coronary atherosclerosis due to lipid-rich plaque, and coronary atherosclerosis due to calcified coronary lesion.

Subcategory code I25.4 differentiates between aneurysms and dissections of the heart. Code I25.42 is included for dissection of the coronary artery. An arterial dissection is characterized by blood coursing within the layers of the arterial wall and is not an aneurysm.

Subcategory I25.82, Chronic total occlusion of coronary artery, is used as an additional code when a patient with coronary atherosclerosis (I25.1-, I25.7-, and I25.81-) also has the complete blockage of a coronary artery. There is an increased risk of myocardial infarction or death for individuals with chronic total occlusion of a coronary artery. Chronic total occlusion of a coronary artery may be treated with angioplasty or stent placement, which is technically more difficult to perform than an angioplasty or stent placement in a patient with less than total occlusion of a coronary artery.

Subcategory I25.83, Coronary atherosclerosis due to lipid rich plaque, identifies the type of plaque within a coronary artery. This diagnostic information is important to the cardiologist in determining the most appropriate type of stent (drug-eluting or bare metal) to place in the vessel depending on the location and amount of lipid rich plaque present. Code I25.83 is used in addition to a code for the location and type of coronary atherosclerosis (I25.1-, I25.7-, and I25.81-) that exists in the patient.

Check Your Understanding 12.3

Assign diagnosis codes for the following conditions.

1. A patient was admitted for a type 1 ST elevation myocardial infarction (STEMI) involving the left main coronary artery that was followed three days later, while the patient was still in the hospital, by a subsequent type 1 ST elevation (STEMI) of the inferior wall.

2. A patient was admitted for a second STEMI of the anterior wall, two weeks after being hospitalized for a STEMI of the anterior wall that was also treated during the same admission.

3. Non-ST elevation myocardial infarction (NSTEMI) in a patient who had a STEMI six months ago

4. Atherosclerosis of multiple native coronary arteries due to lipid rich plaque of one coronary artery without angina pectoris

5. Demand ischemia Angiospastic angina

Heart Failure (I50)

Heart failure is the heart's inability to contract with enough force to properly pump blood (NHLBI 2019b). This condition may be caused by coronary artery disease (usually in a patient with a previous myocardial infarction), cardiomyopathy, hypertension, or heart valve disease. Sometimes the exact cause of heart failure is not found. Heart failure may develop gradually or occur acutely. Heart failure can involve the heart's left side, right side, or both sides. However, it usually affects the left side first.

Heart failure has the following three effects:

- Pressure in the lungs is increased. Fluid collects in the lung tissue, inhibiting O_2 and CO_2 exchange.

- Kidney function is hampered. Blood does not filter well, and body sodium and water retention increase, resulting in edema.

- Blood is not properly circulated throughout the body. Fluid collects in tissues, resulting in edema of the feet and legs.

Symptoms of heart failure include the following:

- Sudden weight gain, such as three or more pounds a day or five or more pounds a week

- Shortness of breath or difficulty breathing, especially while at rest or when lying flat in bed

- Waking up breathless at night, trouble sleeping, using more pillows

- Frequent dry, hacking cough, especially when lying down

- Increased fatigue and weakness, feeling tired all the time

- Dizziness or fainting

- Swollen feet, ankles, and legs

- Nausea with abdominal swelling, pain, and tenderness

An illustration of the blood flow within the heart and lungs is shown in figure 12.2.

Heart failure causes blood to flow in and out of the heart at a slower rate. At the same time, this causes blood in the veins trying to return to the heart to slow down, and congestion in the body tissues occurs. Patients with heart failure with this congestion have swelling in the

Figure 12.2 Blood flow within the heart and lungs

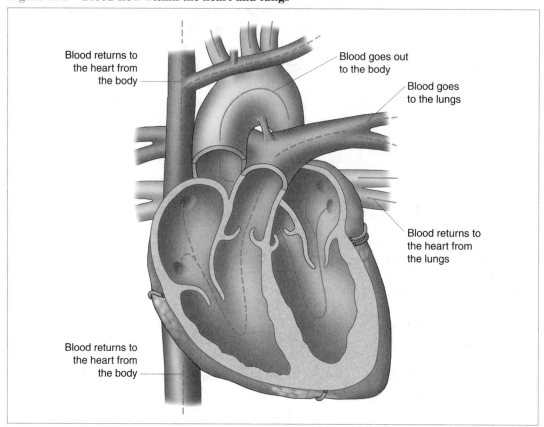

Blood returns to the heart from the body

Blood goes out to the body

Blood goes to the lungs

Blood returns to the heart from the lungs

Blood returns to the heart from the body

© AHIMA

legs, ankles, wrists, and hands. Fluid also collects in the lungs, and the patient will experience shortness of breath, especially pronounced when the person is lying down. Physicians describe the pulmonary congestion as pulmonary edema that must be treated before it produces respiratory distress or respiratory failure. The kidneys' ability to filter and dispose of waste is hampered by heart failure. The body retains water when the kidneys are not functioning properly, and swelling occurs in other parts of the body than strictly the extremities. The same condition may be referred to as **congestive heart failure,** left-sided heart failure, or right-sided heart failure (NHLBI 2019b).

 ICD-10-CM category I50 includes codes that distinguish between unspecified type of heart failure that would include left ventricular failure (I50.1), systolic heart failure (I50.2-), diastolic heart failure (I50.3-), combined systolic and diastolic heart failure (I50.4-), and other forms of heart failure, such as right heart failure (I50.81-), biventricular heart failure (I50.82), high output heart failure (I50.83), end stage heart failure (I50.84), with codes for other and unspecified heart failure (I50.89–I50.9).

Left-Sided Heart Failure

The heart's pumping action moves oxygen-rich blood from the lungs to the left atrium and then on to the left ventricle, which pumps it to the rest of the body. The left ventricle supplies most of the heart's pumping power, so it is larger than the other chambers and essential for normal function. In left-sided or left ventricular (LV) heart failure, the left side of the heart must work harder to pump the same amount of blood.

There are two types of **left-sided heart failure**. Drug treatments are different for the two types.

- Systolic failure: The left ventricle loses its ability to contract normally. The heart cannot pump with sufficient force to push enough blood into circulation.

- Diastolic failure: The left ventricle loses its ability to relax normally (because the muscle has become stiff). The heart cannot properly fill with blood during the resting period between each beat.

In addition to systolic and diastolic failure, the condition may be described as acute or chronic or acute on chronic. The coder must follow the ICD-10-CM Index to Diseases and Injuries carefully. For example, the various types of acute or chronic diastolic heart failure include the entries as follows:

Failure,
    heart,
        diastolic (congestive) (left ventrical) I50.30
            acute (congestive) I50.31
                and (on) chronic (congestive) I50.33
            chronic (congestive) I50.32
                and (on) acute (congestive) I50.33
            combined with systolic (congestive) I50.40
                acute (congestive) I50.41
                    and (on) chronic (congestive) I50.43
                chronic (congestive) I50.42
                    and (on) acute (congestive) I50.43

Right-Sided Heart Failure

The heart's pumping action also moves deoxygenated blood, which returns through the veins to the heart, through the right atrium, and into the right ventricle. The right ventricle then pumps the blood back out of the heart into the lungs to be replenished with oxygen.

Right-sided heart failure usually occurs as a result of left-sided failure. When the left ventricle fails, increased fluid pressure is, in effect, transferred back through the lungs, ultimately damaging the heart's right side. When the right side loses pumping power, blood backs up in the body's veins. This usually causes swelling in the legs and ankles.

    EXAMPLE: The attending physician documented in the discharge summary of his patient's record that the patient was treated for right ventricular heart failure. In the history and physical examination report, the physician used the terminology of right-sided heart failure as the patient's diagnosis. The diagnosis could be coded as follows using the following ICD-10-CM Index to Diseases and Injuries:

        Failure,
        -heart,
        - - right (isolated) (ventricular) I50.810
        - - - acute I50.811
        - - - - and (on) chronic I50.813
        - - - chronic I50.812
        - - - - and acute I50.813
        - - - secondary to left heart failure I50.814

Diagnostic Tests

Several diagnostic tests are important in diagnosing heart failure in a patient. Typical remarks on a chest x-ray indicating heart failure include hilar congestion, "butterfly" or "batwing" appearance of vascular markings, bronchial edema, Kerley B lines signifying chronic elevation of left atrial pressure, and heart enlargement. An echocardiograph measures the amount of blood pumped from the heart with each beat. This measurement is known as the ejection fraction. A normal heart pumps one half (50 percent) or more of the blood in the left ventricle with each heartbeat. With heart failure, the weakened heart may pump 40 percent or less, and less blood is pumped with less force to all parts of the body.

In a patient with heart failure, a urine test shows evidence of heart failure with the presence of slight albuminuria, increased concentration with specific gravity of 1.020, and decreased urine sodium. Laboratory findings may include blood urea nitrogen (BUN) 60 mg/100 mL; acidosis, pH 7.35 due to increased CO_2 in blood from pulmonary insufficiency; and increased blood volume with decrease in chloride, albumin, and total protein.

For most patients, heart failure is a chronic condition, which means it can be treated and managed, but not cured. Usually the patient's management plan consists of medications, such as angiotensin-converting enzyme (ACE) inhibitors; diuretics and digitalis; low-sodium diet; possibly some modifications in daily activities; regular exercise such as walking and swimming; and other changes in lifestyle and health habits such as reducing alcohol consumption and quitting smoking.

Cardiac Arrhythmias and Conduction Disorders (I44–I49)

Cardiac arrhythmias identify disturbances or impairments of the normal electrical activity of heart muscle excitation. ICD-10-CM classifies cardiac arrhythmias to several categories depending on the specific type. Without further specification as to the type of cardiac arrhythmia, code I49.9 may be reported. A discussion of common arrhythmias follows (NHLBI 2019c).

Atrial fibrillation (I48.0–I48.2, I48.9-) is commonly associated with organic heart diseases, such as coronary artery disease, hypertension and rheumatic mitral valve disease, thyrotoxicosis, pericarditis, and pulmonary embolism. Treatment includes pharmacologic therapy (verapamil, digoxin, or propranolol) and cardioversion. Distinctions are made between the types of atrial fibrillation, such as paroxysmal, persistent, chronic, and unspecified types.

Atrial flutter (I48.3–I48.4) is associated with organic heart diseases, such as coronary artery disease, hypertension, and rheumatic mitral valve disease. Treatment is similar to that for atrial fibrillation. Typical and atypical atrial flutters are coded separately.

Ventricular fibrillation (I49.01) involves no cardiac output and is associated with cardiac arrest. Treatment is consistent with that for cardiac arrest.

Paroxysmal tachycardia (I47.0–I47.9) is associated with congenital accessory atrial conduction pathway, physical or psychological stress, hypoxia, hypokalemia, caffeine and marijuana use, stimulants, and digitalis toxicity. Treatment includes pharmacologic therapy (quinidine, propranolol, or verapamil) and cardioversion.

Sick sinus syndrome (SSS) (I49.5) is an imprecise diagnosis with various characteristics. SSS may be diagnosed when a patient presents with sinus arrest, sinoatrial exit block, or persistent sinus bradycardia. This syndrome is often the result of drug therapy, such as digitalis, calcium channel blockers, beta-blockers, sympatholytic agents, or antiarrhythmics. Another presentation includes recurrent supraventricular tachycardias associated with bradyarrhythmias. Prolonged ambulatory monitoring may be indicated to establish a diagnosis of SSS. Treatment includes insertion of a permanent cardiac pacemaker.

Various forms of conduction disorders may be classified in ICD-10-CM. Conduction disorders are disruptions or disturbances in the electrical impulses that regulate the heartbeats.

Wolff-Parkinson-White (WPW) syndrome (I45.6) is caused by conduction from the sinoatrial node to the ventricle through an accessory pathway that bypasses the atrioventricular node. Patients with WPW syndrome present with tachyarrhythmias, including supraventricular tachycardia, atrial fibrillation, or atrial flutter. Treatment includes catheter ablation following electrophysiologic evaluation.

Atrioventricular (AV) heart blocks are classified as first, second, or third degree:

- **First-degree AV block** is associated with atrial septal defects or valvular disease. ICD-10-CM classifies first-degree AV block to code I44.0.

- **Second-degree AV block** is further classified as follows:

  - Mobitz type I (Wenckebach) is associated with acute inferior wall myocardial infarction or with digitalis toxicity. Treatment includes discontinuation of digitalis and administration of atropine. ICD-10-CM classifies Mobitz type I AV block to code I44.1.

  - Mobitz type II is associated with anterior wall or anteroseptal myocardial infarction and digitalis toxicity. Treatment includes temporary pacing and, in some cases, permanent pacemaker insertion, as well as discontinuation of digitalis and administration of atropine. ICD-10-CM classifies Mobitz type II AV block to code I44.1.

- **Third-degree heart block**, also referred to as complete heart block, is associated with ischemic heart disease or infarction, postsurgical complication of mitral valve replacement, digitalis toxicity, and Stokes-Adams syndrome. Treatment includes permanent cardiac pacemaker insertion. ICD-10-CM classifies third-degree heart block to code I44.2. When this type of heart block is congenital in nature, code Q24.6 is reported rather than I44.2.

Without further specification, AV block is reported with code I44.30.

Supraventricular tachycardia is a heart rate over 90 beats per minute triggered by the sinoatrial node, usually in response to exogenous factors, such as fever, exercise, anxiety, stress, pain, thyroid hormone, hypoxia, and dehydration. It may also accompany shock, left ventricular failure, cardiac tamponade, anemia, hyperthyroidism, hypovolemia, pulmonary embolism, and anterior myocardial infarction. Tachycardia is also a response to stimulants such as caffeine, cocaine, or amphetamines. Treatment is geared toward correcting the underlying cause. ICD-10-CM classifies supraventricular tachycardia to code I47.1.

Cardiac Arrest (I46)

Cardiac arrest is the sudden stopping of the heart's pumping function that causes arterial blood pressure to cease and produces either ventricular fibrillation or ventricular standstill. Cardiac arrest usually leads to death unless resuscitation occurs (Dorland 2012, 133). ICD-10-CM includes three codes for cardiac arrest: I46.2, Cardiac arrest due to underlying cardiac condition; I46.8, Cardiac arrest due to other underlying condition; and I46.9, Cardiac arrest, cause unspecified. Under codes I46.2 and I46.3, there is a code first note to code the underlying cardiac or other underlying condition as the first code. The specificity of the type of cardiac arrest is essential for coding; is it due to a cardiac condition or another disease or is the cardiac arrest related to another medical condition or procedure.

There is an Excludes1 note under category I46, Cardiac arrest that cardiogenic shock, R57.0, cannot be assigned with a code from category I46. Other codes are available in other chapters of ICD-10-CM for cardiac arrest complicating abortion—see Abortion, by types, complicated by, cardiac arrest. Other cardiac arrest codes exist for when it occurs in a newborn or when cardiac arrest complicates anesthesia and complicating a delivery. Intraoperative and postprocedural cardiac arrest codes are also available.

Check Your Understanding 12.4

Assign diagnosis codes to the following conditions.

1. Acute on chronic systolic heart failure

2. Combined chronic systolic with diastolic heart failure with end stage heart failure

3. Paroxysmal atrial fibrillation

4. Aortic valve stenosis with insufficiency

5. Tachycardia-bradycardia syndrome

6. Second-degree atrioventricular block

Cerebrovascular Disease (I60–I69)

ICD-10-CM contains very specific codes to identify various forms of **cerebrovascular accidents (CVAs)**. CVAs may also be referred to as a strokes or stroke syndrome. A stroke is a condition with a sudden onset of acute vascular lesions of the brain, such as an infarction from a hemorrhage or an embolism or a thrombosis. It can also be caused by a ruptured aneurysm. The condition causes neurological symptoms such as hemiparesis, vertigo, numbness, aphasia, and dysarthria that may be temporary and resolve as the patient recovers from the stroke. For other patients, these neurological deficits may be permanent (Dorland 2012, 1849). The codes specify whether the condition is a cerebral hemorrhage or infarction due to a thrombosis, embolism, or unspecified occlusion or stenosis in the cerebral vessel. The cerebral infarction codes identify the specific cerebral artery involved and laterality (right or left). Category I69, Sequelae of cerebrovascular disease, contains a lot of codes for very specific conditions that remain after the acute CVA is treated.

The category for late effects of cerebrovascular disease, I69, is titled "Sequelae of cerebrovascular disease"; all subcategory codes are expanded. This expansion involves specifying laterality, changing subcategory titles, making terminology changes, adding sixth characters, and providing greater specificity in general. Late effects of cerebrovascular disease are differentiated by type of stroke (hemorrhage, infarction).

Cerebrovascular disease is an insufficient blood supply to a part of the brain and is usually secondary to atherosclerotic disease, hypertension, or a combination of both.

At the beginning of the Cerebrovascular Disease section, there is a "use additional code" note to identify the presence of

Alcohol abuse and dependence (F10.-)
Exposure to environmental tobacco smoke (Z77.22-)
History of tobacco dependence (Z87.891)
Hypertension (I10–I16)

Occupational exposure to environmental tobacco smoke (Z57.31)
Tobacco dependence (F17.-)
Tobacco use (Z72.0)

ICD-10-CM classifies cerebrovascular disease according to the following types of conditions: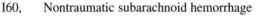

I60,	Nontraumatic subarachnoid hemorrhage
I61,	Nontraumatic intracerebral hemorrhage
I62,	Other and unspecified nontraumatic intracranial hemorrhage
I63,	Cerebral infarction
I65,	Occlusion and stenosis of precerebral arteries, not resulting in cerebral infarction
I66,	Occlusion and stenosis of cerebral arteries, not resulting in cerebral infarction
I67,	Other cerebrovascular disease
I68,	Cerebrovascular disorders in diseases classified elsewhere
I69,	Sequelae of cerebrovascular disease

Carotid Artery Stenosis (I65.2-)

Occlusion and stenosis of precerebral arteries include the carotid artery. An occlusion is an obstruction of the artery. Stenosis is a narrowing of the artery (Dorland 2012, 1310, 1769). The condition may be unilateral or bilateral. The codes for occlusion and stenosis of the carotid artery not resulting in cerebral infarction are codes:

I65.21,	Occlusion and stenosis of right carotid artery
I65.22,	Occlusion and stenosis of left carotid artery
I65.23,	Occlusion and stenosis of bilateral carotid arteries
I65.29,	Occlusion and stenosis of unspecified carotid artery

Cerebral Infarction (I63)

A **cerebral infarction** is an ischemic condition of the brain that produces local brain tissue death. This usually produces neurological deficits in the area of the cerebral arteries where the ischemia is present. The ischemia causes obstruction of the circulation in the cerebral vessels, which causes the tissue to become necrotic. The ischemia is most commonly caused by embolism or thrombosis (Dorland 2012, 934). Category I63 includes occlusion and stenosis of cerebral and precerebral arteries that result in a cerebral infarction. The default code for stroke or CVA is I63.9, Cerebral infarction, unspecified. More specific codes are available when the physician's documentation includes the cause of the stroke (thrombosis or embolism) and the location of the artery where the stroke occurred (vertebral, carotid, cerebral). Laterality is also included in the coding options: right and left or unspecified artery. The specificity of the cerebral infarction can be coded according to the following:

I63.0-,	Cerebral infarction due to thrombosis of precerebral arteries
I63.1-,	Cerebral infarction due to embolism of precerebral arteries
I63.2-,	Cerebral infarction due to unspecified occlusion or stenosis of precerebral arteries
I63.3-,	Cerebral infarction due to thrombosis of cerebral arteries
I63.4-,	Cerebral infarction due to embolism of cerebral arteries
I63.5-,	Cerebral infarction due to unspecified occlusion or stenosis of cerebral arteries
I63.6,	Cerebral infarction due to cerebral venous thrombosis, nonpyogenic
I63.8,	Other cerebral infarction
I63.9,	Cerebral infarction, unspecified

At the time the acute stroke is treated, the conditions resulting from the cerebral infarction or other cerebrovascular events, such as aphasia or hemiplegia, should be coded in addition to the code for the CVA or cerebral infarction as well.

> **EXAMPLE:** A patient was admitted with aphasia and left nondominant side hemiplegia due to an acute CVA. The CVA and the resulting conditions were treated. On discharge, the aphasia had cleared; however, the hemiplegia is still present and will require outpatient physical therapy. Codes include I63.9, the default code for acute CVA; G81.94, Hemiplegia, unspecified affecting left nondominant side; and R47.01, Aphasia.

Sequelae of Cerebrovascular Disease (I69)

Category I69 codes identify sequelae or late effects of cerebrovascular disease, which is usually a cerebral infarction but could be due to any of the conditions classifiable to categories I60 through I67. These conditions are specified as due to the cerebral infarction or as residuals that may occur at any time after the onset of the cerebrovascular disease. In other words,

the conditions identified by the I69 category codes describe the condition that remains in the patient after the acute episode of the cerebral infarction or cerebrovascular disease is over. These conditions may be permanent after the stroke or the condition may remain for a period of time after the acute phase of the illness is over.

The neurologic deficits caused by cerebrovascular disease may be present from the onset or may arise at any time after the onset of the condition classifiable to I60 through I67.

> **EXAMPLE:** A patient is receiving physical therapy for monoplegia of the left leg affecting the nondominant side due to an old cerebral infarction. The code reported would be I69.344, Monoplegia of lower limb following other cerebrovascular disease affecting the left nondominant side.

The coder must be very careful in using the Index to Diseases to code the sequelae conditions because the type of cerebrovascular disease or condition is precise. The particular neurological deficit or remaining condition is specified under the identified cause of the remaining sequelae in the Index. For example, the Index to Diseases and Injuries entries include the following:

Sequelae (of)
        Disease, cerebrovascular
        Hemorrhage, intracerebral
        Infarction, cerebral
        Stroke, NOS
        Each of these subterms is followed with
                Alteration of sensation
                Aphasia
                Apraxia
                And more entries listed alphabetically

The codes under category I69 for sequelae of cerebrovascular disease are a combination of two facts:

1. The cerebrovascular disease responsible for the deficit, such as:

    • Nontraumatic subarachnoid hemorrhage, I69.0

    • Nontraumatic intracerebral hemorrhage, I69.1

- Other nontraumatic intracranial hemorrhage, I69.2

- Cerebral infarction, I69.3

- Other cerebrovascular disease, I69.8

- Unspecified cerebrovascular disease, I69.9

and

2. The type of deficit present such as:

- Unspecified sequelae

- Cognitive deficits

- Speech and language deficits

- Monoplegia of the upper limb

- Monoplegia of the lower limb

- Hemiplegia and hemiparesis

- Other paralytic syndrome

- Apraxia

- Dysphagia

- Facial weakness

- Ataxia

- Other sequelae

When the health record documentation indicates that the patient has a history of a cerebral infarction but no neurological deficits are present, the code Z86.73, Personal history of transient ischemic attack (TIA) and cerebral infarction without residual deficits, should be assigned. In this circumstance, it is incorrect to assign a code from category I69.

The code Z86.73 is located in the Index under "History (personal), stroke without residual deficits, Z86.73" and "History (personal), cerebral infarction, cerebral, without residual deficits Z86.73."

Codes from category I69 may be assigned on a healthcare record with codes from I60 through I67, if the patient has a current stroke and deficits from an old stroke.

> **EXAMPLE:** A patient was admitted with occlusion of cerebral arteries resulting in a cerebral infarction. The patient has a history of previous cerebral infarction one year ago with residual hemiplegia affecting the right dominant side. Codes for this episode of care would be
>
> I63.50, Cerebral artery occlusion, unspecified, with cerebral infarction
>
> I69.351, Hemiplegia and hemiparesis following cerebral infarction affecting right dominant side.

Venous Embolism and Thrombosis (I82)

Very specific codes exist in ICD-10-CM to describe acute and chronic deep and superficial vein thrombosis. The codes identify the specific vessel involved and the right or left side of the body. This same type of detail is also included in the thrombophlebitis and varicose vein codes.

Venous embolism and thrombosis, also referred to as **venous thromboembolism (VTE)**, is an occlusion within the venous system. The terms **deep vein thrombosis (DVT)** and VTE are commonly documented in health records. A DVT is a blood clot in one or more of the deep veins in the body, usually in the lower limbs, that is characterized by pain, swelling, warmth, and redness at the location of the DVT (Dorland 2012, 1921). Venous embolism and thrombosis may also occur in superficial veins. These conditions may occur in the thorax, neck, and upper and lower extremities. The patient with new or acute venous embolism and thrombosis conditions requires the initiation of anticoagulant therapy. The patient with the diagnosis of chronic or old venous embolism and thrombosis continues to receive anticoagulant therapy over a period of time but is no longer in the acute phase of the illness.

Category code I82, Other venous embolism and thrombosis, contains four-, five-, and six-character codes that distinguish between the location of the VTE and the acute versus chronic status of the condition. Under subcategory code I82.5, Chronic embolism and thrombosis of deep veins of lower extremity, is an Exclude1 note that personal history of venous thrombosis and embolism, Z86.718, which describes the VTE condition that has resolved or no longer exists, cannot be used with a code from I82.5-. Another note that appears under subcategory code I82.5 is a "use additional code" note to use, if applicable, Z79.01 for associated long-term (current) use of anticoagulants.

Deep veins in the lower extremity include the femoral, iliac, popliteal, tibial, and other specified and unspecified deep veins of the lower extremity. Superficial veins in the lower extremity include the greater and lesser saphenous vein. Deep veins in the upper extremity include the brachial, radial, and ulnar veins. Superficial veins in the upper extremity include the antecubital, basilica, and cephalic veins.

Specific diagnosis codes for VTEs are as follows:

- Acute embolism and thrombosis of deep veins of lower extremity, I82.4-

- Chronic embolism and thrombosis of deep veins of lower extremity, I82.5-

- Acute embolism and thrombosis of veins of upper extremity, I82.6-

- Chronic embolism and thrombosis of veins of upper extremity, I82.7-

- Embolism and thrombosis of axillary vein, I82.A-

- Embolism and thrombosis of subclavian vein, I82.B-

- Embolism and thrombosis of internal jugular vein, I82.C-

- Embolism and thrombosis of other specified veins, I82.8-

- Embolism and thrombosis of unspecified vein, I82.9-

EXAMPLE: A patient came to the physician's office complaining of pain and swelling in his right leg calf. Upon examination, the physician noted, in addition to the swelling, the presence of warmth and erythema or redness in the calf. The patient had recently returned from a 2000-mile vacation car trip. The patient was sent immediately for a vascular imaging study. Upon reviewing the radiologist's report, the physician documented the diagnosis of deep vein thrombosis of the right calf and the patient was admitted to the hospital. The diagnosis code for this condition is I82.4Z1, acute embolism and thrombosis of unspecified deep veins of right distal lower extremity.

Intraoperative and Postprocedural Circulatory Complications (I97)

Intraoperative and postprocedural circulatory complications can be identified with greater specificity in ICD-10-CM. Instructional notes appear under certain codes to add detail by using an additional code to further describe the condition, for example, using an additional code to identify heart failure or to further specify the disorder. For example, different codes exist for intraoperative and postprocedural complications, such as the following:

- Postcardiotomy syndrome

- Other postprocedural and intraoperative cardiac functional disturbances

- Intraoperative versus postprocedural cardiac arrest

- Postmastectomy lymphedema syndrome

- Postprocedural hypertension

- Postprocedural heart failure

- Intraoperative and postprocedural cerebral infarction

- Accidental puncture or laceration during a circulatory system procedure

- Accidental puncture or laceration of a circulatory system organ during another body system procedure

---

Check Your Understanding 12.5

Assign diagnosis codes to the following conditions.

1. Current cerebral infarction due to thrombosis of right vertebral artery with left non-dominant sided hemiplegia

2. Cerebral infarction due to middle cerebral artery with dysphagia that was a sequela from previous stroke

3. Intraoperative stroke during cardiac surgery

4. Acute deep vein thrombosis (DVT), lower leg, left

5. Thrombosis of right subclavian vein

ICD-10-PCS Procedure Coding for Circulatory System Procedures

This section highlights several cardiovascular procedures that are commonly performed to treat conditions in patients with acute and chronic forms of heart disease. Described in this section are invasive procedures that are performed by Percutaneous and Open approaches.

Measurement and Monitoring (4A0–4B0)

Technically, a **cardiac catheterization** is not a procedure. The catheterization of the heart represents a usual percutaneous approach to gain access to the heart for diagnostic and therapeutic procedures. In ICD-10-PCS, the coder assigns codes for the actual root operations or root types that are performed inside the heart or through the catheter. For example, if an angioplasty is performed, the root operation is Dilation. If only images are taken of the coronary vessels and structure, the imaging is coded. If pressure measurement and sampling is performed, the procedure code is assigned from the Measurement and Monitoring section in ICD-10-PCS.

Through the cardiac catheter, diagnostic tests are used to identify, measure, and verify almost every type of intracardiac condition. The technique includes the passage of a flexible catheter through the arteries or veins into the heart chambers and vessels. The diagnostic procedures determine the size and location of a coronary lesion, evaluate left and right ventricular function, and measure heart pressures.

In addition to serving as a diagnostic tool, therapeutic procedures can be performed through the cardiac catheters. For example, both percutaneous transluminal coronary angioplasties (PTCAs) and intracoronary streptokinase injections can be performed via a cardiac catheter.

Cardiac catheterization is most commonly performed on the left side of the heart, using the Percutaneous approach via the antecubital and femoral vessels. In a right heart catheterization, a catheter is inserted through the femoral or antecubital vein, advanced first into the superior or inferior vena cava, then into the right atrium, the right ventricle, and, finally, into the pulmonary artery. In a left heart catheterization, a catheter enters the body through either the brachial artery or the femoral artery. The catheter is advanced into the aorta, through the aortic valve and then into the left ventricle.

There are two ways to access the correct ICD-10-PCS table for coding cardiac catheterization. First, the coder can use the Index term "Catheterization, heart." The coder will be directed to see the term "Measurement, cardiac A402." The other approach is to access the main term in the ICD-10-PCS Index as "Measurement" with subterms of cardiac, sampling, and pressure for bilateral, left heart, and right heart. The first three characters given are 4A0 (see table 12.1).

Table 12.1.   **ICD-10-PCS Table 4A0**

4 Measurement and Monitoring
A Physiological Systems
0 Measurement

Body System	Approach	Function/Device	Qualifier
2 Cardiac	0 Open 3 Percutaneous 7 Via natural or artificial opening 8 Via natural or artificial opening endoscopic	N Sampling and Pressure	6 Right Heart 7 Left Heart 8 Bilateral

Source: CMS 2019

The ICD-10-PCS code for a left heart catheterization for oxygen sampling and pressure measurements taken on the left side of the heart, usually, the left ventricle is 4A023N7.

Diagnostic Procedures

The following procedures are often performed during a cardiac catheterization:

- Coronary angiography

- Coronary arteriography

- Ventriculography

Coronary Angiography

Coronary angiography can be performed on the right or left side of the heart, or in a combined process including both the right and left sides of the heart. Right-side cardiac angiography is useful in detecting pericarditis and congenital lesions, such as Ebstein's malformation of the tricuspid valve. Left-side cardiac angiography reveals congenital and acquired lesions affecting the mitral valve, including mitral stenosis and mitral regurgitation.

Coronary Arteriography

Coronary arteriography serves as a diagnostic tool in detecting obstruction within the coronary arteries. The following two techniques are used in performing a coronary arteriography:

- The Sones technique uses a single catheter inserted via a brachial arteriotomy.

- The Judkins technique uses two catheters inserted percutaneously through the femoral artery.

Ventriculography

Ventriculography measures stroke volume and ejection fraction. The ejection fraction is the amount of blood ejected from the left ventricle per beat; it is presented as a percentage of the total ventricular volume. An ejection fraction of 60 percent means that 60 percent of the total amount of blood in the left ventricle is ejected with each heartbeat. A normal ejection fraction may be between 55 and 70. An ejection fracture under 40 may be a sign of ventricular dysfunction, heart failure, or cardiomyopathy. A higher ejection fracture of 75 or above may indicate hypertrophic cardiomyopathy exists (AHA 2018).

Coding the Procedures

The imaging modality used for the coronary angiograms, arteriograms, and ventriculograms is fluoroscopy with the root type Fluoroscopy with the appropriate body part for the number and type of coronary arteries imaged. The main term to use in the ICD-10-PCS Index is Fluoroscopy. The subterms under fluoroscopy are as follows:

Artery
    Coronary
        Bypass Graft
            Multiple (B213)
                Laser, Intraoperative (B213)
            Single (B212)
                Laser, Intraoperative (B212)
        Multiple (B211)
            Laser, Intraoperative (B211)
        Single (B210)
            Laser, Intraoperative (B210)

The first three characters for the ICD-10-PCS code for the fluoroscopy entries are B21. The coder locates Table B21 to build the ICD-10-PCS code (see table 12.2).

Table 12.2.   **ICD-10-PCS Table B21**

B Imaging			
2 Heart			
1 Fluoroscopy			
Body Part	**Contrast**	**Qualifier**	**Qualifier**
0 Coronary Artery, Single 1 Coronary Artery, Multiple 2 Coronary Artery Bypass Graft, Single 3 Coronary Artery Bypass Graft, Multiple	0 High Osmolar 1 Low Osmolar Y Other Osmolar	1 Laser	0 Intraoperative
0 Coronary Artery, Single 1 Coronary Artery, Multiple 2 Coronary Artery Bypass Graft, Single 3 Coronary Artery Bypass Graft, Multiple	0 High Osmolar 1 Low Osmolar Y Other Osmolar	Z None	Z None
4 Heart, Right 5 Heart, Left 6 Heart, Right and Left 7 Internal Mammary Bypass Graft, Right 8 Internal Mammary Bypass Graft, Left F Bypass Graft, Other	0 High Osmolar 1 Low Osmolar Y Other Osmolar	Z None	Z None

Source: CMS 2019

The ICD-10-PCS procedure code for a multiple vessel native coronary artery angiography or arteriography using low osmolar contrast material is B2111ZZ. The ICD-10-PCS procedure code for a left ventriculogram using low osmolar contrast material is B2151ZZ.

Percutaneous Transluminal Coronary Angioplasty

Percutaneous transluminal coronary angioplasty (PTCA) is used to relieve obstruction of coronary arteries. PTCA is performed to widen a narrowed area of a coronary artery by employing a balloon-tipped catheter. The catheter is passed to the obstructed area, and the balloon is inflated one or more times to exert pressure on the narrowed area. A thrombolytic agent may be infused into the heart.

A PTCA procedure may also include the insertion of one or more coronary stents. It is possible to insert stents in several different vessels during the same operative episode. It is also possible to insert multiple adjoining or overlapping stents.

The objective of a PTCA is to open or dilate the coronary artery or bypass coronary graft. The root operation in ICD-10-PCS for this procedure is Dilation by definition. The main term in the ICD-10-PCS Index is Dilation with subterms artery, coronary, and then the number of vessels: one, two, three, four, or more. The Index gives the first three digits as "027." To construct the procedure code for the PTCA, the coder accesses Table 027. If the insertion of a coronary artery stent is performed with the angioplasty, the sixth character (device) is used to identify the type of stent: Intraluminal Device, Drug Eluting or Intraluminal Device, or Nondrug Eluting. If the PTCA is performed without the insertion of a stent, there is a value of Z for no device used for the sixth character. The number of codes assigned depends on the number of vessels treated by angioplasty and the number of vessels that have a stent or device inserted. For example, if an angioplasty is performed on one coronary artery and if an angioplasty with the insertion of a stent is performed on a different coronary artery, two codes are assigned because the device value would be different for the two vessels. On the other hand, if an angioplasty is performed on two coronary arteries and neither has a stent inserted, there would be one procedure code assigned. Table 027 is shown in table 12.3. For example, if an angioplasty is performed on the left anterior descending and the right coronary artery without any stent insertion in either vessel, the code assigned would be 02713ZZ. However, if an angioplasty is performed on the left anterior descending and an angioplasty with a plain stent inserted in the right coronary artery, two codes would be assigned: 02703ZZ and 02703DZ.

Table 12.3. **Excerpt from ICD-10-PCS Table 027**

0 Medical and Surgical 2 Heart and Great Vessels 7 Dilation			
Body Part	**Approach**	**Device**	**Qualifier**
0 Coronary Artery, One Artery 1 Coronary Artery, Two Arteries 2 Coronary Artery, Three Arteries 3 Coronary Artery, Four or more arteries	0 Open 3 Percutaneous 4 Percutaneous endoscopic	4 Intraluminal Device, Drug eluting 5 Intraluminal Device, Drug eluting, Two 6 Intraluminal Device, Drug eluting, Three 7 Intraluminal Device, Drug eluting, Four or More D Intraluminal Device E Intraluminal Device, Two F Intraluminal Device, Three G Intraluminal Device, Four or More T Intraluminal Device, Radioactive Z No Device	6 Bifurcation Z No Qualifier

Source: CMS 2019

Coronary Artery Bypass Graft (CABG)

The coronary circulation consists of two main arteries, the right and the left, that are further subdivided into several branches:

> **EXAMPLE:** Right coronary artery
>   Right marginal
>   Right posterior descending
>   Left main coronary artery
>   Left anterior descending branch
>   Diagonal
>   Septal
>   Left circumflex
>   Obtuse marginal
>   Posterior descending
>   Posterolateral

Aortocoronary Bypass or Coronary Artery Bypass Graft

Aortocoronary bypass brings blood from the aorta into the obstructed coronary artery using a segment of the saphenous vein or a segment of the internal mammary artery for the graft. The procedure is commonly referred to as coronary artery bypass graft(s) or by the abbreviation CABG, pronounced "cabbage."

The following three surgical approaches are used in CABG procedures:

- Aortocoronary bypass uses the aorta to bypass the occluded coronary artery.

- Internal mammary-coronary artery bypass uses the internal mammary artery to bypass the occluded coronary artery.

- Abdominal-coronary artery bypass uses an abdominal artery.

Internal mammary-coronary artery bypass is accomplished by loosening the distal end of the internal mammary artery from its normal position and attaching the internal mammary artery distal to the blockage in order to bring blood from the subclavian artery directly to the occluded coronary artery. Codes are selected based on whether one or both internal mammary arteries are used, regardless of the number of coronary arteries involved.

An **abdominal-coronary artery bypass** procedure involves harvesting an abdominal artery, commonly the gastroepiploic, and creating an anastomosis between the abdominal artery, and a coronary artery distal to the occluded portion.

The root operation for coronary artery bypass procedures is Bypass. The body part value identifies the number of coronary arteries bypassed to, and the qualifier identifies the vessel bypassed from or the vessel that is the source of the blood flow to the bypassed vessel. The device character identifies the tissue used as the bypass. If a saphenous vein is used as the bypass tissue, the harvesting of the saphenous vein is coded as an Excision procedure based on the side (left or right) from which it was harvested. The main term used in the ICD-10-PCS Index is Bypass with subterms of artery, coronary, and one, two, three, or four or more arteries. The three-digit character is 021, as shown in table 12.4.

Table 12.4. **Excerpt from ICD-10-PCS Table 021**

0 Medical and Surgical **2 Heart and Great Vessels** **1 Bypass**			
Body Part	**Approach**	**Device**	**Qualifier**
0 Coronary Artery, One artery 1 Coronary Artery, Two arteries 2 Coronary Artery, Three arteries 3 Coronary Artery, Four or more arteries	0 Open	8 Zooplastic Tissue 9 Autologous Venous Tissue A Autologous Arterial Tissue J Synthetic Substitute K Nonautologous Tissue Substitute	3 Coronary Artery 8 Internal Mammary, Right 9 Internal Mammary, Left C Thoracic Artery F Abdominal Artery W Aorta
0 Coronary Artery, One artery 1 Coronary Artery, Two arteries 2 Coronary Artery, Three arteries 3 Coronary Artery, Four or more arteries	0 Open	Z No Device	3 Coronary Artery 8 Internal Mammary, Right 9 Internal Mammary, Left C Thoracic Artery F Abdominal Artery
0 Coronary Artery, One Artery 1 Coronary Artery, Two Arteries 2 Coronary Artery, Three Arteries 3 Coronary Artery, Four or More Arteries	3 Percutaneous	4 Intraluminal Device, Drug-eluting D Intraluminal Device	4 Coronary Vein

Table 12.4. **Excerpt from ICD-10-PCS Table 021** *(continued)*

0 Medical and Surgical 2 Heart and Great Vessels 1 Bypass			
Body Part	**Approach**	**Device**	**Qualifier**
0 Coronary Artery, One Artery 1 Coronary Artery, Two Arteries 2 Coronary Artery, Three Arteries 3 Coronary Artery, Four or More Arteries	4 Percutaneous Endoscopic	4 Intraluminal Device, Drug-eluting D Intraluminal Device	4 Coronary Vein
0 Coronary Artery, One Artery 1 Coronary Artery, Two Arteries 2 Coronary Artery, Three Arteries 3 Coronary Artery, Four or More Arteries	4 Percutaneous Endoscopic	8 Zooplastic Tissue 9 Autologous Venous Tissue A Autologous Arterial Tissue J Synthetic Substitute K Nonautologous Tissue Substitute	3 Coronary Artery 8 Internal Mammary, Right 9 Internal Mammary, Left C Thoracic Artery F Abdominal Artery W Aorta

Source: CMS 2019

For example, using table 12.4, if a triple coronary artery bypass is performed with two aortocoronary bypass grafts and one left internal mammary artery bypass using a left saphenous vein and cardiopulmonary bypass, the procedure is coded as

> 021109W for the double-vessel aortocoronary bypass using saphenous vein grafts
> 02100Z9 for the single-vessel left internal mammary artery bypass

Using other Index and Table entries, the other two procedure codes to be assigned are

> 06BQ0ZZ for Excision of greater left saphenous vein for bypass material
> 5A1221Z for Bypass, cardiopulmonary

Cardiac Pacemakers

A cardiac pacemaker has the following three basic components:

- The **pulse generator** is the pacing system that contains the pacemaker battery (power source) and the electronic circuitry.

- The **pacing lead** carries the stimulating electricity from the pulse generator to the stimulating electrode.

- The **electrode** is the metal portion of the lead that comes in contact with the heart (NHLBI 2019d).

There are different types of pacemakers:

- Single-chamber pacemakers use a single lead that is placed in the right atrium or the right ventricle.

- Dual-chamber pacemakers use leads that are inserted into both the atrium and the ventricle.

- Rate-responsive pacemakers have a pacing rate modality that is determined by physiological variables other than the atrial rate.

- Cardiac resynchronization pacemakers without a defibrillator (CRT-P) is also known as a biventricular pacing device without internal cardiac defibrillator.

ICD-10-PCS Coding of Pacemakers

ICD-10-PCS classifies the placement of cardiac pacemakers by coding the insertion of each lead into one or more of the chambers of the heart and the insertion of the generator in the subcutaneous tissue.

For example, the insertion of a dual-chamber cardiac pacemaker with leads inserted into the right atrium and right ventricle and the generator implanted in left chest subcutaneous tissue is coded as follows. A simple illustration of a pacemaker is shown in figure 12.3.

Figure 12.3.   **Cardiac pacemaker**

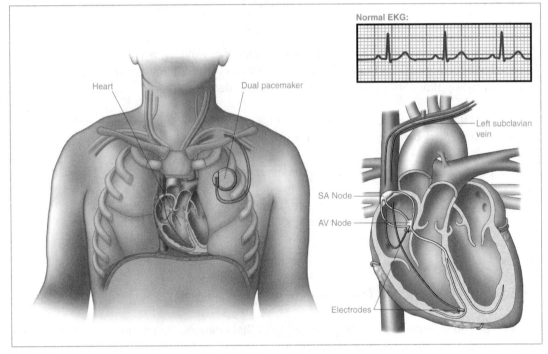

© AHIMA

The root operation Insertion is used to code all three procedures. Codes for all three procedures are required because the insertion of each lead is coded separately, and the insertion of the pacemaker generator is coded separately. Leads are inserted percutaneously into the right atrium and right ventricle. The device value for both leads is J, Cardiac Lead, Pacemaker. There is no qualifier value for either code. The body part value for the pacemaker generator insertion is Subcutaneous Tissue and Fascia, Chest. The approach for this procedure is Open. The device value is Pacemaker, Dual Chamber, and there is no qualifier for this code. For example, the codes for insertion of the pacemaker device are as follows:

02H63JZ, Insertion of device in, Atrium, right (device is J for Cardiac Lead, Pacemaker)
02HK3JZ, Insertion of device in Ventricle, right (device is J for Cardiac Lead, Pacemaker)
0JH606Z, Insertion of device in, Subcutaneous Tissue and Fascia, Chest (device is 6 for Pacemaker, Dual Chamber)

Automatic Implantable Cardioverter-Defibrillators

The **automatic implantable cardioverter-defibrillator (AICD)** is a special type of pacemaker that proves effective for patients with recurring, life-threatening dysrhythmias, such as ventricular tachycardia or fibrillation (NHLBI 2019e).

The AICD is an electronic device consisting of a pulse generator and three leads. The pulse generator is implanted under the patient's skin, usually in the shoulder area. The first lead senses heart rate at the right ventricle; the second lead, sensing morphology and rhythm, defibrillates at the right atrium; the third lead defibrillates at the apical pericardium. The AICD can be programmed to suit each patient's needs, and it uses far less energy than an external defibrillator.

The insertion of an AICD is coded similarly to the coding of cardiac pacemaker; however, the device value is different. For an AICD the device value is K for Cardiac Lead, Defibrillator in ICD-10-PCS Table 02H for insertion of device in (location). The insertion of the AICD generator in the subcutaneous tissue such as the chest has device values of 8 or 9 for the type of defibrillator generator used.

ICD-10-CM and ICD-10-PCS Review Exercises: Chapter 12

Assign the correct ICD-10-CM diagnosis codes and ICD-10-PCS procedure codes to the following.

1. Cerebral infarction with left nondominant hemiparesis and dysphasia

   _____

2. Postinfarction pericarditis

   _____

3. Chronic atrial fibrillation; essential hypertension

   _____

4. Coronary artery disease in autologous vein bypass graft

   _____

5. Venous thrombosis of greater saphenous vein, right leg

   _____

6. Thoracic aortic aneurysm

   _____

7. Mitral valve insufficiency

   _____

(Continued on next page)

ICD-10-CM and ICD-10-PCS Review Exercises: Chapter 12 *(continued)*

8. Acute type 1 myocardial infarction (STEMI) of anterior wall

9. Subacute bacterial endocarditis secondary to *Staphylococcus aureus*; ventricular tachycardia

10. Coronary artery disease with unstable angina with documented spasm, no history of coronary artery bypass surgery

11. Arteriosclerosis of left thigh native arteries with ulcerative breakdown of skin only

12. End-stage renal disease (ESRD) with hypertension

13. Inflamed varicose veins of the left lower extremity with development of calf ulcer

14. Myocardial infarction secondary to demand ischemia

15. PROCEDURE: Coronary artery bypass graft (CABG) using four saphenous veins for aortocoronary bypass with cardiopulmonary bypass

16. PROCEDURE: Placement of dual chamber cardiac pacemaker and leads to the right ventricle and right atrium

17. PROCEDURE: Percutaneous transluminal coronary angioplasty, three vessels, no stents

18. PROCEDURE: Percutaneous insertion of central venous catheter infusion device, left subclavian vein

19. PROCEDURE: Ablation, right atrium, percutaneous (MAZE procedure)

20. PROCEDURE: PTCA, via femoral approach, two vessels with insertion of non-drug-eluting stent into same two vessels

References

Alaeddini, J. 2018. Medscape. Angina Pectoris. http://emedicine.medscape.com/article/150215-overview.

American Association for Clinical Chemistry (AACC). 2019. Lab Tests Online: ASO, Antistreptolysin O Test. https://labtestsonline.org/understanding/analytes/aso/tab/test.

American Heart Association (AHA). 2018. Ejection Fraction Heart Failure Measurement. https://www.heart.org/en/health-topics/heart-failure/diagnosing-heart-failure/ejection-fraction-heart-failure-measurement.

Bisognano, J. D. 2017. Medscape. Malignant Hypertension. http://emedicine.medscape.com/article/241640-overview.

Centers for Disease Control and Prevention (CDC), National Center for Health Statistics (NCHS). 2019. *ICD-10-CM Official Guidelines for Coding and Reporting*, 2020. http://www.cdc.gov/nchs/icd/icd10cm.htm.

Centers for Medicare and Medicaid Services (CMS). 2019. *ICD-10-PCS Official Guidelines for Coding and Reporting*, 2020. http://www.cms.gov/Medicare/Coding/ICD10/.

Dorland, W.A.N., ed. 2012. *Dorland's Illustrated Medical Dictionary*, 32nd ed. Philadelphia: Elsevier Saunders.

Madhur, M. S. 2019. Medscape. Hypertension. http://emedicine.medscape.com/article/241381-overview.

National Heart, Lung and Blood Institute (NHLBI). 2019a. What Is a Heart Attack? https://www.nhlbi.nih.gov/health/health-topics/topics/heartattack.

National Heart, Lung and Blood Institute (NHLBI). 2019b. What Is Heart Failure? http://www.nhlbi.nih.gov/health/health-topics/topics/hf.

National Heart, Lung and Blood Institute (NHLBI). 2019c. What Is an Arrhythmia? http://www.nhlbi.nih.gov/health/health-topics/topics/arr.

National Heart, Lung and Blood Institute (NHLBI). 2019d. What Is a Pacemaker? http://www.nhlbi.nih.gov/health/health-topics/topics/pace.

National Heart, Lung and Blood Institute (NHLBI). 2019e. How Does an Implantable Cardioverter Defibrillator Work? http://www.nhlbi.nih.gov/health/health-topics/topics/icd/howdoes.

Riaz, K. 2014. Medscape. Hypertensive Heart Disease. http://emedicine.medscape.com/article/162449-overview#a1.

Tan, W. 2019. Medscape. Unstable Angina. http://emedicine.medscape.com/article/159383-overview.

U.S. National Library of Medicine. MedLine Plus (NLM). 2019a. Mitral Stenosis. https://www.nlm.nih.gov/medlineplus/ency/article/000175.htm.

U.S. National Library of Medicine. MedLine Plus (NLM). 2019b. Sydenham Chorea. https://www.nlm.nih.gov/medlineplus/ency/article/001358.htm.

Weinberg, G. A. 2019. Rheumatic Fever. Merck Manual Consumer Version. http://www.merckmanuals.com/home/children-s-health-issues/miscellaneous-bacterial-infections-in-infants-and-children/rheumatic-fever.

Chapter 13

Diseases of the Respiratory System (J00–J99)

Learning Objectives

At the conclusion of this chapter, you should be able to do the following:

- Describe the organization of the conditions and codes included in Chapter 10 of ICD-10-CM, Diseases of the Respiratory System (J00–J99)

- Specify the ICD-10-CM codes used to describe bronchitis

- Identify the ICD-10-CM codes used to describe asthma

- Summarize the various conditions that may be described as forms of chronic obstructive pulmonary disease

- Apply the ICD-10-CM coding and sequencing rules for assigning respiratory failure codes

- Assign ICD-10-CM codes for diseases of the respiratory system

- Assign ICD-10-PCS codes for procedures related to diseases of the respiratory system

Key Terms

Acute bronchitis
Acute exacerbation
Asthma
Bronchiectasis
Bronchiolitis
Bronchitis
Chronic bronchitis
Chronic obstructive pulmonary disease (COPD)

Emphysema
Endoscopy
Influenza
Mechanical ventilation
Respiratory failure
Status asthmaticus
Viral pneumonia

Overview of ICD-10-CM Chapter 10: Diseases of the Respiratory System

Chapter 10 includes categories J00–J99 arranged in the following blocks:

J00–J06	Acute upper respiratory infections
J09–J18	Influenza and pneumonia
J20–J22	Other acute lower respiratory infections
J30–J39	Other diseases of upper respiratory tract
J40–J47	Chronic lower respiratory diseases
J60–J70	Lung diseases due to external agents
J80–J84	Other respiratory diseases principally affecting the interstitium
J85–J86	Suppurative and necrotic conditions of the lower respiratory tract
J90–J94	Other diseases of the pleura
J95	Intraoperative and postprocedural complications and disorders of respiratory system, not elsewhere classified
J96–J99	Other diseases of the respiratory system

Code titles in the respiratory system chapter of ICD-10-CM reflect current terminology used in pulmonary medicine. For example, asthma codes include the descriptors of mild intermittent, mild persistent, moderate persistent, and severe persistent. Emphysema codes include descriptors for panlobular and centrilobular emphysema. Influenza and acute bronchitis codes include the manifestations of these diseases in one code.

For example, ICD-10-CM category J43, Emphysema, contains codes with panlobular emphysema and centrilobular emphysema in the titles. ICD-10-CM category J45, Asthma, classifies asthma as mild intermittent, mild persistent, moderate persistent, and severe persistent.

ICD-10-CM provides specificity in the respiratory system chapter codes. For example, ICD-10-CM has individual codes for acute recurrent sinusitis for each sinus. Subcategory J10.8, Influenza due to other identified influenza virus with other manifestations, has been expanded to reflect the manifestations of the influenza. Category J20, Acute bronchitis, has been expanded to reflect the causes of the acute bronchitis (CDC 2019).

Coding Guidelines and Instructional Notes for ICD-10-CM Chapter 10

At the beginning of Chapter 10, the following instructional guideline appears: "When a respiratory condition is described as occurring in more than one site and is not specifically indexed, it should be classified to the lowest anatomic site" (CDC 2019). For example, tracheobronchitis is classified to bronchitis in J40, Bronchitis, not specified as acute or chronic.

An additional instructional note also appears at the beginning of Chapter 10 that instructs the coding professional to use an additional code, where applicable, to identify

- exposure to environmental tobacco smoke (Z77.22),

- exposure to tobacco smoke in the perinatal period (P96.81),

- history of tobacco dependence (Z87.891),

- occupational exposure to environmental tobacco smoke (Z57.31),

- tobacco dependence (F17.-), or

- tobacco use (Z72.0).

Since these instructional notes appear at the beginning of the chapter, they should be followed when assigning any code from this chapter.

Some of the codes in Chapter 10 include notes indicating that an additional code should be assigned or an associated condition should be sequenced first. The following are examples of the instructional notes:

- Use additional code to identify the infectious agent

- Use additional code to identify the virus

- Code first any associated lung abscess

- Code first the underlying disease

- Use additional code to identify other conditions such as tobacco use or exposure

In the Tabular, there is a note under category J44 to code also the type of asthma, if applicable (J45.-). There is also an Excludes2 note under category J45 for asthma with chronic obstructive pulmonary disease. By definition, when an Excludes2 note appears under a code, it is acceptable to use both the code and the excluded code together if the patient has both conditions at the same time.

The NCHS has published chapter-specific guidelines for Chapter 10 in the *ICD-10-CM Official Guidelines for Coding and Reporting*. The coding student should review all of the coding guidelines for Chapter 10 of ICD-10-CM, which appear in an ICD-10-CM code book or on the CDC website (CDC 2019) or in appendix F of this textbook.

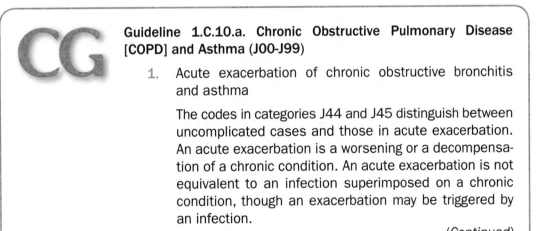

Guideline 1.C.10.a. Chronic Obstructive Pulmonary Disease [COPD] and Asthma (J00-J99)

1. Acute exacerbation of chronic obstructive bronchitis and asthma

The codes in categories J44 and J45 distinguish between uncomplicated cases and those in acute exacerbation. An acute exacerbation is a worsening or a decompensation of a chronic condition. An acute exacerbation is not equivalent to an infection superimposed on a chronic condition, though an exacerbation may be triggered by an infection.

(Continued)

(Continued)

Guideline I.C.10.b. Acute Respiratory Failure

1. Acute respiratory failure as principal diagnosis

    A code from subcategory J96.0, Acute respiratory failure, or subcategory J96.2, Acute and chronic respiratory failure, may be assigned as a principal diagnosis when it is the condition established after study to be chiefly responsible for occasioning the admission to the hospital, and the selection is supported by the Alphabetic Index and Tabular List. However, chapter-specific coding guidelines (such as obstetrics, poisoning, HIV, newborn) that provide sequencing direction take precedence.

2. Acute respiratory failure as secondary diagnosis

    Respiratory failure may be listed as a secondary diagnosis if it occurs after admission, or if it is present on admission, but does not meet the definition of principal diagnosis.

3. Sequencing of acute respiratory failure and another acute condition

    When a patient is admitted with respiratory failure and another acute condition, (e.g., myocardial infarction, cerebrovascular accident, aspiration pneumonia), the principal diagnosis will not be the same in every situation. This applies whether the other acute condition is a respiratory or nonrespiratory condition. Selection of the principal diagnosis will be dependent on the circumstances of admission. If both the respiratory failure and the other acute condition are equally responsible for occasioning the admission to the hospital, and there are no chapter-specific sequencing rules, the guideline regarding two or more diagnoses that equally meet the definition for principal diagnosis may be applied in these situations.

    If the documentation is not clear as to whether acute respiratory failure and another condition are equally responsible for occasioning the admission, query the provider for clarification.

Guideline I.C.10.c. Influenza due to certain identified influenza viruses

Code only confirmed cases of influenza due to certain identified influenza viruses (category J09), and due to other identified influenza virus (category J10). This is an exception to the hospital inpatient guideline Section II, H. (Uncertain Diagnosis).

In this context, "confirmation" does not require documentation of positive laboratory testing specific for avian or other novel influenza A or other identified influenza virus. However, coding should be based on the provider's diagnostic statement that the patient has avian influenza, or other novel influenza A, for category J09, or has another particular identified strain of influenza, such as H1N1 or H3N2, but not identified as novel or variant, for category J10.

If the provider records "suspected" or "possible" or "probable" avian influenza, or novel influenza, or other identified influenza, then the appropriate influenza code from category J11, Influenza due to unidentified influenza virus, should be assigned. A code from category J09, Influenza due to certain identified influenza viruses, should not be assigned nor should a code from category J10, Influenza due to other identified influenza virus.

Guideline I.C.10.d. Ventilator associated Pneumonia

1. **Documentation of Ventilator associated Pneumonia**

   As with all procedural or postprocedural complications, code assignment is based on the provider's documentation of the relationship between the condition and the procedure.

   Code J95.851, Ventilator associated pneumonia, should be assigned only when the provider has documented ventilator associated pneumonia (VAP). An additional code to identify the organism (e.g., Pseudomonas aeruginosa, code B96.5) should also be assigned. Do not assign an additional code from categories J12-J18 to identify the type of pneumonia.

   Code J95.851 should not be assigned for cases where the patient has pneumonia and is on a mechanical ventilator and the provider has not specifically stated that the pneumonia is ventilator-associated pneumonia. If the documentation is unclear as to whether the patient has a pneumonia that is a complication attributable to the mechanical ventilator, query the provider.

2. **Ventilator associated Pneumonia Develops after Admission**

   A patient may be admitted with one type of pneumonia (e.g., code J13, Pneumonia due to Streptococcus pneumonia) and subsequently develop VAP. In this instance, the principal diagnosis would be the appropriate code from categories J12–J18 for the pneumonia diagnosed at the time of admission. Code J95.851, Ventilator associated pneumonia, would be assigned as an additional diagnosis when the provider has also documented the presence of ventilator associated pneumonia.

Coding Diseases of the Respiratory System in ICD-10-CM Chapter 10

Chapter 10 of ICD-10-CM contains codes for a wide variety of pulmonary conditions, ranging from acute upper respiratory infections, pneumonia, influenza, as well as diseases of the lower respiratory tract including chronic lung diseases and diseases acquired from exposure to external substances. Intraoperative and postprocedural complications are also available to be coded in this chapter. Figure 13.1 is a diagram of the respiratory track including the trachea, bronchi, and lungs.

Figure 13.1. **Diagram of the respiratory track**

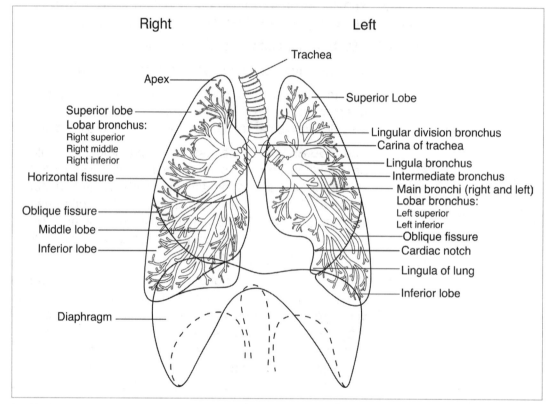

Acute Upper Respiratory Infections (J00–J06)

The codes in this section are used to describe acute infections of the sites within the upper respiratory tract, including the nose, sinuses, pharynx, tonsils, larynx, and trachea. A use additional code note (B95–B97) to identify the infectious agent appears under the categories of acute sinusitis (J01), acute pharyngitis (J02), acute tonsillitis (J03), acute laryngitis and tracheitis (J04), and acute obstructive laryngitis and epiglottis (J05) to include the codes for such infectious organisms as *Streptococcus*, *Staphylococcus*, and other bacterial and viral organisms that can be identified as the cause of the acute upper respiratory conditions.

One three-character code, J00, is used to identify the classification of acute nasopharyngitis or the common cold, which may also be described as acute rhinitis. An Excludes1 listing of conditions under this category reminds the coder what conditions cannot be coded with acute nasopharyngitis. However, the Excludes2 note identifies conditions that can exist concurrently with acute nasopharyngitis and can be coded, for example, chronic pharyngitis and chronic rhinitis.

> **EXAMPLE:** The physician documents at the end of an office visit that the 25-year-old female patient has a common cold or acute nasopharyngitis that was treated. The patient also is known to have vasomotor rhinitis that is also being treated on an ongoing basis. The diagnosis codes assigned for this visit are as follows:
> J00 Acute nasopharyngitis [common cold]
> J30.0 Vasomotor rhinitis
> Note: There is an Excludes2 note under code J00 that list vasomotor rhinitis to indicate that both conditions can be coded at the same time.

Influenza (J09–J11)

Influenza is an acute viral infection of the respiratory tract. It produces symptoms of inflammation of the nasal mucosa, pharynx, and conjunctiva; headache; myalgia; and often fever and chills (Dorland 2012, 937). Influenza is classified with ICD-10-CM diagnosis codes to describe the type of influenza virus and the respiratory conditions it produces. The three categories of codes are as follows:

J09,	Influenza due to certain identified influenza virus
	Includes avian and bird influenza A/H5N1 and swine influenza viruses
J10,	Influenza due to other identified influenza virus
	Includes novel (2009) H1N1 and novel influenza A/H1N1 viruses
J11,	Influenza due to unidentified influenza virus
	Includes influenza when the type of virus is not or cannot be identified

Influenza Due to Certain Identified Influenza Virus

Avian influenza virus is a highly contagious disease of wild and domesticated birds caused by *avian influenza virus* (Dorland 2012, 937). Avian influenza disease has not been reported in humans in the United States. It has however been reported in United States poultry, but not transmitted to humans as of yet. It has been identified in other parts of the globe with various body system complications (CDC 2015). The subcategory code J09.X includes here are as follows:

J09.X1,	Influenza due to identified novel influenza A virus with pneumonia.
	Code also, if applicable, associated lung abscess or other specified type of pneumonia
J09.X2,	Influenza due to identified novel influenza A virus with other respiratory manifestations
	The respiratory manifestations coded here are laryngitis, pharyngitis and other upper respiratory symptoms.
	The coder is reminded to use an additional code, if applicable, for associated pleural effusion and sinusitis.
J09.X3,	Influenza due to identified novel influenza A virus with gastrointestinal manifestations
	"Intestinal flu" or viral gastroenteritis would not be coded with J09.X3 according to the Excludes1 note that follows this code. Instead "intestinal flu" is coded as A08.-.

Influenza Due to Other Identified Influenza Virus (J10)

Novel H1N1 influenza virus was a flu virus of swine origin that first caused illness in Mexico and the United States in 2009. It was thought to spread the same way that regular seasonal influenza viruses are spread, mainly through coughing and sneezing by people who are sick with the virus. It produced flu-like symptoms, including fever, cough, sore throat, headaches, body aches, fatigue, and chills. During 2009 to 2010, more than 70 countries had reported cases of novel influenza A (H1N1) infection, and there were ongoing community level outbreaks of novel H1N1 in multiple parts of the world. For this reason, it was classified as a pandemic by the United States' Centers for Disease Control and Prevention (CDC 2009). By 2010, the pandemic was considered over, and the H1N1 virus that caused that pandemic is now a regular human flu virus and continues to circulate seasonally worldwide (CDC 2009).

The Alphabetic Index of Diseases and Injuries includes the following direction on how to code this condition.

EXAMPLE: Influenza
Novel (2009) H1N1 influenza (see also Influenza, due to, identified novel influenza A virus) NEC J10.1
Novel influenza A/H1N1 (see also Influenza, due to, identified novel influenza A virus) NEC J10.1

The subcategory codes included here are as follows:

J10.00,   Influenza due to other identified influenza virus with unspecified type of pneumonia

J10.01,   Influenza due to other identified influenza virus with the same other identified influenza virus pneumonia

J10.08,   Influenza due to other identified influenza virus with other specified type of pneumonia

Two instruction notes included here are "Code also associated lung abscess, if applicable (J85.1)" under subcategory J10.0, Influenza due to other identified influenza virus with pneumonia and "Code also other specified type of pneumonia" under code J10.08 for influenza with other specified type of pneumonia.

Other subcategory codes for the other identified influenza virus J10 codes are as follows:

J10.1,   Influenza due to other identified influenza virus with other respiratory manifestations

J10.2,   Influenza due to other identified influenza virus with gastrointestinal manifestations

J10.81–J10.89,   Influenza due to other identified influenza virus with encephalopathy, myocarditis, otitis media and other manifestations

Two instruction notes appear with the J10.8X codes: "use additional code for any associated perforated tympanic membrane (H72.-)" with the code for influenzal otitis media and "use additional codes to identify the manifestations" to specify what other manifestations or conditions are caused by the influenza virus.

Influenza Due to Unidentified Influenza Virus (J11)

The conditions coded to category J11 are respiratory, gastrointestinal, and other body system manifestations that are viral in nature, but the exact type of influenza virus cannot be identified. The subcategory codes of J11.0–J11.89 follow the pattern seen in the subcategories J11:

J11.0X,	Influenza due to unidentified influenza virus with pneumonia
J11.1,	Influenza due to unidentified influenza virus with other respiratory manifestations
J11.2,	Influenza due to unidentified influenza virus with gastrointestinal manifestations
J11.8X,	Influenza due to unidentified influenza virus with other manifestations

Pneumonia (J12–J18)

The category and subcategory codes in Chapter 10 of ICD-10-CM include codes for pneumonia with the following specific categories and subcategories identifying the underlying organisms or site:

J12,	Viral pneumonia, not elsewhere classified
J13,	Pneumonia due to *Streptococcus pneumoniae*
J14,	Pneumonia due to *Haemophilus influenzae*
J15,	Bacterial pneumonia, not elsewhere classified
J16,	Pneumonia due to other infectious organisms, not elsewhere classified
J17,	Pneumonia in diseases classified elsewhere
J18,	Pneumonia, unspecified organism

Viral Pneumonia (J12)

Viral pneumonia is a highly contagious disease affecting both the trachea and the bronchi of the lungs. Inflammation destroys the action of the cilia and causes hemorrhage. Isolation of the virus is difficult, and x-rays do not reveal any pulmonary changes. The types of viruses causing pneumonia specified in this category include adenovirus, respiratory syncytial virus (RSV), parainfluenza virus, SARS-associated corona virus, and other specified viruses (Dorland 2012, 1474).

Category J12, Viral pneumonia, is subdivided to fourth-character subcategories that identify the specific virus. When this condition is associated with influenza, a code first note appears under this category heading to direct the coder to code first the associated influenza, if applicable, with codes in the range of J09.X1, J10.0-, and J11.0-. When this condition occurs with a lung abscess, the coder is reminded to code also associated abscess, if applicable, with J85.1.

Depending on the type of virus causing the pneumonia, the ICD-10-CM Alphabetic Index to Diseases and Injuries provides the following directions:

Pneumonia
    Viral J12.9
        Adenoviral J12.0
        Congenital P23.0
        Human metapneumovirus J12.3
        Parainfluenza J12.2
        Respiratory syncytial J12.19.2015
        SARS-associated coronavirus J12.61
        Specified J12.89

> **EXAMPLE:** The patient was discharged from the hospital following treatment of adenoviral pneumonia that was complicated with the development of a lung abscess during the long hospital stay.
> J12.0, Adenoviral pneumonia
> J85.1, Abscess of lung with pneumonia

Two diagnosis codes are assigned as directed by the "code also associated abscess, if applicable, J85.1" as it appears under category J12, Viral Pneumonia, not elsewhere classified. The Alphabetic Index to Diseases and Injuries also provides an entry for abscess, lung, with pneumonia, J85.1. Under code J85.1, Abscess of lung with pneumonia, a "code also the type of pneumonia" note appears.

Pneumonia Due to Streptococcus pneumoniae (J13)

Category J13, Pneumonia due to *Streptococcus pneumoniae*, describes pneumonia caused by this specific pneumococcal bacteria. Physicians may document this disease as bronchopneumonia due to *S. pneumoniae* as well. The bacteria lodge in the alveoli and cause an inflammation. If the pleura are involved, the irritated surfaces rub together and cause painful breathing. On examination, pleural friction can be heard. A chest x-ray demonstrates a consolidation of the lungs that results from pus forming in the alveoli and replacing the air (Dorland 2012, 1474). Physicians may describe the same condition as pneumococcal pneumonia. When this condition is associated with influenza, a code first note appears under this category heading to direct the coder to code first the associated influenza, if applicable, with codes in the range of J09.X1, J10.0-, and J11.0-. When this condition occurs with a lung abscess, the coder is reminded to code also associated abscess, if applicable, with J85.1.

> **EXAMPLE:** Three physicians treated the patient in the hospital for pneumonia. The attending physician documented pneumococcal pneumonia. The critical care physician documented bronchopneumonia due to *Streptococcus pneumoniae*. The pulmonologist described the condition as *Streptococcus pneumoniae* pneumonia. All three descriptions of the patient's pneumonia are coded in ICD-10-CM as J13, Pneumonia due to Streptococcal pneumonia.

Pneumonia Due to Hemophilus influenzae (J14)

Pneumonia due to *Hemophilus influenzae* is a bacterial pneumonia caused by an infection with the *Hemophilus influenzae* organism and is seen mainly in young children and debilitated adults (Dorland 2012, 1472). Category J14, Pneumonia due to *Hemophilus influenzae* or bronchopneumonia due to *H. influenzae*, is classified with this three-character code. When this condition is associated with influenza, a code first note appears under this category heading to direct the coder to code first the associated influenza, if applicable, with codes in the range of J09.X1, J10.0-, and J11.0-. When this condition occurs with a lung abscess, the coder is reminded to code also associated abscess, if applicable, with J85.1.

> **EXAMPLE:** The child was treated in the hospital for pneumonia due to *H. influenzae*
> The Alphabetic Index provides two entries to identify the correct code of J14 for this patient:
>
> Pneumonia, *Hemophilus* influenza, J14
> Pneumonia, in (due to) *H. influenzae*, J14

Bacterial Pneumonia, Not Elsewhere Classified (J15)

In ICD-10-CM, category J15 is used to code types of pneumonia that are not due to *Streptococcus pneumoniae* of *Haemophilus influenzae*. Category J15, Bacterial pneumonia, not elsewhere classified, is subdivided to fourth- and fifth-character subcategories that identify specific bacteria, such as *Klebsiella pneumoniae* (J15.0), *Pseudomonas* (J15.1), *Staphylococcus* (J15.20–J15.212), *Streptococcus* B (J15.3, J15.4), and other specified types of pneumonia. Bacteria is a common cause of pneumonia in adults. Gram staining is a rapid and cost-effective method for diagnosing bacterial pneumonia, if a good sputum sample is available (Dorland 2012, 1472).

> **EXAMPLE:** The elderly patient was treated in the hospital for acute bacterial *Klebsiella* pneumonia of the right upper lobe. The Alphabetic Index entry provides the correct code of J15.0 as follows:
>
> Pneumonia, in (due to), *Klebsiella* (pneumonia) J15.0
> Pneumonia, *Klebsiella* J15.0

Pneumonia Due to Other Infectious Organisms, Not Elsewhere Classified (J16)

Category J16, Pneumonia due to other infectious organisms, not elsewhere classified, is used to identify organisms other than bacteria that cause pneumonia. For example, chlamydial pneumonia is coded with subcategory J16.0. This is not a sexually transmitted disease but instead is an infectious organism that is airborne after a person carrying the organism has coughed and another person inhales the bacteria. When this type of pneumonia is associated with influenza, a "code first" note appears under this category heading to direct the codes to code first the associated influenza, if applicable, with codes in the range of J09.X1, J10.0-, and J11.0-. When this condition occurs with a lung abscess, the coder is reminded to code also associated abscess, if applicable, with J85.1.

> **EXAMPLE:** The young-adult patient returns to the physician's office for a follow-up visit to evaluate him for resolution of the mild pneumonia. He was treated for pneumonia at home that was found to be due to chlamydial pneumoniae. The condition is coded to J16.0, Chlamydial pneumonia.

Pneumonia in Diseases Classified Elsewhere (J17)

Category J17, Pneumonia in diseases classified elsewhere, is a three-character code intended to identify that this type of pneumonia is the result or complication of another disease. This code is set in italic type and thus not meant to be listed first or as a single code. In addition, instructional notations in this category direct coders to code first the underlying disease, such as Q fever, rheumatic fever, or schistosomiasis. A lengthy Excludes1 note appears under category J17 to identify various types of pneumonia that have specific ICD-10-CM codes and cannot be used with category code J17.

> **EXAMPLE:** The physician's final diagnosis for the hospitalized child was "Pneumonia in rheumatic fever." The two codes required to classify this condition are sequenced in the following order: (1) Rheumatic fever, I00; (2) Pneumonia in diseases classified elsewhere, J17

Pneumonia, Unspecified Organism (J18)

Category J18, Pneumonia, unspecified organism, is subdivided at the fourth-character level to classify conditions that are not specified by the physician as being caused by a particular bacteria, virus, or other organism. Nonspecific diagnoses of pneumonia that are coded here are as follows:

J18.0, Bronchopneumonia
J18.1, Lobar pneumonia
J18.2, Hypostatic pneumonia
J18.8, Other pneumonia, unspecified organism
J18.9, Pneumonia

A lengthy Excludes1 note appears under category J18 to identify various types of pneumonia that have specific ICD-10-CM codes and cannot be used with category code J18.

Check Your Understanding 13.1

Assign diagnosis codes to the following conditions.

1. Acute streptococcal tonsillitis
2. Influenza with pneumonia
3. Acute upper respiratory viral infection
4. Pneumonia due to methicillin-resistant *Staphylococcus aureus* (MRSA)
5. Acute sinusitis, pansinusitis

Other Acute Lower Respiratory Infections (J20–J22)

The conditions of the other part of the lower respiratory tract, the bronchus, is classified with codes from J20–J22 in ICD-10-CM.

Acute Bronchitis

Bronchitis is an inflammation of the bronchi and can be acute or chronic in nature. **Acute bronchitis** is an inflammation of the tracheobronchial tree with a short and more or less severe course. It is often due to exposure to cold, inhalation of irritant substances, or acute infections. **Chronic bronchitis** is a condition associated with prolonged exposure to nonspecific bronchial irritants and is accompanied by mucus hypersecretion and certain structural changes in the bronchi. Usually associated with cigarette smoking, one form of bronchitis is characterized clinically by a chronic productive cough (Dorland 2012, 252). ICD-10-CM provides separate codes to describe acute and chronic bronchitis and acute bronchiolitis.

The following types of acute conditions of bronchitis are classified:

J20.0, Acute bronchitis due to *Mycoplasma pneumoniae*
J20.1, Acute bronchitis due to *Haemophilus influenzae*
J20.2, Acute bronchitis due to *Streptococcus*
J20.3, Acute bronchitis due to coxsackievirus
J20.4, Acute bronchitis due to parainfluenza virus

J20.5,   Acute bronchitis due to respiratory syncytial virus
J20.6,   Acute bronchitis due to rhinovirus
J20.7,   Acute bronchitis due to echovirus
J20.8,   Acute bronchitis due to other specified virus
J20.9,   Acute bronchitis, unspecified

Acute bronchiolitis is classified according to the organisms that cause this disease. **Bronchiolitis** is an acute inflammatory disease of the bronchioles that is usually caused by a viral infection. Although it may occur in persons of any age, severe symptoms are usually only evident in young infants. The larger airways of older children and adults better accommodate mucosal edema associated with this condition.

Bronchiolitis most often affects children under the age of two years, with a peak occurrence in infants aged three to six months. Acute bronchiolitis is the most common cause of lower respiratory tract infection in the first year of life. It is generally a self-limiting condition and is most commonly associated with RSV (Maraga 2018).

The following types of acute conditions of bronchiolitis are classified:

J21.0,   Acute bronchiolitis due to respiratory syncytial virus
J21.1,   Acute bronchiolitis due to human metapneumovirus
J21.8,   Acute bronchiolitis due to other specified organisms
J21.9,   Acute bronchiolitis, unspecified or stated as "bronchiolitis"

Other Diseases of the Upper Respiratory Tract (J30–J39)

This section identifies chronic conditions of body parts within the upper respiratory system. Almost all of the categories in this section include the instructional note "use additional code, where applicable" to direct the coder to assign an additional code for exposure to environmental tobacco smoke (Z77.22), exposure to tobacco smoke in the perinatal period (P96.81), history of tobacco dependence (Z87.891), occupational exposure to environmental tobacco smoke (Z57.31), tobacco dependence (F17.-), and tobacco use (Z72.0). The categories within this section include the following:

J30,   Vasomotor and allergic rhinitis
        Subcategories include allergic rhinitis due to pollen and food.
J31,   Chronic rhinitis, nasopharyngitis and pharyngitis
        Subcategories include chronic rhinitis and chronic pharyngitis.
J32,   Chronic sinusitis
        Codes in this category identify the sinus involved, such as maxillary, frontal, ethmoidal, and sphenoidal, and simple terminology such as chronic sinusitis.
J33,   Nasal polyp
        Polyp of the nasal cavity and the sinuses are included here.
J34,   Other and unspecified disorders of nose and nasal sinuses
        Conditions classified here include cyst and mucocele of nose and nasal sinuses, deviated nasal septum, and nasal mucositis among others.
J35,   Chronic diseases of tonsils and adenoids
        The most commonly occurring conditions coded here are chronic tonsillitis, chronic adenoiditis, and hypertrophy of tonsils and adenoids.
J36,   Peritonsillar abscess
        This three-character code is strictly for peritonsillar abscess with a note to "use additional code (B95–B97) to identify the infectious agent."

J37,   Chronic laryngitis and laryngotracheitis
        Only two subcategory codes are included here for chronic laryngitis and chronic laryngotracheitis.
J38,   Diseases of vocal cords and larynx, not elsewhere classified
        Frequently occurring conditions that would be classified with J38 category codes include vocal cord paralysis, vocal cord nodules, laryngeal spasm or cellulitis or abscess of vocal cords or larynx.
J39,   Other diseases of upper respiratory tract
        Every condition can be classified with an ICD-10-CM code. This category is intended to provide a code for all the other and unspecified diseases of the respiratory tract that are not appropriately coded to categories J30–J38.

Chronic Lower Respiratory Disease (J40–J47)

Conditions classified in this group of categories are chronic pulmonary conditions, such as chronic bronchitis, emphysema, asthma, chronic obstructive pulmonary disease (COPD), and bronchiectasis.

Chronic Bronchitis

Chronic bronchitis is a condition associated with prolonged exposure to nonspecific bronchial irritants and is accompanied by mucus hypersecretion and certain structural changes in the bronchi. Usually associated with cigarette smoking, one form of bronchitis is characterized clinically by a chronic productive cough (Kleinschmidt 2018).

Code J40, Bronchitis, not specified as acute or chronic, is assigned when the specific type of bronchitis is not documented in the health record. If the physician documented only "bronchitis," this is the code assigned. However, it must be noted that code J40 is intended to reflect a chronic lung disease. When the primary care physician in her office or the emergency department physician writes "bronchitis" as a final diagnosis for an outpatient visit for a child, adolescent, or young adult, the physician probably means the patient has an acute type of bronchitis. However, the physician must be asked to clarify the type of bronchitis to assign a different code; no assumptions should be made based on the age of the patient.

Chronic bronchitis is included in the section titled "Chronic Obstructive Pulmonary Disease and Allied Conditions." Category J41, Simple and mucopurulent chronic bronchitis, contains subcategories including simple chronic bronchitis (J41.0), mucopurulent chronic bronchitis (J41.1), and mixed simple and mucopurulent chronic bronchitis (J41.8).

EXAMPLE: The patient is seen in the physician's office for ongoing treatment of what the physician documents as "Smokers' bronchitis." The Alphabetic Index to Disease and Injuries in ICD-10-CM classifies the condition to code J41.0 by using the entry of:
Bronchitis, smokers' J41.0

Emphysema

Emphysema is a specific type of chronic obstructive pulmonary disease (COPD). Emphysema is defined pathologically as an abnormal permanent enlargement of air spaces down to the terminal bronchioles, accompanied by the destruction of alveolar walls without obvious fibrosis. Emphysema frequently occurs in association with chronic bronchitis. Patients who have been diagnosed as having COPD have either an emphysema form of COPD or a chronic bronchitis type of COPD. There are at least two different morphological types of emphysema, that is, centriacinar or centrilobular, and panacinar or panlobular (Boka 2016).

Centriacinar emphysema begins in the respiratory bronchioles and spreads peripherally. Also termed centrilobular emphysema, this form is associated with long-standing cigarette smoking and predominantly involves the upper half of the lungs.

Panacinar, or panlobular, emphysema destroys the entire alveolus uniformly and is predominant in the lower half of the lungs. Panacinar emphysema generally is observed in patients with homozygous alpha-1-antitrypsin (AAT) deficiency. In people who smoke, focal panacinar emphysema at the lung bases may accompany centriacinar emphysema.

The subcategory codes for emphysema are as follows:

J43.0,   Unilateral pulmonary emphysema (MacLeod's syndrome)
J43.1,   Panlobular emphysema
J43.2,   Centrilobular emphysema
J43.8,   Other emphysema
J43.9,   Emphysema, unspecified

Chronic Obstructive Pulmonary Disease (COPD)

Chronic obstructive pulmonary disease (COPD) is a diffuse obstruction of the smaller bronchi and bronchioles that results in coughing, wheezing, shortness of breath, and disturbances of gas exchange. Exacerbations of COPD, such as episodes of increased shortness of breath and cough, often are treated on an outpatient basis. More severe exacerbations, such as an infection, usually result in admission to the hospital (Kleinschmidt 2018).

When acute bronchitis is documented with COPD, code J44.0, Obstructive chronic bronchitis with acute bronchitis, should be assigned. Code J44.1 is used when the medical record includes documentation of COPD with exacerbation or acute exacerbation, without mention of acute bronchitis.

Code J44.9 is an unspecified form of COPD. The diagnosis of COPD does not identify what type of chronic obstructive pulmonary disease the patient has. Sometimes physicians use COPD as a shortcut diagnosis, and other times the diagnosis of COPD is used because the patient has several forms of COPD, such as chronic bronchitis, obstructive asthma, or emphysema. Code J44.9 is an unspecified form of COPD and should not be used if the documentation from the provider is more specific as to what type of chronic obstructive pulmonary disease is present in the patient.

Instructional notes appear under category J44 to remind the coder to "code also" the type of asthma, if applicable, J45.-. There is another instruction to "use additional code" where applicable notes appear to direct the coder to assign an additional code for exposure to environmental tobacco smoke (Z77.22), history of tobacco dependence (Z87.891), occupational exposure to environmental tobacco smoke (Z57.31), tobacco dependence (F17.-), and tobacco use (Z72.0).

ICD-10-CM classifies COPD to the following codes:

J44.0,   Chronic obstructive pulmonary disease with acute lower respiratory infection
     Code also to identify the infection
J44.1,   Chronic obstructive pulmonary disease with (acute) exacerbation
     This may be documented as decompensated COPD.
J44.9,   Chronic obstructive pulmonary disease, unspecified
     Chronic obstructive airway disease NOS
     Chronic obstructive lung disease NOS

Asthma

Asthma is a condition marked by recurrent attacks of paroxysmal dyspnea, with wheezing due to spasmodic contraction of the bronchi. In some cases, it is an allergic manifestation in sensitized persons. The term reactive airway disease is considered synonymous with asthma (NLM 2018).

The inclusion terms that appear under the category heading of J45, Asthma, include allergic (predominantly) asthma, allergic bronchitis, allergic rhinitis with asthma, atopic asthma, extrinsic allergic asthma, hay fever with asthma, idiosyncratic asthma, intrinsic nonallergic asthma, and nonallergic asthma.

Conditions that are not classified to category J45, Asthma, are included in the Excludes1 listing of codes such as detergent asthma, eosinophilic asthma, lung diseases due to external agents, miner's asthma, wheezing NOS, and wood asthma. The Excludes2 note includes conditions that can be coded with asthma J45 category codes, specifically:

Asthma with chronic obstructive pulmonary disease (J44.9)
Chronic asthmatic (obstructive) bronchitis (J44.9)
Chronic obstructive asthma (J44.9)

The terminology used to describe asthma in ICD-10-CM reflects the current clinical classification of asthma. The terms included in the codes to describe asthma are mild, intermittent, and three degrees of persistent—mild persistent, moderate persistent, and severe persistent (see table 13.1). Intrinsic asthma (nonallergic) and extrinsic (allergic) are both classified to J45.909, Unspecified asthma, uncomplicated, if not further specified.

Table 13.1. **Asthma severity terms**

Asthma severity	Frequency of daytime symptoms
Intermittent	Less than or equal to 2 times per week
Mild persistent	More than 2 times per week
Moderate persistent	Daily. May restrict physical activity
Severe persistent	Throughout the day. Frequent severe attacks limiting ability to breathe

Source: Kaliner et al. 2015

Fourth- and Fifth-Character Subcategories

ICD-10-CM classifies asthma to the type and severity that includes asthma with acute exacerbation or status asthmaticus or identifies the type of asthma without those complications. In addition to mild intermittent, mild persistent, moderate persistent, and severe persistent, ICD-10-CM provides codes for other forms of asthma, such as exercise-induced bronchospasm and cough variant asthma. The following subcategories describe the specific types of asthma along with the clinical status:

J45.2,   Mild intermittent asthma
       J45.20,   Mild intermittent asthma, uncomplicated
       J45.21,   Mild intermittent asthma with (acute) exacerbation
       J45.22,   Mild intermittent asthma with status asthmaticus
J45.3,   Mild persistent asthma
       J45.30,   Mild persistent asthma, uncomplicated
       J45.31,   Mild persistent asthma with (acute) exacerbation
       J45.32,   Mild persistent asthma with status asthmaticus

J45.4,	Moderate persistent asthma	
	J45.40,	Moderate persistent asthma, uncomplicated
	J45.41,	Moderate persistent asthma with (acute) exacerbation
	J45.42,	Moderate persistent asthma with status asthmaticus
J45.5,	Severe persistent asthma	
	J45.50,	Severe persistent asthma, uncomplicated
	J45.51,	Severe persistent asthma with (acute) exacerbation
	J45.52,	Severe persistent asthma with status asthmaticus
J45.9,	Other and unspecified asthma	
	J45.90,	Unspecified asthma
	J45.901,	Unspecified asthma with (acute) exacerbation
	J45.902,	Unspecified asthma with status asthmaticus
	J45.909,	Unspecified asthma, uncomplicated
	J45.99,	Other asthma
	J45.990,	Exercise-induced bronchospasm
	J45.991,	Cough variant asthma
	J45.998,	Other asthma

Fifth- and Sixth-Character Codes

The fifth-digit subclassifications describe whether the patient was in status asthmaticus or suffered what may be described as an exacerbation or acute exacerbation of the asthma.

An **acute exacerbation**, or with exacerbation, is an increase in the severity of the disease or any of its signs or symptoms, such as wheezing or shortness of breath (Dorland 2012, 656).

Status asthmaticus is an acute asthmatic attack in which the degree of bronchial obstruction is not relieved by usual treatments such as epinephrine or aminophylline. A patient in status asthmaticus fails to respond to therapy administered during an asthmatic attack. This is a life-threatening complication that requires emergency care and, most likely, inpatient hospitalization (Dorland 2012, 1767).

> **EXAMPLE:** Two patients were seen in the emergency department. The first patient had moderate persistent asthma with acute exacerbation. The younger patient was given inhalation treatments with medications and had a complete resolution of his symptoms within a short period of time. The older patient was seen acutely ill with severe persistent asthma with status asthmaticus and was admitted to the critical care unit for intensive respiratory treatments to prevent respiratory failure. These two patients would be coded differently, for example, using the Alphabetic Index to Diseases and Injuries:
>
> 1. Asthma, moderate persistent, with, exacerbation (acute) J45.41
> 2. Asthma, severe persistent, with, status asthmaticus J45.52

Bronchiectasis

Bronchiectasis is a chronic, congenital, or acquired disease characterized by irreversible dilation of the bronchi as a consequence of inflammatory disease or obstruction. The incidence of bronchiectasis has decreased with the widespread use of antibiotics and immunizations in pediatrics. In adults, the condition may develop following a necrotizing pneumonia or lung abscess (NHLBI 2018a).

Category J47 codes are as follows:

J47.0, Bronchiectasis with acute lower respiratory infection

J47.1, Bronchiectasis with (acute) exacerbation

J47.9, Bronchiectasis, uncomplicated

Check Your Understanding 13.2

Assign diagnosis codes to the following conditions.

1. Acute bronchiolitis due to RSV

2. Chronic tonsillitis and adenoiditis

3. Mild persistent asthma with acute exacerbation

4. Chronic obstructive lung disease with emphysema

5. Chronic obstructive pulmonary disease with asthma

Lung Diseases Due to External Agents (J60–J70)

Categories in this section describe lung diseases that are caused by external factors, including chemical, organic, and inorganic substances. Numerous external agents cause lung disease; many of these are long-term conditions and may be incurable. Many of these conditions may be referred to as occupational lung disorders because the individuals acquire the conditions as part of their occupation or employment. For example, what is commonly referred to as "Black Lung Disease" is a hazard of working in coal mines and inhaling carbon particles and is classified in ICD-10-CM with code J60 for Coal worker's pneumoconiosis. Hypersensitivity pneumonitis is a disease of the lungs that become inflamed by breathing in foreign substances, such as dust, mold, and chemicals or substances known as antigens. Most people who breathe in these substances do not develop hypersensitivity pneumonitis. Inhaling mold, hay, straw, and grain over the long term can lead to hypersensitivity pneumonia. That is why hypersensitivity pneumonitis may also be called "farmer's lung" as farm workers often work in dusty environments and inhale the antigens of mold, hay, stray, and grain that damage their lungs (NHLBI 2018b).

The categories of lung diseases due to external agents are as follows:

J60, Coal worker's pneumoconiosis

J61, Pneumoconiosis due to asbestos and other mineral fibers

J62, Pneumoconiosis due to dust-containing silica

J63, Pneumoconiosis due to other inorganic dusts
       Includes aluminosis, bauxite fibrosis, berylliosis, graphite fibrosis, siderosis, stannosis

J64, Unspecified pneumoconiosis

J65, Pneumoconiosis associated with tuberculosis

J66, Airway disease due to specific organic dust
       Includes byssinosis, flax-dresser's disease, cannabinosis

J67, Hypersensitivity pneumonitis due to organic dust
       Includes farmer's lung, bagassosis, bird fancier's lung, suberosis, malt worker's lung, mushroom-worker's lung, maple bark stripper's lung, and air conditioner and humidifier lung

J68, Respiratory conditions due to inhalation of chemicals, gases, fumes, and vapors

J69,   Pneumonitis due to solids and liquids
        The most commonly coded condition from this category is aspiration pneumonia, J69.0.

J70,   Respiratory conditions due to other external agents
        Instructional notes under this category's codes include "Use additional code (W88–W90, X93.0-) to identify the external cause" or "Use additional code for adverse effect, if applicable, to identify drug (T36–T50 with fifth or sixth characters 5)."

Other Categories to Classify Diseases of the Respiratory System

Other sections of ICD-10-CM codes included in Chapter 10, Diseases of the Respiratory System, are as follows:

J80–J84,   Other respiratory disease principally affecting the interstitium
J85–J86,   Suppurative and necrotic conditions of the lower respiratory tract
J90–J94,   Other diseases of the pleura

The conditions in Sections J80–J84 are conditions that affect the interstitium of small areas, spaces, or gaps within the lung tissue (Stedman 2012, 886). Acute respiratory distress syndrome in an adult or child is an interstitial and alveolar pulmonary edema that is thought to develop within a short period of time after some type of damage to the lungs has occurred (Dorland 2012, 1820). Code J80 is also used to classify adult hyaline membrane disease in which the lining of the lungs is covered with a glassy membrane (Stedman 2012, 803). Acute and chronic pulmonary edema or the accumulation of watery fluid in the cells of the lungs is also classified here. Pulmonary edema is usually a consequence of another disease, such as heart failure or mitral stenosis (Dorland 2012, 1398).

J80–J84,   Other respiratory diseases principally affecting the interstitium
            The more commonly coded conditions from this section include the following:
            J80,   Acute respiratory distress syndrome
            J81.0,   Acute pulmonary edema
            J81.1,   Chronic pulmonary edema
            J84.10,   Pulmonary fibrosis

Conditions within categories J85–J86 are suppurative (pus-forming) and necrotic (pathologic death of cells) diseases that occur in the lungs or thorax usually as a consequence of an inflammation or infection in the tissue.

EXAMPLE: J85–J86,   Suppurative and necrotic conditions of the lower respiratory tract
                The conditions in this section that are coded frequently include the following:
                J85.1,   Abscess of the lung with pneumonia
                J86.9,   Pyothorax without fistula

Diseases of the pleura are classified to the codes within the Sections J90–J94. Codes within this section have notes appearing with them to code first the underlying condition, such as a neoplasm or influenza. Some of these conditions exist because the patient has another serious illness. For example, pleural effusion or excess fluid in the pleural space may be caused by heart failure, hypoalbuminemia, or it may be the result of a metastatic neoplasm, Hodgkin's disease, AIDS, or lupus syndromes. Pleural effusion may be caused by rheumatoid disease, acute pancreatitis, and postcardiac injury syndromes; in other words, there is usually an underlying condition that causes the fluid to accumulate (Beers and Berkow 2000, 643).

EXAMPLE:

J90–J94,	Other disease of the pleura
	The commonly coded conditions in this section include
J90,	Pleural effusion
J91.0,	Malignant pleural effusion
J93.0,	Spontaneous tension pneumothorax
J93.11,	Primary spontaneous pneumothorax
J93.82,	Other or persistent air leak
J94.2,	Hemothorax and hemopneumothorax

Intraoperative and Postprocedural Complications and Disorders of Respiratory System, Not Elsewhere Classified (J95)

Procedural complication codes are included in category J95 to identify specific respiratory complications such as the following:

J95.00–J95.09,	Tracheostomy complications such as hemorrhage, infections, malfunction of the stoma or tracheoesophageal fistula formation
J95.1–J95.3,	Acute and chronic pulmonary insufficiency following thoracic surgery and nonthoracic surgery, that is, the result of surgery within the chest cavity or other body cavities
J95.811–J95.812,	Postprocedural pneumothorax and air leak that occurs after surgery within the thoracic cavity
J95.851,	Ventilator-associated pneumonia that is a serious type of bacterial, viral, or fungal pneumonia that can occur in patients breathing with a ventilator that is usually caused by aspiration of secretions or stomach contents

 Other complications in this category include intraoperative and postprocedural, hematoma, seroma, and accidental puncture or laceration. Again, the complication can be identified as occurring during a respiratory system procedure or as complicating another body system procedure.

Other Diseases of the Respiratory System (J96–J99)

The commonly coded conditions in this section of codes include acute and chronic respiratory failure and acute bronchospasm.

Respiratory Failure (J96)

Respiratory failure is the inability of the respiratory system to supply adequate oxygen to maintain proper metabolism or to eliminate carbon dioxide (CO_2). Respiratory failure is the consequence of another illness, such as acute and chronic heart and lung diseases, sepsis, trauma, or poisonings. The patient's respiratory system is unable to maintain the necessary levels of oxygen for life and is unable to expel the accumulating carbon dioxide that damages tissues and organs (Dorland 2012, 678). ICD-10-CM classifies different forms of respiratory failure to the following codes in category J96, Respiratory failure, not elsewhere classified:

J96.0,	Acute respiratory failure	
	J96.00,	Acute respiratory failure, unspecified whether with hypoxia or hypercapnia
	J96.01,	Acute respiratory failure with hypoxia
	J96.02,	Acute respiratory failure with hypercapnia
J96.1,	Chronic respiratory failure	
	J96.10,	Chronic respiratory failure, unspecified whether with hypoxia or hypercapnia
	J96.11,	Chronic respiratory failure with hypoxia
	J96.12,	Chronic respiratory failure with hypercapnia
J96.2,	Acute and chronic respiratory failure	
	J96.20,	Acute and chronic respiratory failure, unspecified whether with hypoxia or hypercapnia
	J96.21,	Acute and chronic respiratory failure with hypoxia
	J96.22,	Acute and chronic respiratory failure with hypercapnia
J96.9,	Respiratory failure, unspecified	
	J96.90,	Respiratory failure, unspecified, unspecified whether with hypoxia or hypercapnia
	J96.91,	Respiratory failure, unspecified, with hypoxia
	J96.92,	Respiratory failure, unspecified, with hypercapnia

The code for respiratory failure is assigned when documentation in the health record supports its use. It may be due to, or associated with, other respiratory conditions such as pneumonia, chronic bronchitis, or COPD. Respiratory failure also may be due to, or associated with, nonrespiratory conditions such as myasthenia gravis, congestive heart failure, myocardial infarction, or CVA. Arterial blood gases may be useful in diagnosing respiratory failure; however, normal values may vary from person to person depending on individual health status. Coders should not assume the condition of respiratory failure exists based solely on laboratory and radiology test findings.

Coding and Sequencing of Acute Respiratory Failure

The coding and sequencing of acute respiratory failure presents many challenges to both the new and the experienced clinical coder. Various coding rules and guidelines must be considered.

Acute respiratory failure, codes J96.00–J96.02, may be assigned as a principal or secondary diagnosis depending on the circumstances of the inpatient admission. Chapter-specific coding guidelines (obstetrics, poisoning, HIV, newborn) provide specific sequencing direction. Respiratory failure may be listed as a secondary diagnosis. In addition, if respiratory failure occurs after admission, it may be listed as a secondary diagnosis.

When a patient is admitted in acute respiratory failure with another acute condition, the principal diagnosis will not be the same in every situation. There is not one respiratory failure coding rule. This is true whether or not the other acute condition is a respiratory or nonrespiratory condition. Selection of the principal diagnosis will depend on the circumstances of the admission. If both the respiratory failure and the other acute condition are equally responsible for the patient's admission to the hospital, and there are no chapter-specific sequencing rules, the guideline regarding two or more diagnoses that equally meet the definition for principal diagnosis may be applied. If the documentation is not clear as to whether the acute respiratory failure and another condition are equally responsible for occasioning the admission, the physician must be asked for clarification.

Respiratory failure is a life-threatening condition that is always caused by an underlying condition. It may be caused by diseases of the circulatory system, respiratory system, central nervous system, peripheral nervous system, respiratory muscles, and chest wall muscles. The primary goal of the treatment of acute respiratory failure is to assess the severity of underlying disease and to correct the inadequate oxygen delivery and tissue hypoxia.

The following are examples of the appropriate coding and sequencing of acute respiratory failure in association with the underlying disease.

EXAMPLE 1: A patient with chronic myasthenia gravis suffers an acute exacerbation and develops acute respiratory failure. The patient is admitted to the hospital to treat the respiratory failure.

Principal diagnosis: J96.00, Acute respiratory failure
Secondary diagnosis: G70.00, Myasthenia gravis with (acute) exacerbation

EXAMPLE 2: A patient with emphysema develops acute respiratory failure. The patient is admitted to the hospital for treatment of the respiratory failure.

Principal diagnosis: J96.00, Acute respiratory failure
Secondary diagnosis: J43.9, Emphysema

EXAMPLE 3: A patient with congestive heart failure is brought to the emergency department in acute respiratory failure. The patient is intubated and admitted to the hospital. The physician documents that acute respiratory failure is the reason for the admission.

Principal diagnosis: J96.00, Acute respiratory failure
Secondary diagnosis: I50.9, Congestive heart failure

In example 3, the physician has stated that the reason for the admission is to treat the respiratory failure. If the documentation is not clear regarding whether the congestive heart failure or the acute respiratory failure was the reason for admission, the coder should ask the physician for clarification.

EXAMPLE 4: A patient with asthma in status asthmaticus develops acute respiratory failure and is admitted to the hospital for treatment of the acute respiratory failure.

Principal diagnosis: J96.00, Acute respiratory failure
Secondary diagnosis: J45.902, Asthma, unspecified, with status asthmaticus

EXAMPLE 5: A patient is admitted to the hospital during the postpartum period as a result of developing a thromboembolism or pulmonary blood clot leading to respiratory failure.

Principal diagnosis: O88.23, Thromboembolism in the puerperium
Secondary diagnosis: J96.00, Acute respiratory failure

Example 5 is one of a chapter-specific guideline. The obstetric code is sequenced first because chapter 11 (obstetric) codes have sequencing priority over codes from other ICD-10-CM chapters (Guideline Section I.C.15.a.).

EXAMPLE 6: A patient who is diagnosed as having overdosed on crack cocaine is admitted to the hospital with respiratory failure.

Principal diagnosis: T40.5X1A, Poisoning by crack cocaine, initial
Secondary diagnosis: J96.00, Acute respiratory failure

Example 6 of a chapter-specific guideline. The poisoning code is sequenced first because a chapter-specific guideline (Section I.C.19.5.(b)) provides sequencing directions specifying that the poisoning code is listed first, followed by a code for the manifestation of the poisoning. In example 6, the respiratory failure is a manifestation of the poisoning or overdose.

EXAMPLE 7: A patient is admitted with respiratory failure due to *Pneumocystis carinii* pneumonia, which is associated with AIDS.

Principal diagnosis: B20, Human immunodeficiency virus (HIV) disease
Secondary diagnosis: J96.00, Acute respiratory failure; B59, Pneumocystosis

In example 7, the AIDS code (B20) is listed as the principal diagnosis with the respiratory failure and pneumonia listed as secondary diagnoses according to the chapter-specific guidelines regarding HIV-related conditions. In this case, the pneumocystosis is the HIV-related condition that caused the respiratory failure. The guidelines in Section I.C.1.a.2.a state that if a patient is admitted for an HIV-related condition, the principal diagnosis should be B20, AIDS, followed by additional diagnosis codes for all reported HIV-related conditions.

EXAMPLE 8: A patient is admitted to the hospital with severe *Staphylococcus aureus*, methicillin susceptible, sepsis, and acute respiratory failure.

Principal diagnosis: A41.01, Methicillin Susceptible *Staphylococcus aureus* septicemia
Secondary diagnosis: R65.20, Severe sepsis; J96.00, Acute respiratory failure

Bronchospasm (J98.01)

Bronchospasm is the spasmodic contraction of smooth muscle in the walls of the bronchi and bronchioles that cause narrowing of the lumen and obstructs breathing (Stedman 2012, 249). Acute bronchospasm is coded in ICD-10-CM with code J98.01. However, acute bronchospasm is frequently a symptom of another respiratory condition. The Excludes1 note under code J98.01 states that this code for bronchospasm is not coded if bronchospasm is specified as follows:

Acute bronchiolitis with bronchospasm (J21.-)
Acute bronchitis with bronchospasm (J20.-)
Bronchospasm with asthma (J45.-)
Exercise-induced bronchospasm (J45.990)

Check Your Understanding 13.3

Assign diagnosis codes to the following conditions.

1. Aspiration pneumonia due to gastric secretions
2. Malignant pleural effusion due to carcinoma of right lung
3. Idiopathic pulmonary fibrosis
4. Acute and chronic respiratory failure with hypercapnia
5. Complication (hemorrhage) of tracheostomy stoma

ICD-10-PCS Coding for Procedures Related to the Respiratory System

Procedures performed on the sites in the respiratory system are included in the tables from 0B1–0BY. Like procedures in other body systems, in order to code respiratory procedures, the coder needs to know the definition of root operations and the anatomy of the respiratory tract to identify the body parts.

The procedures performed on the sites in the respiratory system appear in the ICD-10-PCS code book in tables that start with the two characters 0 and 8 followed by five characters representing root operation, body part, approach, device, and qualifier:

Character 1 is Value 0—Medical and Surgical
Character 2 is Value B—Respiratory

Root Operation

Character 3 of the Medical and Surgical ICD-10-PCS codes is the root operation. The root operations that represent the objectives of procedures for surgical treatment of the diseases of the Respiratory system are shown in table 13.2.

Table 13.2. **Root operations for procedures on body parts within the Respiratory system**

Bypass: Altering the route of passage of the contents of a tubular body part
Change: Taking out or off a device from a body part and putting back an identical or similar device in or on the same body part without cutting or puncturing the skin or a mucous membrane.
Destruction: Physical eradication of all or a portion of a body part by the direct use of energy, force, or a destructive agent
Dilation: Expanding the orifice or lumen of a tubular body part
Drainage: Taking or letting out fluids and/or gases from a body part
Excision: Cutting out or off, without replacement, a portion of a body part
Extirpation: Taking or cutting out solid matter from a body part
Extraction: Pulling or stripping out or off all or a portion of a body part by the use of force
Fragmentation: Breaking solid matter in a body part into pieces

Insertion: Putting in a nonbiological appliance that monitors, assists, performs, or prevents a physiological function but does not physically take the place of the body part
Inspection: Visually and/or manually exploring a body part
Occlusion: Completely closing an orifice or the lumen of a tubular body part
Reattachment: Putting back in or on all or a portion of a separated body part to its normal location or other suitable location
Release: Freeing a body part from an abnormal physical constraint by cutting or by the use of force
Removal: Taking out or off a device from a body part
Repair: Restoring, to the extent possible, a body part to its normal anatomic structure and function
Replacement: Putting in or on a biological or synthetic material that physically takes the place and/or function of all or a portion of a body part
Reposition: Moving to its normal location, or other suitable location, all or a portion of a body part
Resection: Cutting out or off, without replacement, all of a body part
Supplement: Putting in or on biological or synthetic material that physically reinforces and/or augments the function of a portion of a body part
Restriction: Partially closing an orifice or the lumen of a tubular body part
Revision: Correcting, to the extent possible, a portion of a malfunctioning device or the position of a displaced device
Transplantation: Putting in or on all or a portion of a living body part taken from another individual or animal to physically take the place and/or function of all or a portion of a similar body part

Source: CMS 2019

Body Part

Character 4 identifies the body part involved in the procedure. The body parts in ICD-10-PCS have individual values that include laterality, for example, as shown in table 13.3.

Table 13.3.   **Body parts and values included in the ICD-10-PCS codes for the Respiratory system**

0—Tracheobronchial tree
1—Trachea
2—Carina
3—Main Bronchus, right
4—Upper Lobe Bronchus, right
5—Middle Lobe Bronchus, right
6—Lower Lobe Bronchus, right
7—Main Bronchus, left
8—Upper Lobe Bronchus, left

(Continued)

9—Lingula Bronchus
B—Lower Lobe Bronchus, left
C—Upper Lung Lobe, right
D—Middle Lung Lobe, right
F—Lower Lung Lobe, right
G—Upper Lung Lobe, left
H—Lung Lingula
J—Lower Lung Lobe, left
K—Lung, right
L—Lung, left
M—Lungs, bilateral
N—Pleura, right
P—Pleura, left
Q—Pleura
T—Diaphragm

Source: CMS 2019

Approach

Character 5 identifies the approach used in the procedure. The approach for procedures performed on organs within the Respiratory system is shown in table 13.4.

Table 13.4. **Approaches, definitions, and values included in the ICD-10-PCS codes for the Respiratory system**

Open (0): Cutting through the skin or mucous membrane and any other body layers necessary to expose the site of the procedure
Percutaneous (3): Entry, by puncture or minor incision, of instrumentation through the skin or mucous membrane and any other body layers necessary to reach the site of the procedure
Percutaneous endoscopic (4): Entry, by puncture or minor incision, of instrumentation through the skin or mucous membrane and any other body layers necessary to reach and visualize the site of the procedure.
Via Natural or Artificial Opening (7): Entry of instrumentation through a natural or artificial external opening to reach the site of the procedure
Via Natural or Artificial Opening Endoscopic (8): Entry of instrumentation through a natural or artificial external opening to reach and visualize the site of the procedure
External (X): Procedures performed directly on the skin or mucous membrane and procedures performed indirectly by the application of external force through the skin or mucous membrane

Source: CMS 2019

Device

Character 6 identifies if a device remains in the patient's body after the procedure is concluded. The devices used to code procedures performed on organs within the Respiratory system are limited to a few devices, as shown in table 13.5.

Table 13.5. **Devices and values included in the ICD-10-PCS codes for the Respiratory system**

0—Drainage Device
1—Radioactive Element
2—Monitoring Device
3—Infusion Device
7—Autologous Tissue Substitute
C—Extraluminal Device
D—Intraluminal Device
E—Intraluminal Device, Endotracheal Airway
F—Tracheostomy Device
G—Intraluminal Device, Endobronchial Valve
J—Synthetic Substitute
K—Nonautologous Tissue Substitute
M—Diaphragmatic Pacemaker Lead
Y—Other Device
Z—No Device

Source: CMS 2019

Qualifier

Character 7 is a qualifier that specifies an additional attribute of the procedure, if applicable. The qualifier characters used to code procedures performed on organs within the Respiratory system are limited to the values shown in table 13.6. The qualifier value of X for diagnostic procedure is available for the root operations Drainage, Excision, and Extraction.

Table 13.6. **Qualifiers used to code procedures within the Respiratory system**

0—Allogeneic
1—Syngeneic
2—Zooplastic
4—Cutaneous
6—Esophagus
X—Diagnostic
Z—No Qualifier

Source: CMS 2019

Specific Procedures Performed in the Respiratory System

This section describes the ICD-10-PCS coding of several of the commonly performed respiratory procedures, that is, closed endoscopic biopsy, other endoscopic procedures, and mechanical ventilation.

Closed Endoscopic Biopsy

Endoscopy is a procedure that involves a visual inspection of any cavity of the body or an organ by the means of an endoscope. An endoscope is an instrument for examining the interior of a body cavity or organ (Dorland 2012, 620). Unlike most other medical imaging devices, endoscopes are inserted directly into the organ. An endoscope can consist of a rigid or flexible tube with a light delivery system to illuminate the organ or object under inspection. There is a lens attached to the tube transmitting the image from the lens to the viewer through an eyepiece. There is an additional tube to allow the entry of medical instruments. In the respiratory tract, the two types of endoscopies performed are via the nose (rhinoscopy) and via the mouth (bronchoscopy) to the lower respiratory tract.

 A closed endoscopic biopsy of the respiratory system is the excision of tissue for diagnostic purposes through a bronchoscope in the respiratory system. By ICD-10-PCS definition, a Biopsy is an excision or cutting out or off, without replacement, a portion of a body part. For the Respiratory system, Excision procedures are coded according to table 13.7 (CMS 2019).

Table 13.7.   **ICD-10-PCS Table 0BB**

0 Medical and Surgical B Respiratory System B Excision			
Body Part	**Approach**	**Device**	**Qualifier**
1 Trachea 2 Carina 3 Main Bronchus, Right 4 Upper Lobe Bronchus, Right 5 Middle Lobe Bronchus, Right 6 Lower Lobe Bronchus, Right 7 Main Bronchus, Left 8 Upper Lobe Bronchus, Left 9 Lingula Bronchus B Lower Lobe Bronchus, Left C Upper Lung Lobe, Right D Middle Lung Lobe, Right F Lower Lung Lobe, Right G Upper Lung Lobe, Left H Lung Lingula J Lower Lung Lobe, Left K Lung, Right L Lung, Left M Lungs, Bilateral	0 Open 3 Percutaneous 4 Percutaneous Endoscopic 7 Via Natural or Artificial Opening 8 Via Natural or Artificial Opening Endoscopic	Z No Device	X Diagnostic Z No Qualifier
N Pleura, Right P Pleura, Left	0 Open 3 Percutaneous 4 Percutaneous Endoscopic 8 Via Natural or Artificial Opening Endoscopic	Z No Device	X Diagnostic Z No Qualifier
T Diaphragm	0 Open 3 Percutaneous 4 Percutaneous Endoscopic	Z No Device	X Diagnostic Z No Qualifier

Source: CMS 2019

When coding closed endoscopic biopsies, the specific site where the excision is made, including the laterality, is required:

0BBK4ZX, Thoracoscopic lung biopsy, right
0BB78ZX, Closed [bronchoscopic] biopsy of left main bronchus
0BBG8ZX, Closed [bronchoscopic] biopsy of lung, upper lung lobe
0BBN4ZX, Thoracoscopic pleural biopsy, right

Endoscopic Procedures in the Respiratory System

Because many lesions in the respiratory tract can be removed by endoscopic means that do not require opening the chest, ICD-10-PCS provides codes for this type of procedure. For example:

0BB68ZZ, Bronchoscopic excision of lesion or tissue of bronchus, lower lobe bronchus, right
0BBG8ZZ, Bronchoscopic excision of lesion or tissue of lung, upper lung lobe, left
0BBG4ZZ, Thoracoscopic lobectomy of lung, upper lung lobe, left

The difference in the examples above is the type of endoscopy performed: bronchoscopy or thoracoscopy. The bronchoscopy is performed with the Via Natural or Artificial Opening Endoscopic approach (through the mouth). The thoracoscopy is performed through a Percutaneous Endoscopic approach.

Mechanical Ventilation

Mechanical ventilation is clinically indicated for patients with apnea, acute respiratory failure, and impending acute respiratory failure. Invasive mechanical ventilation pumps air into the patient's lungs even when there is no attempt by the patient to breathe on his or her own (Braunwald et al. 2001, 1526).

Mechanical ventilation is coded to the Extracorporeal Assistance and Performance section in ICD-10-PCS. Mechanical ventilation is provided via an invasive interface, such as endotracheal intubation or tracheostomy. Endotracheal intubation requires the placement of the tracheal tube, either orally or nasally. Assign code 0BH17EZ, Insertion of endotracheal airway into trachea, via natural or artificial opening, or code 0BH18EZ, Insertion of endotracheal airway into trachea, via natural or artificial opening endoscopic.

On the other hand, insertion of an endotracheal tube in order to maintain an airway in patients who are unconscious or unable to breathe on their own is the central objective of the procedure. Therefore, insertion of an endotracheal tube as an end in itself is coded to the root operation Insertion and the device Endotracheal Airway (CMS 2019).

The ICD-10-PCS procedure codes for mechanical ventilation and related procedures are as follows:

5A1935Z, Mechanical ventilation for less than 24 consecutive hours
5A1945Z, Mechanical ventilation for 24 to 96 consecutive hours
5A1955Z, Mechanical ventilation for greater than 96 consecutive hours
0B110F4, Creation of tracheostomy for use with mechanical ventilation
0BH17EZ, Insertion of endotracheal airway into trachea, via natural or artificial opening
0BH18EZ, Insertion of endotracheal airway into trachea, via natural or artificial opening endoscopic

ICD-10-CM and ICD-10-PCS Review Exercises: Chapter 13

Assign the correct ICD-10-CM diagnosis codes and ICD-10-PCS procedure codes to the following exercises.

1. Patient presents with a high fever, cough, and chest pain. Gram stain of the sputum showed numerous small gram-negative coccobacilli. Diagnosis: *H. influenzae* pneumonia.

   _____

2. Acute respiratory insufficiency due to acute exacerbation of COPD and tobacco dependence

   _____

3. Moderate persistent asthma with acute exacerbation

   _____

4. Hypertrophy of tonsils and adenoids

   _____

5. Chronic asthmatic bronchitis

   _____

6. Panlobular emphysema

   _____

7. *Streptococcus pneumoniae* with associated lung abscess

   _____

8. Novel influenza A with pneumonia

   _____

9. Hay fever due to pollen

   _____

10. Unilateral vocal cord paralysis

    _____

11. Acute pneumothorax

    _____

12. Chronic laryngotracheitis

    _____

13. Acute postprocedural respiratory failure

    _____

14. Black lung disease

    _____

ICD-10-CM and ICD-10-PCS Review Exercises: Chapter 13 (continued)

15. PROCEDURE: Tracheostomy tube exchange

_____

16. PROCEDURE: Thoracoscopic biopsy for diagnostic purposes, right upper lobe of lung

_____

17. PROCEDURE: Laryngoscopy with endoscopic biopsy of the larynx by excision

_____

18. PROCEDURE: Bronchoscopic excision of lesion of right upper lobe of the lung

_____

19. PROCEDURE: Mechanical ventilation for 48 consecutive hours following endotracheal tube intubation

_____

20. PROCEDURE: Thoracotomy with resection of left lower lobe of lung

_____

References

Beers, M. H. and R. Berkow, eds. 2000. *The Merck Manual*, 17th ed. Rahway, NJ: Merck & Co.

Boka, K. 2016. Medscape. Emphysema. http://emedicine.medscape.com/article/298283 -overview#a5.

Braunwald, E., A. Fauci, D. Kasper, S. Hauser, D. Longo, and J. Jameson. 2001. *Harrison's Principles of Internal Medicine*. New York: McGraw-Hill.

Centers for Disease Control and Prevention (CDC), National Center for Health Statistics (NCHS). 2019. *ICD-10-CM Official Guidelines for Coding and Reporting*, 2020. https://www .cdc.gov/nchs/icd/icd10cm.htm and https://www.cdc.gov/nchs/data/icd/10cmguidelines -FY2020_final.pdf.

Centers for Disease Control and Prevention (CDC). 2015. Update: Outbreaks of Avian Influenza A H5 in U.S. Wild and Domestic Birds: Human Health Implications. http://www .cdc.gov/flu/news/outbreaks-h5-human-health.htm.

Centers for Disease Control and Prevention (CDC). 2009. Novel H1N1 Flu: Background on the Situation. http://www.cdc.gov/h1n1flu/background.htm.

Centers for Medicare and Medicaid Services (CMS). 2019. *ICD-10-PCS Official Guidelines for Coding and Reporting*, 2020. https://www.cms.gov/Medicare/Coding/ICD10/2020-ICD -10-PCS.html.

Dorland, W.A.N., ed. 2012. *Dorland's Illustrated Medical Dictionary*, 32nd ed. Philadelphia: Elsevier Saunders.

Kaliner, M. A., H. H. Li, and N. M. Kushnir. 2015. Allergic Asthma: Symptoms and Treatment. World Allergy Organization. http://www.worldallergy.org/professional/allergic _diseases_center/allergic_asthma/.

Kleinschmidt, P. 2018. Medscape. Chronic Obstructive Pulmonary Disease and Emphysema in Emergency Medicine. http://emedicine.medscape.com/article/807143-overview.

Maraga, Nizar F. 2018. Medscape. Bronchiolitis. http://emedicine.medscape.com/article /961963-overview.

National Heart, Lung and Blood Institute (NHLBI). 2018a. What Is Bronchiectasis? http:// www.nhlbi.nih.gov/health/health-topics/topics/brn/.

National Heart, Lung and Blood Institute (NHLBI). 2018b. What Is Hypersensitivity Pneumonia? http://www.nhlbi.nih.gov/health/health-topics/topics/hp.

Stedman, T. 2012. *Stedman's Medical Dictionary for the Health Professions and Nursing,* 7th ed. Philadelphia: Wolters Kluwer/Lippincott Williams & Wilkins.

U.S. National Library of Medicine (NLM). 2018. Asthma. https://www.nlm.nih.gov/medlineplus /asthma.html.

Chapter 14

Diseases of the Digestive System (K00–K95)

Learning Objectives

At the conclusion of this chapter, you should be able to do the following:

- Describe the organization of the conditions and codes included in Chapter 11 of ICD-10-CM, Diseases of the Digestive System (K00–K95)

- Identify the ICD-10-CM codes for the various ulcers of the gastrointestinal tract

- Explain the various types of hernia conditions that can be classified

- Summarize various types of noninfectious enteritis and colitis conditions that can be classified

- Distinguish the ICD-10-CM codes for the various types of gallbladder disease and calculus

- Apply the ICD-10-CM codes for gastrointestinal hemorrhage, and its relationship with other digestive conditions

- Explain the methods of repairing various digestive system hernias

- Give examples of the types of procedures that can be performed endoscopically within the digestive system

- Specify the ICD-10-PCS codes for various types of procedures performed for intestinal resection and anastomosis

- Assign ICD-10-PCS codes for procedures related to diseases of the digestive system

Key Terms

Anastomosis
Bypass
Cholecystitis
Choledocholithiasis

Cholelithiasis
Colostomy
Crohn's disease
Duodenitis

Gastritis
Gastroenteritis
Gastrostomy
Hematemesis
Hernia
Ileostomy
Irreducible hernia
Laparotomy
Melena

Mucositis
Obstruction
Occult blood
Peritonitis
Reducible
Stoma
Strangulated hernia
Supplement
Ulcer

Overview of ICD-10-CM Chapter 11: Diseases of the Digestive System

Chapter 11 includes categories K00–K95 arranged in the following blocks:

K00–K14	Diseases of oral cavity and salivary glands
K20–K31	Diseases of esophagus, stomach and duodenum
K35–K38	Diseases of appendix
K40–K46	Hernia
K50–K52	Noninfective enteritis and colitis
K55–K64	Other diseases of intestines
K65–K68	Diseases of peritoneum and retroperitoneum
K70–K77	Diseases of liver
K80–K87	Disorders of gallbladder, biliary tract and pancreas
K90–K95	Other diseases of digestive system

Chapter 11 of ICD-10-CM contains commonly coded gastrointestinal (GI) conditions that occur in many patients from infections in the mouth and organs in the upper GI tract as well as in the appendix, small bowel, colon, gallbladder, and liver. The organs of the gastrointestinal tract are featured in the diagram in figure 14.1. There are combination codes to describe facts about digestive conditions, for example, if the condition is an acute versus a chronic disease, and whether bleeding is present. In ICD-10-CM, the term "hemorrhage" is used when referring to ulcers while the term "bleeding" is used when classifying gastritis, duodenitis, diverticulosis, and diverticulitis. Note the following examples:

- K25.0, Acute gastric ulcer with hemorrhage

- K29.01, Acute gastritis with bleeding

- K57.31, Diverticulosis of large intestine without perforation or abscess with bleeding

Combination codes for specific sites of hernias in the digestive system also include whether the condition is present with gangrene or obstruction and whether the hernia is present on one side of the body or is a bilateral condition. Other codes identify whether complications exist, for example, whether rectal bleeding, intestinal obstruction, fistula, or abscess is present with ulcerative colitis or regional enteritis. Complications of artificial openings of the digestive system, including colostomy, enterostomy, and gastrostomy infections and malfunctions, are included in the chapter. ICD-10-CM codes exist for intraoperative and postprocedural complications that are specific to the digestive system, such as postprocedural intestinal obstruction. There are also codes for hemorrhages, hematomas, seromas, accidental punctures and lacerations that occur during procedures.

Figure 14.1. Gastrointestinal tract

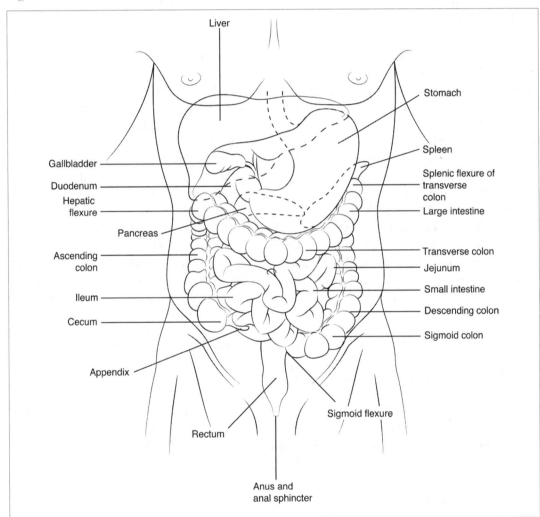

© AHIMA

Coding Guidelines and Instructional Notes for ICD-10-CM Chapter 11

The NCHS has not published chapter-specific guidelines for Chapter 11, Diseases of the Digestive System (K00-K95) in the *ICD-10-CM Official Guidelines for Coding and Reporting for 2020*.

371

There are "use additional code to identify" instructional notes throughout the chapter to identify the use of substances that have an influence on the diseases of the digestive system. For example, under categories K05, Gingivitis and periodontal diseases, and K12, Stomatitis and related lesions, there is a use additional code note to identify the following:

Alcohol abuse and dependence (F10.-)
Exposure to environmental tobacco smoke (Z77.22)
Exposure to tobacco smoke in the perinatal period (P96.81)
History of tobacco dependence (Z87.891)
Occupational exposure to environmental tobacco smoke (Z57.31)
Tobacco dependence (F17.-)
Tobacco use (Z72.0)

Other instructional notes appear under the ulcer of the stomach, duodenum, and other digestive system sites to "use additional code to identify" alcohol abuse and dependence (F10.-). Certain digestive conditions are the result of other diseases. For example, under code K31.84, Gastroparesis, is a note stating "code first underlying disease, if known, such as anorexia nervosa, diabetes mellitus, or scleroderma." For infections in the digestive tract, a "use additional code (B95–B97) to identify infectious agent" note appears with codes. For example, this note appears under category K65, Peritonitis, because the cause of the infection may be known and therefore should be coded. Other codes that identify infections that complicate the artificial openings of the digestive system include "use additional code to specify the type of infection." For example, this note appears under code K94.22, Gastrostomy infection, to instruct the coder to identify when cellulitis of the abdominal way (L03.311) or sepsis (A40-, A41-) is present.

There is an instructional note after the heading of Hernia (K40–K46) stating, "hernia with both gangrene and obstruction is classified to hernia with gangrene" (CDC 2019). This applies to all conditions coded to categories K40 through K46. The includes note that follows states that the codes K40–K46 include acquired hernia, congenital hernia, and recurrent hernia.

Coding Diseases of the Digestive System in ICD-10-CM Chapter 11

Chapter 11 of ICD-10-CM, Diseases of the Digestive System (K00–K95), contains many commonly diagnosed problems that patients experience in their gastrointestinal tract. This section describes the coding of some of these digestive system conditions with ICD-10-CM diagnosis codes.

Diseases of Oral Cavity and Salivary Glands (K00–K14)

In the past, diagnosis coding was not widely used in dentistry. However, the need for dental diagnosis codes has become urgent with the advent of electronic health records and the desire of dentists to track patient conditions with their outcomes. The use of codes also supports the educational and research needs of dentistry. Codes describe types of dental caries, pulpitis, periodontitis, abrasions and erosions, gingival and periodontal disease, and other disorders of teeth and supporting structures. Other codes within this section include diseases of the salivary glands, mouth, lips, and tongue. Figure 14.2 illustrates the anatomical structures within the oral cavity.

Mucositis can occur as an adverse effect of antineoplastic treatment and other medications (AHA 2006, 88). There is redness or ulcerative sores in the soft tissue of the mucosal surfaces throughout the body, resulting in severe pain as well as difficulty in eating, drinking, and taking

Figure 14.2. **Oral cavity**

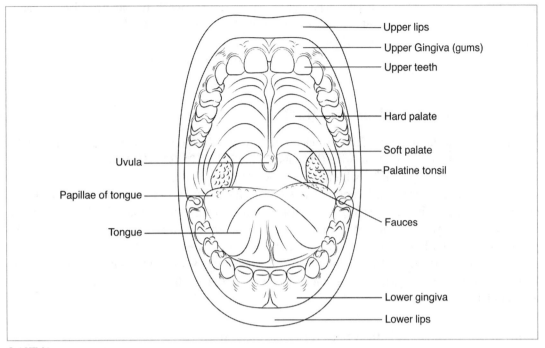

© AHIMA

oral medications. The most common location for mucosal toxicity is the oral cavity. The codes for oral mucositis due to antineoplastic therapy or other drugs are included in the digestive system chapter of ICD-10-CM with code K12.31. Code K12.32 has a "use additional code for adverse effect" direction to identify antineoplastic and immunosuppressive drugs or other drugs (T36–T50) with fifth or sixth character 5.

Gastrointestinal Ulcers (K25–K28)

Ulcers of the gastrointestinal (GI) tract can be found in the following categories:

K25, Gastric ulcer
K26, Duodenal ulcer
K27, Peptic ulcer, site unspecified
K28, Gastrojejunal ulcer

The preceding categories are subdivided to fourth-digit subcategories that describe acute and chronic conditions and the presence of hemorrhage or perforation. An **ulcer** is an erosive or penetrating lesion on the skin or subcutaneous or mucosal tissue, usually with inflammation (Stedman 2012, 1739). The bleeding ulcer or hemorrhage does not have to be actively bleeding at the time of the examination procedure, such as an endoscopy, to use the code for ulcer with hemorrhage. A statement by the physician that bleeding has occurred and it is attributed to the ulcer is sufficient. Each of these categories includes the "use additional code" note to identify the concurrent condition, if applicable, for alcohol abuse and dependence (F10.-).

> **EXAMPLE:** The patient was a 58-year-old male seen in the physician's office for ongoing treatment of his chronic gastric ulcer. At this time, there was no evidence of bleeding by the ulcer. The patient stated he was feeling much better. The physician concluded the patient's alcohol addiction

in remission since he completed the residential treatment program for alcohol dependence. The entries in Alphabetic Index to Diseases and Injuries and the codes for these diagnoses would be

K28.7, Ulcer, gastric, chronic
F10.21, Addiction (see also Dependence), alcohol, alcoholic, with remission

Gastritis and Duodenitis (K29)

Gastritis is the inflammation of the stomach lining, while **duodenitis** is the inflammation of the duodenal portion of the small intestine (Dorland 2012, 762, 572). ICD-10-CM classifies gastritis and duodenitis to category K29, which is subdivided to fourth- and fifth-digit subcategories that describe types of gastritis and duodenitis. The fourth-digit category identifies the severity or etiology of the gastritis, for example, alcoholic gastritis with and without bleeding or chronic atrophic gastritis with or without bleeding. Active bleeding during the current examination or procedure does not have to be present to use the specific code. It may be diagnosed clinically by the physician based on the patient's history or physical examination. An illustration of the Upper Gastrointestinal system is shown in figure 14.3 that includes the esophagus, stomach, and duodenum.

Figure 14.3. Organs within the Upper Gastrointestinal system

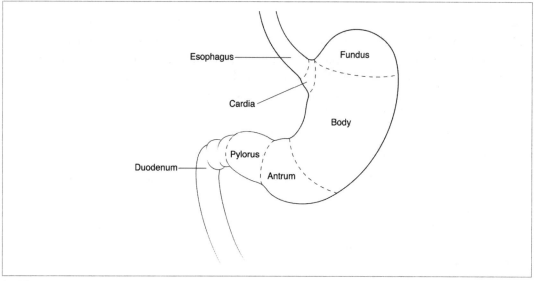

© AHIMA

EXAMPLE: A 40-year-old female was seen in the emergency department (ED) with upper abdominal pain that she has experienced on several occasions, but on this date, the pain did not relent. The patient thinks the pain is related to her stressful job. The patient denies coughing up blood or seeing blood in her stools. The patient was seen by a gastroenterologist during the ED visit, and a simple gastroscopy exam showed mucosal lesions that represent an acute erosive gastritis present in the patient. The patient was given an appointment to see the gastroenterologist in one week and was given prescriptions. The entries in the Alphabetic Index to Disease and Injuries and the codes for this diagnosis would be:

K29.00, Gastritis, acute (erosive)

Acute Appendicitis (K35)

Acute appendicitis is an inflammation of the appendix that can progress to gangrene and perforation of the appendix. Perforation of the appendix contaminates the peritoneal space with enteric bacteria that can result in an abscess formation or generalized peritonitis. Perforation, the presence of an abscess, and the presence of generalized peritonitis are characteristics of appendicitis that surgeons use to describe the severity of the disease and determine the most appropriate treatment and duration of antibiotic treatment. The codes in category K35 make distinctions between perforation and no perforation, gangrenous and non-gangrenous, and perforation with abscess and perforation without abscess:

K35.2-, Acute appendicitis with generalized peritonitis
    K35.20, Acute appendicitis with generalized peritonitis, without abscess
    K35.21, Acute appendicitis with generalized peritonitis, with abscess
K35.3-, Acute appendicitis with localized peritonitis, with and without perforation or gangrene, without and with abscess
    K35.30, Acute appendicitis with localized peritonitis, without perforation or gangrene
    K35.31, Acute appendicitis with localized peritonitis and gangrene, without perforation
    K35.32, Acute appendicitis with perforation and localized peritonitis, without abscess
    K35.33, Acute appendicitis with perforation and localized peritonitis, with abscess
K35.8-, Other and unspecified acute appendicitis without perforation with or without gangrene
    K35.80, Unspecified acute appendicitis
    K35.890, Other acute appendicitis without perforation or gangrene
    K35.891, Other acute appendicitis without perforation, with gangrene

Hernia (K40–K46)

A **hernia** is the protrusion of a loop or knuckle of an organ or tissue through an abdominal opening (Dorland 2012, 848). Many different types of hernias exist, including the following:

- An inguinal hernia is a hernia of an intestinal loop into the inguinal canal. An inguinal hernia may be referred to as direct or indirect, which describes the anatomical location more precisely but cannot be coded as specifically with ICD-10-CM diagnosis codes.

- A femoral hernia is a hernia of a loop of intestine into the femoral canal.

- A hiatal hernia is the displacement of the upper part of the stomach into the thorax through the esophageal opening (hiatus) of the diaphragm.

- A diaphragmatic hernia is the protrusion of an abdominal organ into the chest cavity through a defect in the diaphragm.

- A ventral hernia, or abdominal hernia, is a herniation of the intestine or some other internal body structure through the abdominal wall.

- An incisional hernia is an abdominal hernia at the site of a previously made incision.

- An umbilical hernia is a type of abdominal hernia in which part of the intestine protrudes at the umbilicus and is covered by skin and subcutaneous tissue. This type may also be described as an omphalocele.

- A hernia may be described as **reducible**. This means the physician can manipulate the displaced structure(s) back into normal position.

Codes for different type of hernias of the abdominal cavity are included in the following categories:

K40, Inguinal hernia
K41, Femoral hernia
K42, Umbilical hernia
K43, Ventral hernia
K44, Diaphragmatic (hiatal) hernia
K45, Other abdominal hernia
K46, Unspecified abdominal hernia

A note appears under the category heading that hernia with both gangrene and obstruction is coded as a hernia with gangrene. Hernias are classified by the site or type of hernia; the clinical presentation of the presence of gangrene or obstruction; whether the hernia is unilateral, bilateral, or unspecified as to one- or two-sided; and whether it is a recurrent condition.

ICD-10-CM uses the term **obstruction** to indicate that incarceration, irreducibility, or strangulation is present with the hernia.

- An **irreducible hernia** is also known as an incarcerated hernia. An incarcerated hernia is a hernia of the intestine that cannot be returned or reduced by manipulation; it may or may not be strangulated.

- A **strangulated hernia** is an incarcerated hernia that is so tightly constricted as to restrict the blood supply to the contents of the hernial sac and possibly cause gangrene of the contents, such as the intestine. This represents a medical emergency requiring surgical correction.

EXAMPLE: A 40-year-old male patient was seen in the surgeon's office for a preoperative evaluation prior to his scheduled surgery for a recurrent right-sided inguinal hernia. The patient's preoperative diagnosis is coded as follows with the Alphabetic Index entry of K40.91, Hernia, inguinal, unilateral, recurrent.

Check Your Understanding 14.1

Assign diagnosis codes to the following conditions.

1. Generalized chronic periodontitis, moderate

2. Initial evaluation of oral mucositis due to antineoplastic chemotherapy drug

3. Gastroesophageal reflux with esophagitis

4. Type 1 diabetes mellitus with gastroparesis

5. Acute appendicitis with localized peritonitis

Crohn's Disease [Regional Enteritis] (K50)

Crohn's disease, also known as regional enteritis, is defined as a chronic enteritis or inflammatory disease commonly affecting the distal ileum and, less frequently, other parts of the gastrointestinal tract. The cause is unknown (Stedman 2012, 1442). Crohn's disease is characterized by chronic diarrhea, abdominal pain, fever, anorexia, weight loss, right lower quadrant mass or fullness, and lymphadenitis of the mesenteric nodes.

ICD-10-CM classifies Crohn's disease to category K50, with the fifth and sixth character identifying the specific site affected, such as the small or large intestine. The associated clinical manifestations of rectal bleeding, intestinal obstruction, fistula, or abscess, as well as other complications, are identified with the sixth character under each site. Without further specification as to site and without complication, assign code K50.90 for Crohn's disease.

EXAMPLE: The patient was a 50-year-old female who was hospitalized for treatment of an acute episode of Crohn's disease that she has suffered with the past two years. The final diagnosis for this admission was "Crohn's disease (regional enteritis) of the distal ileum with rectal bleeding." The code for the diagnosis is found in the Alphabetic Index to Diseases and Injuries as follows:

K50.011, Crohn's disease—see Enteritis, regional, ileum—see Enteritis, regional, small intestine, with, rectal bleeding

Gastroenteritis (K52)

Gastroenteritis, an inflammation of the mucous membrane of both the stomach and intestine (Stedman 2012, 683), is characterized by diarrhea, nausea and vomiting, and abdominal cramps. It can be caused by toxins and allergic and dietetic etiology, as well as bacteria, amebae, parasites, viruses, reaction to drugs, or enzyme deficiencies. Allergic reactions as a response to food allergens may manifest as GI reactions, the most common of which are nausea, vomiting, diarrhea, and abdominal cramping. Codes exist in this category to identify the noninfectious origins of gastroenteritis in this category. Gastroenteritis is classified by cause in Chapters 1 and 9 in the Tabular List in Volume 1 of ICD-10-CM. Different forms of gastroenteritis can be described in the following codes:

A02.0, Salmonella gastroenteritis
A08.4, Viral gastroenteritis, NEC
A09, Infectious gastroenteritis
K52.1, Toxic gastroenteritis and colitis
K52.2, Allergic and dietetic gastroenteritis and colitis
K52.9, Noninfectious gastroenteritis and colitis, unspecified
Includes colitis, enteritis, gastroenteritis, ileitis, jejunitis, and sigmoiditis, NOS

Toxic gastroenteritis and colitis, code K52.1, is followed by a "code first" note to identify the toxic agent with a code from the range T51–T66. Another possible cause of toxic gastroenteritis and colitis is the side effect of a drug, which is the reason for the "use additional code for adverse effect" note that also appears under code K52.1.

Under code K52.2, Allergic and dietetic gastroenteritis and colitis, is a "use additional code" note to identify the type of food allergy (Z91.01-, Z91.02-) that caused the bowel inflammation.

EXAMPLE: A 28-year-old female was seen on an urgent basis in her primary care physician's office complaining of nausea, vomiting, diarrhea, and abdominal cramps. The patient does not have a fever. The patient's symptoms started after a party she attended the night before with friends, but none of her friends are ill as a result. The physician documents the diagnosis for the office visit as "acute gastroenteritis, cause unknown, possible food hypersensitivity, food poisoning." The diagnosis for the office visit is coded as follows:

K52.9, Gastroenteritis (acute)
The conditions identified as possible cannot be coded for an outpatient visit per the ICD-10-CM Coding Guidelines, Section IV (CDC 2019).

Peritonitis, Other Disorders of Peritoneum and Disorders of Retroperitoneum (K65–K68)

Peritonitis is inflammation of the peritoneum or the serous membrane lining the abdominopelvic walls and covering the viscera (Dorland 2012, 1418–1419). Peritonitis causes abdominal pain and tenderness, constipation, vomiting, and moderate fever. It may be caused by a bacteria or a virus or caused by other factors, such as ruptured internal organs, trauma, or childbirth. Under the category heading K65, Peritonitis, there is an instructional note to use an additional code (B95–B97) to identify the infectious agent responsible for the infection.

Also, appearing under the category heading is an Excludes1 note that identifies all the conditions that cannot be coded with a category K65 code. For example, acute appendicitis with generalized peritonitis is coded with K35.2- and is not coded with K65, Peritonitis. Under category K65, there is a use additional code (B95-B97) to identify infectious agent, if known. There is a code also note, if applicable, to code diverticular disease of intestine (K57.-).

ICD-10-CM codes distinguish between acute (generalized) peritonitis, code K65.0, and peritoneal abscess, code K65.1. Similarly, a retroperitoneal abscess (K68.19) is coded differently than other forms of retroperitoneal infections (such as K68.9). Spontaneous bacterial peritonitis is coded with K65.2. Choleperitonitis, code K65.3, occurs as the result of bile in the peritoneal cavity. Sclerosing mesenteritis, code K65.4, refers to a number of inflammatory processes involving the mesenteric fat, including fat necrosis and fibrosis. The generic diagnosis of peritonitis is presumed to be bacterial in origin and coded to the unspecified peritonitis code of K65.9. Each condition requires specific treatment. Another commonly occurring condition is peritoneal adhesions. The presence of adhesions could be due to infections or could have developed after a procedure and is coded to K66.0 in the category K66 for other disorders of the peritoneum. If the peritoneal adhesions cause an intestinal obstruction, use codes K56.50–K56.52, intestinal adhesions with partial, complete or unspecified type of obstruction. Peritonitis due to appendicitis or diverticular disease is coded to categories K35, Acute appendicitis, or K57, Diverticular disease of the intestine with combination codes that include both conditions.

> **EXAMPLE:** Two acutely ill patients were treated in the intensive care unit for peritonitis. The first patient had choleperitonitis due to a leakage of bile into the peritoneum. The second patient had generalized peritonitis due to appendicitis with rupture of the appendix. The diagnoses are coded as follows using the Alphabetic Index to Diseases and Injuries entries:
>
> Patient 1 K65.3, Choleperitonitis
> Patient 2 K35.2, Peritonitis, with or following, appendicitis, with perforation or rupture or appendicitis, generalized

Check Your Understanding 14.2

Assign diagnosis codes to the following conditions.

1. Crohn's disease of both small and large intestine with intestinal obstruction
2. Partial intestinal obstruction with adhesions
3. Acute suppurative peritonitis due to *E. coli* from perforation of the intestine
4. Colonic inflammatory bowel disease unclassified (IBDU)
5. Hepatopulmonary syndrome with nonalcoholic portal cirrhosis of the liver

Cholecystitis and Cholelithiasis (K80–K81)

Two categories are available to classify cholecystitis and cholelithiasis: K80, Cholelithiasis and K81, Cholecystitis. Figure 14.4 depicts the organs within the hepatobiliary system and pancreas including the gallbladder, the cystic duct, and the common bile duct.

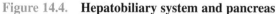

Figure 14.4. **Hepatobiliary system and pancreas**

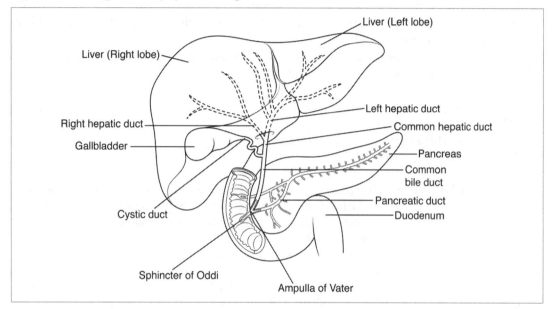

© AHIMA

Cholelithiasis is the presence of one or more calculi (gallstones) in the gallbladder (Dorland 2012, 349). Gallstones tend to be asymptomatic. The most common symptom is biliary colic. More serious complications include cholecystitis, biliary tract obstruction (from stones in the bile ducts or choledocholithiasis), bile duct infection (cholangitis), and gallstone pancreatitis. A diagnosis is usually made by ultrasonography. If cholelithiasis causes symptoms or complications, a cholecystectomy may be necessary.

Choledocholithiasis is the presence of stones in the common bile duct (Dorland 2012, 349). The stones can form in the gallbladder or in the bile ducts. The stones cause biliary colic, biliary obstruction, gallstone pancreatitis, or cholangitis. Cholangitis can lead to stricture, stasis, and choledocholithiasis. The diagnosis is usually made by magnetic resonance cholangiopancreatography (MRCP) or endoscopic retrograde cholangiopancreatography (ERCP). Frequently occurring with the stones is **cholecystitis**, or inflammation of the gallbladder (Dorland 2012, 348).

Category K80 is further divided into the following fifth-character subcategories to describe the existence of calculus or stones in the gallbladder or in the bile ducts or both locations with acute or chronic cholecystitis, and whether or not an obstruction is present:

K80.0-, Calculus of gallbladder with acute cholecystitis
K80.1-, Calculus of gallbladder with other cholecystitis
K80.2-, Calculus of gallbladder without cholecystitis
K80.3-, Calculus of bile duct with cholangitis
K80.4-, Calculus of bile duct with cholecystitis
K80.5-, Calculus of bile duct without cholangitis or cholecystitis
K80.6-, Calculus of gallbladder and bile duct with cholecystitis
K80.7-, Calculus of gallbladder and bile duct without cholecystitis
K80.8, Other cholelithiasis

The coder must be careful in following the Alphabetic Index directions when coding gallbladder disease. For example, if a patient had acute and chronic cholecystitis with cholelithiasis, the coder may access the Index using the diagnosis "cholecystitis." There is a connecting term "with" beneath the main term cholecystitis that is very important to read. The coder must follow the direction when reviewing the Index entry for "Cholecystitis" with "calculus, stones in gallbladder" and follow the direction to see "Calculus, gallbladder, with, cholecystitis." The coder must then go to the main term "calculus, gallbladder" and see the connecting term "with" and find codes following "cholecystitis, acute" and "cholecystitis, chronic." The code to be assigned for acute and chronic cholecystitis with cholelithiasis (without mention of obstruction) is K80.12.

Category K81 contains the following four codes relating to cholecystitis without mention of calculus or stones in the gallbladder or bile duct:

K81.0, Acute cholecystitis
K81.1, Chronic cholecystitis
K81.2, Acute cholecystitis with chronic cholecystitis
K81.9, Cholecystitis, unspecified

> **EXAMPLE:** Two patients were seen in the general surgeon's office for preoperative evaluations prior to their scheduled cholecystectomy and possible common duct exploration. The first patient had proven cholelithiasis with chronic cholecystitis.
>
> The second patient had proven choledocholithiasis with chronic cholecystitis.
>
> The conditions are coded using the Alphabetic Index to Diseases and Injuries with the following index entries:
>
> K80.10, Cholelithiasis—see Calculus, gallbladder, with, cholecystitis, chronic
>
> K80.44, Choledocholithiasis—see Calculus, bile duct, with, cholecystitis, chronic

Gastrointestinal Hemorrhage (K92)

Category K92, Other diseases of the digestive system, includes subcategories for hematemesis (K92.0), melena (K92.1), and unspecified gastrointestinal hemorrhage (K92.2).

 The use of category K92 is limited to cases where a GI bleed is documented, but no bleeding site or cause is identified. A hemorrhage in the GI tract may produce dark black, tarry, clotted stools (also referred to as **melena**) or bright red blood in the stool or vomiting blood (**hematemesis**) (Stedman 2012, 1041 and 754). This is not the same as occult blood, which is invisible and only detected by microscopic examination or by a guaiac test. **Occult blood** is a small amount of blood coming from the GI tract (Stedman 2012, 1184). Occult blood or guaiac-positive stool is reported with ICD-10-CM diagnosis code R19.5, Nonspecific abnormal findings in other body substances, stool contents.

Note the Excludes1 note under the code K92.2. This note identifies a number of GI conditions that can be coded based on the presence of hemorrhage. The use of the K92.2 code is not appropriate when one of the conditions listed under the Excludes1 note is present.

Even though ICD-10-CM includes the combination codes describing a gastrointestinal hemorrhage with a gastrointestinal condition (angiodysplasia, diverticulitis, gastritis, duodenitis, and ulcer), these codes should not be assigned unless the physician identifies a causal relationship.

The coder should not assume a causal relationship between gastrointestinal bleeding and a single finding such as a gastric ulcer, gastritis, diverticulitis, and so on. The physician must identify the source of the bleeding and link the clinical findings from the colonoscopy or upper endoscopy because these findings may be unrelated to the bleeding. Active bleeding does not have to be occurring at the time of the examination or procedure, but it does have to be identified in the patient's history. Two codes should be assigned when the physician states that the GI hemorrhage is unrelated to a coexisting GI condition: one for the GI hemorrhage and one for the GI condition without hemorrhage.

EXAMPLE: Two patients were seen today in the gastroenterology (GI) department for gastrointestinal hemorrhage of unknown origin. After both patients underwent a colonoscopy, diagnoses were established. Patient 1 had no disease found in the lower GI tract, and the physician documented melena as the final diagnosis. Patient 2 was found to have diverticulitis of the large intestine with hemorrhage and that condition was documented as the final diagnosis for the patient. The codes to be assigned for these two patients are as follows, using the Alphabetic Index to Diseases or Injuries:

Patient 1 K92.1, Melena
Patient 2 K57.33, Diverticulitis, intestine, large, with bleeding

Check Your Understanding 14.3

Assign diagnosis codes to the following conditions.

1. Acute and chronic cholecystitis
2. Choledocholithiasis with acute cholecystitis
3. Cholelithiasis with choledocholithiasis with acute cholecystitis with obstruction
4. Acute biliary pancreatitis with necrosis
5. Enterostomy site infection with E. coli sepsis

ICD-10-PCS Procedure Coding for Diseases of the Gastrointestinal System

The procedures performed on the digestive or gastrointestinal system organs appear in the ICD-10-PCS code book in tables that start with the two characters 0 and D followed by five characters representing root operation, body part, approach, device, and qualifier:

Character 1 is Value 0—Medical and Surgical
Character 2 is Value D—Gastrointestinal System

Root Operation

Character 3 of the Medical & Surgical ICD-10-PCS codes is the root operation. The root operations that represent the objectives of procedures for surgical treatment of the diseases of the Gastrointestinal system are shown in table 14.1.

Table 14.1.   Root operations for procedures on body parts within the Gastrointestinal system

Bypass: Altering the route of passage of the contents of a tubular body part
Change: Taking out or off a device from a body part and putting back an identical or similar device in or on the same body part without cutting or puncturing the skin or a mucous membrane
Destruction: Physical eradication of all or a portion of a body part by the direct use of energy, force, or a destructive agent
Dilation: Expanding the orifice or lumen of a tubular body part
Division: Cutting into a body part, without draining fluids and/or gases from the body part, in order to separate or transect a body part
Drainage: Taking or letting out fluids and/or gases from a body part
Excision: Cutting out or off, without replacement, a portion of a body part
Extirpation: Taking or cutting out solid matter from a body part
Extraction: Pulling or stripping out or off all or a portion of a body part by the use of force
Fragmentation: Breaking solid matter in a body part into pieces
Insertion: Putting in a nonbiological appliance that monitors, assists, performs, or prevents a physiological function but does not physically take the place of the body part
Inspection: Visually and/or manually exploring a body part
Occlusion: Completely closing an orifice or the lumen of a tubular body part
Reattachment: Putting back in or on all or a portion of a separated body part to its normal location or other suitable location
Release: Freeing a body part from an abnormal physical constraint by cutting or by the use of force
Removal: Taking out or off a device from a body part
Repair: Restoring, to the extent possible, a body part to its normal anatomic structure and function
Replacement: Putting in or on biological or synthetic material that physically takes the place and/or function of all or a portion of a body part
Reposition: Moving to its normal location, or other suitable location, all or a portion of a body part
Resection: Cutting out or off, without replacement, all of a body part
Supplement: Putting in or on biological or synthetic material that physically reinforces and/or augments the function of a portion of a body part
Restriction: Partially closing an orifice or the lumen of a tubular body part
Revision: Correcting, to the extent possible, a portion of a malfunctioning device or the position of a displaced device
Transfer: Moving, without taking out, all or a portion of a body part to another location to take over the function of all or a portion of a body part
Transplantation: Putting in or on all or a portion of a living body part taken from another individual or animal to physically take the place and/or function of all or a portion of a similar body part

Source: CMS 2019

Body Part

Character 4 identifies the body part involved in the procedure. The body parts in ICD-10-PCS have individual values that include laterality, for example, as shown in table 14.2.

Table 14.2.   **Body parts and values included in the ICD-10-PCS codes for the Gastrointestinal system**

0—Upper intestinal tract
1—Esophagus, upper
2—Esophagus, middle
3—Esophagus, lower
4—Esophagogastric junction
5—Esophagus
6—Stomach
7—Stomach, pylorus
8—Small intestine
9—Duodenum
A—Jejunum
B—Ileum
C—Ileocecal valve
D—Lower intestinal tract
E—Large intestine
F—Large intestine, right
G—Large intestine, left
H—Cecum
J—Appendix
K—Ascending colon
L—Transverse colon
M—Descending colon
N—Sigmoid colon
P—Rectum
Q—Anus
R—Anal sphincter
U—Omentum
V—Mesentery
W—Peritoneum

Source: CMS 2019

Approach

Character 5 identifies the approach used in the procedure. The approach for procedures performed on organs within the Gastrointestinal system is shown in table 14.3.

Table 14.3. **Approaches, definitions, and values included in the ICD-10-PCS codes for the Gastrointestinal system**

Open (0): Cutting through the skin or mucous membrane and any other body layers necessary to expose the site of the procedure
Percutaneous (3): Entry, by puncture or minor incision, of instrumentation through the skin or mucous membrane and any other body layers necessary to reach the site of the procedure
Percutaneous endoscopic (4): Entry, by puncture or minor incision, of instrumentation through the skin or mucous membrane and any other body layers necessary to reach and visualize the site of the procedure
Via Natural or Artificial Opening (7): Entry of instrumentation through a natural or artificial external opening to reach the site of the procedure
Via Natural or Artificial Opening Endoscopic (8): Entry of instrumentation through a natural or artificial external opening to reach and visualize the site of the procedure
Via Natural or Artificial Opening with Percutaneous Endoscopic Assistance (F): Entry by instrumentation through a natural or artificial opening and entry, by puncture or minor incision, of instrumentation through the skin or mucous membrane and any other body layer necessary to aid in the performance of the procedure
External (X): Procedures performed directly on the skin or mucous membrane and procedures performed indirectly by the application of external force through the skin or mucous membrane

Source: CMS 2019

Device

Character 6 identifies if a device remains in the patient's body after the procedure is concluded. The devices used to code procedures performed on organs within the Gastrointestinal system are shown in table 14.4.

Table 14.4. **Devices and values included in the ICD-10-PCS codes for the Gastrointestinal system**

0—Drainage Device
1—Radioactive Element
2—Monitoring Device
3—Infusion Device
7—Autologous Tissue Substitute
B—Intraluminal Device, Airway
C—Extraluminal Device
D—Intraluminal Device
J—Synthetic Substitute
K—Nonautologous Tissue Substitute
L—Artificial Sphincter

| M—Stimulator Lead |
| U—Feeding Device |
| Y—Other Device |
| Z—No Device |

Source: CMS 2019

Qualifier

Character 7 is a qualifier that specifies an additional attribute of the procedure, if applicable. The qualifier characters used to code procedures performed on organs within the gastrointestinal system are the values as shown in table 14.5. Many of the qualifiers are used with the root operation of bypass to indicate the site the bypass was directed to. The qualifier value of X for diagnostic procedure is available for the root operations of Drainage and Excision.

Table 14.5. **Qualifiers used to code procedures within the Gastrointestinal system**

| 0—Allogeneic |
| 1—Syngeneic |
| 2—Zooplastic |
| 3—Vertical |
| 4—Cutaneous |
| 5—Esophagus |
| 6—Stomach |
| 7 - Vagina |
| 8 – Small Intestine |
| 9—Duodenum |
| A—Jejunum |
| B—Ileum |
| E - Cecum |
| H—Cecum |
| K—Ascending Colon |
| L—Transverse Colon |
| M—Descending Colon |
| N—Sigmoid Colon |
| P—Rectum |
| Q—Anus |
| X—Diagnostic |
| Z—No Qualifier |

Source: CMS 2019

ICD-10-PCS Procedure Coding for Diseases of the Hepatobiliary System and Pancreas

A second set of procedures performed for digestive system disorders appear in the ICD-10-PCS book in tables that start with the two characters 0 and F followed by five characters representing root operation, body part, approach, device, and qualifier:

Character 1 is Value 0—Medical and Surgical
Character 2 is Value F—Hepatobiliary System and Pancreas

Root Operation

Character 3 of the Medical & Surgical ICD-10-PCS codes is the root operation. The root operations that represent the objectives of procedures for surgical treatment of the diseases of the Hepatobiliary System and Pancreas are shown in table 14.6.

Table 14.6. **Root operations for procedures on body parts within the Hepatobiliary System and Pancreas**

Bypass: Altering the route of passage of the contents of a tubular body part
Change: Taking out or off a device from a body part and putting back an identical or similar device in or on the same body part without cutting or puncturing the skin or a mucous membrane
Destruction: Physical eradication of all or a portion of a body part by the direct use of energy, force, or a destructive agent
Dilation: Expanding the orifice or lumen of a tubular body part
Division: Cutting into a body part, without draining fluids and/or gases from the body part, in order to separate or transect a body part
Drainage: Taking or letting out fluids and/or gases from a body part
Excision: Cutting out or off, without replacement, a portion of a body part
Extraction: Pulling or stripping out or off all or a portion of a body part by the use of force
Extirpation: Taking or cutting out solid matter from a body part
Fragmentation: Breaking solid matter in a body part into pieces
Insertion: Putting in a nonbiological appliance that monitors, assists, performs, or prevents a physiological function but does not physically take the place of the body part
Inspection: Visually and/or manually exploring a body part
Occlusion: Completely closing an orifice or the lumen of a tubular body part
Reattachment: Putting back in or on all or a portion of a separated body part to its normal location or other suitable location
Release: Freeing a body part from an abnormal physical constraint by cutting or by the use of force
Removal: Taking out or off a device from a body part
Repair: Restoring, to the extent possible, a body part to its normal anatomic structure and function
Replacement: Putting in or on biological or synthetic material that physically takes the place and/or function of all or a portion of a body part

Reposition: Moving to its normal location, or other suitable location, all or a portion of a body part
Resection: Cutting out or off, without replacement, all of a body part
Supplement: Putting in or on biological or synthetic material that physically reinforces and/or augments the function of a portion of a body part
Restriction: Partially closing an orifice or the lumen of a tubular body part
Revision: Correcting, to the extent possible, a portion of a malfunctioning device or the position of a displaced device
Transplantation: Putting in or on all or a portion of a living body part taken from another individual or animal to physically take the place and/or function of all or a portion of a similar body part

Source: CMS 2019

Body Part

Character 4 identifies the body part involved in the procedure. The body parts in ICD-10-PCS have individual values that include laterality, for example, as shown in table 14.7.

Table 14.7. **Body parts and values included in the ICD-10-PCS codes for the Hepatobiliary System and Pancreas**

0—Liver
1—Liver, right lobe
2—Liver, left lobe
4—Gallbladder
5—Hepatic Duct, right
6—Hepatic Duct, left
7—Hepatic Duct, common
8—Cystic Duct
9—Common Bile Duct
B—Hepatobiliary Duct
C—Ampulla of Vater
D—Pancreatic Duct
F—Pancreatic Duct, accessory
G—Pancreas

Source: CMS 2019

Approach

Character 5 identifies the approach used in the procedure. The approach for procedures performed on organs within the Hepatobiliary System and Pancreas are shown in table 14.8.

Table 14.8. **Approaches, definitions, and values included in the ICD-10-PCS codes for the Hepatobiliary System and Pancreas**

Open (0): Cutting through the skin or mucous membrane and any other body layers necessary to expose the site of the procedure
Percutaneous (3): Entry, by puncture or minor incision, of instrumentation through the skin or mucous membrane and any other body layers necessary to reach the site of the procedure

(Continued)

387

Percutaneous endoscopic (4): Entry, by puncture or minor incision, of instrumentation through the skin or mucous membrane and any other body layers necessary to reach and visualize the site of the procedure
Via Natural or Artificial Opening (7): Entry of instrumentation through a natural or artificial external opening to reach the site of the procedure
Via Natural or Artificial Opening Endoscopic (8): Entry of instrumentation through a natural or artificial external opening to reach and visualize the site of the procedure
External (X): Procedures performed directly on the skin or mucous membrane and procedures performed indirectly by the application of external force through the skin or mucous membrane

Source: CMS 2019

Device

Character 6 identifies if a device remains in the patient's body after the procedure is concluded. The devices used to code procedures performed on organs within the Hepatobiliary System and Pancreas are shown in table 14.9.

Table 14.9.   **Devices and values included in the ICD-10-PCS codes for the Hepatobiliary System and Pancreas**

0—Drainage Device
1—Radioactive Element
2—Monitoring Device
3—Infusion Device
7—Autologous Tissue Substitute
C—Extraluminal Device
D—Intraluminal Device
J—Synthetic Substitute
K—Nonautologous Tissue Substitute
Y—Other Device
Z—No Device

Source: CMS 2019

Qualifier

Character 7 is a qualifier that specifies an additional attribute of the procedure, if applicable. The qualifier characters used to code procedures performed on organs within the hepatobiliary system are the values as shown in table 14.10. The qualifier value of X for diagnostic procedure is available for the root operations of Drainage and Excision.

Table 14.10.   **Qualifiers used to code procedures within the Hepatobiliary System and Pancreas**

0—Allogeneic
1—Syngeneic

2—Zooplastic	
3—Duodenum	
4—Stomach	
5—Hepatic Duct, right	
6—Hepatic Duct, left	
7—Hepatic Duct, caudate	
8—Cystic Duct	
9—Common Bile Duct	
B—Small intestine	
C—Large intestine	
F – Irreversible Electroporation	
X—Diagnostic	
Z—No Qualifier Specific	

Source: CMS 2019

Coding of Gastrointestinal Procedures

This section highlights coding for GI procedures such as the following:

- Laparoscopic and open repair of hernia

- Closed endoscopic biopsies and endoscopic excisions of lesions

- Gastrointestinal stoma procedures

- Intestinal resection

- Laparotomy

Laparoscopic and Open Repair of Hernia

There are both surgical and nonsurgical treatments for groin hernias. While nonsurgical repairs of inguinal hernias in adults who are not uncomfortable are acceptable, many patients experience symptoms within one to two years and require surgery (Strand et al. 2018). Hernia repair procedures are performed both by incision (open) and by the laparoscopic technique. Open hernia repairs are performed through an incision with sutured tissue repair. Using synthetic mesh materials to repair the hernia has become fairly standard technique. Laparoscopic hernia repair is a less invasive procedure, with a small incision made to allow a thin, lighted instrument called a laparoscope to be inserted through the incision. Laparoscopic procedures also use mesh that is fixated to the fascia with tacks or sutures to repair the hernia.

The main term "herniorrhaphy" is included in the Index with two root operations listed. Herniorrhaphy with synthetic substitute used for the repair directs the coder to see the root operation Supplement with subterms for anatomical regions for general and lower extremities. The second root operation listed under herniorrhaphy is Repair with subterms for anatomical regions for general and lower extremities. Use the main term "supplement" when synthetic substitute is used and "repair" for all other repairs, along with the subterm for the anatomic

389

location where the hernia is being repaired. The subterms of abdominal wall, diaphragm, femoral region, or inguinal region under supplement give the first three characters 0WU, 0BU, and 0YU for coding. The root operation **Supplement** is defined as "putting in or on biological or synthetic material that physically reinforces or augments the function of a portion of a body part" (CMS 2019). Using the Table 0YU (see table 14.11) for the repair of a laparoscopic right inguinal hernia repair using mesh, the procedure code 0YU54JZ is constructed.

Table 14.11. **Excerpt from Table 0YU for the root operation Supplement**

0 Medical and Surgical Y Anatomical Regions, Lower Extremities U Supplement: Putting in or on biological or synthetic material that physically reinforces or augments the function of a portion of a body part			
Body Part	**Approach**	**Device**	**Qualifier**
5 Inguinal Region, Right 6 Inguinal Region, Left A Inguinal Region, Bilateral	0 Open 4 Percutaneous Endoscopic	7 Autologous Tissue Substitute J Synthetic Substitute K Nonautologous Tissue Substitute	Z No Qualifier

Source: CMS 2019

Closed Endoscopic Biopsies and Endoscopic Excision of Lesions

Closed endoscopic biopsies are common procedures performed on the gastrointestinal tract. A biopsy is taken to determine the pathology of a lesion in a digestive system organ. The main term of Biopsy in the Index refers the coder to the terms "Drainage" or "Excision" with qualifier Diagnostic. The subterms under the main term "Excision" identify the organ where the biopsy was taken. For example, the coding of an esophagoscopy with a biopsy of the middle esophagus would use the main term "Excision" and subterm "esophagus, middle" in the Index and find 0DB2 listed. Table 14.12 contains an excerpt from table 0DB to show how code 0DB28ZX is constructed.

The same table 14.12 shows how an excision of a lesion performed endoscopically would be coded. For example, if an esophagogastroduodenoscopy is performed to excise a lesion of the pylorus of the stomach, the ICD-10-PCS code would be 0DB78ZZ. The qualifier is Z because the excision of a lesion is not a biopsy or diagnostic; instead, it is a therapeutic procedure to remove the lesion.

Table 14.12. **Excerpt from Table 0DB for the root operation Excision**

0 Medical and Surgical D Gastrointestinal System B Excision: Cutting out or off, without replacement, a portion of a body part			
Body Part	**Approach**	**Device**	**Qualifier**
1 Esophagus, Upper 2 Esophagus, Middle 3 Esophagus, Lower 4 Esophagogastric Junction 5 Esophagus 7 Stomach, Pylorus	0 Open 3 Percutaneous 4 Percutaneous Endoscopic 7 Via Natural or Artificial Opening 8 Via Natural or Artificial Opening Endoscopic	Z No Device	X Diagnostic Z No Qualifier

Source: CMS 2019

Gastrointestinal Stoma Procedures

A **stoma** is an artificial opening between two cavities or channels or between a cavity or tube and the exterior (Stedman 2012, 1596). A stoma might also be called an "ostomy" to create a passage to allow for the contents of the gastrointestinal tract to move from the interior to the outside of the body through an opening in the skin.

A **gastrostomy** involves making an incision into the stomach to permit insertion of a synthetic feeding tube. This surgery is performed on patients who are unable to ingest food normally because of stricture or lesion of the esophagus. A **colostomy** is the creation of an artificial opening of the colon through the abdominal wall. It involves bringing a loop of the large intestine out through a small abdominal incision, suturing it to the skin, and opening it. This resulting colostomy provides a temporary channel for the emptying of feces. This procedure is performed to give the bowel a rest following a colon resection. When the bowel is able to return to normal functioning, the loop colostomy is closed. An **ileostomy** is the creation of an opening of the ileum through the abdominal wall. A loop ileostomy involves transposing a segment of the small intestine to the exterior of the body (Stedman 2012, 685, 365, 840).

The root operation **Bypass** is defined as altering the route of passage of the contents of a tubular body part. The root operation Bypass is used to code gastrostomy, colostomy, ileostomy, and other enterostomy. Using either the ICD-10-PCS Index term "Bypass" or the title of the procedure (gastrostomy, colostomy, or ileostomy) leads the coder to Table 0D1 with the following characters to complete the code:

- The fourth character identifies the body part where the ostomy started, for example, the stomach, a part of the colon, or the ileum or other part of the digestive tract.

- The fifth character identifies the approach with the options of Open, Percutaneous Endoscopic, or Via Natural or Artificial Opening Endoscopic.

- The sixth character identifies if a synthetic or tissue substitute is used to create the bypass.

- The seventh character (the qualifier) is intended to identify where the new passage route is directed, for example, if the bypass ends through an opening in the skin, the seventh character is 4 for Cutaneous (skin).

Intestinal Resection

Colorectal surgery is often the treatment of colon cancer or other diseases of the colon, such as ulcerative colitis or Crohn's disease. Colectomy procedures or colon resections remove portions of the large intestine to treat the disease. The procedures can be performed through an incision (open procedure) or done with a laparoscope. Open surgeries can require 6- to 10-inch incisions and are highly invasive procedures that require long recovery periods. Open and other partial excisions of the large intestine are reported with the ICD-10-PCS root operations Excision or Resection to classify such procedures.

The Index contains titles of gastrointestinal procedures and directional notes to see another term in the Index such as hemicolectomy (see Resection), colectomy (see Excision or Resection, gastrointestinal tract), sigmoidectomy (see Excision or Resection), and other similar procedures. The entries direct the coder to either 0DB or 0DT, as shown in table 14.13.

Table 14.13. **Excision and Resection**

Excision	Resection
0 Medical and Surgical	0 Medical and Surgical
D Gastrointestinal System	D Gastrointestinal System
B **Excision**: Cutting out or off, without replacement, a portion of a body part	T **Resection**: Cutting out or off, without replacement, all of a body part

Source: CMS 2019

The fourth character for both Excision and Resection is the body part excised or resected, such as Large Intestine, Right; Large Intestine, Left; Duodenum; Jejunum; Ileum; or Ascending, Descending, Transverse, or Sigmoid Colon, and such. The fifth character identifies the approach, specifically, Open, Percutaneous, Percutaneous Endoscopic, Via Natural or Artificial Opening, or Via Natural or Artificial Opening Endoscopic. A laparoscopic procedure would be the approach of Percutaneous Endoscopic. There is no option for the sixth character or seventh character other than Z, meaning there is no device and no qualifier.

An **anastomosis** is the surgical formation of a channel between tubular structures, such as blood vessels or intestines (Dorland 2012, 75). The anastomosis performed as part of a colon resection would not be coded separately. According to the ICD-10-PCS Official Coding Guidelines, B3.1b, "Procedural steps necessary to reach the operative site and close the operative site, including anastomosis of a tubular body part, are also not coded separately" (CMS 2019).

Laparotomy

A **laparotomy** is an incision into the abdominal cavity (Dorland 2012, 1005). If the laparotomy is for the purposes of opening the cavity, the definitive procedure performed in the cavity is coded with the approach Open. The definitive procedure may be a biopsy, control of postoperative bleeding, drainage, lysis of adhesions (release), or removal of a device. If the laparotomy is for exploratory purposes only, the root operation Inspection is coded with the approach Open.

ICD-10-CM and ICD-10-PCS Review Exercises: Chapter 14

Assign the correct ICD-10-CM diagnosis codes and ICD-10-PCS procedure codes to the following exercises.

1. Recurrent right inguinal hernia with gangrene and obstruction

2. Acute gastric ulcer with hemorrhage and perforation

3. Acute appendicitis with generalized peritonitis and abscess

ICD-10-CM and ICD-10-PCS Review Exercises: Chapter 14 (continued)

4. Diffuse acute infarction of large intestine

5. Chronic duodenal ulcer with hemorrhage; Chronic blood loss anemia

6. The patient is a 65-year-old female who was admitted to the hospital for repair of an incisional hernia. During her preanesthesia evaluation, it was determined that she had both hypertension that was not well controlled and acute on chronic diastolic heart failure. The anesthesiologist and attending physician advised the patient that her surgery would be canceled in order to manage her medical conditions. The patient stayed in the hospital two days for treatment of the heart failure and hypertension and then was discharged with an appointment to see her attending physician in one week to evaluate if and when the hernia surgery can be rescheduled.

7. The patient is a 56-year-old male who was admitted with cellulitis of the abdominal wall due to an infection at the patient's colostomy site. It was determined that the infection was due to enterococcus, and it was treated successfully with intravenous antibiotics. Code the diagnoses only.

8. Chronic alcoholic hepatitis with ascites; Chronic alcoholism

9. Acute and chronic cholecystitis with cholelithiasis

10. Irritable bowel syndrome with diarrhea

11. Rectal polyp

12. Acute and chronic alcohol induced pancreatitis

13. Postgastrectomy malabsorption syndrome

14. Diverticulitis of small intestine with abscess and perforation/rupture with peritonitis

15. PROCEDURE: Laparoscopic cholecystectomy

16. PROCEDURE: Colonoscopy with excision of colon polyp, descending colon and biopsy of sigmoid colon

(Continued on next page)

ICD-10-CM and ICD-10-PCS Review Exercises: Chapter 14 *(continued)*

17. PROCEDURE: Laparotomy with resection of a portion of the jejunum

18. PROCEDURE: Open cholecystectomy with open choledocholithotomy

19. PROCEDURE: Percutaneous needle biopsy of liver

20. PROCEDURE: Left inguinal herniorrhaphy with mesh (synthetic material)

References

American Hospital Association (AHA). 2006. *Coding Clinic for ICD-9-CM*. Fourth Quarter. Chicago: American Hospital Association.

Centers for Disease Control and Prevention (CDC), National Center for Health Statistics (NCHS). 2019 *ICD-10-CM Official Guidelines for Coding and Reporting*, 2020. http://www .cdc.gov/nchs/icd/icd10cm.htm https://www.cdc.gov/nchs/data/icd/10cmguidelines-FY2020 _final.pdf.

Centers for Medicare and Medicaid Services (CMS). 2019. *ICD-10-PCS Official Guidelines for Coding and Reporting*, 2020. http://www.cms.gov/Medicare/Coding/ICD10/.

Dorland, W.A.N., ed. 2012. *Dorland's Illustrated Medical Dictionary*, 32nd ed. Philadelphia: Elsevier Saunders.

Stedman, T. 2012. *Stedman's Medical Dictionary for the Health Professions and Nursing*, 7th ed. Philadelphia: Wolters Kluwer/Lippincott Williams & Wilkins.

Strand, N., D. Feliciano, and M. Hawn. 2018. American College of Surgeons. Groin Hernia: Inguinal and Femoral Repair. https://www.facs.org/~/media/files/education/patient%20ed /groin_hernia.ashx.

Chapter 15

Diseases of the Skin and Subcutaneous Tissue (L00–L99)

Learning Objectives

At the conclusion of this chapter, you should be able to do the following:

- Describe the organization of the conditions and codes included in Chapter 12 of ICD-10-CM, Diseases of the Skin and Subcutaneous Tissue (L00–L99)

- Define and differentiate between the terms *cellulitis* and *abscess*

- Identify the different stages of decubitus or pressure ulcers

- Assign ICD-10-CM codes for diseases of the skin and subcutaneous tissue

- Assign ICD-10-PCS codes for procedures related to diseases of the skin and subcutaneous tissue

Key Terms

Abscess
Actinic keratosis
Cellulitis
Debridement
Decubitus ulcer
Deep tissue pressure injury
Dermatitis
Erythema
Hyperhidrosis
Lymphangitis

Pressure ulcer
Stage 1 pressure injury
Stage 2 pressure injury
Stage 3 pressure injury
Stage 4 pressure injury
Stevens-Johnson syndrome (SJS)
Toxic epidermal necrolysis (TEN)
Unstageable pressure injury
Urticaria

Overview of ICD-10-CM Chapter 12: Diseases of the Skin and Subcutaneous Tissue

Chapter 12 includes categories L00–L99 arranged in the following blocks:

L00–L08	Infections of the skin and subcutaneous tissue
L10–L14	Bullous disorders
L20–L30	Dermatitis and eczema
L40–L45	Papulosquamous disorders
L49–L54	Urticaria and erythema
L55–L59	Radiation-related disorders of the skin and subcutaneous tissue
L60–L75	Disorders of skin appendages
L76	Intraoperative and postprocedural complications of skin and subcutaneous tissue
L80–L99	Other disorders of the skin and subcutaneous tissue

Chapter 12 of ICD-10-CM is organized into blocks of codes for diseases of the skin and subcutaneous tissue that are grouped into similar types of conditions. For example, dermatitis and eczema are separated from urticaria and erythematous conditions. A block of codes for radiation-related disorders of the skin and subcutaneous tissue is included in ICD-10-CM that was not contained in previous classification systems.

The Chapter 12 codes contain specificity for the conditions at the fourth-, fifth-, and sixth-character levels. The specific site where the condition exists is included; for example, parts of the trunk are described as back, chest wall, groin, perineum, and umbilicus. Laterality is also part of the code's description, such as right upper limb, left lower limb, and such. Combination codes are included; for example, the codes for decubitus ulcers represent the site, the laterality, and the stage of the ulcer all in one code. These codes and their determinants will be explained throughout this chapter.

Coding Guidelines and Instructional Notes for ICD-10-CM Chapter 12: Diseases of the Skin and Subcutaneous Tissue

At the beginning of Chapter 12 in ICD-10-CM, a series of conditions listed under an Excludes2 note identifies conditions in other chapters that may be coded with diseases of the skin and subcutaneous tissue. As an example, diseases of the skin and subcutaneous tissue that are connective tissue disorders, viral conditions, or related to endocrine, nutritional, and metabolic diseases are classified to other chapters of ICD-10-CM.

An instruction to "use additional code (B95–B97) to identify infectious agent" follows the heading for the block of codes for infections of the skin and subcutaneous tissue (L00–L08) (CDC 2019).

Instructions for coding dermatitis and eczema are also included in Chapter 12. For example, the note "in this block the terms dermatitis and eczema are used synonymously and interchangeably" is included in the description of conditions classified to categories L20–L30 (CDC 2019). Additionally, the Excludes2 note for categories L20–L30 states

Dermatitis and Eczema (L20–L30)
Excludes2   chronic (childhood) granulomatous disease (D71)
             dermatitis gangrenosa (L08.0)
             dermatitis herpetiformis (L13.0)
             dry skin dermatitis (L85.3)
             factitial dermatitis (L98.1)
             perioral dermatitis (L71.0)
             radiation-related disorders of skin and subcutaneous tissue (L55–L59)
             stasis dermatitis (I87.2)
             (CDC 2019)

Category L23, Allergic contact dermatitis, and category L24, Irritant contact dermatitis, include both Excludes1 and Excludes2 notes that identify what allergic or irritant contact dermatitis conditions can or cannot be coded with conditions classified in categories L23 and L24. For the conditions that are due to drugs in contact with the skin, a "use additional code for adverse effect, if applicable, to identify drug (T36–T50 with fifth or sixth character 5)" appears to direct the coder to use the additional code (CDC 2019).

> **EXAMPLE:**   L23.3, Allergic contact dermatitis due to drugs in contact with skin
> Use additional code for adverse effect, if applicable, to identify drug (T36–T50 with fifth or sixth character 5)
>
> L24.4, Irritant contact dermatitis due to drugs in contact with skin
> Use additional code for adverse effect, if applicable, to identify drug (T36–T50 with fifth or sixth character 5)

Other codes such as L25.1, Unspecified contact dermatitis due to drugs in contact with skin, L27.0 and L27.1 for generalized and localized skin eruption due to drugs and medicaments taken internally, and L43.2, Lichenoid drug reaction, include a similar "use additional code" note relating to the adverse effect of drugs (CDC 2019).

Skin and subcutaneous tissue conditions can be caused by other diseases, and the underlying condition is significant in describing the total clinical situation. Within Chapter 12 of ICD-10-CM, there are codes identified as present "in diseases classified elsewhere." For these conditions, the coder is reminded to "Code first underlying disease" as shown with the following codes:

L14, Bullous disorders in diseases classified elsewhere

L45, Papulosquamous disorders in diseases classified elsewhere

L54, Erythema in diseases classified elsewhere

The NCHS has published chapter-specific guidelines for Chapter 12 in the *ICD-10-CM Official Guidelines for Coding and Reporting*. The coding student should review all of the coding guidelines for Chapter 12 of ICD-10-CM, which appear in an ICD-10-CM code book or on the CDC website (CDC 2019) or in appendix F.

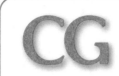

Guideline 1.C.12.a. Pressure ulcer stage codes (L00-L99)

a. **Pressure ulcer stage codes**

1) Pressure ulcer stages

Codes in category L89, Pressure ulcer, identify the site and stage of the pressure ulcer.

The ICD-10-CM classifies pressure ulcer stages based on severity, which is designated by stages 1 to 4, deep pressure injury, unspecified stage and unstageable.

Assign as many codes from category L89 as needed to identify all the pressure ulcers the patient has, if applicable.

See Section I.B.14 for pressure ulcer stage documentation by clinicians other than patient's provider.

2) Unstageable pressure ulcers

Assignment of the code for unstageable pressure ulcer (L89.--0) should be based on the clinical documentation. These codes are used for pressure ulcers whose stage cannot be clinically determined (e.g., the ulcer is covered by eschar or has been treated with a skin or muscle graft). This code should not be confused with the codes for unspecified stage (L89.--9). When there is no documentation regarding the stage of the pressure ulcer, assign the appropriate code for unspecified stage (L89.--9).

3) Documented pressure ulcer stage

Assignment of the pressure ulcer stage code should be guided by clinical documentation of the stage or documentation of the terms found in the Alphabetic Index. For clinical terms describing the stage that are not found in the Alphabetic Index, and there is no documentation of the stage, the provider should be queried.

4) Patients admitted with pressure ulcers documented as healed

No code is assigned if the documentation states that the pressure ulcer is completely healed at the time of admission.

5) Pressure ulcers documented as healing

Pressure ulcers described as healing should be assigned the appropriate pressure ulcer stage code based on the documentation in the medical record. If the documentation does not provide information about the stage of the healing pressure ulcer, assign the appropriate code for unspecified stage.

If the documentation is unclear as to whether the patient has a current (new) pressure ulcer or if the patient is being treated for a healing pressure ulcer, query the provider.

For ulcers that were present on admission but healed at the time of discharge, assign the code for the site and stage of the pressure ulcer at the time of admission.

6) Patient admitted with pressure ulcer evolving into another stage during the admission

If a patient is admitted with a pressure ulcer at one stage and it progresses to a higher stage, two separate codes should be assigned: one code for the site and stage of the ulcer on admission and a second code for the same ulcer site and highest stage reported during the stay.

7) Pressure-induced deep tissue damage

For pressure-induced deep tissue damage or deep tissue pressure injury, assign only the appropriate code for pressure-induced deep tissue damage (L89.--6),

Guideline 1.C.12.b. Non-Pressure Chronic Ulcers

b. **Non-Pressure Chronic Ulcers**

1) Patients admitted with non-pressure ulcers documented as healed

No code is assigned if the documentation states that the non-pressure ulcer is completely healed at the time of admission.

2) Non-pressure ulcers documented as healing

Non-pressure ulcers described as healing should be assigned the appropriate non-pressure ulcer code based on the documentation in the medical record. If the documentation does not provide information about the severity of the healing non-pressure ulcer, assign the appropriate code for unspecified severity.

If the documentation is unclear as to whether the patient has a current (new) non-pressure ulcer or if the patient is being treated for a healing non-pressure ulcer, query the provider.

For ulcers that were present on admission but healed at the time of discharge, assign the code for the site and severity of the non-pressure ulcer at the time of admission.

3) Patient admitted with non-pressure ulcer that progresses to another severity level during the admission

If the patient is admitted to an inpatient hospital with a non-pressure ulcer at one severity level and it

(Continued)

(Continued)

progresses to a higher severity level, two separate codes should be assigned: one code for the site and severity of the ulcer on admission and a second code for the same ulcer site and the highest severity level reported during the stay.

See Section I.B.14 for pressure ulcer stage documentation by clinicians other than patient's provider.

Coding Diseases of the Skin and Subcutaneous Tissue in ICD-10-CM Chapter 12

Chapter 12 of ICD-10-CM, Diseases of the Skin and Subcutaneous Tissue (L00–L99), contains specific codes for infections of the skin and subcutaneous tissue, bullous disorders, dermatitis, eczema, papulosquamous disorders, urticaria, erythema, radiation-related skin disorders, pressure ulcers, and nonpressure chronic skin ulcers as well as intraoperative and postprocedural complications of the skin and subcutaneous tissue.

Many codes include laterality, such as L02.522, Furuncle of the left hand, and L03.111, Cellulitis of the right axilla. Codes for unspecified sides of the body, such as L02.639, Carbuncle of unspecified foot, also exist.

Cutaneous Abscess and Cellulitis (L02–L03)

Cellulitis is an acute inflammation of a localized area of subcutaneous tissue (Stedman 2012, 296–297). Predisposing conditions are open wounds, ulcerations, tinea pedis, and dermatitis, but these conditions need not be present for cellulitis to occur. Physical findings of cellulitis reveal red, hot skin with edema at the site of the infection. The area is tender, and the skin surface has a *peau d'orange* (skin of an orange) appearance with ill-defined borders. Nearby lymph nodes often become inflamed.

A cutaneous or subcutaneous **abscess** is a circumscribed collection of purulent material or pus appearing in an acute or chronic localized infection, caused by tissue destruction and associated with swelling, pain, and other signs of inflammation, such as erythema (Stedman 2012, 7). These abscesses usually follow skin trauma, and the organisms isolated are typically bacterial infection indigenous to the skin of the involved area. Abscesses may occur internally in tissues, organs, and confined spaces. An abscess begins as cellulitis. Cellulitis will clear within a few days with antibiotic treatment. Although drainage of abscesses may occur spontaneously, some abscesses may require incision and drainage, and possibly antibiotic therapy.

Lymphangitis is the inflammation of lymphatic vessels or channels of the lymph system (Dorland 2012, 1083). These lymph vessels are located superficially under the skin. *Streptococcus* bacteria are the common cause of lymphangitis. The bacteria usually invade the lymph vessels through openings in the skin caused by abrasions, lacerations, or skin infections. Symptoms of lymphangitis include warm, tender, red streaks on the affected area. The lymph vessels are warm, tender, and enlarged near the original injury, which could be a minor skin wound. It is important to treat lymphangitis quickly as there is the possibility that bacteria could spread quickly through the lymph system to other parts of the body. A related term that is used to describe a similar inflammation is lymphadenitis, that is, an inflammation of the one or more lymph nodes. Given the similar spelling of the two conditions, coders must be careful not to confuse and code the two conditions incorrectly.

ICD-10-CM classifies cellulitis and acute lymphangitis to the category code L03. The category code is subdivided to fourth-character subcategories that identify the site, such as finger and toe, other parts of limb, face and neck, trunk, and other sites. Within the fourth character, there are the fifth-character codes that separate the two conditions—a set of codes for cellulitis and another set for lymphangitis. The sixth-character code identifies the condition, cellulitis or lymphangitis, and the anatomic site including laterality. An additional code should be assigned to identify the organism involved.

EXAMPLE: Cellulitis of the left upper arm due to *Streptococcus*: L03.114, Cellulitis of left upper limb; B95.5, Unspecified *Streptococcus* as the cause of diseases classified elsewhere

Dermatitis and Eczema (L20–L30)

A note under block L20–L30, Dermatitis and eczema, indicates that in this block, the terms "dermatitis" and "eczema" are used synonymously and interchangeably. **Dermatitis** is an inflammation of the skin (Dorland 2012, 494). There is no single test to diagnose dermatitis. The diagnosis is determined by the appearance of the skin and a thorough medical history. Treatment of the condition depends on the severity and identified cause. Medications may be prescribed to control the itchy nature of it, as well as drugs to control secondary infections. ICD-10-CM classifies dermatitis and eczema according to its cause or clinical type in categories L20–L27 (CDC 2018) as follows:

L20—Atopic dermatitis
Atopic dermatitis is a noninfectious chronic skin inflammation characterized by itchy, inflamed skin usually in individuals who also have asthma or hay fever.

L21—Seborrheic dermatitis
Seborrheic dermatitis is an inflammation of unknown cause that appears on the scalp, eyebrows, and behind the ears as well as on the body that presents with varying degrees of redness, scaling, and itchiness. In its mildest form, it is known as dandruff.

L22—Diaper dermatitis
Diaper dermatitis is also known as diaper rash, which is skin irritation cause by prolonged dampness from urine, feces, and sweat in contact with the baby's skin.

L23—Allergic contact dermatitis
This is a skin inflammation or a localized reaction of redness, itching, and possibly blisters that is due to contact between the skin and an allergy-producing substance that may be a naturally occurring or manufactured substance. Common allergens are metals in jewelry or objects a person comes in contact with, adhesives, cosmetics, drugs in contact with the skin, dyes, certain chemical products like plastic or rubber, food in contact with the skin, plants, and animals.

L24—Irritant contact dermatitis
Irritant contact dermatitis is similar to allergic contact dermatitis in its presentation of redness, blisters, and itching, but the substance is more likely chemical products that produce irritation such as detergents, oils, greasers, and solvents; it also can be caused by cosmetics, other chemical products, food, and plants that come in contact with the skin.

L25—Unspecified contact dermatitis
Category L25 is for use when the diagnosis of allergic or irritant contact dermatitis cannot be made, but the cause may be specified as cosmetics, chemical products, dyes, food, or plants in contact with the skin as well as the possibility that the substance is not identified but its presentation is consistent with contact dermatitis.

L26—Exfoliative dermatitis
This form of the disease produces a generalized exfoliation or shedding, peeling, or scaling of skin. Another exfoliative disease is exfoliative neonatorum dermatitis or Ritter's disease, a serious condition affecting young children and coded with L00.

L27—Dermatitis due to substances taken internally
The substances taken internally can be drugs and medications, ingested food, and other substances taken internally. An instructional note is included under the codes for generalized and localized skin eruptions due to drugs and medicaments to use an additional code for adverse effect, if applicable, to identify the drug (T36–T50 with fifth or sixth character 5).

Check Your Understanding 15.1

Answer the following questions or assign diagnosis codes to the following conditions.

1. According to the *Official Guidelines for Coding and Reporting* for Chapter 12 of ICD-10-CM, how should a pressure ulcer that has been described by the healthcare provider as "healing" be coded?

2. According to the *Official Guidelines for Coding and Reporting* for Chapter 12 of ICD-10-CM, what is the difference between an "unstageable" pressure ulcer and a pressure ulcer that is "unspecified" as to the stage?

3. Bullous pemphigoid

4. Allergic contact dermatitis due to rubber

5. Periorbital cellulitis

Urticaria and Erythema (L49–L54)

Urticaria is the vascular reaction in the upper dermis. It may be transient in nature. It is an area of localized edema caused by dilatation and increase capillary permeability with wheals. It is also called hives (Dorland 2012, 2011). Physicians suspect hives or urticaria to be due to hypersensitivity to food or drugs and insect bites among other triggers. Urticaria develops when natural chemicals including histamines are released in the skin as an allergic reaction to something but can also occur due to a nonallergic cause such as an autoimmune disease. Urticaria usually resolves quickly in less than 24 hours. The best treatment is to find the cause and eliminate contact with it. Persistent urticaria is usually treated with over-the-counter antihistamine topical ointments or creams. When hives or urticaria are present with swelling of the lips, tongue, or throat or any other symptoms that are accompanied by respiratory problems, emergency medical care is warranted (ACAAI 2018).

Erythema is redness of the skin due to capillary dilation (Dorland 2012, 643). Erythematous conditions are skin disorders relating to or marked by erythema. A number of distinct disorders are included in categories L51–L53. Erythema multiforme is an acute eruption of macules, papules, or subepidermal vesicles presenting in a multiform appearance. The characteristic lesions appear over the dorsal aspect of the hands and forearms. Its origin may be allergic or drug sensitivity, or it may be caused by herpes simplex infection. The eruption may be self-limited (erythema multiforme minor) or recurrent, or it could run a severe and possibly fatal course (erythema multiforme major).

Stevens-Johnson syndrome (SJS) is a bullous form of erythema multiforme that may be extensive over the body and produce serious subjective symptoms and possibly death (Dorland

2012, 1849). **Toxic epidermal necrolysis (TEN)** may also occur with SJS. TEN is a syndrome in which large portions of skin become intensely erythematous with epidermal necrolysis. The skin peels off the body in the manner of a second-degree burn. This condition is usually seen in adults as a severe reaction to a drug, although it may be caused by infections, neoplastic disease, or chemical exposure. Its source may also be unknown (Dorland 2012, 1234). Codes are available to describe SJS (code L51.1), SJS with TEN (L51.3), and TEN (L51.2).

If erythema multiforme is caused by an adverse effect of a drug, an instructional note reminds the coder to use additional code to identify the drug (T36–T50 with fifth or sixth character 5). Erythema multiforme produces other physical manifestations. An instructional note appears under the category L51 to use additional code(s) to assign codes for such conditions as arthropathy, conjunctivitis, corneal ulcer, and other conditions of the eye that erythema multiforme can produce.

Erythema nodosum is the single condition classified with category code L52. Category L53, Other erythematous conditions, is separated at the fourth-character level into other forms of erythema. Toxic erythema (L53.0) may be caused by a drug or toxin poisoning or as a result of an adverse effect of a drug. A "code first" note for the poisoning and a "use additional code" note to identify the drug producing the adverse effect of toxic erythema remind the coder to assign the applicable codes.

Category code L49 identifies exfoliation due to erythematous conditions according to extent of body surface involved. Subcategory codes L49.0–L49.9 are used to describe the percentage of body surface that has the exfoliation. A "code first" note appears within the category to direct the coder to code first the erythematous condition causing the exfoliation, such as Ritter's disease, staphylococcal scalded skin syndrome, SJS with or without TEN overlap, or toxic epidermal necrolysis.

> **EXAMPLE:** The allergist examines the patient in the office for two skin conditions and diagnoses the patient as having idiopathic urticaria of both forearms and erythema nodosum of the right lower leg. The codes are L50.1, idiopathic urticaria and L52, erythema nodosum. Neither condition includes the anatomical site of the body where the skin condition occurs.

Radiation-Related Disorders of the Skin and Subcutaneous Tissue (L55–L59)

Codes in this block of codes are skin conditions or skin damage that was caused by radiation such as solar factors, ultraviolet light, and nonionizing radiation. The sun is the major source of ultraviolet light damage to skin. Tanning bed lamps also produce ultraviolet light responsible for tanning and the resulting skin damage from overexposure.

Category L55, Sunburn, includes four-character codes to identify first-degree (L55.0), second-degree (L55.1), and third-degree sunburns (L55.2). An unspecified code for "sunburn" with no degree specified exists with L55.9.

Category L56 classifies other acute skin changes due to ultraviolet radiation. A "use additional" code note appears under the category heading to assign a code from W89 or X32 to identify the source of the ultraviolet radiation such as exposure to man-made visible and ultraviolet light or exposure to sunlight. Conditions that are coded to this category are solar urticaria (L56.3) and disseminated superficial actinic porokeratosis (DSAP) (L56.5).

Skin damage can also be produced by chronic exposure to ultraviolet light radiation. Category code L57 contains codes for skin changes from this chronic exposure. The most common condition that is coded in this category is actinic keratosis (L57.0). **Actinic keratosis** is a sharply outlined, red or skin-colored, flat or elevated, thick growth that sometimes develops into a cutaneous horn or gives rise to squamous cell carcinoma of the skin (Dorland 2012, 982). These growths usually affect the middle-aged or elderly person, especially those with fair skin, and are the result of long-term sun exposure (Skin Cancer Foundation 2018).

> **EXAMPLE:** The patient has two red, flat, thick skin growths on each side of her face on her temples. The physician diagnoses both conditions as "senile keratosis" and advises the patient to avoid sun exposure and apply sunscreen to the face and body when exposed to sun. The patient receives a referral to see a dermatologist in her office for a consultation for the senile or actinic keratosis as diagnoses today. The ICD-10-CM diagnosis code written on the referral form is L57.0, Actinic or solar keratosis.

Disorders of Skin Appendages (L60–L75)

Categories L60–L75 contain some of the more commonly diagnosed and treated skin and nail conditions. Nail disorders such as ingrowing nail, oncolysis, and nail dystrophy are individual codes within category L60. Forms of alopecia and conditions involving hair loss are identified with codes in categories L65–L66. Hair color, hair shaft abnormalities, and excessive hair (hypertrichosis and hirsutism) are disorders coded with category codes L67–L68.

Some of the more frequently occurring and treated skin conditions that are treated in physicians' offices and ambulatory settings are contained in categories L70 for different types of acne, L71 for rosacea and rhinophyma, and L72 for follicular cysts of skin and subcutaneous tissue. Epidermal, pilar, trichodermal, and sebaceous cysts are examples of follicular cysts commonly excised in an outpatient setting when the cyst becomes enlarged or infected.

Eccrine sweat and apocrine sweat gland disorders are classified with codes from categories L74 and L75. Primary focal hyperhidrosis of the axilla, face, palms, and soles are coded with six-character codes L74.510–L74.513. **Hyperhidrosis** is excessive or profuse sweating or perspiration where the exact cause is unknown and can occur spontaneously (Stedman 2012, 814). Topical preparations help reduce the sweating, and botulinum toxin (Botox) injections also decrease sweat secretion.

> **EXAMPLE:** A 16-year-old male patient was seen in the dermatologist office for ongoing treatment of acne vulgaris that was responding to treatment. The diagnosis code for this visit would be L70.0, acne vulgaris.

Check Your Understanding 15.2

Assign diagnosis codes to the following conditions.

1. Primary focal hyperhidrosis, soles of feet
2. Inflamed seborrheic keratosis
3. Alopecia areata
4. Pilar cyst of the scalp
5. Acquired disseminated superficial actinic porokeratosis (DSAP)

Pressure Ulcer (L89)

Category L89, Pressure ulcer, contains combination codes that identify the site, the laterality, as well as the stage of the pressure ulcer. Pressure ulcers may also be documented by a physician or a wound care provider as a decubitus ulcer or bed sore. No code is assigned in ICD-10-CM if the documentation states that the pressure ulcer is completely healed. For all the codes in category L89, Pressure ulcer, there is a note to "Code first any associated gangrene (I96)" (CDC 2019).

The codes for pressure ulcers are very specific:

- Category L89 for pressure ulcers is a three-character category code.

- Each of the four-character codes identifies the anatomic site, such as elbow, back, hip, buttocks, contiguous sites of the back, ankle, heel, and other sites.

- Each of the five-character codes for each anatomic site identifies if the site is the right side of the body, left side, or unspecified side.

- Each of the six-character codes for each of the anatomic sites with its laterality identified includes the stage of the ulcer.

- Individual codes are mostly six characters long with five-character codes for pressure ulcers of unspecified sites (CDC 2018).

Examples of these codes follow:

L89.001,	Pressure ulcer of unspecified elbow stage 1
L89.132,	Pressure ulcer of right lower back, stage 2
L89.223,	Pressure ulcer of left hip, stage 3
L89.314,	Pressure ulcer of right buttock, stage 4
L89.520,	Pressure ulcer of left ankle, unstageable

Pressure ulcers, or **decubitus ulcers,** are caused by ischemic hypoxia caused by prolonged pressure on the skin in one position. The sore or ulcer may become infected with components of the skin and gastrointestinal flora. The ulceration of tissue usually is at the location of a bony prominence that has been subjected to pressure against the skin by an external object such as lying in bed, sitting in a wheelchair, or pressure from a cast or splint. The most frequent sites for a pressure ulcer are the sacrum, buttock, elbows, heels, outer ankles, inner knees, hips, shoulder blades, and occipital bone of the head. Other sites may be involved depending on the patient's position in bed or in a sitting position. Patients at high risk for developing pressure ulcers are the elderly, patients of any age who are immobile and debilitated from their chronic diseases, or patients who are in bed for an extended period of time to recover from a severe injury. Patients may have more than one pressure ulcer, located at different sites on the body. Pressure ulcers may extend into deeper tissue including muscle and bone. The ulcers may also be referred to as decubitus ulcers, pressure necrosis, pressure sores, or bedsores (Mosby 2017, 1087).

The depth of the ulcer is identified by stages 1 through 4. The National Pressure Ulcer Advisory Panel (NPUAP) updated the definitions of the staging system in 2016. A pressure ulcer may be documented as a pressure injury. The updated staging system includes the following definitions:

A pressure ulcer may be referred to in documentation as a pressure injury or pressure ulcer/injury. A pressure injury is localized damage to the skin and/or underlying soft tissue usually over a bony prominence or related to a medical or other device. The injury can present as intact skin or an open ulcer and may be painful. The injury occurs as a result of intense and/or prolonged pressure or pressure in combination with shear. The tolerance of soft tissue for pressure and shear may also be affected by microclimate, nutrition, perfusion, co-morbidities and condition of the soft tissue.

Stage 1 Pressure Injury: Non-blanchable erythema of intact skin

Intact skin with a localized area of non-blanchable erythema, which may appear differently in darkly pigmented skin. Presence of blanchable erythema or changes in sensation, temperature, or firmness may precede visual changes. Color changes do not include purple or maroon discoloration; these may indicate deep tissue pressure injury.

Stage 2 Pressure Injury: Partial-thickness skin loss with exposed dermis

Partial-thickness loss of skin with exposed dermis. The wound bed is viable, pink or red, moist, and may also present as an intact or ruptured serum-filled blister. Adipose (fat) is not visible and deeper tissues are not visible. Granulation tissue, slough and eschar are not present. These injuries commonly result from adverse microclimate and shear in the skin over the pelvis and shear in the heel. This stage should not be used to describe moisture associated skin damage (MASD) including incontinence associated dermatitis (IAD), intertriginous dermatitis (ITD), medical adhesive related skin injury (MARSI), or traumatic wounds (skin tears, burns, abrasions).

Stage 3 Pressure Injury: Full-thickness skin loss

Full-thickness loss of skin, in which adipose (fat) is visible in the ulcer and granulation tissue and epibole (rolled wound edges) are often present. Slough and/or eschar may be visible. The depth of tissue damage varies by anatomical location; areas of significant adiposity can develop deep wounds. Undermining and tunneling may occur. Fascia, muscle, tendon, ligament, cartilage and/or bone are not exposed. If slough or eschar obscures the extent of tissue loss this is an Unstageable Pressure Injury.

Stage 4 Pressure Injury: Full-thickness skin and tissue loss

Full-thickness skin and tissue loss with exposed or directly palpable fascia, muscle, tendon, ligament, cartilage or bone in the ulcer. Slough and/or eschar may be visible. Epibole (rolled edges), undermining and/or tunneling often occur. Depth varies by anatomical location. If slough or eschar obscures the extent of tissue loss this is an Unstageable Pressure Injury.

Unstageable Pressure Injury: Obscured full-thickness skin and tissue loss

Full-thickness skin and tissue loss in which the extent of tissue damage within the ulcer cannot be confirmed because it is obscured by slough or eschar. If slough or eschar is removed, a Stage 3 or Stage 4 pressure injury will be revealed. Stable eschar (i.e. dry, adherent, intact without erythema or fluctuance) on the heel or ischemic limb should not be softened or removed.

Deep Tissue Pressure Injury (DTPI): Persistent non-blanchable deep red, maroon or purple discoloration

Intact or non-intact skin with localized area of persistent non-blanchable deep red, maroon, purple discoloration or epidermal separation revealing a dark wound bed or blood-filled blister. Pain and temperature change often precede skin color changes. Discoloration may appear differently in darkly pigmented skin. This injury results from intense and/or prolonged pressure and shear forces at the bone-muscle interface. The wound may evolve rapidly to reveal the actual extent of tissue injury, or may resolve without tissue loss. If necrotic tissue, subcutaneous tissue, granulation tissue, fascia, muscle or other underlying structures are visible, this indicates a full thickness pressure injury (Unstageable, Stage 3 or Stage 4). Do not use DTPI to describe vascular, traumatic, neuropathic or dermatologic conditions.

The National Pressure Ulcer Advisory Panel (NPUAP) updated the definitions of the staging system in 2016 is used with permission of the National Pressure Ulcer Advisory Panel, 2016. Website reference accessed August 2019: https://npuap.org/page/pressureinjurystages

CODING EXAMPLE: The elderly, bedridden patient has four pressure ulcers: stage 3 of the sacral region, stage 2 of the heels of feet bilaterally, and stage 2 of the right elbow. The pressure ulcers would be coded as L89.153 for the stage 3 sacral region, L89.612 for stage 2 of right heel, L89.622 for stage 2 of left heel, and L89.012 for stage 2 of right elbow.

As of October 1, 2019, ICD-10-CM has been expanded to include codes for deep tissue pressure injury (DTPI). Previously, DTPI conditions were coded as an unstageable pressure injury. However, the usual approach to care for unstageable wounds is for the provider to debride the wound in order to determine the extent, and stage the wound once the wound could be seen or probed. DTPI in its early stages is not debrided; hence the code for unstageable wounds does not denote the problem. Deep tissue pressure injury is located in the ICD-10-CM Index as damage, deep tissue, pressured-induced – see also L89 with final character of .6 for each site listed or under the main term of injury, pressure, injury – see Ulcer, pressure, by site.

Non-Pressure Chronic Ulcer of Lower Limb, Not Elsewhere Classified (L97)

A patient may have a chronic ulcer of the skin of the lower limbs as a sole problem or the ulcer may be the result of another condition. A code from L97 may be used as a principal or first-listed code if no underlying condition is documented as the cause of the ulcer. An important note under category L97 instructs the coder to "code first" any of the following underlying conditions (CDC 2019):

- Any associated gangrene (I96)
- Atherosclerosis of the lower extremities (I70.23-, I70.24-, I70.33-, I70.34-, I70.43-, I70.44-, I70.53-, I70.54-, I70.63-, I70.64-, I70.73-, I70.74-)
- Chronic venous hypertension (I87.31-, I87.33-)
- Diabetic ulcers (E08.621, E08.622, E09.621, E09.622, E10.621, E10.622, E11.621, E11.622, E13.621, E13.622)
- Postphlebitic syndrome (I87.01-, I87.03-)
- Postthrombotic syndrome (I87.01-, I87.03-)
- Varicose ulcer (I83.0-, I83.2-)

Individual codes in category L97 include (1) the site; (2) the laterality of (a) right, (b) left, or (c) unspecified; and (3) the severity of the ulcer identified as (a) limited to breakdown of skin, (b) fat layer exposed, (c) muscle involvement with or without necrosis of muscle, (d) bone involvement with or without necrosis of bone, or (e) unspecified.

> ## Check Your Understanding 15.3
>
> Assign diagnosis codes to the following conditions.
>
> 1. Pressure ulcer, right heel, stage 2
> 2. Non-pressure chronic ulcer, right heel with skin breakdown only
> 3. Chronic skin ulcer on back with only skin breakdown
> 4. Chronic ulcer, right ankle, with muscle involvement but no necrosis of muscle
> 5. Decubitus ulcer, right buttock, stage 3

ICD-10-PCS Procedure Coding for Diseases of the Skin and Subcutaneous Tissue

Two sections in ICD-10-PCS identify procedures that are performed on the skin and subcutaneous tissue. The procedures performed on the skin and breast appear in the ICD-10-PCS code book in tables that start with the two characters 0 and H followed by five characters representing root operation, body part, approach, device, and qualifier. The second set of procedures appears in the ICD-10-PCS code book in tables that start with two characters 0 and J for subcutaneous tissue and fascia.

Section for the Skin and Breast

Character 1 is Value 0—Medical and Surgical
Character 2 is Value H—Skin and Breast

Root Operation

Character 3 of the Medical & Surgical section of ICD-10-PCS codes is the root operation. The root operations that represent the objectives of procedures for surgical treatment of the diseases of the Skin and Breast are shown in table 15.1.

Table 15.1. **Root operations for procedures on body parts of the Skin and Breast**

Alteration: Modifying the anatomic structure of a body part without affecting the function of the body part
Change: Taking out or off a device from a body part and putting back an identical or similar device in or on the same body part without cutting or puncturing the skin or a mucous membrane.
Destruction: Physical eradication of all or a portion of a body part by the direct use of energy, force, or a destructive agent
Division: Cutting into a body part, without draining fluids and/or gases from the body part, in order to separate or transect a body part
Drainage: Taking or letting out fluids and/or gases from a body part
Excision: Cutting out or off, without replacement, a portion of a body part
Extirpation: Taking or cutting out solid matter from a body part
Extraction: Pulling or stripping out or off all or a portion of a body part by the use of force

Insertion: Putting in a nonbiological appliance that monitors, assists, performs, or prevents a physiological function but does not physically take the place of the body part
Inspection: Visually and/or manually exploring a body part
Reattachment: Putting back in or on all or a portion of a separated body part to its normal location or other suitable location
Release: Freeing a body part from an abnormal physical constraint by cutting or by the use of force
Removal: Taking out or off a device from a body part
Repair: Restoring, to the extent possible, a body part to its normal anatomic structure and function
Replacement: Putting in or on biological or synthetic material that physically takes the place and/or function of all or a portion of a body part
Reposition: Moving to its normal location, or other suitable location, all or a portion of a body part
Resection: Cutting out or off, without replacement, all of a body part
Supplement: Putting in or on biological or synthetic material that physically reinforces and/or augments the function of a portion of a body part
Revision: Correcting, to the extent possible, a portion of a malfunctioning device or the position of a displaced device
Transfer: Moving, without taking out, all or a portion of a body part to another location to take over the function of all or a portion of a body part

Source: CMS 2019

Body Part

Character 4 identifies the body part involved in the procedure. The body parts in ICD-10-PCS have individual values that include laterality, for example, as shown in table 15.2.

Table 15.2.   **Body parts and values included in the ICD-10-PCS codes for the Skin and Breast**

0—Skin, scalp
1—Skin, face
2—Skin, right ear
3—Skin, left ear
4—Skin, neck
5—Skin, chest
6—Skin, back
7—Skin, abdomen
8—Skin, buttock
9—Skin, perineum
A—Skin, inguinal
B—Skin, right upper arm
C—Skin, left upper arm

(Continued)

D—Skin, right lower arm
E—Skin, left lower arm
F—Skin, right hand
G—Skin, left hand
H—Skin, right upper leg
J—Skin, left upper leg
K—Skin, right lower leg
L—Skin, left lower leg
M—Skin, right foot
N—Skin, left foot
P—Skin
Q—Finger nail
R—Toe nail
S—Hair
T—Breast, right
U—Breast, left
V—Breast, bilateral
W—Nipple, right
X—Nipple, left
Y—Supernumerary breast

Source: CMS 2019

Approach

Character 5 identifies the approach used in the procedure. The approach for procedures performed on the Skin and Breast is shown in table 15.3.

Table 15.3. **Approaches, definitions, and values included in the ICD-10-PCS codes for the Skin and Breast**

Open (0): Cutting through the skin or mucous membrane and any other body layers necessary to expose the site of the procedure
Percutaneous (3): Entry, by puncture or minor incision, of instrumentation through the skin or mucous membrane and any other body layers necessary to reach the site of the procedure
Via Natural or Artificial Opening (7): Entry of instrumentation through a natural or artificial external opening to reach the site of the procedure
Via Natural or Artificial Opening Endoscopic (8): Entry of instrumentation through a natural or artificial external opening to reach and visualize the site of the procedure
External (X): Procedures performed directly on the skin or mucous membrane and procedures performed indirectly by the application of external force through the skin or mucous membrane

Source: CMS 2019

Device

Character 6 identifies if a device remains in the patient's body after the procedure is concluded. The devices used to code procedures performed on the Skin and Breast are limited to a few devices as shown in table 15.4.

Table 15.4. **Devices and values included in the ICD-10-PCS codes for the Skin and Breast**

0—Drainage device
1—Radioactive element
7—Autologous tissue substitute
J—Synthetic substitute
K—Nonautologous tissue substitute
N—Tissue expander
Y—Other device
Z—No device

Source: CMS 2019

Qualifier

Character 7 specifies an additional attribute of the procedure, if applicable. The qualifier characters used to code procedures performed on the Skin and Breast are as shown in table 15.5. The qualifier value of X for diagnostic procedure is available for the root operations of Drainage and Excision.

Table 15.5. **Qualifiers used to code procedures for the Skin and Breast**

2 – Cell suspension technique
3—Full thickness
4—Partial thickness
5—Latissimus dorsi myocutaneous flap
6—Transverse rectus abdominis myocutaneous flap
7—Deep inferior epigastric artery perforator flap
8—Superficial inferior epigastric artery flap
9—Gluteal artery perforator flap
D—Multiple
X—Diagnostic
Z—No Qualifier

Source: CMS 2019

ICD-10-PCS Procedure Coding for Diseases of the Subcutaneous Tissues and Fascia

The set of procedures that appears in the ICD-10-PCS code book in tables that start with two characters 0 and J are for subcutaneous tissue and fascia.

Section for the Subcutaneous Tissue and Fascia

Character 1 is Value 0—Medical and Surgical
Character 2 is Value J—Subcutaneous Tissue and Fascia

Root Operation

Character 3 of the Medical & Surgical section of ICD-10-PCS codes is the root operation. The root operations that represent the objectives of procedures for surgical treatment of the diseases of Subcutaneous Tissue and Fascia are shown in table 15.6.

Table 15.6.   **Root operations for procedures on body parts of the Subcutaneous Tissue and Fascia**

Alteration: Modifying the anatomic structure of a body part without affecting the function of the body part
Change: Taking out or off a device from a body part and putting back an identical or similar device in or on the same body part without cutting or puncturing the skin or a mucous membrane
Destruction: Physical eradication of all or a portion of a body part by the direct use of energy, force, or a destructive agent
Division: Cutting into a body part, without draining fluids and/or gases from the body part, in order to separate or transect a body part
Drainage: Taking or letting out fluids and/or gases from a body part
Excision: Cutting out or off, without replacement, a portion of a body part
Extirpation: Taking or cutting out solid matter from a body part
Extraction: Pulling or stripping out or off all or a portion of a body part by the use of force
Insertion: Putting in a nonbiological appliance that monitors, assists, performs, or prevents a physiological function but does not physically take the place of the body part
Inspection: Visually and/or manually exploring a body part
Release: Freeing a body part from an abnormal physical constraint by cutting or by the use of force
Removal: Taking out or off a device from a body part
Repair: Restoring, to the extent possible, a body part to its normal anatomic structure and function
Replacement: Putting in or on biological or synthetic material that physically takes the place and/or function of all or a portion of a body part
Supplement: Putting in or on biological or synthetic material that physically reinforces and/or augments the function of a portion of a body part

Revision: Correcting, to the extent possible, a portion of a malfunctioning device or the position of a displaced device
Transfer: Moving, without taking out, all or a portion of a body part to another location to take over the function of all or a portion of a body part

Source: CMS 2019

Body Part

Character 4 identifies the body part involved in the procedure. The body parts in ICD-10-PCS have individual values that include laterality, for example, as shown in table 15.7.

Table 15.7. **Body parts and values included in the ICD-10-PCS codes for Subcutaneous Tissue and Fascia**

0—Subcutaneous tissue and fascia, scalp
1—Subcutaneous tissue and fascia, face
4—Subcutaneous tissue and fascia, right neck
5—Subcutaneous tissue and fascia, left neck
6—Subcutaneous tissue and fascia chest
7—Subcutaneous tissue and fascia, back
8—Subcutaneous tissue and fascia, abdomen
9—Subcutaneous tissue and fascia, buttock
B—Subcutaneous tissue and fascia, perineum
C—Subcutaneous tissue and fascia, pelvic region
D—Subcutaneous tissue and fascia, right upper arm
F—Subcutaneous tissue and fascia, left upper arm
G—Subcutaneous tissue and fascia, right lower arm
H—Subcutaneous tissue and fascia, left lower arm
J—Subcutaneous tissue and fascia, right hand
K—Subcutaneous tissue and fascia, left hand
L—Subcutaneous tissue and fascia, right upper leg
M—Subcutaneous tissue and fascia, left upper leg
N—Subcutaneous tissue and fascia, right lower leg
P—Subcutaneous tissue and fascia, left lower leg
Q—Subcutaneous tissue and fascia, right foot
R—Subcutaneous tissue and fascia, left foot
S—Subcutaneous tissue and fascia, head and neck

(*Continued*)

| T—Subcutaneous tissue and fascia, trunk |
| V—Subcutaneous tissue and fascia, upper extremity |
| W—Subcutaneous tissue and fascia, lower extremity |

Source: CMS 2019

Approach

Character 5 identifies the approach used in the procedure. The approach for procedures performed on the Subcutaneous Tissue and Fascia are shown in table 15.8.

Table 15.8.   **Approaches, definitions, and values included in the ICD-10-PCS codes for Subcutaneous Tissue and Fascia**

| **Open** (0): Cutting through the skin or mucous membrane and any other body layers necessary to expose the site of the procedure |
| **Percutaneous** (3): Entry, by puncture or minor incision, of instrumentation through the skin or mucous membrane and any other body layers necessary to reach the site of the procedure |
| **External** (X): Procedures performed directly on the skin or mucous membrane and procedures performed indirectly by the application of external force through the skin or mucous membrane |

Source: CMS 2019

Device

Character 6 identifies if a device remains in the patient's body after the procedure is concluded. The devices used to code procedures performed on the Subcutaneous Tissue and Fascia are shown in table 15.9. The qualifier value of X for diagnostic procedure is available for the root operations of Drainage and Excision.

Table 15.9.   **Devices and values included in the ICD-10-PCS codes for Subcutaneous Tissue and Fascia**

| 0—Monitoring Device, Hemodynamic |
| 0—Drainage Device |
| 1—Radioactive Element |
| 2—Monitoring Device |
| 3—Infusion Device |
| 4—Pacemaker, Single Chamber |
| 5—Pacemaker, Single Chamber, Rate Responsive |
| 6—Pacemaker, Dual Chamber |
| 7—Cardiac Resynchronization Pacemaker Pulse Generator |
| 7—Autologous Tissue Substitute |
| 8—Defibrillator Generator |
| 9—Cardiac Resynchronization Pacemaker Defibrillator Pulse Generator |

A—Contractility Modulation Device
B—Stimulator Generator, Single Array
C—Stimulator Generator, Single Array Rechargeable
D—Stimulator Generator, Multiple Array
E—Stimulator Generator, Multiple Array Rechargeable
F – Subcutaneous Defibrillator Lead
H—Contraceptive Device
J—Synthetic Substitute
K—Nonautologous Tissue Substitute
M—Stimulator Generator
N—Tissue expander
P—Cardiac Rhythm Related Device
V—Infusion Device, Pump
W—Vascular Access Device, Totally implantable
X—Vascular Access Device, Tunneled
Y—Other Device
Z—No Device

Source: CMS 2019

Qualifier

Character 7 specifies an additional attribute of the procedure, if applicable. The qualifier characters used to code procedures performed on Subcutaneous Tissue and Fascia are as shown in table 15.10.

Table 15.10.   **Qualifiers used to code procedures on the Subcutaneous Tissue and Fascia**

B—Skin and Subcutaneous Tissue
C—Skin, Subcutaneous Tissue and Fascia
X—Diagnostic
Z—No Qualifier

Source: CMS 2019

Specific Operations on Skin and Subcutaneous Tissue

Commonly performed operations on skin and subcutaneous tissue include excision of skin and subcutaneous lesions and skin grafting as well as the insertion of infusion pumps and totally implantable vascular access devices for chemotherapy or other long-term infusion.

Excision of skin lesions is coded using the root operation Excision or cutting out or off, without replacement, a portion of a body part from the root operation Table 0HB. An excision of skin is usually done for therapeutic purposes to remove a known diseased lesion. A skin biopsy is also a common procedure; however, a biopsy is a diagnostic procedure and would be identified with an Excision ICD-10-PCS code with the qualifier X for Diagnostic.

Table 0HT, for Resection or cutting out or off, without replacement, all of a body part, does not contain the body part of Skin because it is not possible to perform a resection of the skin as all of the skin could not possibly be included. Body parts in the integumentary system that could be resected or completely removed are finger- and toenails, a breast, or a breast nipple. For example, the resection of the left breast would be coded 0HTU0ZZ in the Medical and Surgical section.

Excision of subcutaneous tissue and fascia is coded using the root operation Excision (0JB), but there is no table for Resection of subcutaneous tissue because it is not possible to cut out or off, without replacement, all of that body part, which is the definition of Resection.

Skin grafting is described with the root operation Replacement when a full-thickness or partial-thickness graft is performed on the skin. If a skin substitute is grafted into place on the skin, the root operation Supplement would describe the objective of the procedure, that is, putting in or on biological or synthetic material that physically reinforces or augments the function of a portion of a body part.

Insertion of infusion pumps and totally implantable vascular access devices is coded to the root operation of Insertion for subcutaneous tissue. There is no option to insert a device into the skin. The type of device left in place is identified with the character 6 for the device. The choices for devices implanted in the subcutaneous tissue are an Infusion Pump device, Vascular Access Device Totally Implantable, and Vascular Access Device, Tunneled.

Debridement

Debridement is the removal of foreign material and contaminated or devitalized tissue from, or adjacent to, a traumatic or infected lesion until the surrounding healthy tissue is exposed (Dorland 2012, 473). There is no root operation in ICD-10-PCS of simply the term "debridement."

ICD-10-PCS classifies debridement depending on whether it was identified as excisional or nonexcisional debridement. Following the main term "Debridement" in the ICD-10-PCS Index, the entry of Debridement, excisional sends the coder to the entry for the root operation Excision. If the debridement was described as nonexcisional debridement, the Index sends the coder to the entry for the root operation Extraction. The physician is responsible for describing the debridement as excisional or nonexcisional.

For excisional debridement, the entry in the Index is the main term "Excision," with a subterm of "skin," and it refers the coder to Table 0HB. The code is constructed based on where the excisional procedure is performed on the skin, that is, what body part's skin. A excisional debridement must be documented as excisional by the person who performs the debridement. This procedure may be performed in an operating room, treatment room or at bedside by a provider with training and credentials required for this type of procedure. The entries in the Index for Excision of "subcutaneous tissue and fascia" procedures direct the coder to Table 0JB to select a code for the Excision of subcutaneous tissue for the debridement according to the part body where the surgery is performed.

For nonexcisional debridement, the entry in the Index is the main term "extraction, skin," and it refers the coder to Table 0HD for skin and Table 0JD for subcutaneous tissue and fascia, respectively. Similar to the excisional procedures, the extraction procedures are constructed using the body part where the skin or subcutaneous tissue is removed with a nonexcision debridement procedure. Non-excisional debridement is considered an non-operative procedure such as brushing scrubbing, irrigation or washing of devitalized tissue, necrosis, foreign material or slough. This is pulling or stripping out of tissue. This procedure is likely performed in a treatment room or at bedside, but the location of the procedure on wounds has no influence on whether a procedure is excisional or non-excisional.

ICD-10-CM and ICD-10-PCS Review Exercises: Chapter 15

Assign the correct ICD-10-CM diagnosis and ICD-10-PCS procedure codes to the following exercises.

1. Actinic keratosis, right temple due to exposure to man-made sunlight from a tanning bed (external cause) (initial encounter)

2. Hidradenitis suppurativa, bilateral axilla

3. Localized primary hyperhidrosis of the axilla

4. Stage 4 pressure ulcer of the sacrum

5. Pilonidal cyst with abscess

6. The patient was seen for initial treatment of a fine rash that had developed on the patient's trunk over the last three to four days. The patient was diagnosed with hypertension seven days ago and started on ramipril 10 mg daily. The physician determined the rash to be dermatitis due to the ramipril. The ramipril was discontinued, and the patient was prescribed a new antihypertensive medication, captopril. In addition, the physician prescribed a topical cream for the localized dermatitis.

7. The patient was seen with extensive inflammation and irritation of the skin of both upper eyelids and under her eyebrows that was spreading to her temples and forehead. Upon questioning the patient, the physician learned that she had recently used new eye cosmetics. The physician had examined the patient during a prior visit for cystic acne. The patient's condition was diagnosed as irritant contact dermatitis due to cosmetics. During this visit, the physician also examined the patient's cystic acne on her forehead and jawline. The patient was advised to continue using the medication previously prescribed. The patient was also advised to immediately discontinue use of any makeup on the face and was given a topical medication to resolve the inflammation, which was an adverse effect of the cosmetics.

(Continued on next page)

ICD-10-CM and ICD-10-PCS Review Exercises: Chapter 15 *(continued)*

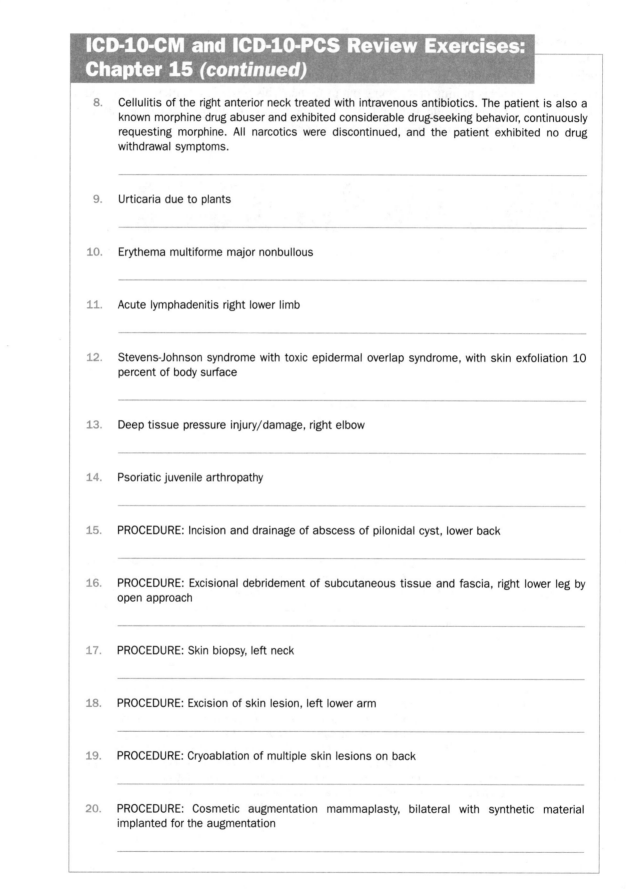

8. Cellulitis of the right anterior neck treated with intravenous antibiotics. The patient is also a known morphine drug abuser and exhibited considerable drug-seeking behavior, continuously requesting morphine. All narcotics were discontinued, and the patient exhibited no drug withdrawal symptoms.

9. Urticaria due to plants

10. Erythema multiforme major nonbullous

11. Acute lymphadenitis right lower limb

12. Stevens-Johnson syndrome with toxic epidermal overlap syndrome, with skin exfoliation 10 percent of body surface

13. Deep tissue pressure injury/damage, right elbow

14. Psoriatic juvenile arthropathy

15. PROCEDURE: Incision and drainage of abscess of pilonidal cyst, lower back

16. PROCEDURE: Excisional debridement of subcutaneous tissue and fascia, right lower leg by open approach

17. PROCEDURE: Skin biopsy, left neck

18. PROCEDURE: Excision of skin lesion, left lower arm

19. PROCEDURE: Cryoablation of multiple skin lesions on back

20. PROCEDURE: Cosmetic augmentation mammaplasty, bilateral with synthetic material implanted for the augmentation

References

American College of Allergy, Asthma, and Immunology (ACAAI). 2018. Hives (Urticaria). http://acaai.org/allergies/types/skin-allergies/hives-urticaria.

Centers for Disease Control and Prevention (CDC), National Center for Health Statistics (NCHS). 2019. *ICD-10-CM Official Guidelines for Coding and Reporting*, 2020. http://www.cdc.gov/nchs/icd/icd10cm.htm or https://www.cdc.gov/nchs/data/icd/10cmguidelines-FY2020_final.pdf.

Centers for Medicare and Medicaid Services (CMS). 2019. *ICD-10-PCS Official Guidelines for Coding and Reporting*, 2020. http://www.cms.gov/Medicare/Coding/ICD10/.

Dorland, W.A.N., ed. 2012. *Dorland's Illustrated Medical Dictionary*, 32nd ed. Philadelphia: Elsevier Saunders.

Mosby. 2017. *Mosby's Pocket Dictionary of Medicine, Nursing, and Health Professions*, 8th ed. St. Louis: Mosby, Inc.

National Pressure Ulcer Advisory Panel. 2016. National Pressure Ulcer Advisory Panel (NPUAP) announces a change in terminology from pressure ulcer to pressure injury and updates the stages of pressure injury. Website accessed July 2019 : https://npuap.org/page/PressureInjuryStages?&hhsearchterms=%22staging%22.

Skin Cancer Foundation. 2018. Actinic Keratosis. http://www.skincancer.org/skin-cancer-information/actinic-keratosis.

Stedman, T. 2012. *Stedman's Medical Dictionary for the Health Professions and Nursing*, 7th ed. Philadelphia: Wolters Kluwer/Lippincott Williams & Wilkins.

Chapter 16

Diseases of the Musculoskeletal System and Connective Tissue (M00–M99)

Learning Objectives

At the conclusion of this chapter, you should be able to do the following:

- Describe the organization of the conditions and codes included in Chapter 13 of ICD-10-CM, Diseases of the Musculoskeletal System and Connective Tissue (M00–M99)

- Summarize the classification of rheumatoid arthritis and osteoarthritis

- Identify the coding of various types of deforming dorsopathies

- Define the two types of *compartment syndrome*

- Explain the classification of different forms of osteoporosis

- Define and differentiate between coding of *pathologic, malunion, nonunion,* and *stress* fractures

- Summarize the classification of different types of osteomyelitis

- Explain the ICD-10-PCS coding of arthroscopic surgery and joint replacement procedures

- Assign ICD-10-CM codes for diseases of the musculoskeletal system and connective tissue

- Assign ICD-10-PCS codes for procedures related to diseases of the musculoskeletal system and connective tissue

Key Terms

Ankylosis	Direct infection of joint
Arthroscope	Felty's syndrome
Compartment syndrome	Indirect infection of joint

Kyphosis
Lordosis
Malunion
Nonunion
Osteoarthritis
Osteomyelitis
Osteoporosis
Pathologic fracture
Polyosteoarthritis
Primary osteoarthritis

Rheumatism
Rheumatoid arthritis
Scoliosis
Secondary osteoarthritis
Spinal stenosis
Spondylopathy
Spondylosis
Stress fracture
Systemic lupus erythematosus (SLE)

Overview of ICD-10-CM Chapter 13: Diseases of the Musculoskeletal System and Connective Tissue

Chapter 13 of ICD-10-CM includes categories M00–M99 arranged in the following blocks:

M00–M02	Infectious arthropathies
M04	Autoinflammatory syndromes
M05–M14	Inflammatory polyarthropathies
M15–M19	Osteoarthritis
M20–M25	Other joint disorders
M26–M27	Dentofacial anomalies [including malocclusion] and other disorders of jaw
M30–M36	Systemic connective tissue disorders
M40–M43	Deforming dorsopathies
M45–M49	Spondylopathies
M50–M54	Other dorsopathies
M60–M63	Disorders of muscles
M65–M67	Disorders of synovium and tendon
M70–M79	Other soft tissue disorders
M80–M85	Disorders of bone density and structure
M86–M90	Other osteopathies
M91–M94	Chondropathies
M95	Other disorders of the musculoskeletal system and connective tissue
M96	Intraoperative and postprocedural complications and disorders of musculoskeletal system, not elsewhere classified
M97	Periprosthetic fracture around internal prosthetic joint
M99	Biomechanical lesions, not elsewhere classified

The codes in Chapter 13 of ICD-10-CM include anatomic specificity and laterality of the condition being classified.

EXAMPLES:	M23.011,	Cystic meniscus, anterior horn of medial meniscus, right knee
	M89.151,	Complete physeal arrest, right proximal femur

Instructional notes indicate that additional codes should be assigned for associated conditions and that underlying conditions should be coded first.

EXAMPLES: Arthritis of right hip due to staphylococcal infection
M00.051,   Staphylococcal arthritis, right hip
Use additional code (B95.61–B95.8) to identify bacterial agent
B95.8,   Unspecified *Staphylococcus* as the cause of diseases classified elsewhere

Arthropathy of left hip due to erythema multiforme
L51.9,   Erythema multiforme, Unspecified
Use additional code to identify associated manifestation, such as:
Arthropathy associated with dermatological disorders (M14.8-)
M14.852,   Arthropathies in other specified diseases classified elsewhere, left hip. Code first underlying disease, such as:
Erythema multiforme (L15.1-)

Another example of specificity in ICD-10-CM is the coding of osteoporosis. The type of osteoporosis including the site of a current pathological fracture is present in one combination code in Chapter 13. Category M80, Osteoporosis with current pathological fracture, combines three facts into one code: the type of osteoporosis, the site of the fracture including laterality, and the episode of care to identify the status of the patient's treatment, for example, initial versus subsequent encounter.

EXAMPLE: Pathological fracture of right humerus due to age-related osteoporosis, initial encounter for fracture
M80.021A,   Age-related osteoporosis with current pathological fracture, right humerus

Some categories and subcategories in diseases of the musculoskeletal system and connective tissue require the use of a seventh character to identify the episode of care, for example, initial encounter for fracture and subsequent encounter for fracture with routine healing, delayed healing, nonunion, or malunion in addition to sequelae of the disease.

EXAMPLE: Patient seen in the physician's office for a subsequent encounter to the stress fracture of the left tibia with routine healing
M84.362D,   Stress fracture, left tibia, subsequent encounter for fracture with routine healing

Coding Guidelines and Instructional Notes for ICD-10-CM Chapter 13

Chapter 13 begins with a note to "use an external cause code following the code for the musculoskeletal condition, if applicable, to identify the cause of the musculoskeletal condition" (CDC 2019). An Excludes2 note identifies the other conditions, such as certain infectious, parasitic, and neoplastic diseases, that can be coded with diseases of the musculoskeletal system and connective tissue.

The first block of codes in the chapter, M00–M02, are for infectious arthropathies, which include arthropathies due to microbiological agents. To assist coding professionals on the correct usage of categories M00–M02, an instructional note in the ICD-10-CM classification provides definitions for direct and indirect infection:

- **Direct infection of joint**, where organisms invade synovial tissue and microbial antigen is present in the joint.

- **Indirect infection of joint**, which may be of two types: a reactive arthropathy, where microbial infection of the body is established but neither organisms nor antigens can be identified in the joint, and a postinfective arthropathy, where microbial antigen is present but recovery of an organism is inconstant and evidence of local multiplication is lacking (CDC 2019).

Instructional notes are added to different categories or subcategories to explain how codes should be assigned.

EXAMPLE:	M21.7,	Unequal limb length (acquired)
		Note: The site used should correspond to the shorter limb.
	M50,	Cervical disc disorders
		Note: Code to the most superior level of disorder.

Includes notes are also used to define terms.

EXAMPLE:	M66,	Spontaneous rupture of synovium and tendon
		Includes: rupture that occurs when a normal force is applied to tissues that are inferred to have less than normal strength.
	M70,	Soft tissue disorders related to use, overuse and pressure
		Includes soft tissue disorders of occupational origin
	M80,	Osteoporosis with current pathological fracture
		Includes osteoporosis with current fragility fracture
	M87,	Osteonecrosis
		Includes avascular necrosis of bone

The NCHS has published chapter-specific guidelines for Chapter 13 in the *ICD-10-CM Official Guidelines for Coding and Reporting*. The coding student should review all of the coding guidelines for Chapter 13 of ICD-10-CM that appear in an ICD-10-CM code book or on the CDC website (CDC 2019) or in appendix F.

CG

Chapter 13: Diseases of the Musculoskeletal System and Connective Tissue (M00-M99)

Guideline I.C.13.a. Site and laterality: Most of the codes within Chapter 13 have site and laterality designations. The site represents the bone, joint or the muscle involved. For some conditions where more than one bone, joint or muscle is usually involved, such as osteoarthritis, there is a "multiple sites" code available. For categories where no multiple site code is provided and more than one bone, joint or muscle is involved, multiple codes should be used to indicate the different sites involved.

Guideline I.C.13.a.1 Bone versus joint: For certain conditions, the bone may be affected at the upper or lower end, (e.g., avascular necrosis of bone, M87, Osteoporosis, M80, M81). Though the portion of the bone affected may be at the joint, the site designation will be the bone, not the joint.

Guideline I.C.13.b. Acute traumatic versus chronic or recurrent musculoskeletal conditions: Many musculoskeletal conditions are a result of previous injury or trauma to a site, or are recurrent conditions. Bone, joint or muscle conditions that are the result of a healed injury are usually found in chapter 13. Recurrent bone, joint or muscle conditions are also usually found in chapter 13. Any current, acute injury should be coded to the appropriate injury code from chapter 19. Chronic or recurrent conditions should generally be coded with a code from chapter 13. If it is difficult to determine from the documentation in the record which code is best to describe a condition, query the provider.

Guideline I.C.13.c. Coding of Pathologic Fractures: 7th character A is for use as long as the patient is receiving active treatment for the fracture. While the patient may be seen by a new or different provider over the course of treatment for a pathological fracture, assignment of the 7th character is based on whether the patient is undergoing active treatment and not whether the provider is seeing the patient for the first time.

7th character, D is to be used for encounters after the patient has completed active treatment for the fracture and is receiving routine care for the fracture during the healing or recovery phase. The other 7th characters, listed under each subcategory

(Continued)

(Continued)

in the Tabular List, are to be used for subsequent encounters for treatment of problems associated with healing, such as malunions, nonunions, and sequelae.

Care for complications of surgical treatment for fracture repairs during the healing or recovery phase should be coded with the appropriate complication codes.

See Section I.C.19. Coding of traumatic fractures.

Guideline I.C.13.d. Osteoporosis: Osteoporosis is a systemic condition, meaning that all bones of the musculoskeletal system are affected. Therefore, site is not a component of the codes under category M81, Osteoporosis without current pathological fracture. The site codes under category M80, Osteoporosis with current pathological fracture, identify the site of the fracture, not the osteoporosis.

Guideline I.C.13.d.1 Osteoporosis without pathological fracture: Category M81, Osteoporosis without current pathological fracture, is for use for patients with osteoporosis who do not currently have a pathologic fracture due to the osteoporosis, even if they have had a fracture in the past. For patients with a history of osteoporosis fractures, status code Z87.310, Personal history of (healed) osteoporosis fracture, should follow the code from M81.

Guideline I.C.d.2 Osteoporosis with current pathological fracture: Category M80, Osteoporosis with current pathological fracture, is for patients who have a current pathologic fracture at the time of an encounter. The codes under M80 identify the site of the fracture. A code from category M80, not a traumatic fracture code, should be used for any patient with known osteoporosis who suffers a fracture, even if the patient had a minor fall or trauma, if that fall or trauma would not usually break a normal, healthy bone.

Coding Diseases of the Musculoskeletal System and Connective Tissue in ICD-10-CM Chapter 13

Chapter 13 of ICD-10-CM, Diseases of the Musculoskeletal System and Connective Tissue (M00–M99), describes many acute and chronic conditions of bones, joints, ligaments, muscles, and intervertebral discs. Another mnemonic is found in this chapter: M codes for

Musculoskeletal. Figure 16.1 shows anterior and posterior views of the bones that constitute the skeletal system of the body.

Figure 16.1. **Bones of the body**

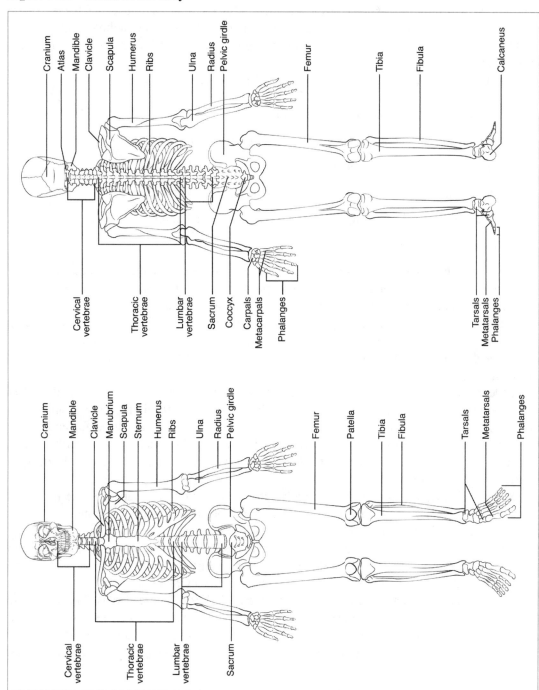

© AHIMA

Most of the codes in Chapter 13 include site and laterality. The site indicates the bone, joint, or muscle involved. For example, there are codes for stress fracture of right tibia (M84.361), rheumatoid bursitis of left shoulder (M06.212), and muscle spasm of back (M62.830).

Seventh Characters

 Some current musculoskeletal conditions in Chapter 13 are the result of a previous injury or trauma to a site, and others are recurrent conditions. Any acute injury is coded using a different chapter in ICD-10-CM. However, some fractures that are included in Chapter 13 are current events. Examples of exceptions are stress fractures (M84.3) and pathological fractures (M84.4–M84.6). These fracture codes require an appropriate seventh character to identify the episode of care.

The following seventh characters are used in Chapter 13:

- A indicates initial encounter for the fracture.

- D indicates subsequent encounter for fracture with routine healing.

- G indicates subsequent encounter for fracture with delayed healing.

- K indicates subsequent encounter for fracture with nonunion.

- P indicates subsequent encounter for fracture with malunion.

- S indicates sequela.

Seventh character A is for use for each encounter where the patient is receiving active treatment for the fracture or condition. While the patient may be seen by a new or different provider over the course of treatment for a fracture, assignment of the seventh character is based on whether the provider is undergoing active treatment and not whether the provider is seeing the patient for the first time. For complication codes, active treatment refers to treatment for the condition described by the code, even though it may be related to an earlier precipitating problem.

Seventh character D is to be used for encounters with the physician or at a facility after the patient has completed active treatment of the condition and is receiving routine care for the condition during the healing or recovery phase. Seventh character G is used for encounters when the patient is seen during a subsequent visit to the physician or at a facility and it determined to have delayed healing of the fracture or for continued management of the delayed healing of the fracture.

Seventh character K is used to describe a subsequent visit by the patient to the physician or at a facility when it is determined there is a failure of normal healing, a nonunion, of the fractured bone or for treatment of the nonunion of the fracture.

Seventh character P is used to describe a subsequent visit by the patient to the physician or at a facility when it is determined there is a malunion of the fracture when the ends of the fracture bone do not align properly resulting in a deformity in the bone.

These seventh characters for the episode of care in ICD-10-CM are also used for traumatic fractures coded in Chapter 19. Code extensions such as the seventh character letters are defined in the *ICD-10-CM Official Guidelines for Coding and Reporting* specifically in chapter-specific guidelines (Chapter 19) for injury, poisoning, and certain other consequences of external causes.

Rheumatoid Arthritis (M05–M06)

Rheumatoid arthritis is a systemic disease that affects the connective tissue in the body. The disease manifests as arthritis involving many joints, especially those in the extremities, arms, and legs. It is a chronic, crippling condition that may become progressively worse leading to joint deformities and overall disability (Stedman 2012, 1465). Periods of remission and exacerbation occur in afflicted patients. Although the exact etiology is unknown, immunologic changes and tissue hypersensitivity, complicated by a cold and damp climate, may have a contributory effect. The synovial membranes are primarily affected. The joints become inflamed, swollen, and painful, as well as stiff and tender. During an active period of rheumatoid arthritis, the patient suffers from malaise, fever, and sweating. Diagrams of the bones and joints in the elbow, wrist, and ankle are shown in figures 16.2, 16.3, and 16.4.

Figure 16.2. **Elbow joint**

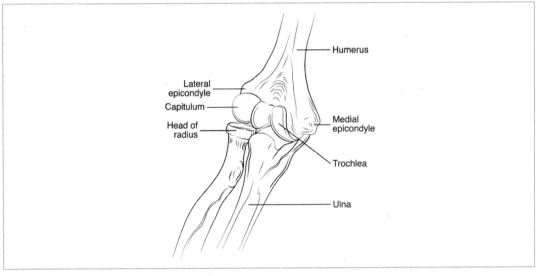

© AHIMA

Figure 16.3. **Wrist joint**

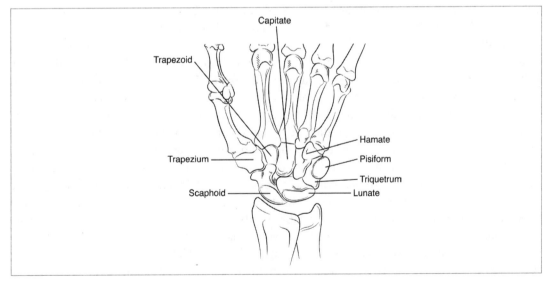

© AHIMA

Figure 16.4. **Ankle joint**

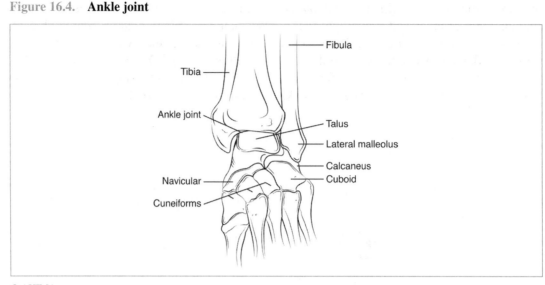

© AHIMA

ICD-10-CM classifies rheumatoid arthritis to the following categories:

M05	Rheumatoid arthritis with rheumatoid factor
M06	Other rheumatoid arthritis
M08	Juvenile arthritis

Category M05 includes **Felty's syndrome** (M05.0-), that is, rheumatoid arthritis with splenoadenomegaly (enlargement of the spleen) and leukopenia (decrease in the number of white blood cells in the circulating blood) (Stedman 2012, 962, 1576). Rheumatoid arthritis may also exist with rheumatoid lung disease (M05.1-). Rheumatoid lung disease is a group of lung conditions that may include any of the following: blockage of the small airways, pleural effusion, pulmonary hypertension, lung nodules, and pulmonary fibrosis (Dorland 2012, 542). Other subcategories in M05 include rheumatoid arthritis with vasculitis, heart disease, myopathy, and polyneuropathy with and without involvement of other organs and systems.

Category M06 classifies rheumatoid arthritis without rheumatoid factor. This category includes bursitis, joint nodule, polyarthropathy, and other specified conditions that are caused by the rheumatoid condition. Juvenile rheumatoid arthritis is classified with category M08.

Subcategories for M08 include juvenile rheumatoid arthritis with systemic onset, which may also be documented as Still's disease. The codes within M06 and M08 include the specific joint and the laterality. Because juvenile arthritis is often associated with other conditions, a "code also" note appears under category M08 to advise the coder to code also any associate condition, such as regional enteritis or ulcerative colitis.

The diagnosis of **rheumatism** can be classified in ICD-10-CM with code M79.0, Rheumatism, unspecified. The medical term of rheumatism is a popular name for any of a variety of disorders marked by inflammation, degeneration, or metabolic derangement of connective tissue structures of the body, especially the joints and related structures, including muscles, bursae, tendons, and fibrous tissue, with pain, stiffness, or limitation of motion. Rheumatism confined to the joints is more precisely called arthritis. While the code is valid, the code is nondescriptive of a patient's condition, and the physician should be asked to be more specific if possible (Dorland 2012, 1639).

> **EXAMPLE:** The patient was seen in the physician's office for treatment of rheumatoid arthritis present in the joints in both hands and both wrists. The diagnoses would be coded as follows:
> M06.841, Rheumatoid arthritis, right hand
> M06.842, Rheumatoid arthritis, left hand
> M06.831, Rheumatoid arthritis, right wrist
> M06.832, Rheumatoid arthritis, left wrist

Osteoarthritis (M15–M19)

Osteoarthritis is the most common type of arthritis. It is a disease of the joints that mainly affects the cartilage in the joint. Cartilage is the tissue that covers the ends of the bones; it glides over each bone, allowing smooth movements and absorbing the shock of motion. However, the cartilage can break down and wear away. When the cartilage is thin or absent, the bones under the cartilage rub together and create friction. The friction causes swelling, pain, and stiffness. This friction leads to deformity of the joint, which loses its normal shape. Bone spurs develop, and pieces of bone or cartilage break off and float in the joint space. This creates more pain and joint damage. Osteoarthritis occurs over time as a person ages, but younger people can acquire osteoarthritis from joint injuries or the stress on joints from certain occupations or playing sports. Osteoarthritis can develop in any joint, but the most common joints it occurs in are the hands, knees, hips, and spine, specifically the neck or low back (NIAMS 2014; Stacy 2016).

Illustrations of the joints that are commonly treated for osteoarthritis are shown in figure 16.5, shoulder joint; figure 16.6, hip joint; and figure 16.7, knee joint.

Figure 16.5. **Shoulder joint**

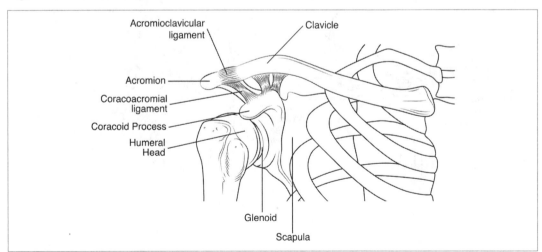

© AHIMA

Figure 16.6. **Hip joint**

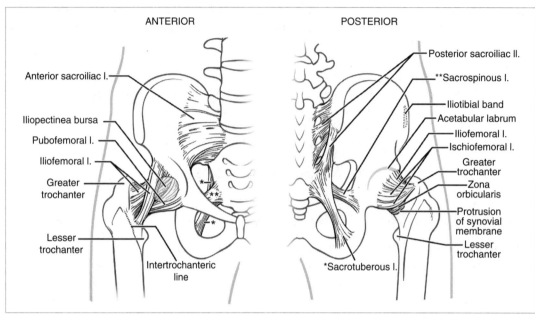

© AHIMA

Figure 16.7. **Knee joint**

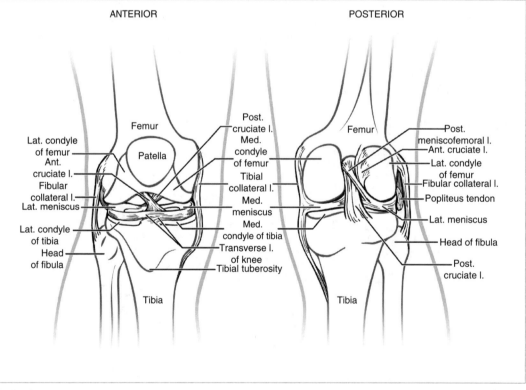

© AHIMA

Categories in this block of codes include **polyosteoarthritis** (M15), which is used to classify arthritis of multiple sites that may be described as generalized arthritis or osteoarthritis. Categories M16, M17, and M18 classify the common sites of the condition in the hip, knee, and carpometacarpal joints. Codes identify bilateral and unilateral conditions with laterality included. The osteoarthritis in these codes is described as primary, secondary, or posttraumatic.

Primary osteoarthritis is not caused by another disease; instead, it is usually related to the aging process but could also be related to unrecognized congenital or developmental defects. Alternatively, it may be idiopathic or have an unknown cause. **Secondary osteoarthritis** is a degenerative disease of the joints that results from a predisposing factor, usually trauma, that damages the cartilage or subchondral bone of the affected joints. Secondary osteoarthritis usually occurs in younger individuals (Derrer 2018).

Check Your Understanding 16.1

Assign diagnosis codes to the following conditions.

1. Rheumatoid arthritis, both hands with rheumatoid factor seropositive. No other organ or system involvement

2. Acute gouty attack, primary type, right knee

3. Posttraumatic osteoarthritis of right knee

4. Recurrent dislocation of patella, left

5. Pain and muscle weakness right shoulder

Systemic Connective Tissue Disorders (M30–M36)

Systemic connective tissue disorders includes autoimmune and collagen vascular disease. It does not include autoimmune disease of a single organ or cell type. The categories here include polyarteritis nodosa and related conditions (M30), other necrotizing vasculopathies (M31), systemic lupus erythematous (M32), dermatopolymyositis (M33), systemic sclerosis or scleroderma (M34), and other systemic involvement of connective tissue (M35).

EXAMPLE Examples of systemic connective tissue disorders are as follows:
M30.0, Polyarteritis nodosa
M31.5, Giant cell arteritis with polymyalgia rheumatic
M32.10, Systemic lupus erythematosus, organ or site involvement unspecified
M33.21, Polymyositis with respiratory involvement
M34.81, Systemic sclerosis with lung involvement
M35.6, Relapsing panniculitis

Systemic Lupus Erythematosus (M32)

Systemic lupus erythematosus (SLE) is a chronic, inflammatory, multisystem disorder of connective tissue disorder involving the skin, joints, kidneys, and serosal membranes. The etiology is unknown but may be an autoimmune disease. SLE produces a variety of conditions including arthritis, nephritis, pleurisy, pericarditis, leukopenia, thrombocytopenia, hemolytic anemia, and a distinctive cell in the blood called LE cells. The condition can exhibit acute manifestations of the disease in a relapse of the disease but also move into remission for periods of time. SLE is not the same condition as discoid lupus erythematosus (L93.0), which is a disease strictly of the skin and subcutaneous tissue, characterized by skin plaques with edema, erythema, scaliness, and skin atrophy surrounded by erythematous borders (Dorland 2012, 1079–1080).

ICD-10-CM classifies SLE that is not specified further to code M32.9. When the diagnosis of SLE is more specific with the specific organ or diagnosis included, subcategory M32.1 is used. Codes to the fifth-character level identify when endocarditis, pericarditis, and lung and renal disease occur as the result of the systemic lupus erythematosus.

EXAMPLE: M32.12, Pericarditis in systemic lupus erythematosus
M32.13, Pleural effusion due to systemic lupus erythematosus
M32.14, Systemic lupus erythematosus with renal disease

Check Your Understanding 16.2

Assign diagnosis codes to the following conditions.

1. Giant cell arteritis with polymyalgia rheumatica

2. Sjögren syndrome with lung involvement

3. Multiple sites of arthropathy in patient with multiple myeloma

4. Systemic lupus erythematosus with endocarditis (Libman-Sacks disease)

5. Kawasaki disease/syndrome

Dorsopathies (M40–M54)

The dorsopathies section (M40–M54) contains codes describing deforming dorsopathies, spondylopathies, and other dorsopathies. The codes are specific to the regions of the cervical, thoracic, lumbar, and sacral spine. Two diagrams of the vertebrae and the vertebral joint are shown in figures 16.8 and 16.9.

Figure 16.8. **Vertebra**

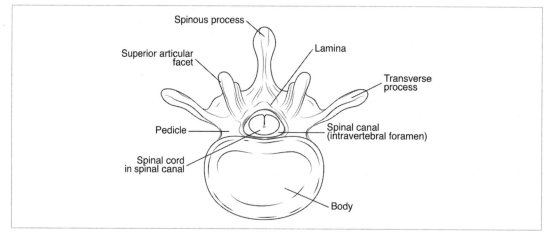

© AHIMA

Figure 16.9. **Posterior view of lumbar vertebral joint**

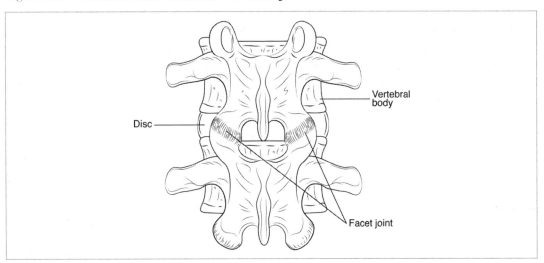

Disc

Vertebral body

Facet joint

© AHIMA

Deforming Dorsopathies (M40–M43)

Conditions within the Deforming Dorsopathies section of codes, as described by the title, are deformities of the back. Three common deformities of the spine are curvatures described in the following paragraph.

Kyphosis (M40.0 to M40.2) is a rounding or outward curve of the thoracic spine that may be described as a hunchback or slouching posture. It can occur at any age but is not usually present at birth. A different form of the condition is adolescent kyphosis, also known as Scheuermann's disease, which is classified to M42.00–M42.19. In adults, kyphosis is usually caused by osteoporotic fracture, injuries to the spine, degenerative arthritis, disc diseases of the spine, or the slipping of one vertebra (spondylolisthesis) (NLM 2019a).

Lordosis (M40.4- to M40.5-) is the inward curvature of the lumbar spine. A layman's term for the condition is swayback. It is an anterior curvature where the abdomen appears to protrude and the buttocks appear more prominent (NLM 2019b).

Scoliosis (M41.0- to M41.9) is a sideways curvature of the spine. In imaging views, the curves may appear S shaped or C shaped. The diagnosis is frequently made in middle school age children and young teenagers and is known to occur in multiple generations of families. For an unknown reason, the curvature is more common in girls than it is in boys. Sometimes the curve is temporary, and growth seems to straighten the spine. Other children benefit from wearing a brace to correct the curvature (NLM 2019c).

> **EXAMPLES:** M41.116, Idiopathic juvenile scoliosis of the lumbar region
> M40.204, Kyphosis of the thoracic region
> M40.57, Lordosis of the lumbosacral region

Spondylopathies (M45–M49)

Spondylopathy is any disorder of the spinal vertebrae (Dorland 2012, 1754). **Ankylosis** is an abnormal immobility and consolidation of a joint due to disease, injury, or surgical procedure (Dorland 2012, 94). **Spondylosis** is ankylosis of the vertebral joint or degenerative spinal changes due to osteoarthritis (Dorland 2012, 1754). Ankylosing spondylitis is a common condition of the spine and is classified with category M45 according to the region of the spine that is involved. Spondylosis is classified by category M47 according to the region (cervical, thoracic, lumbar, lumbosacral) and whether or not it occurs with myelopathy or radiculopathy. Another common spondylopathy is spinal stenosis, which is classified in ICD-10-CM according to the location of the stenosis (M48.00–M48.08). **Spinal stenosis** is a narrowing of the spaces in between the vertebrae of the spine. This narrowing creates pressure on the spinal cord and the nerves and causes pain. Spinal stenosis usually occurs in individuals after the age of 50. Arthritis and scoliosis can cause spinal stenosis (NLM 2019d).

> **EXAMPLES:** M45.2, Ankylosing spondylitis of cervical region
> M47.014, Anterior spinal artery compression syndromes, thoracic region
> M48.07, Spinal stenosis, lumbosacral region

Compartment Syndrome (M79.A-)

A **compartment syndrome** or compartmental syndrome is a serious condition in which increased pressure exists within a muscle compartment. Within in the arms and the legs, layers of fascia separate the muscle groups. Within this fascia, there are confined spaces called compartments. In the compartments, the fascia surrounds the muscles, nerves, and blood vessels to protect them. This fascia is thick and does not expand in order to shield the area. When disease or injury causes swelling in a compartment, there will be increased pressure in the area. This swelling puts pressure on the muscles, nerves, and blood vessels. If the pressure is great enough, blood will be restricted from the compartment. The loss of circulation in the compartment can lead to permanent damage to the muscles and nerves, including necrosis and tissue damage that could lead to an amputation of the limb (NLM 2019e). When the physician determines the compartment pressure is rising, the physician is likely to request a surgical consultation from a surgeon as a fasciotomy to relieve the compartment pressure is often indicated.

Traumatic compartment syndrome occurs when swelling occurs from trauma such as a car accident or a crush injury. Swelling can also be caused by complex fractures and soft tissue injuries due to trauma. Nontraumatic compartment syndrome producing increased pressure within a muscle compartment may also be called long-term or chronic compartment syndrome. This may also be known as exertional compartment syndrome. This is not caused by one traumatic event but rather is caused by repetitive activities such as running or other athletic activities. The pressure in a muscle compartment only increases during the activity. This type of compartment syndrome is most common in the lower leg and forearm but can also occur in the hand, foot, thigh, and upper arm. Other traumatic and nontraumatic forms of compartment syndrome may be caused by external compression or soft tissue swelling such as edema or hematoma. Some specific causes are burns, frostbite, snakebite, postsurgical edema or hemorrhage, hemophilia, and anticoagulant therapy (NLM 2019e).

Nontraumatic compartment syndrome is coded based on its location in the body, that is, M79.A1- for upper extremity, M79.A2- for lower extremity, M79.A3 for abdomen, and M79. A8- for other sites. Traumatic compartment syndrome is recognized as an early complication of trauma and is coded within the injury section of ICD-10-CM. Specific codes exist in the range of T79.A- depending on the location of the compartment syndrome following trauma.

> **EXAMPLES:** T79.A21, Traumatic compartment syndrome of right lower leg
> M79.A2, Non-traumatic compartment syndrome of right lower leg

---

Check Your Understanding 16.3

Assign diagnosis codes to the following conditions.

1. Spinal stenosis of lumbar region with neurogenic claudication
2. Juvenile scoliosis, idiopathic type, of thoracolumbar spine
3. Nontraumatic compartment syndrome, right lower leg
4. Cervical disc disorder with radiculopathy at C4–C5 level
5. Sciatica with lumbago due to intervertebral disc disorder, lumbosacral region

---

Osteoporosis (M80–M81)

Osteoporosis is the reduction in the quantity of bone or atrophy of skeletal tissue. Osteoporosis occurs in postmenopausal women and elderly men and results in the bone trabeculae becoming scanty, thin, and without osteoclastic resorption. This reduction in bone mineral density can lead to fractures that occur with only minimal trauma (Stedman 2012, 1218).

Category M80, Osteoporosis with current pathological fracture, includes osteoporosis with current fragility fracture. Category M80.0- is age-related osteoporosis with current pathological fracture. Category M80.8- is other osteoporosis with current pathological fracture. Category M80 codes are combination codes that identify the type of osteoporosis such as age-related or other types including drug-induced, idiopathic, osteoporosis of disuse, post-oophorectomy, postsurgical malabsorption, and posttraumatic osteoporosis. The individual codes include site and laterality of the pathological fracture that is present with the osteoporosis. These are pathological fractures as the bone breaks as a result of the osteoporotic nature of the bone. The sites of the fracture may occur at the shoulder, humerus, forearm, hand, femur, lower leg, or ankle and foot. If the patient has a major osseous defect occurring with the osteoporosis, an additional code is used from the series of codes in M89.7-. If there is a drug responsible for inducing the osteoporosis, an additional code for adverse effect to identify the drug (T36–T50 with fifth or sixth character 5) is used with the codes for drug-induced osteoporosis (M80.8-).

Codes in the M80 category require a seventh character to identify the episode of care and if there is another condition occurring with the osteoporosis and pathological fracture. The seventh character options are as follows:

A	Initial encounter for fracture
D	Subsequent encounter for fracture with routine healing
G	Subsequent encounter for fracture with delayed healing
K	Subsequent encounter for fracture with nonunion
P	Subsequent encounter for fracture with malunion
S	Sequela

Malunion of a fracture refers to a fracture that was reduced, but the bone ends did not align properly during the healing process (Stedman 2012, 1011). A malunion is often diagnosed during the healing stages and requires surgical intervention.

Nonunion of a fracture is the failure of the bone ends to align or heal (Stedman 2012, 1167). This usually requires a reopening of the fracture site, with some type of internal fixation and bone grafting performed. Nonunion fractures are often more difficult to treat than a malunion.

The condition of strictly osteoporosis with a current pathological fracture is classified with codes in category M81. The type of osteoporosis is identified at the fourth-character level: age-related osteoporosis, localized osteoporosis, and other osteoporosis that may be drug-induced, idiopathic, osteoporosis of disuse, post-oophorectomy, postsurgical malabsorption, and posttraumatic osteoporosis. The "use additional code" note that appears at the heading of M81 reminds the coder to use a code for any major osseous defect (M89.7-) or personal history of (healed) osteoporosis fracture (Z87.310) if applicable.

EXAMPLE: Two patients were seen in the orthopedic surgeon's office for a follow-up exam following treatment for pathological fractures due to age-related osteoporosis that occurred several weeks ago. Radiology examinations were taken of both patients' fracture sites. The first patient was diagnosed with a malunion of the distal tibia on the left leg and scheduled for an open reduction in the next week. The second patient was diagnosed with a nonunion of the distal radius of the right arm that was treated with a closed reduction six weeks ago. The second patient was scheduled for the insertion of a bone stimulator to the right arm the next day. The diagnoses for these two patients are as follows:

First patient, M80.062P, Age-related osteoporosis with current pathological fracture, left lower leg, subsequent encounter for fracture with malunion.

Second patient, M80.031K, Age-related osteoporosis with current pathological fracture, right forearm, subsequent encounter for fracture with nonunion.

Pathologic and Stress Fractures (M84.3–M84.6)

Pathologic fractures and **stress fractures** are breaks in a bone as a result of disease or repetitive force. These are not traumatic fractures that are the result of an injury or trauma. Coders must be cautious not to confuse the pathologic and stress fractures with the traumatic injuries that cause bones to fracture, which are coded with the traumatic fracture injury codes in ICD-10-CM. A pathologic fracture is a break in the bone due to weakening of the bone structure due to disease, such as a neoplastic tumor (metastatic carcinoma of the bone) or osteoporosis or other bone diseases such as osteomalacia or osteomyelitis (Dorland 2012, 743). In the Alphabetic Index, pathologic fractures are located under the main term, Fracture, pathological.

Stress fractures occur because of repetitive or unusual stress on a bone, such as the fractures that soldiers or athletes who walk or run repeatedly suffer as a result (Dorland 2012, 743). When a stress fracture is first suspected, x-rays are often negative. Days or weeks may pass before the fracture line is visible. However, a presumptive diagnosis is necessary to begin prompt treatment. The terms stress reaction, fatigue fracture, and march fracture are synonymous with stress fracture. ICD-10-CM codes in the range of M84.30–M84.38 identify the site and laterality of the bone that has the stress fracture. In the Alphabetic Index, stress fractures are located under the main term Fracture, traumatic, stress.

Codes in the M84.3- range require a seventh character to identify the episode of care and if there is another condition occurring with the osteoporosis and pathological fracture. The seventh-character options are as follows:

A	Initial encounter for fracture
D	Subsequent encounter for fracture with routine healing
G	Subsequent encounter for fracture with delayed healing
K	Subsequent encounter for fracture with nonunion
P	Subsequent encounter for fracture with malunion
S	Sequela

Pathologic fractures are also classified to several subcategories of M84:

M84.4-	Pathological fracture, not elsewhere classified
M84.5-	Pathological fracture in neoplastic disease
M84.6-	Pathological fracture in other disease

These types of fractures occur in existing diseases such as cancer of the bone and other conditions that can weaken the bone. Pathologic fractures are often spontaneous in nature; however, minor injuries can result in a fracture because the bone is already weakened. Pathologic fractures are reported with subcategory codes from M84.4-, M84.5-, and M84.6- depending on the known or unknown cause. The codes are used as long as the condition is treated and reported with the specific seventh character to indicate the episode of care and if there is a problem with a bone's healing.

> **EXAMPLE:**   M84.363A, Stress fracture, right fibula, initial encounter
> M84.563A, Pathologic fracture, right fibula due to neoplastic disease of bone, initial encounter

Osteomyelitis (M86)

Osteomyelitis is an infection of the bone affecting the metaphyseal area of the long bones caused by bacteria. The bacteria can enter the bone through the bloodstream and at a weakened area. A puncture wound can allow bacteria to spread to a nearby bone. If the patient has a direct injury when the patient has an open fracture, bacteria can invade the bone. Finally, direct contamination of the bone can occur during a joint replacement surgery or open repair of fractures. Most often, osteomyelitis affects the long bones of the legs, the humerus, and vertebrae. Diabetic patients may develop osteomyelitis in the bones of their feet from foot ulcers (Mayo Clinic 2015).

Category M86, Osteomyelitis, is further subdivided to fourth-digit subcategories that describe acute, subacute, or chronic osteomyelitis. The fifth- and sixth-character subclassifications identify the bone involved and its laterality. Codes are also included for unspecified anatomic sites. Two "use additional code" notes appear at the heading of category M86 to remind the coder to use an additional code to identify an infectious agent (B95–B97) or major osseous defect (M89.7-).

> **EXAMPLE:**   Acute osteomyelitis of the tarsus bone in the right foot, due to methicillin susceptible *Staphylococcus aureus* as cause of the disease
> M86.171, Acute osteomyelitis, right ankle and foot
> B95.61, Methicillin susceptible *Staphylococcus aureus* infection as the cause of diseases classified elsewhere

Check Your Understanding 16.4

Assign diagnosis codes to the following conditions.

1. Postmenopausal osteoporosis with pathological fracture, right tarsus of foot

2. Stress fracture of right tibia, emergency room visit for initial treatment

3. Post-oophorectomy osteoporosis

4. Pathological fracture, right radius, follow-up visit, normal healing

5. Major osseous defect, right femur due to osteolysis

ICD-10-PCS Procedure Coding for Musculoskeletal System Procedures

The procedures performed on the structures of the musculoskeletal system appear in the ICD-10-PCS code book in multiple sets of tables that start with the two characters representing the section, followed by five characters representing root operation, body part, approach, device, and qualifier. Operations on the many parts of the musculoskeletal systems are common procedures. ICD-10-PCS contains a large number of procedure codes based on the different parts of the Musculoskeletal system.

The eight sections that describe procedures treating musculoskeletal conditions are as follows:

> Section for Muscles
> > Character 1 is Value 0—Medical and Surgical
> > Character 2 is Value K—Muscles
> Section for Tendons
> > Character 1 is Value 0—Medical and Surgical
> > Character 2 is Value L—Tendons
> Section for Bursae and Ligaments
> > Character 1 is Value 0—Medical and Surgical
> > Character 2 is Value M—Bursae and Ligaments
> Section for Head and Facial Bones
> > Character 1 is Value 0—Medical and Surgical
> > Character 2 is Value N—Head and Facial Bones
> Section for Upper Bones
> > Character 1 is Value 0—Medical and Surgical
> > Character 2 is Value P—Upper Bones
> Section for Lower Bones
> > Character 1 is Value 0—Medical and Surgical
> > Character 2 is Value Q—Lower Bones
> Section for Upper Joints
> > Character 1 is Value 0—Medical and Surgical
> > Character 2 is Value R—Upper Joints
> Section for Lower Joints
> > Character 1 is Value 0—Medical and Surgical
> > Character 2 is Value S—Lower Joints

Source: CMS 2019

The root operations for the various types of procedures that can be performed on bones, joints, muscles, tendons, and ligaments are shown in table 16.1.

Table 16.1.   **Root operations for musculoskeletal procedures**

Site	Root Operations
Muscles 0K2–0KX	Change, Destruction, Division, Drainage, Excision, Extirpation, Insertion, Inspection, Reattachment, Release, Removal, Repair, Replacement, Reposition, Resection, Supplement, Revision, Transfer
Tendons 0L2–0LX	Change, Destruction, Division, Drainage, Excision, Extirpation, Extraction, Insertion, Inspection, Reattachment, Release, Removal, Repair, Replacement, Reposition, Resection, Supplement, Revision, Transfer
Bursae and Ligaments 0M2–0MX	Change, Destruction, Division, Drainage, Excision, Extirpation, Extraction, Insertion, Inspection, Reattachment, Release, Removal, Repair, Reposition, Resection, Supplement, Revision, Transfer
Head and Facial Bones 0N2–0NW	Change, Destruction, Division, Drainage, Excision, Extirpation, Extraction, Insertion, Inspection, Release, Removal, Repair, Replacement, Reposition, Resection, Supplement, Revision
Upper Bones 0P2–0PW	Change, Destruction, Division, Drainage, Excision, Extirpation, Extraction, Insertion, Inspection, Release, Removal, Repair, Replacement, Reposition, Resection, Supplement, Revision
Lower Bones 0Q2–0QW	Change, Destruction, Division, Drainage, Excision, Extirpation, Extraction, Insertion, Inspection, Release, Removal, Repair, Replacement, Reposition, Resection, Supplement, Revision
Upper Joints 0R2–0RW	Change, Destruction, Drainage, Excision, Extirpation, Fusion, Insertion, Inspection, Release, Removal, Repair, Replacement, Reposition, Resection, Supplement, Revision
Lower Joints 0S2–0SW	Change, Destruction, Drainage, Excision, Extirpation, Fusion, Insertion, Inspection, Release, Removal, Repair, Replacement, Reposition, Resection, Supplement, Revision

Source: CMS 2019

Example of a Section for ICD-10-PCS Musculoskeletal Procedure Coding

To demonstrate the structure of the ICD-10-PCS tables for the coding of procedures on the Musculoskeletal system disorders, the following describes the section for lower bones.

Section for Lower Bones

Character 1 is Value 0—Medical and Surgical
Character 2 is Value Q—Lower Bones

Root Operation

Character 3 of the Medical and Surgical section ICD-10-PCS codes is the root operation. The root operations that represent the objectives of procedures for surgical treatment of the diseases of the lower bones are shown in table 16.2.

Table 16.2. **Root operations for procedures on Lower Bones**

Change: Taking out or off a device from a body part and putting back an identical or similar device in or on the same body part without cutting or puncturing the skin or a mucous membrane.
Division: Cutting into a body part, without draining fluids and/or gases from the body part, in order to separate or transect a body part
Drainage: Taking or letting out fluids and/or gases from a body part
Excision: Cutting out or off, without replacement, a portion of a body part
Extirpation: Taking or cutting out solid matter from a body part
Extraction: Pulling or stripping out or off all or a portion of a body part by the use of force
Insertion: Putting in a nonbiological appliance that monitors, assists, performs, or prevents a physiological function but does not physically take the place of the body part
Inspection: Visually and/or manually exploring a body part
Release: Freeing a body part from an abnormal physical constraint by cutting or by the use of force
Removal: Taking out or off a device from a body part
Repair: Restoring, to the extent possible, a body part to its normal anatomic structure and function
Replacement: Putting in or on biological or synthetic material that physically takes the place and/or function of all or a portion of a body part
Reposition: Moving to its normal location, or other suitable location, all or a portion of a body part
Resection: Cutting out or off, without replacement, all of a body part
Supplement: Putting in or on biological or synthetic material that physically reinforces and/or augments the function of a portion of a body part
Revision: Correcting, to the extent possible, a portion of a malfunctioning device or the position of a displaced device

Source: CMS 2019

Body Part

Character 4 identifies the body part involved in the procedure. The body parts in ICD-10-PCS have individual values that include laterality, for example, as shown in table 16.3.

Table 16.3. **Body parts and values included in the ICD-10-PCS codes for the Lower Bones**

0—Lumbar vertebra
1—Sacrum
2—Pelvic bone, right
3—Pelvic bone, left
4—Acetabulum, right
5—Acetabulum, left
6—Upper femur, right
7—Upper femur, left

8—Femoral shaft, right
9—Femoral shaft, left
B—Lower femur, right
C—Lower femur, left
D—Patella, right
F—Patella, left
G—Tibia, right
H—Tibia, left
J—Fibula, right
K—Fibula, left
L—Tarsal, right
M—Tarsal, left
N—Metatarsal, right
P—Metatarsal, left
Q—Toe Phalanx, right
R—Toe Phalanx, left
S—Coccyx
Y—Lower Bone

Source: CMS 2019

Approach

Character 5 identifies the approach used in the procedure. The approach for procedures performed on the lower bones are shown in table 16.4.

Table 16.4. **Approaches, definitions, and values included in the ICD-10-PCS codes for the Lower Bones**

Open (0): Cutting through the skin or mucous membrane and any other body layers necessary to expose the site of the procedure
Percutaneous (3): Entry, by puncture or minor incision, of instrumentation through the skin or mucous membrane and any other body layers necessary to reach the site of the procedure
Percutaneous Endoscopic (4): Entry, by puncture or minor incision, of instrumentation through the skin or mucous membrane and any other body layers necessary to reach and visualize the site of the procedure
External (X): Procedures performed directly on the skin or mucous membrane and procedures performed indirectly by the application of external force through the skin or mucous membrane

Source: CMS 2019

Device

Character 6 identifies if a device remains in the patient's body after the procedure is concluded. The devices used to code procedures performed on the lower bones are shown in table 16.5.

Table 16.5. **Devices and values included in the ICD-10-PCS codes for the Lower Bones**

0—Drainage Device
4—Internal Fixation Device
5—External Fixation Device
6—Internal Fixation Device, Intramedullary
7—Autologous Tissue Substitute
7 – Internal Fixation Device, Intramedullary Limb Lengthening
8—External Fixation Device, Limb Lengthening
B—External Fixation Device, Monoplanar
C—External Fixation Device, Ring
D—External Fixation Device, Hybrid
J—Synthetic Substitute
K—Nonautologous Tissue Substitute
M—Bone Growth Stimulator
Y—Other Device
Z—No Device

Source: CMS 2019

Qualifier

Character 7 is a qualifier that specifies an additional attribute of the procedure, if applicable. The qualifier characters used to code procedures performed on the lower bones are as shown in table 16.6. The qualifier value of X for diagnostic procedure is available for the root operations of Drainage and Excision.

Table 16.6. **Qualifiers used to code procedures on the Lower Bones**

2—Sesamoid Bone(s) 1st Toe
X—Diagnostic
Z—No Qualifier

Source: CMS 2019

Specific Procedures Performed on the Musculoskeletal System

Two types of commonly performed orthopedic procedures, or procedures performed on the musculoskeletal system, include arthroscopic procedures and joint replacement procedures.

Arthroscopic Surgery

An **arthroscope** is an endoscope for examining the interior of a joint and for carrying out diagnostic and therapeutic procedures within the joint (Dorland 2012, 158). Very small instruments are used with the arthroscope to perform surgical procedures on a joint, such as the repair or removal of tissue or to take a biopsy. Arthroscopic surgery is commonly performed on most joints, including the knee, shoulder, wrist, and ankle. Arthroscopic surgery is often performed on an outpatient basis, and these procedures cause less damage to the body, minimize pain and scarring, and allow a faster recovery than do open joint procedures involving an arthrotomy.

The fifth character in an ICD-10-PCS code is the approach. An arthroscopic approach is identified by using the value of 4 for Percutaneous Endoscopic. If the procedure is strictly an arthroscopy with no additional procedure performed, the root operation is Inspection of the joint. According to the root operations defined in ICD-10-PCS, Inspection is "visually and/or manually exploring a body part" (CMS 2018). When a more definitive procedure is performed through an arthroscope, only the definitive procedure code is assigned using the root operation that identifies the objective of the procedure. For example, if a patient had an arthroscopic excisional debridement of the right hip joint, the root operation would be Excision or cutting out or off, without replacement, a portion of a body part. This is coded with 0SB as shown in table 16.7.

Table 16.7. **Arthroscopic excisional debridement of right hip joint**

Character	Code	Explanation
Section	0	Medical and Surgical
Body System	S	Lower Joints
Root Operation	B	Excision
Body Part	9	Hip Joint, Right
Approach	4	Percutaneous Endoscopic
Device	Z	No Device
Qualifier	Z	No Qualifier

Source: CMS 2019

Joint Replacement

The removal and replacement of a diseased joint with a device is a joint replacement. This is coded in ICD-10-PCS with the root operation Replacement, defined as "putting in or on biological or synthetic material that physically takes the place and/or function of all or a portion of a body part" (CMS 2018). Lower joint replacement codes start with the three characters 0SR, and upper joint replacement codes have the first three characters of 0RR. When coding a total hip replacement or when only the acetabular surface or the femoral surface is replaced, the body part replaced is identified with character 4 for the right- or left-sided joint. The joint device left in place is identified with character 6 for the device.

The choices for hip joint replacement devices are the following values, seen in table 16.8.

Table 16.8. **Devices for hip joint replacement**

0 – Synthetic Substitute, Polyethylene
1—Synthetic Substitute, Metal
2—Synthetic Substitute, Metal on Polyethylene

(Continued)

3—Synthetic Substitute, Ceramic
4—Synthetic Substitute, Ceramic on Polyethylene
6—Synthetic Substitute, Oxidized Zirconium on Polyethylene
7—Autologous Tissue Substitute
E—Articulating spacer
K—Nonautologous Tissue Substitute
J—Synthetic Substitute

Source: CMS 2019

The choices for the knee replacement devices are included in table 16.9.

Table 16.9.   **Devices used for knee replacement**

6—Synthetic Substitute, Oxidized Zirconium on Polyethylene
7—Autologous Tissue Substitute
E—Articulating Spacer
J—Synthetic Substitute
K—Nonautologous Tissue Substitute
L—Synthetic Substitute, Unicondylar Medial
M—Synthetic Substitute, Unicondylar Lateral
N—Synthetic Substitute, Patellofemoral

Source: CMS 2019

The choices for the shoulder replacement device are seen in table 16.10.

Table 16.10.   **Devices used for shoulder replacement**

0—Synthetic Substitute, Reverse Ball and Socket
7—Autologous Tissue Substitute
J—Synthetic Substitute
K—Nonautologous Tissue Substitute

Source: CMS 2019

For both hip and knee joint replacements, the seventh character (qualifier) identifies how the device is secured in place. The choices for lower joint replacement qualifiers are seen in table 16.11.

Table 16.11.   **Lower joint replacement qualifiers**

9—Cemented
A—Uncemented
Z—No Qualifier (when there is no statement of cemented or uncemented)

Source: CMS 2019

For the shoulder joint replacement, the seventh character (qualifier) identifies the surface of the joint replaced. The choices for upper joint replacement qualifiers are seen in table 16.12.

Table 16.12. **Upper joint replacement qualifiers**

6—Humeral Surface
7—Glenoid Surface
Z—No Qualifier

Source: CMS 2019

ICD-10-CM and ICD-10-PCS Review Exercises: Chapter 16

Assign the correct ICD-10-CM diagnosis codes or ICD-10-PCS procedure codes to the following exercises.

1. Seropositive rheumatoid arthritis, both hips

2. Juvenile rheumatoid arthritis, only occurring in both ankles

3. Patient has left upper lobe carcinoma, diagnosed over five years ago but is seen now for a fracture of the shaft of the right femur. During this admission, the patient was diagnosed with metastatic bone cancer (from the lung), and this fracture is a result of the metastatic disease. This patient's lung cancer was treated with radiation, and there is no longer evidence of an existing primary malignancy.

4. Patient with senile osteoporosis is seen with a complaint of severe back pain with no history of trauma. X-rays revealed pathological compression fractures of several lumbar vertebrae.

5. Lumbar intervertebral disc degeneration with radiculitis described as sciatica

6. Posttraumatic osteoarthritis, both knees

7. Spondylosis with myelopathy lumbar region

8. Chondromalacia of patella, right knee

(*Continued on next page*)

ICD-10-CM and ICD-10-PCS Review Exercises: Chapter 16 *(continued)*

9. Systemic lupus erythematosus with pericarditis

10. Acute osteomyelitis, toes of right foot due to *Staphylococcus aureus*

11. Postlaminectomy syndrome

12. Kyphosis due to age-related osteoporosis, thoracic region

13. Ruptured Baker's cyst of knee

14. Derangement of anterior horn of medial meniscus due to old injury, right knee

15. PROCEDURE: Right hip replacement using uncemented Oxidized zirconium on polyethylene device prosthesis

16. PROCEDURE: Left knee replacement using cemented unicondylar synthetic prosthesis, medial side

17. PROCEDURE: Open revision of left hip replacement metal prosthesis, existing metal prosthesis was repaired but not replaced

18. PROCEDURE: Laminectomy of lumbosacral disc L5–S1

19. PROCEDURE: Arthroscopic partial medial meniscectomy right knee

20. PROCEDURE: Arthrotomy with removal of right hip metal prosthesis due to internal joint infection and insertion of spacer device in the right hip for the next 8 weeks of antibiotic therapy

References

Centers for Disease Control and Prevention (CDC), National Center for Health Statistics (NCHS). 2019. *ICD-10-CM Official Guidelines for Coding and Reporting,* 2020. http://www.cdc.gov/nchs/icd/icd10cm.htm or https://www.cdc.gov/nchs/data/icd/10cmguidelines-FY2020_final.pdf.

Centers for Medicare and Medicaid Services (CMS). 2019. *ICD-10-PCS Official Guidelines for Coding and Reporting,* 2020. http://www.cms.gov/Medicare/Coding/ICD10/.

Derrer, D. T. 2018. Osteoarthritis Health Center. WebMD. http://www.webmd.com/osteoarthritis/guide/osteoarthritis-causes.

Dorland, W.A.N., ed. 2012. *Dorland's Illustrated Medical Dictionary,* 32nd ed. Philadelphia: Elsevier Saunders.

Mayo Clinic. 2015. Osteomyelitis. http://www.mayoclinic.org/diseases-conditions/osteomyelitis/basics/definition/con-20025518.

National Institute of Arthritis and Musculoskeletal and Skin Diseases (NIAMSD). 2014. National Institutes of Health. What Is Osteoarthritis? http://www.niams.nih.gov/Health_Info/Osteoarthritis/osteoarthritis_ff.pdf.

Stacy, G. S. 2016. Primary Osteoarthritis Imaging. Medscape. http://emedicine.medscape.com/article/392096-overview.

Stedman, T. 2012. *Stedman's Medical Dictionary for the Health Professions and Nursing,* 7th ed. Philadelphia: Wolters Kluwer/Lippincott Williams & Wilkins.

U.S. National Library of Medicine (NLM). 2019a. MedlinePlus. Kyphosis. https://www.nlm.nih.gov/medlineplus/ency/article/001240.htm.

U.S. National Library of Medicine (NLM). 2019b. MedlinePlus. Lordosis. https://www.nlm.nih.gov/medlineplus/ency/article/003278.htm.

U.S. National Library of Medicine (NLM). 2019c. MedlinePlus. Scoliosis. https://www.nlm.nih.gov/medlineplus/scoliosis.html.

U.S. National Library of Medicine (NLM). 2019d. MedlinePlus. Spinal Stenosis. https://www.nlm.nih.gov/medlineplus/spinalstenosis.html.

U.S. National Library of Medicine (NLM). 2019e. MedlinePlus. Compartment Syndrome. https://www.nlm.nih.gov/medlineplus/ency/article/001224.htm.

Chapter 17

Diseases of the Genitourinary System (N00–N99)

Learning Objectives

At the conclusion of this chapter, you should be able to do the following:

- Describe the organization of the conditions and codes included in Chapter 14 of ICD-10-CM, Diseases of the Genitourinary System (N00–N99)

- Provide examples of the types of conditions considered to be chronic kidney disease

- Define the term cystitis and describe the various ICD-10-CM codes that are available to classify these conditions

- Explain the term enlarged prostate and identify the associated urinary conditions that can be coded

- Review the types of female genital tract disorders that can be classified using ICD-10-CM codes

- Translate the abbreviations CIN I, CIN II, CIN III, VIN I, VIN II, and VIN III

- Identify the options for coding various types of menopause states in ICD-10-CM

- Assign ICD-10-CM codes for diseases of the genitourinary system

- Assign ICD-10-PCS codes for procedures related to the diseases of the genitourinary system

Key Terms

Acute kidney failure
Benign bladder neck obstruction (BNO)
Benign prostatic hypertrophy
Cervical dysplasia
Cervical intraepithelial neoplasia (CIN)
Chronic kidney disease (CKD)
Cystitis
Endometriosis
Enlarged prostate

Female genital prolapse
Gross hematuria
Hematuria
Lower urinary tract symptoms (LUTS)
Menopause
Microscopic hematuria
Nontraumatic acute kidney injury (AKI)
Vulvar intraepithelial neoplasia (VIN)

Overview of ICD-10-CM Chapter 14: Diseases of the Genitourinary System

Chapter 14 includes categories N00–N99 arranged in the following blocks:

N00–N08	Glomerular diseases
N10–N16	Renal tubulo-interstitial diseases
N17–N19	Acute kidney failure and chronic kidney disease
N20–N23	Urolithiasis
N25–N29	Other disorders of kidney and ureter
N30–N39	Other diseases of the urinary system
N40–N53	Diseases of the male genital organs
N60–N65	Disorders of breast
N70–N77	Inflammatory diseases of female pelvic organs
N80–N98	Noninflammatory disorders of female genital tract
N99	Intraoperative and postprocedural complications and disorders of genitourinary system, not elsewhere classified

As indicated by the blocks of codes in Chapter 14, ICD-10-CM contains codes for the urinary system, male and female reproductive systems, disorders of the breast, and complications occurring in the intraoperative and postoperative periods. When ICD-10-CM was developed, the terminology for genitourinary conditions was updated to reflect current medical practice. Specificity was added to the code descriptions including the identification of the patient's gender to correctly code posttraumatic urethral stricture.

Genitourinary disorders in diseases classified elsewhere have been placed in their own category at the end of each block of Chapter 14. For example, one category, N08, Glomerular disorders in diseases classified elsewhere, is used to identify glomerulonephritis, nephritis, and nephropathy in diseases classified elsewhere.

Advances in medical treatment prompt changes in Chapter 14. For example, given what has been identified about the causes and treatment for male erectile dysfunction in recent years, ICD-10-CM includes category N52 with subcategories to identify the different causes of the erectile dysfunction.

Coding Guidelines and Instructional Notes for ICD-10-CM Chapter 14

Throughout Chapter 14 are Includes notes that help to clarify the types of disorders that are classified to the various categories.

EXAMPLES: N00 Acute nephritis syndrome
Includes: acute glomerular disease
acute glomerulonephritis
acute nephritis

N71 Inflammatory disease of uterus, except cervix
Includes: endo(myo)metritis
metritis
myometritis
pyometra
uterine abscess

Examples of instructional notes available throughout the chapter indicate that additional coding should be performed as follows:

- N00–N08, Glomerular diseases—Code also any associated kidney failure (N17–N19)

- N10, Acute tubulo-interstitial nephritis and many other infections—Use additional code (B95–B97) to identify infectious agent

- N17, Acute kidney failure—Code also associated underlying condition

- N18, Chronic kidney disease (CKD)—

  Code first any associated:

  ○ diabetic chronic kidney disease (E08.22, E09.22, E10.22, E11.22, E13.22)

  ○ hypertensive chronic kidney disease (I12.-, I13.-)

  Use additional code to identify kidney transplant status, if applicable (Z94.0)

- N30, Cystitis—Use additional code to identify infectious agent (B95–B97)

- N31, Neuromuscular dysfunction of bladder, NEC—Use additional code to identify any associated urinary incontinence (N39.3–N39.4-)

- N33, Bladder disorders in diseases classified elsewhere—Code first underlying disease, such as: schistosomiasis (B65.0–B65.9)

  ○ This type of note appears with other categories in Chapter 14 for other disorders in diseases classified elsewhere.

- N40.1, Benign prostatic hyperplasia with lower urinary tract symptoms (LUTS)—Use additional code for associated symptoms, when specified:

  ○ incomplete bladder emptying (R39.14)

  ○ nocturia (R35.1)

  ○ straining on urination (R39.16)

  ○ urinary frequency (R35.0)

  ○ urinary hesitancy (R39.11)

  ○ urinary incontinence (N39.4-)

  ○ urinary obstruction (N13.8)

  ○ urinary retention (R33.8)

- ○ urinary urgency (R39.15)

- ○ weak urinary stream (R39.12)

- N46.12, Oligospermia due to extratesticular causes

- ○ Code also associated cause

- N99.0, Postprocedural (acute) (chronic) kidney failure

- ○ Use additional code for type of kidney disease (CDC 2019)

ICD-10-CM includes a note stating that menopausal and other perimenopausal disorders due to naturally occurring (age-related) menopause and perimenopause are classified to category N95 (CDC 2019). Other inclusion terms appear under Chapter 14 categories to explain the other diagnoses that would be classified with the category or the code, for example:

- N19, Unspecified kidney failure—includes uremia, NOS

- N28.0, Ischemia and infarction of kidney—includes renal artery embolism, obstruction, occlusion, thrombosis

- N40, Benign prostatic hyperplasia—includes BPH, enlarged prostate, nodular prostate

Includes notes appear throughout Chapter 14 to confirm all the terminology for diseases that are included in various categories (CDC 2019). For example, the following sections and categories include the other terminology that may be more commonly seen in health records:

- N03, Chronic nephritic syndrome—includes chronic glomerulonephritis and chronic nephritis

- N10–N16, Renal tubulo-interstitial diseases—includes pyelonephritis

- N70, Salpingitis and oophoritis—includes tubo-ovarian abscess and pyosalpinx

- N97, Female infertility—includes female sterility or inability to achieve a pregnancy

Excludes1 notes identify conditions that cannot be coded with category codes in Chapter 14, for example:

- N02, Recurrent and persistent hematuria with minor globular abnormality—excludes acute cystitis with hematuria or hematuria NOS or hematuria not associated with specified morphologic lesions

- N43, Hydrocele and spermatocele—excludes congenital hydrocele

- N81, Female genital prolapse—excludes genital prolapse complicating pregnancy, labor or delivery, prolapse and hernia of ovary and fallopian tube or prolapse of vaginal vault after hysterectomy

- N92, Excessive, frequent and irregular menstruation—excludes postmenopausal bleeding and precocious puberty (menstruation)

Excludes2 notes identify other conditions that can be coded with category codes in Chapter 14, for example:

- N39, Other disorders of urinary system—can be coded with hematuria

- N83, Noninflammatory disorders of ovary, fallopian tube and broad ligament—can be coded with hydrosalpinx (CDC 2019)

The NCHS has published chapter-specific guidelines for Chapter 14 in the *ICD-10-CM Official Guidelines for Coding and Reporting*. The coding student should review all of the coding guidelines for Chapter 14 of ICD-10-CM, which appear in an ICD-10-CM code book or on the CDC website (CDC 2019) or in appendix F.

CG

Chapter 14: Diseases of Genitourinary System (N00-N99)

Guideline I.C.14.a.1. Stages of chronic kidney disease (CKD): The ICD-10-CM classifies CKD based on severity. The severity of CKD is designated by stages 1-5. Stage 2, code N18.2, equates to mild CKD; stage 3, code N18.3, equates to moderate CKD; and stage 4, code N18.4, equates to severe CKD. Code N18.6, End stage renal disease (ESRD), is assigned when the provider has documented end-stage-renal disease (ESRD).

If both a stage of CKD and ESRD are documented, assign code N18.6 only.

Guideline I.C.14.a.2. Chronic kidney disease and kidney transplant status: Patients who have undergone kidney transplant may still have some form of chronic kidney disease (CKD) because the kidney transplant may not fully restore kidney function. Therefore, the presence of CKD alone does not constitute a transplant complication. Assign the appropriate N18 code for the patient's stage of CKD and code Z94.0, Kidney transplant status. If a transplant complication such as failure or rejection or other transplant complication is documented, see section I.C.19.g for information on coding complications of a kidney transplant. If the documentation is unclear as to whether the patient has a complication of the transplant, query the provider.

Coding Guideline I.C.14.a.3. Chronic kidney disease with other conditions: Patients with CKD may also suffer from other serious conditions, most commonly diabetes mellitus and hypertension. The sequencing of the CKD code in relationship to codes for other contributing conditions is based on the conventions in the Tabular List.

Coding Diseases of the Genitourinary System in ICD-10-CM Chapter 14

A variety of common conditions in the urinary system and the reproductive systems of men and women are classified with Chapter 14 codes. The frequently coded diseases are discussed in this chapter. Figure 17.1 is an illustration of the structure of the human kidney for reference during the discussion that follows about urinary system disorders.

Figure 17.1. **Kidney**

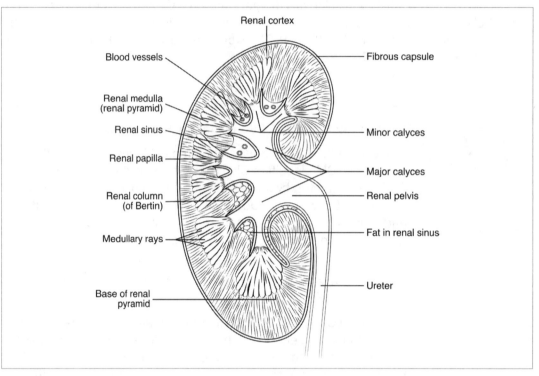

© AHIMA

Recurrent and Persistent Hematuria (N02)

Hematuria is the presence of blood or red blood cells in the urine. Hematuria can be a symptom of an undiagnosed disease, or hematuria can be present with another condition in the genitourinary tract. If the cause of hematuria has not been identified, symptom codes are used. For example, **gross hematuria** (R31.0) is the presence of blood in the urine in sufficient quantity to be visible to the naked eye. **Microscopic hematuria** (R31.1, R31.21–R31.29) is the presence of blood cells in the urine visible only under the microscope. The code R31.9 is used if only the symptom of hematuria is documented (Dorland 2012, 843).

Hematuria can be caused by a number of underlying urinary conditions, including urinary tract infections, benign prostatic hypertrophy, and kidney and ureteral calculi. In patients with certain risk factors, hematuria is a cardinal sign of bladder cancer. These patients require more intensive workup than do the primary hematuria patients. Patients presenting with hematuria who are at high risk for bladder cancer have other distinct risk factors: currently smoking or history of tobacco use, voiding dysfunction, personal history of urinary tract infections, and personal history of irradiation. Bladder cancer is generally associated with environmental or occupational factors and less often familial or inherited.

If the physician describes the patient's hematuria as recurrent, persistent, or idiopathic, the condition is classified to Chapter 14 category code N02, Recurrent and persistent hematuria.

The subcategories of N02 identify whether glomerular lesions, glomerulonephritis, or other morphological changes are present in the kidney.

EXAMPLE: The coding of the presence of hematuria depends on how the condition is documented, for example:
R31.1, Benign hematuria
R31.21, Asymptomatic Microscopic hematuria
N02.9, Persistent hematuria—see hematuria, idiopathic
N02.7, Recurrent hematuria with diffuse crescentic glomerulonephritis

Acute Kidney Failure and Chronic Kidney Disease (N17–N19)

Renal failure and renal insufficiency represent a range of disease processes that occur when the kidneys have problems eliminating metabolic products from the blood. These problems can be caused by various underlying conditions such as hypertension and diabetes, or they may affect patients with a single kidney or those with a family history of kidney disease. There are both acute and chronic kidney diseases that are classified with different codes in ICD-10-CM. An illustration of the urinary system with the adrenal gland, kidney, ureter, urinary bladder, and urethra is shown in figure 17.2.

Figure 17.2. **Diagram of the urinary system**

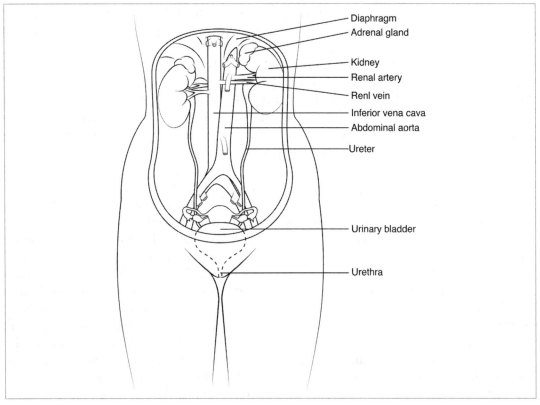

© AHIMA

Proper terminology, as used in ICD-10-CM, is **chronic kidney disease (CKD)**, rather than the vague terms of chronic renal failure and chronic renal insufficiency. CKD has five stages based on the glomerular filtration rate (GFR). But the coder cannot code the chronic kidney disease stage based on the lab result for the GFR as the stage must be documented by the physician or provider in order to be coded. The codes for CKD are:

N18.1, Chronic kidney disease, stage 1 with GFR of 90 or more
N18.2, Chronic kidney disease, stage 2 (mild) with GFR of 60–89
N18.3, Chronic kidney disease, stage 3 (moderate) with GFR of 30–59
N18.4, Chronic kidney disease, stage 4 (severe) with GFR of 15–29
N18.5, Chronic kidney disease, stage 5 with GFR of less than 15
N18.6, End stage renal disease or chronic kidney disease requiring dialysis

Care of patients with CKD stages 4 and 5 is intensive and complicated. For any patient, the goal is to slow the progression of CKD or better prepare the patient for renal replacement therapy. The GFR is a laboratory test to measure kidney function. Specifically, it estimates how much blood passes through the glomeruli of the kidney each minute. Glomeruli are the filters in the kidneys that eliminate waste from the blood (Martin 2019). According to the National Kidney Foundation, the GFR is the best test to measure the patient's level of kidney function and determine the patient's stage of kidney disease. The physician calculates the GFR based on the results of the patient's blood creatinine test, patient's age, body size, and gender. If the GFR number is low, the kidneys are not functioning well as they should. As the kidney disease gets worse, the GFR number goes down. By measuring the GFR along with other clinical factors, the physician can better detect kidney disease early in its progress and take measures at slowing the kidney's loss of function (NKF 2018).

Chronic renal insufficiency is a form of CKD classified with code N18.9, Chronic kidney disease, unspecified. Also included in this unspecified code are the diagnoses of chronic renal disease and chronic renal failure. A specific form of CKD and chronic renal insufficiency should not be coded in the same record. Renal insufficiency or acute renal insufficiency, a vague but different condition from CKD, is classified to code N28.9, Disorder of kidney and ureter, unspecified, with other nonspecific descriptions such as acute renal disease or renal disease unspecified. These forms of chronic kidney disease develop gradually in the patient over time, often associated with hypertension or diabetes. The condition may be controlled but generally is irreversible.

Acute kidney failure, or acute renal failure, is also described as **nontraumatic acute kidney injury (AKI)**. Symptoms include oliguria or anuria with hyperkalemia and pulmonary edema. AKI is a syndrome that results in a sudden decrease in kidney function or kidney damage in a short period of time. AKI causes waste products to collect in the blood making it difficult for the kidneys to keep a balance of fluids in the body. The build-up of fluids affects the heart, lungs, brain, and other organs from functioning properly. AKI can lead to chronic kidney disease, heart disease, and death. Even a mild episode of AKI can have long-lasting effects on the patient's health. Physicians may identify acute kidney failure with more specificity by referring to it as prerenal, intrarenal, or postrenal, which more specifically identifies underlying causes such as congestive heart failure (prerenal), acute nephritis or nephrotoxicity (intrarenal), or obstruction of urine flow out of the kidneys (postrenal). Acute kidney failure typically develops over a short period of time as part of another illness and is generally reversible; it is corrected as the underlying disease is treated or controlled. Major causes of AKI include decreased blood flow to the kidneys from hypotension, blood or fluid loss, heart attack, heart failure, use of certain drugs, severe allergic reactions, burns, injuries, and major surgery. Other causes are kidney disease, such as acute glomerulonephritis, tubular necrosis, sepsis, and blockage in the urinary tract, such as an enlarged prostate, kidney stones,

and blood clots in the urinary tract. Acute kidney failure or acute renal failure is assigned to category N17, with the fourth character identifying the type of necrosis present (NKF 2019).

EXAMPLE: N17.9, Acute kidney injury
Index: Injury, kidney, acute (nontraumatic)

N17.9, Acute kidney failure
Index: Failure, kidney, acute—see also Failure, renal acute

N17.0, Acute renal failure with tubular necrosis
Index: Failure, renal, acute, with, tubular necrosis

Check Your Understanding 17.1

Assign diagnosis codes to the following conditions.

1. Nephrotic syndrome with focal and segmental glomerular lesions

2. Hydropyonephrosis due to proteus infection

3. Multiple calculi in kidney and right ureter

4. Hypertensive cardiorenal disease with mild chronic kidney disease, stage 2 without heart failure

5. Persistent hematuria with glomerular lesion, membranous type

---

Cystitis (N30)

Cystitis is an inflammation of the urinary bladder (Dorland 2012, 463). Most common in women, this condition is often recurrent. Most cases are due to a vaginal infection that extends through the urethra to the bladder. Cystitis in men is due to urethral or prostatic infections or catheterizations. Symptoms include burning or painful urination, urinary urgency and frequency, nocturia, suprapubic pain, and lower back pain. A cross-section diagram of the bladder is shown in figure 17.3.

Figure 17.3.   **Urinary bladder**

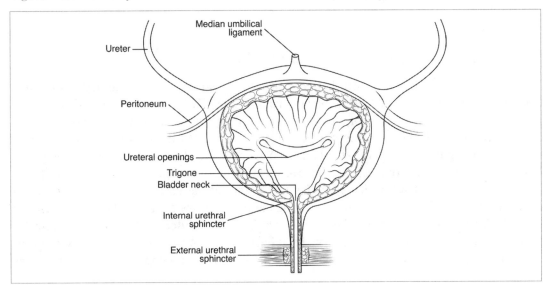

A diagnosis of cystitis is made by obtaining a urine specimen from the bladder by either catheterization or a clean-catch midstream sample. A bacterial colony count of greater than 1,000 colonies/mL in a catheterized specimen indicates cystitis, as does a bacterial count of greater than 100,000/mL in a midstream sample. Urine also may be positive for pyuria and hematuria. Therapy with antibiotics is prescribed for uncomplicated infections. The coder should not arbitrarily record an additional diagnosis on the basis of an abnormal laboratory finding alone, for example, bacteria present in a urine culture. If the specific diagnosis is not clearly stated in the health record, the physician should always be queried.

ICD-10-CM classifies cystitis to category N30, with the fourth-character subcategories describing type, severity, and location. The codes also identify whether or not hematuria is present with cystitis. An instruction at the beginning of this category advises that an additional code is used to identify the infectious agent (B95–B97). The options for coding cystitis in ICD-10-CM are as follows:

N30.00	Acute cystitis without hematuria
N30.01	Acute cystitis with hematuria
N30.10	Interstitial cystitis (chronic) without hematuria
N30.11	Interstitial cystitis (chronic) with hematuria
N30.20	Other chronic cystitis without hematuria
N30.21	Other chronic cystitis with hematuria
N30.30	Trigonitis without hematuria
N30.31	Trigonitis with hematuria
N30.40	Irradiation cystitis without hematuria
N30.41	Irradiation cystitis with hematuria
N30.80	Other cystitis without hematuria
N30.81	Other cystitis with hematuria
N30.90	Cystitis, unspecified without hematuria
N30.91	Cystitis, unspecified with hematuria

Benign Prostatic Hyperplasia (N40)

The diagnosis of **benign prostatic hypertrophy** may also be stated as **enlarged prostate**, benign prostatic hyperplasia (BPH), or nodular prostate. The terminology of BPH may be found in health records in place of the diagnosis of enlarged prostate, but the two descriptions are synonymous. It is a condition commonly occurring in men by the age of 60 years, as part of the normal aging process. By age 80, about 80 percent of men have an enlarge prostate gland. However, only about half of these men have any symptoms due to their enlarged prostate (NKF 2015). The prostate gland, which encircles the urethra at the base of the bladder, becomes enlarged and presses on the urethra, obstructing the flow of urine from the bladder and causing difficulty urinating. This may also be described as **benign bladder neck obstruction (BNO)**. Symptoms of an enlarged prostate may be referred to as **lower urinary tract symptoms (LUTS)** and include incomplete bladder emptying, nocturia, straining on urination, urinating more often or frequency, having to get up at night to urinate or nocturia, unable to start urinating or hesitancy, incontinence, obstruction, retention, urgency, or weak urinary stream. Straining to void may rupture veins of the prostate, causing hematuria. The ICD-10-CM codes distinguish between benign prostatic hyperplasia or nodular prostate with and without lower urinary tract symptoms.

A diagnosis of a benign prostatic hyperplasia or an enlarged prostate is made by a rectal examination that finds the prostate enlarged and with a rubbery texture. Urinalysis shows WBC, RBC, albumin, bacteria, and blood. Cystoscopy reveals the extent of enlargement. A postvoiding cystogram shows the amount of residual urine in the bladder, and the physician can decide how much the prostate is blocking the urine stream. Treatments for a benign prostatic hyperplasia include medications such as alpha-blockers to relax the muscle tissue in the prostate to relieve the blockage or testosterone that can shrink the prostate when the symptoms are severe enough to be troubling to the patient or if the function of the urinary tract is affected or if there are complications such as bleeding, kidney infections, or kidney damage. Surgery removes some of the enlarged prostate tissue to relieve the symptoms. Other treatments use electric current or thermal therapy to reduce the prostate gland's size (NKF 2015).

ICD-10-CM classifies benign prostatic hyperplasia or nodular prostate to category N40. Some forms of the disease may be indicative of the need for further testing due to the increased risk for prostatic cancer. The enlargement of the prostate often produces the symptom of urinary obstruction or the inability to urinate. The urinary obstruction is the problem that typically brings the patient to the physician or to the hospital emergency department.

Category N40 is expanded to the fourth-character subcategory level to describe the type of enlargement and whether or not lower urinary tract symptoms are present.

> **EXAMPLE** N40.0, Benign prostatic hyperplasia without urinary tract symptoms
> N40.1, Benign prostatic hyperplasia with lower urinary tract symptoms
> N40.2, Nodular prostate without lower urinary tract symptoms
> N40.3, Nodular prostate with lower urinary tract symptoms

Under each of the codes with lower urinary tract symptoms, a directional note states, "Use additional code for associated symptoms, when specified." Additional codes are used when the patient also has incomplete bladder emptying (R39.14), nocturia (R35.1), straining on urination (R39.16), urinary frequency (R35.0), urinary hesitancy (R39.11), urinary incontinence (N39.4-), urinary obstruction (N13.8), urinary retention (R33.8), urgency (R39.15), or weak urinary stream (R39.12) with the diagnosis of enlarged or nodular prostate.

Check Your Understanding 17.2

Assign diagnosis codes to the following conditions.

1. Overactive bladder, detrusor muscle hyperactivity, cause undetermined with female stress incontinence

2. Benign prostatic hyperplasia with urinary frequency, urgency and nocturia

3. Urethral bullous stricture in a male patient

4. Inguinal hernia, left side with hydrocele (male)

5. Bacterial epididymitis due to acute *E. coli* bladder infection

Disorders of Breast (N60–N65)

Disorders such as gynecomastia, fibrocystic disease, inflammatory disease, and solitary cyst of the breast are included in this section. A breast lump or breast mass is classified to category code N63, Unspecified lump in breast. An image of the structures of the breast is shown in figure 17.4.

Figure 17.4. **Structures within the breast**

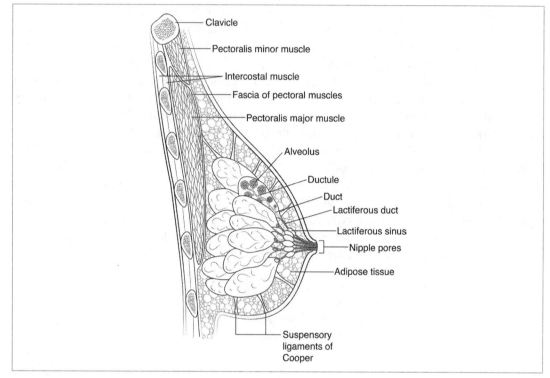

© AHIMA

Certain signs and symptoms of breast disease, such as mastodynia, induration of breast, and nipple discharge, are included in category N64, rather than in Chapter 18 of ICD-10-CM, with other symptoms, signs, and abnormal findings. Neoplasms of the breast are classified in Chapter 2, Neoplasms, in ICD-10-CM.

Specific codes describe conditions of the breast related to staged breast reconstruction following full or partial mastectomy due to breast disease or trauma. Codes identify the various stages for which a breast reconstruction encounter may occur or distinguish between the disorders of reconstructed breasts and native breasts. Specific conditions requiring reconstruction may be described with codes in the range of N64.81–N64.89 for ptosis, hypoplasia, capsular contracture, and other specified disorders of the breast. Deformity or disproportion of reconstructed breast is identified with ICD-10-CM codes N65.0–N65.1.

EXAMPLE N60.01, Solitary cyst of right breast
N60.11 and N60.12, Diffuse cystic mastopathy of both breasts
N61, Acute mastitis
N64.4, Mastodynia

Check Your Understanding 17.3

Assign diagnosis codes to the following conditions.

1. Lump in breast, female, right side, upper outer quadrant

2. Acute mastitis of right breast with abscess

3. Diffuse fibrocystic disease of both breasts

4. Mammary duct ectasia, left breast, female

5. Induration of right breast with nipple discharge and mastodynia

Inflammatory Disease of Female Pelvic Organs (N70–N77)

This section includes infections of the female pelvic organs such as acute salpingitis, endometritis, acute and chronic parametritis, and pelvic cellulitis. The note at the beginning of several category codes in this section states "Use additional code (B95–B97) to identify infectious agent" (CDC 2019). When there is a known bacteria or virus that is causing the infection, it is important to report it as a secondary code.

> **EXAMPLE:** Acute salpingitis; organism involved—*Streptococcus.*
> This can be classified with the codes N70.01, Acute salpingitis, and B95.5, Unspecified streptococcus as the cause of diseases classified elsewhere.

Codes in category N70, Salpingitis and oophoritis, distinguish between acute and chronic forms of the conditions. Acute salpingitis and oophoritis is classified to N70.0-, and chronic salpingitis and oophoritis is classified to N70.1-. The unspecified form of salpingitis and oophoritis is classified with another set of subcategory codes.

Other categories exist in this block of codes to identify inflammatory diseases that are the result of another disease. For example, under category N74, Female pelvic inflammatory disorders in diseases classified elsewhere, there is a "code first underlying disease" note. This same direction also appears with codes N77.0, Ulceration of vulva in diseases classified elsewhere, and N77.1, Vaginitis, vulvitis and vulvovaginitis in diseases classified elsewhere. An illustration of the cavities within the female body is shown in figure 17.5, including the pelvic cavity where many of the female disorders discussed in this chapter are located.

Noninflammatory Disorders of Female Genital Tract (N80–N98)

This section includes conditions such as the following:

- **Endometriosis**, N80. This condition occurs when endometrial glands or the lining of the uterus is present outside the uterine cavity. For example, endometriosis can be diagnosed in the ovary, fallopian tube, pelvic peritoneum, rectovaginal septum and vagina, intestine, and other sites (Stedman 2012, 552–553). ICD-10-CM provides a specific code for the common sites of endometriosis as well as an unspecified code, N80.9. Many women suffer from the effects of endometriosis, and it is one of the most common causes of infertility in women.

- **Female genital prolapse**, N81. Prolapse is the sinking of an organ or other part of the body. For example, the prolapse of a uterus is the downward movement of the uterus due to laxity and atony of the muscular and fascial structures of the pelvic floor. Other organs that can prolapse are the vagina, bladder, rectum, and urethra (Stedman 2012, 553). There are codes in this category for urethrocele, cystocele, uterovaginal prolapse, vaginal enterocele, rectocele, and other weakening of tissue and pelvic muscle wasting.

- Fistulae involving female genital tract, N82

- Noninflammatory disorders of the ovary, fallopian tube, and broad ligament, N83. Commonly occurring conditions classified to this category are follicular cyst or ovary, corpus luteum cyst, torsion of the ovary and fallopian tube, hematosalpinx, and hematoma of broad ligament. Ovarian cysts of a variety of types are the most common pelvic masses diagnosed in women.

- Polyp of female genital tract, N84. Polyps that occur in the corpus uteri, cervix uteri, vagina, vulva, and other parts of the female genital tract are classified here.

- Other inflammatory disorders of the uterus, except cervix, N85. The more commonly occurring conditions that would be coded with category N85 codes are benign endometrial hyperplasia and endometrial hyperplasia neoplasia or that with atypia. These conditions frequently make a hysterectomy a medical necessity.

Figure 17.5. Body cavities in the female body

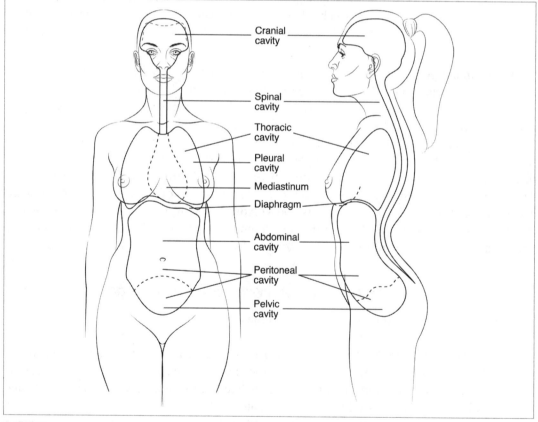

© AHIMA

Other gynecological conditions described in this chapter of ICD-10-CM include the following:

- Other noninflammatory disorders of the cervix uteri, vagina, vulva, and perineum

- Disorders of menstruation

- Infertility

- Complications associated with artificial fertilization

EXAMPLE	N81.2, First degree prolapse of the uterus Index: Prolapse, uterus, first degree
	N81.2, Incomplete prolapse of vagina with prolapse of uterus Index: Prolapse, vagina, with prolapse of uterus, incomplete
	N83.1, Hemorrhagic corpus luteum cyst Index: Cyst, corpus, luteum (hemorrhagic)
	N84.0, Endometrial polyp Index: Polyp, endometrium
	N85.4, Retroversion of uterus and cervix Index: Retroversion, cervix—see Retroversion, uterus (cervix)

Dysplasia of Cervix Uteri (N87) and Vulva (N90.0–N90.4)

Codes N87.0 through N87.9 describe mild dysplasia of the cervix or cervical intraepithelial neoplasia. Mild **cervical dysplasia** or **cervical intraepithelial neoplasia** I (CIN I) as a diagnosis is assigned code N87.0. Likewise, the diagnosis of moderate dysplasia of the cervix (CIN II) is assigned code N87.1. There is a code available, N87.9, for an unspecified form of cervical dysplasia. However, if the condition is described as carcinoma *in situ* of the cervix, severe cervical dysplasia, or cervical intraepithelial neoplasia III (CIN III), it is classified in category D06, Carcinoma in situ of cervix.

Codes N90.0 through N90.1 describe **vulvar intraepithelial neoplasia** I and II (VIN I and VIN II). These conditions are also known as N90.0, mild dysplasia of vulva; N90.1, moderate dysplasia of vulva; N90.3, unspecified form of dysplasia; and N90.4, other leukoplakia of vulva. If the condition is described as carcinoma *in situ* of the vulva, severe dysplasia of vulva, or vulvar intraepithelial neoplasia III (VIN III), code D07.1 is used to classify the disease. The Alphabetic Index entry used to locate the codes for these conditions is the term "dysplasia, cervix" or "dysplasia, vulva."

EXAMPLES:	N87.0, Mild cervical dysplasia or CIN I N87.1, Moderate cervical dysplasia or CIN II N90.0, Mild vulvar dysplasia or VIN grade I N90.1, Moderate vulvar dysplasia or VIN grade II

Check Your Understanding 17.4

Assign diagnosis codes to the following conditions.

1. Acute female pelvic peritonitis

2. Acute bacterial vaginosis, infectious organism not identified

3. Endometrial hyperplasia with atypia

4. Vulvar intraepithelial neoplasia (VIN) grade II

5. Cystocele with urethrocele, midline

Menopause

The diagnosis given by a healthcare provider of **menopause** or menopausal syndrome often needs to be more specific. Menopause is defined as occurring 12 months after the last menstrual period in the woman and marks the end of menstrual cycles. Menopause can happen when a woman is in her 40s or 50s, but the average age is 51 in the United States. Menopause is a natural biological process (Mayo Clinic 2017). ICD-10-CM includes several options for coding. Codes exist for both symptomatic menopausal syndrome and asymptomatic menopausal status. The symptoms a woman may experience with menopause are hot flashes or flushing, sleeplessness, night sweats, headache, and a lack of concentration, and in some women, there are mood changes such as anxiety or feelings of sadness and loss (Mayo Clinic 2017). Subcategory code N95.1, Menopausal and female climacteric states, includes a "use additional code for associated symptoms" note to direct the coder to assign other codes to describe the menopausal symptoms the woman is experiencing.

Menopause occurs either as the result of the natural aging process or as an artificially induced menopause after a hysterectomy when the uterus and ovaries are removed or after other treatments such as chemotherapy or radiation therapy. There is no treatment for menopause except to relieve the signs and symptoms, for example, with hormone therapy to reduce hot flashes, with vaginal estrogen to reduce vaginal dryness, low-dose antidepressants when needed, and medications to prevent or treat osteoporosis that is known to occur in postmenopausal women (Mayo Clinic 2017). For coding, it is necessary to know if the patient has asymptomatic, premature due to surgery or radiation, or symptomatic menopause as different codes are available. The fact that the woman is experiencing symptoms because of the menopausal process or is asymptomatic is required to code the status correctly.

EXAMPLES: The patient who has a menopausal disorder or symptoms associated with artificial or postsurgical menopause may be coded with the following:

E89.41,   Symptomatic postprocedural ovarian failure
N95.1,   Menopause and female climacteric states

The patient who is menopausal as a result of having her ovaries removed surgically but who is asymptomatic may be coded with either:

E89.40,   Asymptomatic postprocedural ovarian failure
Z90.721 or Z90.722, Acquired absence of ovaries (unilateral) (bilateral)

The patient who has a menopausal disorder or symptoms associated with age-related or naturally occurring menopause may be coded with the following:

E28.39, Other primary ovarian failure
N95.1, Menopausal and female climacteric states

The patient who has premature menopause, that is, earlier in life than typically experienced by most women but not due to a procedure, may or may not have symptoms. This person would be diagnosed with a form of ovarian failure and coded with the following:

E28.310, Symptomatic premature menopause
E28.319, Asymptomatic premature menopause

The patient who is postmenopausal as a result of the natural or age-related process and is asymptomatic is coded with the following:

Z78.0, Asymptomatic menopausal state

Intraoperative and Postprocedural Complications and Disorders of Genitourinary System, Not Elsewhere Classified (N99)

The chapter ends with the intraoperative and postprocedural complications of the genitourinary system like those found in the preceding chapters. Postprocedural conditions that are classified with category N99 codes are as follows:

N99.0	Postprocedural (acute) (chronic) kidney failure
N99.110–N99.115, N99.12	Postprocedural urethral stricture
N99.2	Postprocedural adhesions of vagina
N99.3	Prolapse of vaginal vault after hysterectomy
N99.4	Postprocedural pelvic peritoneal adhesions
N99.510–N99.538	Complications of stoma of urinary tract
N99.61–N99.62	Intraoperative hemorrhage and hematoma of a genitourinary system organ or structure complicating a procedure
N99.71–N99.72	Accidental puncture and laceration of a genitourinary system organ or structure during a procedure
N99.81–N99.89	Other intraoperative and postprocedural complication and disorders of the genitourinary tract

Complications of cystostomy and other external stoma of the urinary system are found in the range of codes N99.510–N99.538. The types of complications of the cystostomy or other external stoma that could be coded are hemorrhage or infection at the site or malfunction of the stoma. The Alphabetic Index to Diseases and Injuries have Index entries for the name of the complication or the term "complication" and the subterms intraoperative, postoperative, postprocedural, or surgical procedure.

EXAMPLE: N99.71, Accidental laceration of ureter during hysterectomy (genitourinary procedure)
Index: Complication, accidental puncture or laceration during a procedure (of)—see Complications, intraoperative (intraprocedural) puncture of laceration [Ureter is a genitourinary system structure.]

Check Your Understanding 17.5

Assign diagnosis codes to the following conditions.

1. Symptomatic menopause

2. Premenstrual tension syndrome

3. Excessive menstruation with irregular cycles

4. Postprocedural acute kidney failure

5. Stenosis of urinary tract stoma, continent type

ICD-10-PCS Procedure Coding for Genitourinary System Procedures

Procedures related to the genitourinary system would include procedures on the Urinary system, Female Reproductive system, and Male Reproductive system. ICD-10-PCS contains a large number of procedure codes based on the different parts of these body systems. The root operations for the various types of procedures that can be performed are shown in table 17.1. Like procedures in other body systems, in order to code genitourinary procedures, the coder needs to know the definition of root operations and the anatomy to identify the body parts.

Table 17.1.   **Genitourinary system root operations**

Root Operations and (Third) Character Root Operation Value	Root Operations and (Third) Character Root Operation Value	Root Operations and (Third) Character Root Operation Value
Urinary System	**Female Reproductive System**	**Male Reproductive System**
Bypass (1)	Bypass (1)	Bypass (1)
Change (2)	Change (2)	Change (2)
Destruction (5)	Destruction (5)	Destruction (5)
Dilation (7)	Dilation (7)	Dilation (7)
Division (8)	Division (8)	Drainage (9)
Drainage (9)	Drainage (9)	Excision (B)
Excision (B)	Excision (B)	Extirpation (C)
Extirpation (C)	Extirpation (C)	Insertion (H)
Extraction (D)	Extraction (D)	Inspection (J)
Fragmentation (F)	Fragmentation (F)	Occlusion (L)
Insertion (H)	Insertion (H)	Reattachment (M)
Inspection (J)	Inspection (J)	Release (N)
Occlusion (L)	Occlusion (L)	Removal (P)
Reattachment (M)	Reattachment (M)	Repair (Q)
Release (N)	Release (N)	Replacement (R)
Removal (P)		

Root Operations and (Third) Character Root Operation Value	Root Operations and (Third) Character Root Operation Value	Root Operations and (Third) Character Root Operation Value
Urinary System	Female Reproductive System	Male Reproductive System
Repair (Q) Replacement (R) Reposition (S) Resection (T) Supplement (U) Restriction (V) Revision (W) Transplantation (Y)	Removal (P) Repair (Q) Reposition (S) Resection (T) Supplement (U) Restriction (V) Revision (W) Transplantation (Y)	Reposition (S) Resection (T) Supplement (U) Revision (W) Transfer (X)

Source: CMS 2019

Body parts include laterality, for example, right and left kidneys, and bilateral for such organs as the ovary, fallopian tube, seminal vesicle, spermatic cord, epididymis, vas deferens, and such. The approach for these procedures is frequently endoscopic through a natural orifice, such as the vagina and urethra, as well as percutaneous (for example, laparoscopic). Robotic-assisted prostatic and uterine procedures are becoming more common. An additional code is used to designate that the procedure was robotic assisted. The Index entry for robotic-assisted procedure directs the coder to Table 8E0 in ICD-10-PCS. A code is constructed based on the relevant body region; the sixth character designates the method as a robotic-assisted procedure.

Example of a Section for ICD-10-PCS Genitourinary Procedure Coding

To demonstrate the structure of the ICD-10-PCS tables for the coding of procedures on the genitourinary system disorders, the section for Urinary system is described as follows.

Section for Urinary System

> Character 1 is Value 0—Medical and Surgical
> Character 2 is Value T—Urinary System

Root Operation

Character 3 of the Medical and Surgical section of ICD-10-PCS codes is the root operation. The root operations that represent the objectives of procedures for surgical treatment of the diseases in the Urinary system are shown in table 17.2.

Table 17.2.   **Root operations for procedures on the Urinary system**

Bypass: Altering the route of passage of the contents of a tubular body part
Change: Taking out or off a device from a body part and putting back an identical or similar device in or on the same body part without cutting or puncturing the skin or a mucous membrane
Destruction: Physical eradication of all or a portion of a body part by the direct use of energy, force or a destructive agent
Dilation: Expanding an orifice or the lumen of a tubular body part
Division: Cutting into a body part, without draining fluids and/or gases from the body part, in order to separate or transect a body part

(Continued)

Drainage: Taking or letting out fluids and/or gases from a body part
Excision: Cutting out or off, without replacement, all or a portion of a body part
Extirpation: Taking or cutting out solid matter from a body part
Extraction: Pulling or stripping out or off all or a portion of a body part by the use of force
Fragmentation: Breaking solid matter in a body part into pieces
Insertion: Putting in a nonbiological appliance that monitors, assists, performs, or prevents a physiological function but does not physically take the place of the body part
Inspection: Visually and/or manually exploring a body part
Occlusion: Completely closing an orifice or the lumen of a tubular body part
Reattachment: Putting back in or on all or a portion of a separated body part to its normal location or other suitable location
Release: Freeing a body part from an abnormal physical constraint by cutting or by the use of force
Removal: Taking out or off a device from a body part
Repair: Restoring, to the extent possible, a body part to its normal anatomic structure and function
Replacement: Putting in or on biological or synthetic material that physically takes the place and/or function of all or a portion of a body part
Reposition: Moving to its normal location, or other suitable location, all or a portion of a body part
Resection: Cutting out or off, without replacement, all of a body part
Supplement: Putting in or on biological or synthetic material that physically reinforces and/or augments the function of a portion of a body part
Restriction: Partially closing an orifice or the lumen of a tubular body part
Revision: Correcting, to the extent possible, a portion of a malfunctioning device or the position of a displaced device
Transplantation: Putting in or on all or a portion of a living body part taken from another individual or animal to physically take the place and/or function of all or a portion of a similar body part

Source: CMS 2019

Body Part

Character 4 identifies the body part involved in the procedure. The body parts in ICD-10-PCS have individual values that include laterality, for example, as shown in table 17.3.

Table 17.3. **Body parts and values included in the ICD-10-PCS codes for Urinary system**

0—Kidney, right
1—Kidney, left
2—Kidneys, bilateral
3—Kidney Pelvis, right
4—Kidney Pelvis, left
5—Kidney
6—Ureter, right
7—Ureter, left
8—Ureters, bilateral

9—Ureter
B—Bladder
C—Bladder neck
D—Urethra

Source: CMS 2019

Approach

Character 5 identifies the approach used in the procedure. The approach for procedures performed on organs within the Urinary system is shown in table 17.4.

Table 17.4. **Approaches, definitions, and values included in the ICD-10-PCS codes for the Urinary system**

Open (0): Cutting through the skin or mucous membrane and any other body layers necessary to expose the site of the procedure
Percutaneous (3): Entry, by puncture or minor incision, of instrumentation through the skin or mucous membrane and any other body layers necessary to reach the site of the procedure
Percutaneous Endoscopic (4): Entry, by puncture or minor incision, of instrumentation through the skin or mucous membrane and any other body layers necessary to reach and visualize the site of the procedure
Via Natural or Artificial Opening (7): Entry of instrumentation through a natural or artificial external opening to reach the site of the procedure
Via Natural or Artificial Opening Endoscopic (8): Entry of instrumentation through a natural or artificial external opening to reach and visualize the site of the procedure
External (X): Procedures performed directly on the skin or mucous membrane and procedures performed indirectly by the application of external force through the skin or mucous membrane

Source: CMS 2019

Device

Character 6 identifies if a device remains in the patient's body after the procedure is concluded. The devices used to code procedures performed in the Urinary system are shown in table 17.5.

Table 17.5. **Devices and values included in the ICD-10-PCS codes in the Urinary system**

0—Drainage Device
2—Monitoring Device
3—Infusion Device
7—Autologous Tissue Substitute
C—Extraluminal Device
D—Intraluminal Device
J—Synthetic Substitute
K—Nonautologous Tissue Substitute

(*Continued*)

| L—Artificial Sphincter |
| M—Stimulator Lead |
| Y—Other Device |
| Z—No Device |

Source: CMS 2019

Qualifier

Character 7 is a qualifier that specifies an additional attribute of the procedure, if applicable. The qualifier characters used to code procedures performed on the Urinary system are as shown in table 17.6. The qualifier value of X for diagnostic procedure is available for the root operations of Drainage and Excision.

Table 17.6. **Qualifiers used to code procedures on the Urinary system**

| 0—Allogeneic |
| 1—Syngeneic |
| 2—Zooplastic |
| 3—Kidney Pelvis, right |
| 4—Kidney Pelvis, left |
| 6—Ureter, right |
| 7—Ureter, left |
| 8—Colon |
| 9—Colocutaneous |
| A—Ileum |
| B—Bladder |
| C—Ileocutaneous |
| D—Cutaneous |
| X—Diagnostic |
| Z—No Qualifier |

Source: CMS 2019

Hemodialysis and Renal Replacement Therapy

Hemodialysis and renal replacement therapy may be performed for patients with conditions that produce renal failure that may be coded from this chapter. The amount of time the dialysis is performed is not the important factor for coding purposes. The type of dialysis is what should be coded. Intermittent hemodialysis is the conventional treatment usually performed for ESRD, three times a week, for less than six hours per session. Two other forms of hemodialysis are referred to as renal replacement therapy (RRT). These are performed on patients with acute kidney injury or acute renal failure and delivered to critically ill patients. Prolonged intermittent renal replacement therapy (PIRRT), also called SLED (sustained low efficiency dialysis) or EDD (extended daily dialysis), is performed for 6–18 hours per day and is a gentler form of dialysis on very ill patients. The second type is continuous renal replacement therapy (CRRT), also called CVVH (continuous veno-venous hemofiltration) or CCVHD (continuous veno-venous hemodialysis) or CVVHDF (continuous veno-venous hemodiafiltration), and is performed for at least 18 hours a day and is the slowest and gentlest hemodialysis for patients who have acute kidney injury that has resulted in hemodynamic instability. They would not be able to tolerate the other forms of dialysis. The hemodialysis and renal replacement therapy codes are included in the Extracorporeal or Systemic Assistance and Performance tables for the Urinary body system with the 5th character identifying the duration or type of filtration, that is dialysis or renal replacement therapy:

5A1D70Z for intermittent hemodialysis
5A1D80Z for prolonged intermittent renal replacement therapy
5A1D90Z for continuous renal replacement therapy

Generally, the hospital can decide how often to code the procedures on a hospitalized patient. Usually the practice is to code the intermittent hemodialysis one time for each patient receiving it, no matter how many days it is done. The practice may be coded one time per admission for each type of dialysis or renal replacement therapy instead of coding when it is performed, for example, every day during a hospital stay.

ICD-10-CM and ICD-10-PCS Review Exercises: Chapter 17

Assign the correct ICD-10-CM diagnosis codes or ICD-10-PCS procedure codes to the following exercises.

1. Chronic nephritic syndrome with diffuse membranous glomerulonephritis with symptoms of proteinuria and hematuria

2. Patient complained of frequent urination with pain and was diagnosed with acute suppurative cystitis, with hematuria due to *E. coli*

3. Breast asymmetry between native breast and reconstructed breast

4. This male patient complained of lower abdominal pain and the inability to urinate over the past 24 hours. After study, the patient was diagnosed as having acute kidney failure due to acute tubular necrosis, caused by a urinary obstruction. The urinary obstruction was a result of the patient's benign prostatic hypertrophy. The patient was treated with medications, and the acute kidney failure was resolved prior to discharge

(*Continued on next page*)

ICD-10-CM and ICD-10-PCS Review Exercises: Chapter 17 (continued)

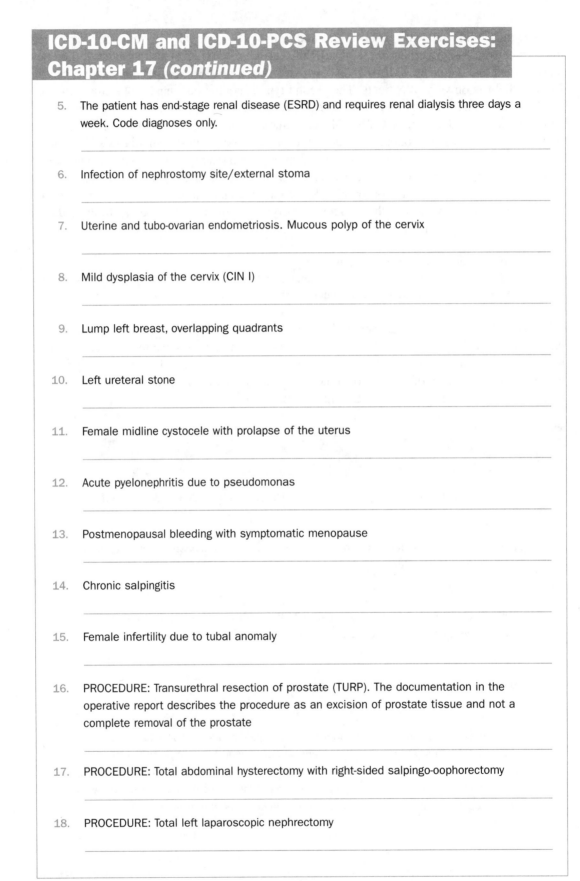

5. The patient has end-stage renal disease (ESRD) and requires renal dialysis three days a week. Code diagnoses only.

6. Infection of nephrostomy site/external stoma

7. Uterine and tubo-ovarian endometriosis. Mucous polyp of the cervix

8. Mild dysplasia of the cervix (CIN I)

9. Lump left breast, overlapping quadrants

10. Left ureteral stone

11. Female midline cystocele with prolapse of the uterus

12. Acute pyelonephritis due to pseudomonas

13. Postmenopausal bleeding with symptomatic menopause

14. Chronic salpingitis

15. Female infertility due to tubal anomaly

16. PROCEDURE: Transurethral resection of prostate (TURP). The documentation in the operative report describes the procedure as an excision of prostate tissue and not a complete removal of the prostate

17. PROCEDURE: Total abdominal hysterectomy with right-sided salpingo-oophorectomy

18. PROCEDURE: Total left laparoscopic nephrectomy

ICD-10-CM and ICD-10-PCS Review Exercises: Chapter 17 *(continued)*

19. PROCEDURE: Anterior colporrhaphy by vaginal approach

   _____

20. PROCEDURE: Lithotripsy (ESWL) to destroy left renal pelvis calculus

   _____

References

Centers for Disease Control and Prevention (CDC), National Center for Health Statistics (NCHS). 2019. *ICD-10-CM Official Guidelines for Coding and Reporting*, 2020. http://www.cdc.gov/nchs/icd/icd10cm.htm or https://www.cdc.gov/nchs/data/icd/10cmguidelines -FY2020_final.pdf.

Centers for Medicare and Medicaid Services (CMS). 2019. *ICD-10-PCS Official Guidelines for Coding and Reporting*, 2020. http://www.cms.gov/Medicare/Coding/ICD10/.

Dorland, W.A.N., ed. 2012. *Dorland's Illustrated Medical Dictionary*, 32nd ed. Philadelphia: Elsevier Saunders.

Martin, L.J. MedlinePlus. 2019. Glomerular Filtration Rate. https://www.nlm.nih.gov /medlineplus/ency/article/007305.htm.

Mayo Clinic. 2017. Menopause. http://www.mayoclinic.org/diseases-conditions/menopause /basics/definition/con-20019726.

National Kidney Foundation (NFK). 2019. Acute Kidney Injury (AKI). https://www.kidney.org /atoz/content/AcuteKidneyInjury.

National Kidney Foundation (NKF). 2018. Glomerular Filtration Rate (GFR). https://www .kidney.org/atoz/content/gfr.

National Kidney Foundation (NFK). 2015. Benign Prostate Disease. https://www.kidney.org /atoz/content/benignprostate.

Stedman, T. 2012. *Stedman's Medical Dictionary for the Health Professions and Nursing*, 7th ed. Philadelphia: Wolters Kluwer/Lippincott Williams & Wilkins.

Chapter 18

Pregnancy, Childbirth and the Puerperium (O00–O9A)

Learning Objectives

At the conclusion of this chapter, you should be able to do the following:

- Describe the organization of the conditions and codes included in Chapter 15 of ICD-10-CM, Pregnancy, Childbirth and the Puerperium (O00–O9A)

- Summarize the different ICD-10-CM categories used to classify the diagnosis of abortion

- Distinguish the terms of *missed abortion* and *threatened abortion*

- Define the term *pregnancy* and apply the weeks of gestation to determine what are preterm, term, and postterm pregnancies

- Explain the term *ectopic pregnancy* and how the condition is classified

- Define the term *normal delivery* and describe the procedures that can be performed with a normal delivery

- Identify the ICD-10-CM category Z37 codes and describe the circumstances in which these codes are used with a delivery code

- Give examples of the ICD-10-PCS procedure codes used to identify delivery procedures

- Assign diagnosis codes for Chapter 15 of ICD-10-CM

- Assign ICD-10-PCS procedure codes for obstetric conditions

Key Terms

Abortion (procedure)
Complete abortion
Delivery (procedure)
Drainage (procedure)
Ectopic pregnancy
Elderly pregnant female

Elective termination of pregnancy
Failed attempted termination of pregnancy
First trimester
Hyperemesis gravidarum
Incomplete abortion
Insufficient antenatal care

Missed abortion
Normal delivery
Outcome of delivery
Preterm labor
Preterm pregnancy
Postpartum
Postterm pregnancy
Pregnancy
Pregnancy state, incidental
Prolonged pregnancy

Puerperium
Recurrent pregnancy loss
Second trimester
Spontaneous abortion
Term pregnancy
Third trimester
Threatened abortion
Weeks of gestation
Young pregnant female

Overview of ICD-10-CM Chapter 15: Pregnancy, Childbirth and the Puerperium

Chapter 15 of ICD-10-CM includes categories O00–O9A arranged in the following blocks:

O00–O08	Pregnancy with abortive outcome
O09	Supervision of high-risk pregnancy
O10–O16	Edema, proteinuria and hypertensive disorders in pregnancy, childbirth and the puerperium
O20–O29	Other maternal disorders predominantly related to pregnancy
O30–O48	Maternal care related to the fetus and amniotic cavity and possible delivery problems
O60–O77	Complications of labor and delivery
O80, O82	Encounter for delivery
O85–O92	Complications predominantly related to the puerperium
O94–O9A	Other obstetric conditions, not elsewhere classified

In ICD-10-CM Chapter 15, terminology is descriptive of what obstetric condition is intended to be represented by the obstetric code. Codes for elective (legal or therapeutic) abortions are classified with the abortion codes in Chapter 15. Complications of induced termination of pregnancy are found in category O04. In comparison, the elective abortion without complication code Z33.2 is included in Chapter 21 of ICD-10-CM, which includes factors influencing health status and contact with health services. Chapter 15 also identifies the trimester of pregnancy in which the condition occurred at the fifth- and sixth-character levels. Figure 18.1 shows a detailed diagram of the female reproductive system including the peritoneal and pelvic cavities.

ICD-10-CM requires the use of a seventh character to identify the fetus to which certain complication codes apply. One of the seventh characters is assigned to certain codes in ICD-10-CM Chapter 15 as directed in the tabular list. The seventh character of 0 is used for a single gestation or when a multiple gestation exists but the fetus cannot be specified as the cause of the maternal condition described by the code. The seventh characters of 1 through 9 are for patients with multiple gestations and used to identify the fetus that is responsible for the condition identified by the code. For example, code O64.1XX2 would be used to state that fetus 2 has caused the obstructed labor due to breech presentation in a pregnant patient with multiple gestations. In summary, the seventh character of 0 is used for all pregnancies with a single gestation. The seventh character of 0 may be used when the patient is pregnant with twins, triplets, or the like but which fetus is responsible for the condition cannot be identified. If the pregnant woman has a condition that can be attributed to one of the multiple fetuses she is carrying, the seventh characters of 1 through 9 are used to identify fetus 1, 2, 3 or similarly fetus A, B, or C, as identified by the attending physician as responsible for the condition.

Figure 18.1. **Female Reproductive system including the peritoneal and pelvic cavities**

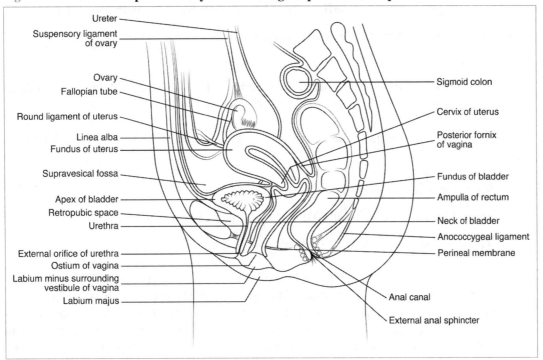

© AHIMA

| | EXAMPLE: | O32, | Maternal care for malpresentation of fetus |

                      One of the following seventh characters is to be assigned to each code under category O32.

                      0—not applicable or unspecified
                      1—fetus 1
                      2—fetus 2
                      3—fetus 3
                      4—fetus 4
                      5—fetus 5
                      9—other fetus

Coding Guidelines and Instructional Notes for ICD-10-CM Chapter 15

At the beginning of Chapter 15 are notes that provide instructions for coding professionals. Codes from this chapter are for use only on maternal records, never on newborn records. For example, Z37.0, Single live birth, is the only outcome of delivery code appropriate for use with O80.

Pregnancy is defined as the state of a female after conception until the birth of the child. Normal pregnancies are intrauterine, and the duration of the pregnancy from conception to delivery is approximately 266 days from the time of fertilization of the oocyte until birth or 288 days from the last normal menstrual period until birth (Dorland 2012, 1509).

The following weeks of gestation are to be used in determining preterm, term, postterm and prolonged pregnancies:

- Preterm: Delivery before 37 completed weeks of gestation. The patient is in her 37th week of pregnancy or an earlier week of pregnancy when the delivery occurs.

- Term: Delivery between 38 and 40 completed weeks of gestation.

- Postterm: Delivery between 41 and 42 completed weeks of gestation.

- Prolonged: Delivery occurs when the pregnancy has advanced beyond 42 completed weeks of gestation. The patient is in her 43rd or later week of pregnancy.

Trimesters are counted from the first day of the last menstrual period. They are defined as follows:

- **First trimester**—less than 14 weeks 0 days

- **Second trimester**—14 weeks 0 days to less than 28 weeks 0 days

- **Third trimester**—28 weeks 0 days until delivery

Assignment of the trimester should be based on the provider's documentation of the trimester or the provider's documentation of the number of weeks of gestation for the current admission or encounter. The provider's documentation of the number of weeks may be used to assign the appropriate code to identify the trimester. The coder should not attempt to identify the trimester or the weeks of gestation according to the stated date of the patient's last menstrual period.

The puerperium, or the **postpartum**, period begins immediately after the third stage of labor when the delivery has occurred until the involution of the uterus is complete, which is normally for 6 weeks or 42 days (Dorland 2012, 1552). A postpartum complication is any complication occurring in the woman who has delivered within the six-week period following delivery.

When the delivery occurs during the current admission and the ICD-10-CM diagnosis code for the patient's condition or obstetrical complication includes the option of "in childbirth" in addition to codes for first, second, or third trimester, the code for "in childbirth" should be assigned.

Another note appears at the start of Chapter 15 that instructs the coder to use an additional code from category Z3A, Weeks of gestation, to identify the specific week of the pregnancy.

The NCHS has published chapter-specific guidelines for Chapter 15 in the *ICD-10-CM Official Guidelines for Coding and Reporting*. The coding student should review all of the coding guidelines for Chapter 15 of ICD-10-CM, which appear in an ICD-10-CM code book or on the CDC website (CDC 2019) or in appendix F.

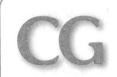

Chapter 15: Pregnancy, Childbirth, and the Puerperium (O00-O0A)

Guideline I.C.15.a. General Rules for Obstetric Cases

Guideline I.C.15.a.1. Codes from Chapter 15 and sequencing priority: Obstetric cases require codes from Chapter 15, codes in the range O00–O9A, Pregnancy, Childbirth, and the Puerperium. Chapter 15 codes have sequencing priority over codes from other chapters. Additional codes from other chapters may be used in conjunction with Chapter 15 codes to further specify conditions. Should the provider document that the pregnancy is incidental to the encounter, then code Z33.1, Pregnant state, incidental, should be used in place of any Chapter 15 codes. It is the provider's responsibility to state that the condition being treated is not affecting the pregnancy.

Guideline I.C.15.a.2. Chapter 15 codes used only on the maternal record: Chapter 15 codes are to be used only on the maternal record, never on the record of the newborn.

Guideline I.C.15.a.3. Final character for trimester: The majority of codes in Chapter 15 have a final character indicating the trimester of pregnancy. The timeframes for the trimesters are indicated at the beginning of the chapter. If trimester is not a component of a code it is because the condition always occurs in a specific trimester, or the concept of trimester of pregnancy is not applicable. Certain codes have characters for only certain trimesters because the condition does not occur in all trimesters, but it may occur in more than just one.

Assignment of the final character for trimester should be based on the provider's documentation of the trimester (or number of weeks) for the current admission/encounter. This applies to the assignment of trimester for pre-existing conditions as well as those that develop during or are due to the pregnancy. The provider's documentation of the number of weeks may be used to assign the appropriate code identifying the trimester.

Whenever delivery occurs during the current admission, and there is an "in childbirth" option for the obstetric complication being coded, the "in childbirth" code should be assigned.

Guideline I.C.15.a.4. Selection of trimester for inpatient admissions that encompass more than one trimester: In instances when a patient is admitted to a hospital for complications of pregnancy during one trimester and remains in the hospital into a subsequent trimester, the trimester character for the antepartum complication code should be assigned on the basis of the trimester when the complication developed, not the trimester of the discharge. If the condition developed prior to the current admission/encounter or represents a pre-existing

(Continued)

(Continued)

condition, the trimester character for the trimester at the time of the admission/encounter should be assigned.

Guideline I.C.15.a.5. Unspecified trimester: Each category that includes codes for trimester has a code for "unspecified trimester." The "unspecified trimester" code should rarely be used, such as when the documentation in the record is insufficient to determine the trimester and it is not possible to obtain clarification.

Guideline I.C.15.a.6. Seventh (7th) character for Fetus Identification: Where applicable, a 7th character is to be assigned for certain categories (O31, O32, O33.3 - O33.6, O35, O36, O40, O41, O60.1, O60.2, O64, and O69) to identify the fetus for which the complication code applies.

Assign 7th character "0":

- For single gestations

- When the documentation in the record is insufficient to determine the fetus affected and it is not possible to obtain clarification.

- When it is not possible to clinically determine which fetus is affected.

Guideline I.C.15.b. Selection of OB Principal or First-listed Diagnosis

Guideline I.C.15.b.1. Routine outpatient prenatal visits: For routine outpatient prenatal visits when no complications are present, a code from category Z34, Encounter for supervision of normal pregnancy, should be used as the first-listed diagnosis. These codes should not be used in conjunction with Chapter 15 codes.

Guideline I.C.15.b.2. Supervision of high-risk pregnancy: Codes from category O09, Supervision of high-risk pregnancy, are intended for use only during the prenatal period. For complications during the labor and delivery episode as a result of a high-risk pregnancy, assign the applicable complication codes from Chapter 15. If there are no complications during the labor or delivery episode, assign O80, Encounter for full-term uncomplicated delivery.

For routine prenatal outpatient visits for patients with high-risk pregnancies, a code from category O09, Supervision of high-risk pregnancy, should be used as the first-listed diagnosis. Secondary Chapter 15 codes may be used in conjunction with these codes if appropriate.

Guideline I.C.15.b.3. Episodes when no delivery occurs: In episodes when no delivery occurs, the principal diagnosis should correspond to the principal complication of the pregnancy which necessitated the encounter. Should more than one complication exist, all of which are treated or monitored, any of the complication codes may be sequenced first.

Guideline I.C.15.b.4. When a delivery occurs: When an obstetric patient is admitted and delivers during that admission, the condition that prompted the admission should be sequenced as the principal diagnosis. If multiple conditions prompted the admission, sequence the one most related to the delivery as the principal diagnosis. A code for any complication of the delivery should be assigned as an additional diagnosis. In cases of cesarean delivery, if the patient was admitted with a condition that resulted in the performance of a cesarean procedure, that condition should be selected as the principal diagnosis. If the reason for the admission/encounter was unrelated to the condition resulting in the delivery, the condition related to the reason for the admission/encounter should be selected as the principal diagnosis.

Guideline I.C.15.b.5. Outcome of delivery: A code from category Z37, Outcome of delivery, should be included on every maternal record when a delivery has occurred. These codes are not to be used on subsequent records or on the newborn record.

Guideline I.C.15.c. Pre-existing conditions versus conditions due to the pregnancy: Certain categories in Chapter 15 distinguish between conditions of the mother that existed prior to pregnancy (pre-existing) and those that are a direct result of pregnancy. When assigning codes from Chapter 15, it is important to assess if a condition was pre-existing prior to pregnancy or developed during or due to the pregnancy in order to assign the correct code.

Categories that do not distinguish between pre-existing and pregnancy-related conditions may be used for either. It is acceptable to use codes specifically for the puerperium with codes complicating pregnancy and childbirth if a condition arises postpartum during the delivery encounter.

Guideline I.C.15.d. Pre-existing hypertension in pregnancy: Category O10, Pre-existing hypertension complicating pregnancy, childbirth and the puerperium, includes codes for hypertensive heart and hypertensive chronic kidney disease. When assigning one of the O10 codes that includes hypertensive heart disease or hypertensive chronic kidney disease, it is necessary to add a secondary code from the appropriate hypertension category to specify the type of heart failure or chronic kidney disease.

See Section I.C.9. Hypertension.

Guideline I.C.15.e. Fetal Conditions Affecting the Management of the Mother

Guideline I.C.15.e.1. Codes from categories O35 and O36: Codes from categories O35, Maternal care for known or suspected fetal abnormality and damage, and O36, Maternal care for other fetal problems, are assigned only when the fetal condition

(Continued)

(Continued)

is actually responsible for modifying the management of the mother, i.e., by requiring diagnostic studies, additional observation, special care, or termination of pregnancy. The fact that the fetal condition exists does not justify assigning a code from this series to the mother's record.

Guideline I.C.15.e.2. In utero surgery: In cases when surgery is performed on the fetus, a diagnosis code from category O35, Maternal care for known or suspected fetal abnormality and damage, should be assigned identifying the fetal condition. Assign the appropriate procedure code for the procedure performed.

No code from Chapter 16, the perinatal codes, should be used on the mother's record to identify fetal conditions. Surgery performed in utero on a fetus is still to be coded as an obstetric encounter.

Guideline I.C.15.f. HIV Infection in Pregnancy, Childbirth and the Puerperium: During pregnancy, childbirth or the puerperium, a patient admitted because of an HIV-related illness should receive a principal diagnosis from subcategory O98.7-, Human immunodeficiency [HIV] disease complicating pregnancy, childbirth and the puerperium, followed by the code(s) for the HIV-related illness(es).

Patients with asymptomatic HIV infection status admitted during pregnancy, childbirth, or the puerperium should receive codes of O98.7- and Z21, Asymptomatic human immunodeficiency virus [HIV] infection status.

Guideline I.C.15.g. Diabetes mellitus in pregnancy: Diabetes mellitus is a significant complicating factor in pregnancy. Pregnant women who are diabetic should be assigned a code from category O24, Diabetes mellitus in pregnancy, childbirth, and the puerperium, first, followed by the appropriate diabetes code(s) (E08-E13) from Chapter 4.

Guideline I.C.15.h. See section I.C.4.a.3, Diabetes mellitus and the use of insulin and oral hypoglycemics.

See section I.C.4.a.3 for information on the long term use of insulin and oral hypoglycemic.

Guideline I.C.15.i. Gestational (pregnancy induced) diabetes: Gestational (pregnancy induced) diabetes can occur during the second and third trimester of pregnancy in women who were not diabetic prior to pregnancy. Gestational diabetes can cause complications in the pregnancy similar to those of pre-existing diabetes mellitus. It also puts the woman at greater risk of developing diabetes after the pregnancy. Codes for gestational diabetes are in subcategory O24.4, Gestational diabetes mellitus. No other code from category O24, Diabetes mellitus in pregnancy, childbirth, and the puerperium, should be used with a code from O24.4.

The codes under subcategory O24.4 include diet controlled, insulin controlled, and controlled by oral hypoglycemic drugs. If a patient with gestational diabetes is treated with both diet and insulin, only the code for insulin-controlled is required. If a patient with gestational diabetes is treated with both diet and oral hypoglycemic medications, only the code for "controlled by oral hypoglycemic drugs" is required. Code Z79.4, Long-term (current) use of insulin or code Z79.84, Long-term (current) use of oral hypoglycemic drugs, should not be assigned with the codes from subcategory O24.4.

An abnormal glucose tolerance in pregnancy is assigned a code from subcategory O99.81, Abnormal glucose complicating pregnancy, childbirth, and the puerperium.

Guideline I.C.15.j. Sepsis and septic shock complicating abortion, pregnancy, childbirth and the puerperium: When assigning a Chapter 15 code for sepsis complicating abortion, pregnancy, childbirth, and the puerperium, a code for the specific type of infection should be assigned as an additional diagnosis. If severe sepsis is present, a code from subcategory R65.2, Severe sepsis, and code(s) for associated organ dysfunction(s) should also be assigned as additional diagnoses.

Guideline I.C.15.k. Puerperal sepsis: Code O85, Puerperal sepsis, should be assigned with a secondary code to identify the causal organism (e.g., for a bacterial infection, assign a code from category B95–B96, Bacterial infections in conditions classified elsewhere). A code from category A40, Streptococcal sepsis, or A41, Other sepsis, should not be used for puerperal sepsis. If applicable, use additional codes to identify severe sepsis (R65.2-) and any associated acute organ dysfunction.

Guideline I.C.15.l. Alcohol, tobacco and drug use during pregnancy, childbirth and the puerperium

Guideline I.C.15.l.1. Alcohol use during pregnancy, childbirth and the puerperium: Codes under subcategory O99.31, Alcohol use complicating pregnancy, childbirth, and the puerperium, should be assigned for any pregnancy case when a mother uses alcohol during the pregnancy or postpartum. A secondary code from category F10, Alcohol related disorders, should also be assigned to identify manifestations of the alcohol use.

Guideline I.C.15.l.2. Tobacco use during pregnancy, childbirth and the puerperium: Codes under subcategory O99.33, Smoking (tobacco) complicating pregnancy, childbirth, and the puerperium, should be assigned for any pregnancy case when a mother uses any type of tobacco product during the pregnancy or postpartum. A secondary code from category F17, Nicotine dependence should also be assigned to identify the type of nicotine dependence.

(Continued)

(Continued)

Guideline I.C.15.I.3 Drug use during pregnancy, childbirth and the puerperium: Codes under subcategory O99.32, Drug use complicating pregnancy, childbirth, and the puerperium, should be assigned for any pregnancy case when a mother uses drugs during the pregnancy or postpartum. This can involve illegal drugs, or inappropriate use or abuse of prescription drugs. Secondary code(s) from categories F11-F16 and F18-F19 should also be assigned to identify manifestations of the drug use.

Guideline I.C.15.m. Poisoning, toxic effects, adverse effects and underdosing in a pregnant patient: A code from subcategory O9A.2, Injury, poisoning and certain other consequences of external causes complicating pregnancy, childbirth, and the puerperium, should be sequenced first, followed by the appropriate injury, poisoning, toxic effect, adverse effect or underdosing code, and then the additional code(s) that specifies the condition caused by the poisoning, toxic effect, adverse effect or underdosing.

See Section I.C.19. Adverse effects, poisoning, underdosing and toxic effects.

Guideline I.C.15.n. Normal Delivery, Code O80

Guideline I.C.15.n.1. Encounter for full term uncomplicated delivery: Code O80 should be assigned when a woman is admitted for a full-term normal delivery and delivers a single, healthy infant without any complications antepartum, during the delivery, or postpartum during the delivery episode. Code O80 is always a principal diagnosis. It is not to be used if any other code from Chapter 15 is needed to describe a current complication of the antenatal, delivery, or postnatal period. Additional codes from other chapters may be used with code O80 if they are not related to or are in any way complicating the pregnancy.

Guideline I.C.15.n.2. Uncomplicated delivery with resolved antepartum complication: Code O80 may be used if the patient had a complication at some point during the pregnancy, but the complication is not present at the time of the admission for delivery.

Guideline I.C.15.n.3. Outcome of delivery for O80 Z37.0, Single live birth, is the only outcome of delivery code appropriate for use with O80.

Guideline I.C.15.o. The Peripartum and Postpartum Periods

Guideline I.C.15.o.1. Peripartum and Postpartum periods: The postpartum period begins immediately after delivery and continues for six weeks following delivery. The peripartum period is defined as the last month of pregnancy to five months postpartum.

Guideline I.C.15.o.2. Peripartum and postpartum complication: A postpartum complication is any complication occurring within the six-week period.

Guideline I.C.15.o.3. Pregnancy-related complications after 6 week period: Chapter 15 codes may also be used to describe pregnancy-related complications after the peripartum or postpartum period if the provider documents that a condition is pregnancy related.

Guideline I.C.15.o.4. Admission for routine postpartum care following delivery outside hospital: When the mother delivers outside the hospital prior to admission and is admitted for routine postpartum care and no complications are noted, code Z39.0, Encounter for care and examination of mother immediately after delivery, should be assigned as the principal diagnosis.

Guideline I.C.15.o.5. Pregnancy associated cardiomyopathy: Pregnancy associated cardiomyopathy, code O90.3, is unique in that it may be diagnosed in the third trimester of pregnancy but may continue to progress months after delivery. For this reason, it is referred to as peripartum cardiomyopathy. Code O90.3 is only for use when the cardiomyopathy develops as a result of pregnancy in a woman who did not have pre-existing heart disease.

Guideline I.C.15.p. Code O94, Sequelae of complication of pregnancy, childbirth, and the puerperium

Guideline I.C.15.p.1. Code O94: Code O94, Sequelae of complication of pregnancy, childbirth, and the puerperium, is for use in those cases when an initial complication of a pregnancy develops a sequelae requiring care or treatment at a future date.

Guideline I.C.15.p.2. After the initial postpartum period: This code may be used at any time after the initial postpartum period.

Guideline I.C.15.p.3. Sequencing of Code O94: This code, like all sequela codes, is to be sequenced following the code describing the sequelae of the complication.

Guideline I.C.15.q. Termination of Pregnancy and Spontaneous abortions

Guideline I.C.15.q.1. Abortion with Liveborn Fetus: When an attempted termination of pregnancy results in a liveborn fetus, assign code Z33.2, Encounter for elective termination of pregnancy and a code from category Z37, Outcome of Delivery.

Guideline I.C.15.q.2. Retained Products of Conception following an abortion: Subsequent encounters for retained products of conception following a spontaneous abortion or elective termination of pregnancy, without complications are assigned O03.4, Incomplete spontaneous abortion without complication, or codes O07.4, Failed attempted termination of pregnancy without complication. This advice is appropriate even when the patient was discharged previously with a discharge diagnosis

(Continued)

(Continued)

of complete abortion. If the patient has a specific complication associated with the spontaneous abortion or elective termination of pregnancy in addition to retained products of conception, assign the appropriate complication code (e.g., O03.-, O04.-, O07.-) instead of code O03.4 or O07.4

Guideline I.C.15.q.3. Complications leading to abortion: Codes from Chapter 15 may be used as additional codes to identify documented complications of the pregnancy in conjunction with codes in categories O04, O07 and O08.

Guideline I.C.15.r. Abuse in a pregnant patient: For suspected or confirmed cases of abuse of a pregnant patient, a code(s) from subcategories O9A.3, Physical abuse complicating pregnancy, childbirth, and the puerperium, O9A.4, Sexual abuse complicating pregnancy, childbirth, and the puerperium, and O9A.5, Psychological abuse complicating pregnancy, childbirth, and the puerperium, should be sequenced first, followed by the appropriate codes (if applicable) to identify any associated current injury due to physical abuse, sexual abuse, and the perpetrator of abuse.

See Section I.C.19. Adult and child abuse, neglect and other maltreatment.

Coding Pregnancy, Childbirth and the Puerperium in ICD-10-CM Chapter 15

Codes in Chapter 15, Pregnancy, Childbirth and the Puerperium, are in the range of O00 (letter O, digit zero, digit zero) to O9A. One way to remember this is to identify that the letter O codes are for Obstetrics. As the note specifies at the beginning of the chapter, codes from Chapter 15 are used only on maternal records and never on newborn infant records. The note also specifies that codes from this chapter are for use for conditions related to or aggravated by the pregnancy, childbirth, or by the puerperium (maternal causes or obstetric causes).

The majority of codes in Chapter 15 have a final character indicating the woman's trimester of pregnancy, that is, first, second, or third trimester. Assignment of the final character for trimester should be based on the trimester for the current admission or encounter. Whenever delivery occurs during the current admission and there is an "in childbirth" option for the obstetric complication being coded, the "in childbirth" code should be assigned.

Use of the Alphabetic Index for Chapter 15 Codes

Locating the correct ICD-10-CM code for an obstetrical condition requires careful use of the Alphabetic Index. Several key main terms are used. The main term "Pregnancy" is used to identify whether the patient is experiencing a normal pregnancy or having a condition or complication that is influencing her treatment and outcome. The main term "Pregnancy"

includes the nonessential modifiers of single or uterine. A directional note follows the main term Pregnancy advising the coder to also see the main terms of Delivery and Puerperal.

Alphabetic Index Main Term Pregnancy and Subterms

Beneath the main term of pregnancy are subterms in alphabetic sequence, such as abdominal (ectopic), ampullar, biochemical, and so on. The subterm of "complicated by (care of) (management affected by)" is following by another long list of subterms in alphabetic order, for example, abnormal, abnormality; abruption placentae; abscess or cellulitis; and so on. Important subterms to reference under "complicated by" include pre-existing conditions and complications that develop during the pregnancy. For example, common conditions that exist in the pregnant woman are included as subterms, such as anemia, diabetes, fetal (maternal care for), hypertension, preterm labor, vomiting, and so on. The codes that appear under the main term of pregnancy can be applied to the patient's record during the pregnancy as well as at the time of delivery.

Another important subterm is "ectopic pregnancy" that refers the coder to the subterm "ectopic under pregnancy." An ectopic pregnancy is when the products of conception or the pregnancy is located outside the normal location of the uterus, for example, within the fallopian tube (Stedman 2012, 525). In the Alphabetic Index to Diseases and Injuries, the coder can find the code for type of ectopic pregnancy that exists, for example, abdominal, tubal, or ovarian, as well as complications that can develop as the result of an ectopic pregnancy as included under "pregnancy, ectopic, complicated by."

The subterm "examination, (normal)" is to be used by the coder to find a code describing the encounter for a pregnant female who is examined during a first pregnancy or other specified pregnancy. A directional note appears under examination referring the code for a high-risk pregnancy examination, the coder should refer to the main term of pregnancy, supervision of high risk.

When a patient experiences maternal care for a fetal condition, the coder should refer to the main term of Pregnancy, complicated by, fetal. Entries here describe when the management of the pregnant female is affected by a fetal condition, such as chromosomal abnormalities, fetal death, excessive growth of the fetus, growth retardation of the fetus, or other fetal problems. Several of these entries lead to a code in the categories O35 and O36 that are only assigned when the fetal condition is responsible for a change in the management of the pregnant female, such as additional testing or observation as well as performing a termination of the pregnancy, for example, the termination of the pregnancy due to the chromosomal abnormalities of the fetus.

Alphabetic Index Main Term Delivery and Subterms

A second important main term is "Delivery (childbirth) (labor)." Subterms beneath the main term delivery describe the type of delivery or the clinical factors that had an influence on the type of delivery that occurred. Coders are likely to use this main term when coding a record for the hospital when the delivery occurs or for the physician/provider who care for the patient during the admission. The main term "Delivery (childbirth) (labor)" has several subterms beneath it in alphabetic order. The subterms with "cesarean (for)" describe the reason(s) for the cesarean delivery. Such terms are breech presentation, failed induction of labor, malposition or malpresentation, planned, occurring after 37 completed weeks of gestation but before 39 completed weeks gestation due to (spontaneous) onset of labor, previous cesarean delivery, prolonged labor, transverse presentation, and the like. Another important subterm under delivery is "complicated, by" that includes a long list of conditions that can complicate a delivery, such as cord around neck, delayed following rupture of membranes, hemorrhage, laceration of perineum, obstructed labor, placenta problems, prolonged labor, uterine inertia, and the like. Other subterms under delivery, in alphabetic sequence, include forceps, normal, precipitate, preterm, spontaneous, and uncomplicated. Multiple conditions such as these can exist in the same patient that necessitate multiple codes to be used.

Other Alphabetic Index Main Terms Subterms

Of note, there are no entries under the main term "Labor" to describe complications or conditions related to the labor. Instead, refer the coder to the main term "Delivery." Conditions that develop during the postpartum period can also be coded. The main term "Postpartum" refers the coder to the main term "Puerperal." The main term of Puerperal or Puerperium includes subterms that describe conditions with the onset during the postpartum period. Such subterms include conditions of abscess, diabetes, disruption, fever, hemorrhage, infection, sepsis, and so on.

Coders may also find it useful to use the pregnant woman's medical condition as a main term and look for a connecting term that associated the medical condition with a pregnancy. For example, the main terms of anemia, diabetes, hypertension, and fever all include subterms that describe it as complicating the pregnancy or occurring following the pregnancy. When the patient is pregnant, the combination code for the pregnancy with the medical (often pre-existing condition) must be used instead of simply using the code for the medical condition.

Summary of Main Terms and Subterms

To summarize the use of the Alphabetic Index to Diseases and Injuries for coding the maternal conditions related to the pregnancy, the important main terms and subterms are as follows:

Delivery (childbirth)(labor)
  arrested active phase
  cesarean for…
  completely normal care
  complicated by…
  delayed NOS
  forceps, low following failed vacuum extraction
  missed
  normal
  obstructed
  precipitate
  preterm
  spontaneous
  term pregnancy
  uncomplicated
  vaginal following previous cesarean delivery

Pregnancy (single)(uterine)—see also Delivery and Puerperal
  abdominal
  ampullar
  biochemical
  broad ligament
  cervical
  chemical
  complicated NOS

complication by…
concealed
continuing following…
corneal
ectopic….
examination…
extrauterine
fallopian
false
hidden
high-risk
incidental finding
interstitial
intraligamentous
intraperitoneal
isthmian
mesometric
molar…
multiple…
mural
normal…
ovarian
postmature
post-term
prenatal care only…
prolonged
quadruplet
quintuplet
sextuplet
supervision of…
triplet
tubal
twin
unwanted
weeks of gestation

Labor—see Delivery
Puerperal, puerperium (complicated by, complications)
  There is an extensive list of puerperal conditions, with some important entries such as
  abscess
  hemorrhage
  infection

Another option to locate an ICD-10-CM diagnosis code for pregnant woman is to locate the pregnant woman's medical condition as it appears alphabetically in the Index connected to the pregnancy state, for example:

Anemia, complicating pregnancy
Diabetes, complicating pregnancy
Diabetes, gestational
Eclampsia
Fever, puerperal
Gestational
Hypertension, complicating childbirth, pregnancy, puerperium

Hypertension, gestational
Post-term, pregnancy
Pre-eclampsia
Premature, birth or delivery or labor or rupture of membranes
Prolonged, gestation or labor or pregnancy

Check Your Understanding 18.1

Assign diagnosis codes to the following conditions.

1. Triplet pregnancy, trichorionic/triamniotic, second trimester, 18 weeks, undelivered

2. Vaginal delivery, uncomplicated, single liveborn infant, 39 weeks

3. Eclampsia complicating the puerperium

4. Pre-existing essential hypertension complicated pregnancy, 27 weeks, undelivered

5. Pregnancy complicated by chorioamnionitis, third trimester (34 weeks), undelivered, single gestation

---

Pregnancy-Related Codes in ICD-10-CM Chapter 21

Codes from other chapters in ICD-10-CM are used to describe conditions and factors related to reproduction. One block of codes in Chapter 21, Factors influencing health status and contact with health services includes Z30–Z39, Persons encountering health services in circumstances related to reproduction. These codes are used to describe reasons for healthcare services for the pregnant female or for services for men and women seeking reproductive health services. The categories are described in the following sections.

Z30 Encounter for Contraceptive Management

Codes in this category are used to describe encounters of care for initial prescription of contraceptives, natural family planning, and other general counseling and advice on contraception. Other codes represent visits for surveillance of contraceptives and other contraceptive management visits, including for the male for an encounter for postvasectomy sperm count. The Alphabetic Index entry for locating these codes is "contraception, contraceptive."

> **EXAMPLE:** The 20-year-old female is seen in her physician's office for an examination and receipt of her initial prescription for contraceptive pills: Z30.011, Encounter for initial prescription for contraceptive pills.

Z31 Encounter for Procreative Management

Codes in this category identify when procreative management services are provided. These services include encounters for fertility testing, genetic testing for men and women seeking procreative services, and genetic counseling. Code Z31.83 is used for the visit when an assisted reproductive fertility procedure is performed. The Alphabetic Index entries for locating these codes includes "encounter" or "test, tests, testing (for)" or "management."

> **EXAMPLE:** The 30-year-old male was seen in the physician's office for fertility testing and submitting a specimen for a sperm count: Z31.41, Encounter for fertility testing.

Z32 Encounter for Pregnancy Test and Childbirth and Childcare Instruction

The codes in this category identify an encounter for a pregnancy test and encounters for childbirth education and child care education. The codes for the pregnancy testing identify if the test result was positive, negative, or the result unknown. Codes for these types of office visits typically are found in the Alphabetic Index under the main term "encounter, pregnancy test."

> **EXAMPLE:** The 28-year-old female was seen in the office of her primary care physician for the purposes of a pregnancy test as she missed her last menstrual period. The patient was told the pregnancy test was negative, and she was given an appointment for the following week to investigate the reasons for the missed period: Z32.02, Encounter for pregnancy test, result negative.

Z33 Pregnant State

Code Z33.1, **Pregnant state, incidental**, would be assigned as an additional code only if a pregnant patient was seen for a reason unrelated to the pregnancy. It is the physician's responsibility to document that the pregnancy is in no way complicating the reason for the visit or the nonobstetrical condition currently being treated. However, it is not a common occurrence for the physician to state the pregnancy is unaffected, no matter how minor the injury or condition. For this reason, a code from Chapter 15 in ICD-10-CM is more frequently used than Z33.1. Code Z33.1 is indexed under the main term "Pregnancy, incidental finding" in the Alphabetic Index. There is an Excludes1 note under code Z33.1 to remind the coder that complications of pregnancy (codes O00–O9A) cannot be used with code Z33.1 as the codes for the pregnancy complications should be used when present and the code for pregnant state is omitted.

> **EXAMPLE:** The patient is seen in the emergency department for the initial visit for a sprained left wrist; the physician documents that the patient is pregnant, but specifically states the pregnancy is incidental to the encounter: S63.502A, Sprains and strains of unspecified site of wrist; Z33.1, Pregnant state, incidental.

The ICD-10-CM code for an uncomplicated elective termination of pregnancy (Z33.2) is found in Chapter 21, Factors influencing health status and contact with health services, not with the OB codes found in Chapter 15. An **elective termination of pregnancy**, or an elective abortion, is the intentional ending of a pregnancy by a medical or surgical procedure. There is an Excludes1 note following code Z33.2 that directs the coder that the conditions of early fetal death with retention of dead fetus, late fetal death, or spontaneous abortion cannot be assigned with code Z33.2.

Z34 Encounter for Supervision of Normal Pregnancy

For routine prenatal outpatient visits when there is no complication present, a code from category Z34 for the encounter for supervision of normal pregnancy is used as the first-listed code. If the prenatal outpatient visit is to manage a high-risk pregnancy, a code from Chapter 15 category O09, Supervision of high-risk pregnancy, is used as the first-listed code. The high-risk pregnancy supervision codes are in the obstetric code chapter and not in the equivalent Z code chapter, where the Z34 codes are located.

A category Z34 code is assigned for supervision of a pregnancy. Code Z34.0, Supervision of normal first pregnancy, uses a fifth character identifying the first, second, third, or unspecified trimester. Z34.8 is a similar code, but it is for supervision of other normal pregnancy than the first pregnancy. The trimester of the pregnancy is identified by the fifth character. Supervision of normal subsequent pregnancies is generally used in outpatient settings and for routine prenatal visits.

When a complication of the pregnancy is present, the code for that condition is assigned rather than a code from category Z34. These codes are not used with any other pregnancy code in Chapter 15 of ICD-10-CM because the Z34 code indicates the patient is pregnant and healthy, whereas the Chapter 15 codes indicate an obstetrical problem or condition exists. Codes in category Z34 are indexed under "Pregnancy, supervision (of) (for)" in the Index to Diseases and Injuries.

> **EXAMPLE:** The 25-year-old female is seen in her obstetrician's office during her 35th week of gestation for supervision of her first pregnancy that appears to be uncomplicated: Z34.03, Encounter for supervision of normal first pregnancy, third trimester.

Z36 Encounter for Antenatal Screening of Mother

Codes in category Z36, are used to describe the encounter for antenatal or prenatal screening of the pregnant female. Screening tests are performed for preventive measures and not necessarily because the mother is experiencing symptoms or problems. The Alphabetic Index entry of "screening, antenatal, of mother" directs the coder to entry of "encounter, antenatal screening" with a list of choices for the types of screenings leading to the category code Z36.

> **EXAMPLE:** The 32-year-old female is seen in her primary care physician's office for a laboratory tests to be completed for chromosomal anomalies: Z36.0, Encounter for antenatal screening for chromosomal anomalies.

Z3A Weeks of Gestation

A code from category Z3A is for use only on the maternal record. The Alphabetic Index entries used to locate this code is "pregnancy, weeks of gestation." The Z3A code is used to indicate the **weeks of gestation** of the pregnancy. The gestation period is the duration of the pregnancy. The weeks of gestation indicate the length of the pregnancy measured in completed weeks. Normal pregnancies are intrauterine and the duration of the pregnancy from conception to delivery is approximately 266 days from the time of fertilization of the oocyte until birth or 288 days from the last normal menstrual period until birth (Dorland 2012, 1509). The Z3A code for the weeks of gestation is used in addition to a code from Chapter 15 to identify the condition or complication of the pregnancy or childbirth. The "code first" note that appears under category Z3A states code first complications of pregnancy, childbirth, and the puerperium, O09-O9A. The ICD-10-CM chapter specific coding guidelines for Chapter 21 (Z00-99), part (11) state the category Z3A codes are not assigned for pregnancies with abortive outcome (O00–O08), elective terminations of pregnancy, nor for conditions that occur during the puerperium. The fifth-character level of the code identifies the individual specific week of gestation starting at 8 weeks through 42 weeks of gestation with other codes for shorter or longer periods of gestation. Table 18.1 is an example of some of the relevant codes.

Table 18.1. Example of the Z3A category codes for weeks of gestation

Z3A.00	Weeks of gestation of pregnancy not specified
Z3A.01	Less than 8 weeks of gestation of pregnancy
Z3A.08	8 weeks of gestation of pregnancy
Z3A.20	20 weeks of gestation of pregnancy
Z3A.38	38 weeks of gestation of pregnancy
Z3A.42	42 weeks of gestation of pregnancy
Z3A.49	Greater than 42 weeks of gestation of pregnancy

Z37 Outcome of Delivery

Outcome of delivery codes (Z37.0–Z37.9) are intended for use as an additional code to identify the outcome of delivery on the mother's record. It is not for use on the newborn record. These codes exclude stillbirth (P95), which would be assigned to the record of a stillborn infant if a record was created for the stillborn. The **outcome of delivery** codes identify the status of the infant, single, twin, or other multiple births, and whether the infant was liveborn or stillborn. The Alphabetic Index entry to locate these codes is the main term "outcome of delivery."

EXAMPLE: The patient is a 26-year-old female who was discharged from the hospital on day 2 after experiencing a completely normal delivery during her 39th week of gestation with the birth of a healthy live female infant: O80, Delivery, completely normal case; Z3A.39, Pregnancy, weeks of gestation, 39 weeks; and Z37.0, Outcome of delivery, single, liveborn

Z39 Encounter for Maternal Postpartum Care and Examination

Code Z39.0 is assigned when the pregnant female delivers a baby outside the hospital and is admitted for care and observation in uncomplicated cases. If the mother delivers outside the hospital and is admitted for care of a pregnancy condition or complication, there is an Excludes1 note that states: care for postpartum complication—see Alphabetic Index. Two other frequently used codes in this category are code Z39.1, Encounter for care and examination of the lactating mother (which is also applicable to supervision of lactation), and code Z39.2, which is used for an encounter for a routine postpartum follow-up visit for a woman who delivered in the previous six weeks. The Alphabetic Index entries to locate these codes include the main terms "Care, postpartum" and "Admission, postpartum observation."

EXAMPLE: The patient is a 33-year-old female who was discharged from the hospital one day after admission for care following the delivery of her son in her family's car on the way to the hospital and was brought to the hospital by paramedics in an ambulance: Z39.0, Encounter for care and examination of mother immediately after delivery.

Pregnancy with Abortive Outcome (O00–O08)

Codes within this block of codes represent the diseases and conditions of the woman who experiences a pregnancy that does not produce a liveborn or stillborn infant. The pregnancies described by these codes end before the completion of 20 weeks of gestation.

The main term "abortion (complete)(spontaneous)" is used to locate the appropriate code. The Alphabetic Index entries for various types of abortions include:

Abortion (complete)(spontaneous)

    with retained productions of conception—see abortion, incomplete
    attempted (elective)(failed)
       complicated by
          followed by subterms describing the complication
    complicated by (describing complications following a spontaneous abortion)
    failed—see abortion, attempted
    habitual or recurrent
    incomplete (spontaneous)
       complicated by
          followed by subterms describing the complication
    induced (encounter for) [with code Z33.2 for elective abortion]
       complicated by
       followed by subterms describing the complication
    missed
    spontaneous—see abortion (complete)(spontaneous)
    threatened
       threatened
       tubal

These Index entries lead the coder to categories O02, O03, O04, and O07 with fourth and fifth characters identifying the specific condition or complication. There is a note at the start of Chapter 15 of ICD-10-CM to "use additional code from category Z3A, weeks of gestation, to identify the specific week of pregnancy." According to ICD-10-CM Coding and Reporting Guidelines, section I.C.21.c.11, the use of category Z3A, Weeks of gestation, codes should not be used for pregnancies with abortive outcomes (categories O00–O08), elective termination of pregnancy (code Z33.2), nor for postpartum conditions, as category Z3A is not applicable to these conditions (CDC 2019).

Ectopic Pregnancy (O00)

An **ectopic pregnancy** is when the products of conception or the pregnancy is located outside the normal location of the uterus, for example, within the fallopian tube (Stedman 2012, 525.) An ectopic pregnancy is a pregnancy arising from implantation of the ovum outside the uterine cavity. About 98 percent of ectopic pregnancies are tubal (occurring in the fallopian tube). Other sites include the peritoneum or abdominal viscera, ovary, or cervix (Sivalingam et al. 2011). Figure 18.2 is a diagram of the locations of implantation for ectopic pregnancies within the fallopian tube.

Figure 18.2. **Ectopic pregnancy areas of implantation**

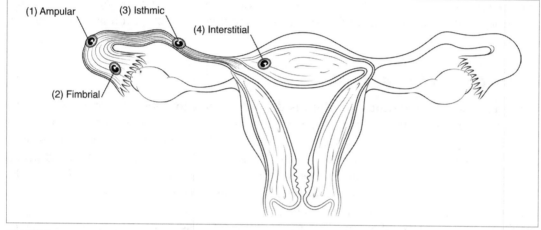

© AHIMA

ICD-10-CM classifies ectopic pregnancy to category O00, with fourth digits identifying the site of the ectopic pregnancy: abdominal, tubal, ovarian, or another site. The 5th character for the ectopic pregnancy codes identify is the ectopic pregnancy is present without or with an intrauterine pregnancy. The 6th character identifies if the tubal or ovarian pregnancy is present on the right side or the left side. An unspecified code O00.90–O00.91 is used for the rare occasions when the site of the ectopic pregnancy is not specified. A "use additional code" note appears under the category heading to use a code from category O08, Complication following ectopic and molar pregnancy, to identify any associated complication. Complications that may occur with an ectopic pregnancy are infection, hemorrhage, embolism, shock, renal failure, metabolic disorders, damage to pelvic organs, or other specified conditions.

> **EXAMPLE:** The 38-year-old woman was discharged from the hospital following treatment for a ruptured right tubal ectopic pregnancy (without intrauterine pregnancy) with resulting renal failure: O00.101, Tubal pregnancy; O08.4, Renal failure following ectopic and molar pregnancy.

Missed Abortion (O02.1)

A **missed abortion** occurs when the fetus has died before completion of 20 weeks' gestation, with retention in the uterus. The death is indicated by cessation of growth, hardening of the uterus, loss of size of the uterus, and absence of fetal heart tones after they have been heard on previous examinations (Dorland 2012, 4). The ICD-10-CM Tabular includes a description of a missed abortion under code O02.1 as early fetal death before completion of 20 weeks of gestation with retention of dead fetus (CDC 2019).

A woman with a missed abortion may develop disseminated intravascular coagulation (DIC), a bleeding disorder that occurs when the blood is lacking the elements needed for blood clotting (Dorland 2012, 376) and progressive hypofibrinogenemia or the lack of fibrinogen in the blood that produces coagulation of blood (Stedman 2012, 629). Massive bleeding may occur when delivery is finally completed in the patient with DIC. During this time, symptoms of pregnancy disappear. For the patient without complications like DIC, once the missed abortion treatment is complete, a brownish vaginal discharge may occur.

Missed abortions should be completed by physician intervention as soon as a diagnosis with Doppler ultrasound or other methods is certain. A common method of terminating the pregnancy involves the insertion of laminaria stents to dilate the cervix followed by a suction D&C.

Spontaneous Abortion (O03)

The diagnosis of **spontaneous abortion** is defined as the expulsion or extraction from the uterus of all or part of the products of conception: an embryo or a nonviable fetus weighing less than 500 grams (Puscheck 2018). The spontaneous abortion occurs without a medical or surgical intervention to cause it. When a fetus's weight cannot be determined, an estimated gestation of less than 20 completed weeks is considered an abortion in ICD-10-CM. The procedure also known as abortion is more precisely described as a dilation and curettage, dilation and evacuation, or aspiration curettage.

Coders frequently confuse the clinical condition of missed abortion with spontaneous abortion. A missed abortion is a nonviable intrauterine pregnancy that has been retained within the uterus without spontaneous abortion. Typically, no symptoms exist beside amenorrhea, and the patient finds out that the pregnancy stopped developing earlier when a fetal heartbeat is not observed or heard at the appropriate time (Puscheck 2018). In contrast to a spontaneous abortion, no products of conception, fetal parts, or tissue is expelled from the uterus when the patient has a missed abortion. All of the uterine contents remain in the uterus. When a spontaneous abortion occurs, the woman experiences one or more of the classic symptoms of a pregnancy loss, such as uterine contractions, uterine hemorrhage, dilation of the cervix, and presentation or expulsion of all or part of the products of conception.

The fourth characters used with category O03 indicate the presence or absence of a complication arising during an admission or an encounter for a spontaneous abortion. The fourth-digit subcategories are classified as follows:

O03.0,	Genital tract and pelvic infection following incomplete spontaneous abortion
	Endometritis
	Oophoritis
	Parametritis
	Pelvic peritonitis
	Salpingitis
	Salpingo-oophoritis
O03.1,	Delayed or excessive hemorrhage following incomplete spontaneous abortion
	Afibrinogenemia
	Defibrination syndrome
	Hemolysis
	Intravascular hemolysis

O03.2,   Embolism following incomplete spontaneous abortion
Air embolism
Amniotic fluid embolism
Blood-clot embolism
Embolism NOS
Fat embolism
Pulmonary embolism
Pyemic embolism
Septic or septicopyemic embolism
Soap embolism

O03.3,   Other and unspecified complications following incomplete spontaneous abortion
Circulatory collapse
Shock
Renal failure
Metabolic disorders
Damage to pelvic organs
Other venous complication
Cardiac arrest
Sepsis
Urinary tract infection

O03.4,   Incomplete spontaneous abortion without complication

O03.5,   Genital tract and pelvic infection following complete or unspecified spontaneous abortion

O03.6,   Delayed or excessive hemorrhage following complete or unspecified spontaneous abortion

O03.7,   Embolism following complete or unspecified spontaneous abortion

O03.8,   Other and unspecified complications following complete or unspecified spontaneous abortion

O03.9,   Complete or unspecified spontaneous abortion without complication

ICD-10-CM uses the following definitions for complete and incomplete spontaneous abortions:

- A **complete abortion** is the expulsion of all of the products of conception from the uterus prior to the episode of care (CDC 2019).

- An **incomplete abortion** is the expulsion of some, but not all, of the products of conception from the uterus. If placenta or secundines remain, the abortion is considered incomplete. A subsequent admission for retained products of conception following a spontaneous abortion or elective termination of pregnancy are assigned the appropriate code from category O03, spontaneous abortion, or codes O07.4, failed attempted termination of pregnancy without complication and Z33.2, encounter for elective termination of pregnancy. This advice is appropriate even when the patient was discharged previously with a discharged diagnosis of complete abortion. A review of the pathology report will confirm a complete or an incomplete abortion (CDC 2019).

Complications Following (Induced) Termination of Pregnancy (O04)

Category O04, Complications following (induced) termination of pregnancy is used when a complication occurs after the abortion itself was completed during a previous admission. According to the Excludes1 note that appears in category O04, these codes are not used during an encounter for elective termination of pregnancy that is uncompleted or during an encounter when a failed attempted termination of pregnancy occurs. The subcategories classify the complications classifiable to the fourth-digit level:

O04.5, Genital tract and pelvic infection following (induced) termination of pregnancy
O04.6, Delayed or excessive hemorrhage following (induced) termination of pregnancy
O04.7, Embolism following (induced) termination of pregnancy
O04.8, (Induced) termination of pregnancy with other and unspecified complications
Shock
Renal failure
Metabolic disorder
Damage to pelvic organs
Other venous complication
Cardiac arrest
Urinary tract infection
Other complications
Unspecified complications

EXAMPLE: The patient was discharged from the hospital following treatment for pelvic peritonitis that developed following the elective termination of pregnancy that she had five days ago at an outpatient center: O04.82, Abortion, induced, complicated by renal failure. (Index: Complications, following termination of pregnancy—see Abortion).

Check Your Understanding 18.3

Assign diagnosis codes to the following conditions:

1. Ectopic tubal pregnancy, right side, treated, that occurred with concurrent intrauterine pregnancy

2. Missed abortion

3. Sepsis following induced termination of pregnancy, termination, current episode

4. Incomplete hydatidiform mole

5. Incomplete spontaneous abortion with urinary tract infection

Failed Attempted Termination of Pregnancy (O07)

Category O07, **Failed attempted termination of pregnancy**, is used when an attempted abortion fails and the pregnancy continues. The failed termination may not produce any complications (O07.4). However, other fourth-character subcategory codes are used when a complication occurs. According to the Excludes1 note that appears in category O07, these codes are not used during an encounter for treatment of an incomplete spontaneous abortion (O03.0-). The subcategories classify the complications classifiable to the fourth-digit level.

O07.0, Genital tract and pelvic infection following failed attempted termination of pregnancy
O07.1, Delayed or excessive hemorrhage following failed attempted termination of pregnancy
O07.2, Embolism following failed attempted termination of pregnancy

O07.3-,   (Induced) termination of pregnancy with other and unspecified complications
          Shock
          Renal failure
          Metabolic disorder
          Damage to pelvic organs
          Other venous complication
          Cardiac arrest
          Sepsis
          Urinary tract infection
          Other complications
O07.4,   Failed attempted termination of pregnancy without complication

> **EXAMPLE:** The patient is seen in her obstetrician's office for a postoperative visit following an elective termination of pregnancy three days ago. During this visit, it was determined that the procedure was a failed attempted abortion, and the patient remained pregnant with apparently no complications: O07.4, Failed attempted termination of pregnancy, without complication.

Complications Following Ectopic and Molar Pregnancy (O08)

Category O08, Complications following ectopic and molar pregnancy, is used when a complication occurs with an ectopic and molar pregnancy. According to the note that appears in category O08, these codes are used with categories O00–O02 to identify any associated complications. The subcategories classify the complications classifiable to the fourth-digit level. The main terms used in the Alphabetic Index to locate these codes are "pregnancy, ectopic" and "pregnancy, molar."

O08.0,   Genital tract and pelvic infection following ectopic and molar pregnancy
          Endometritis
          Oophoritis
          Parametritis
          Pelvic peritonitis
          Salpingitis
          Salpingo-oophoritis
O08.1,   Delayed or excessive hemorrhage following ectopic and molar pregnancy
          Afibrinogenemia
          Defibrination syndrome
          Hemolysis
          Intravascular hemolysis
O08.2,   Embolism following ectopic and molar pregnancy
          Air embolism
          Amniotic fluid embolism
          Blood-clot embolism
          Embolism NOS
          Fat embolism
          Pulmonary embolism
          Pyemic embolism
          Septic or septicopyemic embolism
          Soap embolism
O08.3,   Shock following ectopic and molar pregnancy
          Circulatory collapse
          Shock

O08.4,   Renal failure following ectopic and molar pregnancy

O08.5,   Metabolic disorders following ectopic and molar pregnancy

O08.6,   Damage to pelvic organs and tissues following ectopic and molar pregnancy

O08.7,   Other venous complications following an ectopic and molar pregnancy

O08.8-,   Other complications following an ectopic and molar pregnancy

         Cardiac arrest

         Sepsis

         Urinary tract infection

         Other complications

O08.9,   Unspecified complications following an ectopic and molar pregnancy

> **EXAMPLE:** The patient is a 34-year-old female who was discharged from the hospital following treatment for a complete hydatidiform mole with complicating by a urinary tract infection: O01.0, Incomplete hydatidiform mole; O08.83, Urinary tract infection following an ectopic or molar pregnancy. [Index: Mole, hydatidiform; Complication, following, ectopic or molar pregnancy]

Supervision of High-Risk Pregnancy (O09)

The codes from category O09, Supervision of high-risk pregnancy, are used only during the perinatal period and not at the time of delivery. For complications during labor and delivery admission that are a result of the high-risk pregnancy, pregnancy complication codes from Chapter 15 are assigned instead of the O09 codes. If there are no complications during the labor and delivery admission, the code O80 for full-term uncomplicated delivery is assigned (CDC 2018). Code O09.3-, Supervision of pregnancy with **insufficient antenatal care**, may be assigned to patients who had little or no prenatal care. Healthcare providers must define insufficient prenatal care and consistently capture this code for the information to be valuable. Codes within the O09.5- (**elderly pregnant females**, 35 years or older at the expected date of delivery) and O09.6- (**young pregnant females**, younger than 16 years old at expected date of delivery) subcategories identify patients whose age and current pregnancies put them at a high risk for problems and thus make them worthy of close monitoring. Codes O09.81- and O09.82- identify the fact that the patient is pregnant as a result of assisted reproductive technology or is pregnant with a history of an in utero procedure during a previous pregnancy. The sixth-character level identifies the first, second, third, or unspecified trimester of pregnancy when the supervision occurred. However, if the elderly primigravida or multigravida woman has a completely normal delivery and the patient's diagnosis is advanced maternal age with no other problems, the diagnosis code of O80, Encounter for full-term uncomplicated delivery is the principal diagnosis.

The O09 category codes are indexed under the main terms "Pregnancy, supervision (of) (for), high risk" in the Alphabetic Index.

> **EXAMPLE:** Pregnancy, first trimester with history of infertility:
> O09.01, Supervision of pregnancy with history of infertility, first trimester

Threatened Abortion (O20.0)

A **threatened abortion** is characterized by bleeding of intrauterine origin occurring before the 20th completed week of gestation, with or without uterine colic, without expulsion of the products of conception, and without dilation of the cervix (Puscheck 2018). ICD-10-CM category O20 states that hemorrhage occurs before the completion of 20 weeks. The physician may also document the condition as an intrauterine hemorrhage due to a threatened abortion. When a physician describes the patient's condition as a threatened abortion, it means the loss of the pregnancy is prevented and the patient remains pregnant at the end of the admission or encounter. The Alphabetic Index entries of "abortion" or "threatened" may be used to locate the codes in category O20.

> **EXAMPLE:** The patient is a 30-year-old female who is 16 weeks pregnant who comes to the Emergency Department (ED) of the hospital complaining of vaginal bleeding but does not describe uterine contractions. After evaluation and consultation with the patient's obstetrician, the ED physician receives an order from the obstetrician to place the patient into the Obstetric Observation unit for further monitoring. The diagnosis written by the ED is threatened: O20.0, Threatened abortion.

Recurrent Pregnancy Loss (O26.20–O26.23 and N96)

A **recurrent pregnancy loss**, also known as a habitual or recurrent abortion, is the spontaneous expulsion of a dead or nonviable fetus in two or more pregnancies at any gestational age. Coding assignments for this condition include the following:

- If the recurrent spontaneous abortion is current, that is, the patient's admission or encounter is for an abortion, ICD-10-CM offers direction to the spontaneous abortion code (category O03).

- If the current hospital admission or encounter involves a pregnancy, assign code O26.20–O26.23, Pregnancy care for patient with recurrent pregnancy loss, with the trimester of pregnancy identified if known.

- If the current hospital admission or encounter does not involve a pregnancy, assign code N96, Recurrent pregnancy loss. During an admission or encounter that does not involve pregnancy care, there is likely an investigation or care of a nonpregnant woman with a history of recurrent pregnancy loss.

Check Your Understanding 18.4

Assign diagnosis codes to the following conditions.

1. Left ruptured tubal pregnancy (without intrauterine pregnancy) complicated by kidney kidney failure, treated during this admission

2. Prenatal visit for supervision of elderly primigravida, 40 years old, during the 28th week- of gestation (third trimester)

3. A pregnant female, 15-week gestation, with hemorrhage due to threatened abortion, pregnancy continued

4. Excessive 30-pound weight gain in pregnancy, 24 weeks of pregnancy

5. Varicose veins of lower legs during second trimester of pregnancy, 15 weeks

---

Pregnancy

Pregnancy is defined as the state of a female after conception until the birth (delivery) of the child. Normal pregnancies are intrauterine, and the duration of pregnancy from conception to delivery is about 266 days. As stated earlier, the following guidelines may be used in determining preterm, term, and postterm pregnancies:

- **Preterm**: Delivery before 37 completed weeks of gestation (patient is in her 37th or earlier week of pregnancy)

- **Term**: Delivery between 38 and 40 completed weeks of gestation

- **Postterm**: Delivery between 41 and 42 completed weeks of gestation

- **Prolonged**: Delivery for a pregnancy that has advanced beyond 42 completed weeks of gestation (patient is in her 43rd or later week of pregnancy)

The postpartum period, or **puerperium**, begins immediately after delivery and continues for six weeks. In the Alphabetic Index to Diseases and Injuries, long listings of conditions appear under the following main terms: Pregnancy, Delivery, and Puerperium/Puerperal/Postpartum.

Indentations are often used in the Alphabetic Index under these main terms, so extreme care should be taken in locating and selecting the appropriate code.

Figure 18.3 displays a diagram of the anatomy of a pregnant female with products of conception contained within the uterus, that is, the fetus, placenta, amniotic sac, and umbilical cord.

Figure 18.3.   Products of conception

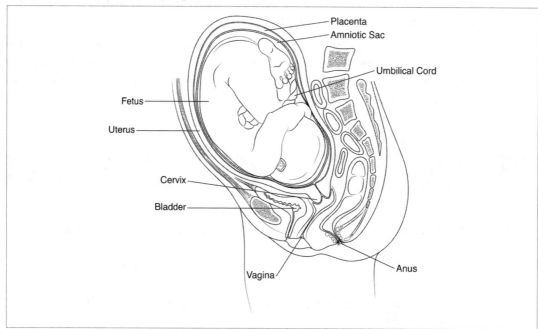

© AHIMA

Encounter for Delivery (O80 and O82)

Two categories are available to describe an uncomplicated **normal delivery** and an encounter for cesarean delivery when there is no mention of the reason for the cesarean delivery.

Encounter for Full-Term Uncomplicated Delivery (O80)

Category O80 is used when the pregnant female has a full-term uncomplicated delivery described as the following:

- Full-term, single, liveborn infant

- Spontaneous, cephalic, vaginal delivery

- Delivery requiring minimal or no assistance, with or without episiotomy, without fetal manipulation (that is, rotation version) or instrumentation (forceps)

ICD-10-CM Coding Guidelines 15.b.2 reminds the coder that codes from category O09, Supervision of high-risk pregnancy, are only used during the prenatal period and not at the time of the delivery. For example, if the physician documents the woman has having "advanced maternal age" but no other complications of the pregnancy and has a completely normal delivery, the principal diagnosis code of O80, Encounter for full-term uncomplicated delivery is assigned.

Code O80 is used as a single diagnosis code and is not to be used with any other code from Chapter 15. An additional code to indicate the outcome of delivery, Z37.0, Single live birth, must be used with code O80. Every woman who has a delivery must have a code from the appropriate procedure classification. For example, an ICD-10-PCS procedure code for the vaginal or cesarean delivery would be used for an inpatient admission, and a CPT procedure code would be used for an outpatient healthcare encounter or for a provider's professional fee billing. Even if the woman delivers the infant at home or on the way to the hospital and expels the placenta after being admitted to the hospital, the delivery of the placenta is coded 10E0XZZ, Delivery of products of conception. ICD-10-PCS considers both the infant and the placenta as products of conception. A diagnosis code can capture the fact the baby was born outside the hospital.

Encounter for Cesarean Delivery Without Indication (O82)

Code O82 is used when the pregnant female has a cesarean delivery without the indication or the reason for the cesarean delivery documented in the health records. Usually when there is no indication for the cesarean delivery documented in the record, the physician should be queried for an explanation or reason for the cesarean delivery. This code is not expected to be used for all encounters for a cesarean delivery. There is always a reason for a cesarean delivery. The diagnosis code O82 means there was no stated reason in the record for the cesarean delivery to be performed. When the reason for the surgical delivery is documented in the health record, the condition must be coded instead of code O82. When the documentation in the record is not clear as to the reason for the cesarean delivery, the physician should be asked for clarification of the obstetrical condition that prompted this type of delivery. When code O82 is used, an additional code Z37.0 is used to indicate the outcome of delivery.

Outcome of Delivery (Z Codes)

The outcome of delivery, as indicated by a code from category Z37, should be included on all maternal delivery records. This is always an additional, not a principal, diagnosis code used to reflect the number and status of babies delivered. Many hospitals rely on these codes to provide more information on obstetrical outcomes. Code Z37 is referenced in the Alphabetic Index to Diseases and Injuries under the main term "Outcome of delivery."

> **EXAMPLE:**   Encounter for full-term uncomplicated delivery: O80, Normal delivery; Z37.0, Outcome of delivery, single live birth

Obstetrical and Nonobstetrical Complications

Many pre-existing conditions, including diabetes, hypertension, and anemia, may affect or complicate the pregnancy or its management. In addition, the pregnancy may aggravate the pre-existing condition.

For this reason, if the pregnancy aggravates the pre-existing or nonobstetrical condition or vice versa, the condition is reclassified to Chapter 15 of ICD-10-CM. The categories representing such conditions are as follows:

- Edema, proteinuria, and hypertensive disorders in pregnancy, childbirth, and the puerperium (O10–O16)

- Other maternal disorders predominantly related to pregnancy (O20–O29)

- Maternal care related to the fetus and amniotic cavity and possible delivery problems (O30–O48)

- Complications of labor and delivery (O60–O77)

- Complications predominantly related to the puerperium (O85–O92)

- Other obstetric conditions, not elsewhere classified (O94–O9A)

Pre-existing Hypertension (O10)

Category O10, Pre-existing hypertension complicating pregnancy, childbirth, and the puerperium, provides specific subcategories for the type of hypertensive disease. The Alphabetic Index entries of "pregnancy, complicated by hypertension" refers the coder to "hypertension, complicating pregnancy" and "pregnancy, hypertensive," which are used to locate these codes:

O10.0,   Pre-existing essential hypertension complicating pregnancy, childbirth and the puerperium
- This code represents any condition in I10, Essential (primary) hypertension specified as a reason of obstetric care during pregnancy, childbirth, or the puerperium. No additional code is required to identify the hypertension.

O10.1,   Pre-existing hypertensive heart disease complicating pregnancy, childbirth and the puerperium
- This code represents any condition in I11, Hypertensive heart disease specified as a reason of obstetric care during pregnancy, childbirth or the puerperium. An additional code from I11 is required to identify the type of hypertensive heart disease.

O10.2,   Pre-existing hypertensive chronic kidney disease complicating pregnancy, childbirth and the puerperium
- This code represents any condition in I12, Hypertensive chronic kidney disease specified as a reason of obstetric care during pregnancy, childbirth or the puerperium. An additional code from I12 is required to identify the type of hypertensive chronic kidney disease.

O10.3,   Pre-existing hypertensive heart and chronic kidney disease complicating pregnancy, childbirth and the puerperium
- This code represents any condition in I13, Hypertensive heart and chronic kidney disease specified as a reason of obstetric care during pregnancy, childbirth or the puerperium. An additional code from I13 is required to identify the type of hypertensive heart and chronic kidney disease.

O10.4,   Pre-existing secondary hypertension complicating pregnancy, childbirth and the puerperium
- This code represents any condition in I15, Secondary hypertension specified as a reason of obstetric care during pregnancy, childbirth or the puerperium. An additional code from I15 is required to identify the type of secondary hypertension.

O10.9,   Unspecified pre-existing hypertension complicating pregnancy, childbirth and the puerperium

> **EXAMPLE:**   The patient is a 33-year-old woman in her 30th week of gestation who was evaluated in her obstetrician's office for her second pregnancy with pre-existing essential hypertension: O10.913, Pre-existing hypertension complicating pregnancy; Z3A.30, Pregnancy, weeks of gestation, 30 weeks

Other Forms of Hypertension, Pre-eclampsia, and Eclampsia (O11–O16)

Other forms of hypertensive disease with pre-eclampsia as well as gestational hypertension, pre-eclampsia, eclampsia, and other material hypertension are classified with categories O11–O16. Gestational hypertension is hypertension that did not exist in the woman prior to the pregnancy, but instead the hypertension was pregnancy induced (Dorland 2012, 896). Pre-eclampsia is the presence of hypertension and proteinuria with or without coexisting systematic abnormalities involving the kidneys, liver, or blood in a pregnant woman. Eclampsia, which is considered a complication of severe pre-eclampsia, is commonly defined as new onset of grand mal seizure activity and/or unexplained coma during pregnancy or postpartum in a woman with signs or symptoms of pre-eclampsia. It typically occurs during or after the 20th week of gestation or in the postpartum period. Ten percent of all pregnancies are complicated by hypertension. Eclampsia and pre-eclampsia account for about half of these cases worldwide and have been recognized and described for years despite the general lack of understanding of the disease (Ross 2019). Alphabetic Index entries of "pregnancy, complicated, by, eclampsia or edema or pre-eclampsia or eclampsia" are used to assign these diagnosis codes. The main terms "pre-eclampsia" and "eclampsia" may also be referenced for coding of these categories as described in the following manner:

O11,   Pre-existing hypertension with pre-eclampsia
         This category requires an additional code from O10, Pre-existing hypertension compli-
         cating pregnancy, childbirth and the puerperium.

O12,   Gestational [pregnancy-induced] edema and proteinuria without hypertension

O13,   Gestational [pregnancy-induced] hypertension without significant proteinuria

O14,   Pre-eclampsia

O15,   Eclampsia

O16,   Unspecified maternal hypertension

EXAMPLE: The patient is a 32-year-old female in her 26th week of pregnancy
who is seen in her obstetrician's office for continued monitoring of her
mild pre-eclampsia. The patient did not have hypertension prior to this
pregnancy: O14.02, Mild to moderate pre-eclampsia, second trimester;
Z3A.26, Pregnancy, weeks of gestation, 26th week.

Excessive Vomiting in Pregnancy (O21)

Hyperemesis is excessive vomiting. **Hyperemesis gravidarum** is severe morning sickness
or excessive nausea and vomiting experienced during the early weeks of pregnancy by some
women (Dorland 2012). Category O21, Excessive vomiting in pregnancy, provides specific
subcategories; therefore, additional codes are not required unless ICD-10-CM notations
instruct otherwise. For example, code O21.8, Other vomiting complicating pregnancy, has the
note to "Use additional code to specify the cause." The Alphabetic Index entries of "pregnancy,
complicated by, vomiting" or "hyperemesis" are used to assign the correct code. The codes in
the category that do not require an additional code are the following:

O21.0,   Mild hyperemesis gravidarum
         This code represents excessive vomiting in pregnancy starting before the end of the 20th
         week of gestation.

O21.1,   Hyperemesis gravidarum with metabolic disturbance
         The metabolic disturbances included in this code with excessive vomiting are
         carbohydrate depletion, dehydration, or electrolyte imbalance starting before the end
         of the 20th week of gestation.

O21.2,   Late vomiting of pregnancy
         This code represents excessive vomiting in pregnancy starting after the 20th completed
         week of pregnancy.

O21.9,   Vomiting of pregnancy, unspecified

Late Pregnancy (O48)

Two codes exist to identify women who are beyond 40 completed weeks of gestation, as this
may be the primary reason for the obstetrical services being rendered. A pregnancy is not
considered a prolonged pregnancy until it extends after 42 completed weeks. Women in this
group are considered potentially high risk for pregnancy complications.

Subcategory O48.0 is used to describe postterm pregnancy or pregnancy over 40
completed weeks to 42 completed weeks of gestation. Subcategory O48.1 is used to describe
prolonged pregnancy or pregnancy that has advanced beyond 42 completed weeks of gestation.
The Alphabetic Index entries to locate these codes are "pregnancy, post-term or postmature or
prolonged."

Preterm Labor With or Without Delivery (O60)

Category O60, **Preterm labor**, is defined as the onset (spontaneous) of labor before 37 completed weeks of gestation. Codes exist in ICD-10-CM for preterm labor without delivery (O60.0X) and preterm delivery with preterm delivery (O60.1X) and term delivery with preterm labor (O60.2X). In addition to category O60, a code to describe the outcome of delivery (Z37) must be assigned.

However, when the delivery of a liveborn infant occurs as the result of an attempted elective abortion, it is coded as an encounter for elective termination of pregnancy, Z33.2 with a code from category Z37 for the outcome of delivery. If the preterm labor occurred prior to the completion of 20 weeks of pregnancy and infant was not liveborn, the spontaneous abortion would likely be the diagnosis provided by the physician.

> **EXAMPLE:**   Preterm labor with preterm delivery, 27 weeks of gestation, resulting in liveborn fetus: O60.12X0, Preterm labor second trimester with preterm delivery; Z3A.27, Weeks of gestation 27; and Z37.0, Outcome of delivery, single live birth.

> **EXAMPLE:**   Elective termination of pregnancy resulting in liveborn, first trimester, 8 weeks: Z33.2, Encounter for elective termination of pregnancy; Z3A.08, weeks of gestation, 8 and Z37.0, Outcome of delivery, single live birth.

Puerperal Sepsis (O85) and Other Puerperal Infection (O86)

Category O85, Puerperal sepsis, includes the most serious manifestations of major postpartum infection including postpartum sepsis, puerperal peritonitis, and puerperal pyemia. This condition occurs during the 6 weeks or 42 days following delivery. The coder should use an additional code (B95–B97) to identify the known infectious agent responsible for the infection. In addition, if the patient also has severe sepsis, an additional code is used for severe sepsis without septic shock (R65.20) or severe sepsis with septic shock (R65.21). Any organ failure or other systemic complication that is present would also be coded with the severe sepsis and the puerperal sepsis codes. The Alphabetic Index entries to locate puerperal sepsis would be the main terms of "puerperal, sepsis" or "sepsis, puerperal."

Category O86, Other puerperal infection, identifies localized infections that occur during the postpartum period, such as the following in table 18.2:

Table 18.2.   **Examples from category O86, Other puerperal infection**

O86.0-	Infection of obstetric surgical wound with 5th characters for superficial incisional site, deep incisional site, organ and space site, sepsis and other surgical site
O86.1-	Other infection of genital tract following delivery including cervicitis, endometritis, vaginitis and other infection of the genital tract
O86.2-	Urinary tract infection following delivery and infection of kidney or bladder
O86.4	Pyrexia of unknown origin following delivery
O86.8-	Other specified puerperal infections, such as puerperal septic thrombophlebitis and other specified puerperal infection

Venous Complications and Hemorrhoids in the Puerperium (O87)

Category O87, Venous complications and hemorrhoids in the puerperium, is subdivided to identify the types of venous conditions or complications. Under subcategory O87.1, Deep phlebothrombosis in the puerperium, an additional code is required to identify the deep vein thrombosis that exists. In addition, a code for associated long-term (current) use of anticoagulants is used with code O87.1, if applicable. The venous conditions can be referenced in the Alphabetic Index under various terms such as hemorrhoids, complicating pregnancy or the puerperium or thrombophlebitis, puerperal, postpartum or childbirth.

EXAMPLE: The patient is seen in her obstetrician's office two weeks after delivering a healthy female infant but is complaining of leg pain and swelling. The physician diagnoses the patient's problem as puerperal phlebitis and begins therapeutic measures to treat the condition: O87.0, Superficial thrombophlebitis in the puerperium.

Check Your Understanding 18.5

Assign diagnosis codes to the following conditions.

1. Pregnancy, delivered, 38 weeks, complicated by pre-existing hypertensive heart disease, noted at time of childbirth, single liveborn infant delivered

2. Post-term pregnancy, delivered, single liveborn infant, 41 weeks of gestation

3. Mild pre-eclampsia, third trimester, undelivered, 30 weeks

4. Pregnancy, delivered, 38 completed weeks, full term, following premature rupture of membranes with onset of labor more than 24 hours following rupture, single liveborn infant

5. Preterm labor, halted without delivery, 34 weeks

6. Puerperal cystitis (bladder infection)

7. Puerperal septic thrombophlebitis

8. Obstructed labor due to breech presentation, delivered by cesarean delivery, single liveborn infant, 39 weeks of pregnancy

9. Scheduled second cesarean delivery due to previous low transverse cesarean delivery, 38 weeks, single liveborn infant, no complications

10. Twin pregnancy, delivered, dichorionic/diamniotic, both liveborn infants, 35 weeks of pregnancy, preterm with spontaneous onset of labor (According to physician, unable to determine which fetus caused preterm labor)

ICD-10-PCS Procedure Coding for the Obstetrics Section

Specific procedure coding guidelines exist for coding procedures in the Obstetrics section. These guidelines can be found in the *Official ICD-10-PCS Guidelines for Coding and Reporting* on the CMS website (CMS 2019) for current year ICD-10-PCS.

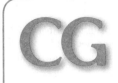

C.1. Products of Conception: Procedures performed on the Products of Conception are coded to the Obstetrics section. Procedures performed on the pregnant female other than the products of conception are coded to the appropriate root operation in the Medical and Surgical section.

EXAMPLE: Amniocentesis is coded to the products of conception body part in the Obstetrics section. Repair of obstetric urethral laceration is coded to the Urethra body part in the Medical and Surgical section.

C.2. Procedures Following Delivery or Abortion: Procedures performed following a delivery or abortion for curettage of the endometrium or evacuation of retained products of conception are all coded in the Obstetrics section, to the root operation Extraction and the body part Products of Conception, Retained. Diagnostic or therapeutic dilation and curettage performed during times other than the postpartum or post-abortion period are all coded in the Medical and Surgical section, to the root operation Extraction and the body part Endometrium.

Coding Note: The products of conception refer to all components of pregnancy, including fetus, embryo, amnion, umbilical cord and placenta. There is no differentiation of the products of conception based on gestational age.

Assigning ICD-10-PCS Procedure Codes for Obstetrics

The Obstetrics section for procedure coding is a distinct group of procedure codes that begin with the character of 1 (numeric one). This section follows the same conventions established in the Medical and Surgical section with all seven characters retaining the same meaning. The second character, 0 (zero), represents the body system Pregnancy.

Character 1 is Value 1—Obstetrics Section
Character 2 is Value 0—Pregnancy

Root Operation

Character 3 of the ICD-10-PCS codes is the root operation. The root operations that represent the objectives of procedures for obstetrics are shown in table 18.3.

Table 18.3. **Root operations for procedures for Obstetrics**

Change: Taking out or off a device from a body part and putting back an identical or similar device in or on the same body part without cutting or puncturing the skin or a mucous membrane.
In the Obstetrics section, the device most likely to be changed is a monitoring electrode via the natural or artificial opening of the pregnancy female.

(Continued)

Drainage: Taking or letting out fluids and/or gases from a body part

In the Obstetrics section, the qualifier used with the root operation. Drainage identifies the substance that is drained from the products of conception, specifically fetal blood, fetal spinal fluid, or amniotic fluid. Examples of procedures coded to the root operation. Drainage in the Obstetrics section are amniocentesis and percutaneous fetal spinal tap

Abortion: Artificially terminating a pregnancy

This root operation is a new root operation that only appears here in the Obstetrics section. It is subdivided according to whether an additional device such as a laminaria or abortifacient is used, or whether the abortion was performed by mechanical means. If either a laminaria or abortifacient is used, the approach is Via Natural or Artificial Opening. All other abortion procedures are those done by mechanical means; that is, the products of conception are physically removed using instrumentation, and the device value is Z, No Device. An example of an abortion procedure is a transvaginal abortion using vacuum aspiration

Extraction: Pulling or stripping out or off all or a portion of a body part by the use of force

Cesarean deliveries are coded in this section to the root operation Extraction as well as forceps and vacuum-assisted deliveries. A 7th character of 9 is used for the manual extraction of a placenta after a delivery.

Delivery: Assisting the passage of the products of conception from the genital canal

This root operation is a new root operation that only appears here in the Obstetrics section. It is used only to report manually assisted vaginal delivery.

Insertion: Putting in a nonbiological appliance that monitors, assists, performs, or prevents a physiological function but does not physically take the place of the body part, that is within the products of conception, such as an insertion of a monitoring electrode.

Inspection: Visually and/or manually exploring a body part, that is, the products of conception

Removal: Taking out or off a device from a body part, that is, from the products of conception, such as a monitoring electrode.

Repair: Restoring, to the extent possible, a body part to its normal anatomic structure and function, that is within the products of conception such as repairing an organ within the fetus.

Reposition: Moving to its normal location, or other suitable location, all or a portion of a body part, that is within the products of conception

Resection: Cutting out or off, without replacement, all of a body part, the products of conception

Transplantation: Putting in or on all or a portion of a living body part taken from another individual or animal to physically take the place and/or function of all or a portion of a similar body part, within the products of conception such as transplanting an organ within the fetus.

Source: CMS 2019

Body Part

Character 4 identifies the body part involved in the procedure. For the majority of the codes, the body part is "products of conception." Products of conception are defined as the intrauterine tissue that result from the fertilization of the ovum with sperm and include the fetus, placenta, amniotic sac, amniotic fluid, and umbilical cord (Kuehn and Jorwic 2018). If a procedure is performed on a body part of the pregnant female patient, other than the uterus and the products of conception, the body part for that procedure is coded to the appropriate body part value in the Medical Surgical section; for example, an episiotomy performed on the woman's perineum (Kuehn and Jorwic 2018). Retained products of conception would be used as the body part when the procedure is directed at extracting the retained products of conception after an incomplete spontaneous abortion has occurred. Ectopic products of conception would be used as the body part when the procedure is directed at extracting or resecting the products of conception from a location outside of the uterus, such as within a fallopian tube.

The body parts in ICD-10-PCS have individual values, as shown in table 18.4.

Table 18.4.   **Body parts and values included in the ICD-10-PCS codes for Obstetric procedures**

0—Products of Conception
1—Products of Conception, retained
2—Products of Conception, ectopic

Source: CMS 2019

Approach

Character 5 identifies the approach used in the procedure. The approaches for Obstetric procedures are shown in table 18.5.

Table 18.5.   **Approaches included in the ICD-10-PCS codes for Obstetric procedures**

Open (0): Cutting through the skin or mucous membrane and any other body layers necessary to expose the site of the procedure
Percutaneous (3): Entry, by puncture or minor incision, of instrumentation through the skin or mucous membrane and any other body layers necessary to reach the site of the procedure
Percutaneous Endoscopic (4): Entry, by puncture or minor incision, of instrumentation through the skin or mucous membrane and any other body layers necessary to reach and visualize the site of the procedure
Via Natural or Artificial Opening (7): Entry of instrumentation through a natural or artificial external opening to reach the site of the procedure
Via Natural or Artificial Opening Endoscopic (8): Entry of instrumentation through a natural or artificial external opening to reach and visualize the site of the procedure
External (X): Procedures performed directly on the skin or mucous membrane and procedures performed indirectly by the application of external force through the skin or mucous membrane

Source: CMS 2019

Device

Character 6 identifies if a device was involved. For example, a monitoring device may be placed on the fetus's scalp during labor to monitor the fetus's vital signs. The devices used to code obstetric procedures are shown in table 18.6.

Table 18.6.   **Devices and values included in the ICD-10-PCS Obstetric procedure codes**

3—Monitoring Device
Y—Other Device
Z—No Device

Source: CMS 2019

Qualifier

Character 7 is a qualifier that specifies an additional attribute of the procedure, if applicable. The qualifier characters used to code Obstetric procedures are as shown in table 18.7.

Table 18.7.   **Qualifiers used to code Obstetric procedures**

0—High
1—Low
2—Extraperitoneal
3—Low Forceps
4—Mid Forceps
5—High Forceps
6—Vacuum
7—Internal version
8—Other
9—Fetal Blood or Manual
A—Fetal Cerebrospinal Fluid
B—Fetal Fluid, other
C—Amniotic Fluid, therapeutic
D—Fluid, other
E—Nervous system
F—Cardiovascular system
G—Lymphatics and Hemic
H—Eye
J—Ear, Nose and Sinus
K—Respiratory system
L—Mouth and Throat
M—Gastrointestinal system
N—Hepatobiliary and Pancreas
P—Endocrine system
Q—Skin
R—Musculoskeletal system
S—Urinary system
T—Female Reproductive system
U—Amniotic Fluid, diagnostic
V—Male Reproductive system
W—Laminaria

| X—Abortifacient |
| Y—Other Body System |
| Z—No Qualifier |

Source: CMS 2019

ICD-10-CM and ICD-10-PCS Review Exercises: Chapter 18

Assign the correct ICD-10-CM diagnosis codes or ICD-10-PCS procedure codes to the following exercises.

1. The patient is a 40-year-old G2 P1 female who is 26 weeks pregnant and being seen for gestational hypertension. Other than being an elderly, multigravida patient, she is not having any other problems during this pregnancy.

2. A 16-week pregnancy with mild hyperemesis and urinary tract infection, caused by E. coli bacteria

3. Patient returns to the office with breast pain. The patient is a 24-year-old female who is three weeks postpartum. Final diagnosis documented as postpartum breast abscess.

4. Delivery of single liveborn infant, full-term, vaginal delivery by cephalic presentation, 40 weeks of gestation

5. Normal full-term vaginal delivery by cephalic presentation, 38 weeks of gestation, elderly multigravida with gestational diabetes that is controlled by oral antidiabetic drugs, single liveborn infant

6. Full-term twin pregnancy (dichorionic/diamniotic) with vaginal delivery, complicated by first-degree perineal laceration, 39 weeks of pregnancy, both liveborn infants

7. Postpartum office visit, five days after discharge, with partial lactation failure

8. False labor with Braxton Hicks contractions, 32 weeks of pregnancy, undelivered

9. Office visit for pregnant female, 19 weeks of gestation, with cervical incompetence complicating pregnancy. Surgical consent signed for cervical cerclage procedure to be performed the following day at the ambulatory surgery center.

(Continued on next page)

ICD-10-CM and ICD-10-PCS Review Exercises: Chapter 18 *(continued)*

10. Pregnancy delivered, single liveborn, vaginal delivery following prolonged first stage of labor, 38 weeks of gestation

   _____

11. Quadruplet pregnancy, first trimester, with equal number of chorions and amnions to the number of fetuses (Quadra or four), 10 weeks gestation

   _____

12. Spontaneous incomplete abortion, 11 weeks

   _____

13. Intraabdominal abscess, within the organ and space site, following cesarean delivery, 2 weeks postpartum, admitted for treatment of the infection of the obstetric surgical wound

   _____

14. Severe pre-eclampsia in pregnancy, second trimester, 26 weeks, undelivered

   _____

15. Pregnancy, 32 weeks, placenta previa without hemorrhage, undelivered

   _____

16. PROCEDURE: Low cervical cesarean delivery

   _____

17. PROCEDURE: Manually assisted delivery

   _____

18. PROCEDURE: Manual extraction of retained placenta after delivery

   _____

19. PROCEDURE: Induced abortion by laminaria

   _____

20. PROCEDURE: Treatment of incomplete spontaneous abortion by dilation and curettage (extraction) of retained products of conception

   _____

References

Centers for Disease Control and Prevention (CDC), National Center for Health Statistics (NCHS). 2019. *ICD-10-CM Official Guidelines for Coding and Reporting*, 2020. http://www.cdc.gov/nchs/icd/icd10cm.htm or https://www.cdc.gov/nchs/data/icd/10cmguidelines-FY2020_final.pdf.

Centers for Medicare and Medicaid Services (CMS). 2019. *ICD-10-PCS Official Guidelines for Coding and Reporting*, 2020. http://www.cms.gov/Medicare/Coding/ICD10/.

Dorland, W.A.N., ed. 2012. *Dorland's Illustrated Medical Dictionary*, 32nd ed. Philadelphia: Elsevier Saunders.

Kuehn, L. and T. Jorwic. 2018. *ICD-10-PCS: An Applied Approach*, 2018. Chicago: AHIMA.

Puscheck, E. E. 2018. Medscape. Early Pregnancy Loss. http://reference.medscape.com /article/266317-overview#a6.

Ross, M. G. 2019. Medscape. Eclampsia. http://emedicine.medscape.com/article/253960 -overview.

Sivalingam, V. N., W. C. Duncan, E. Kirk, L. A. Shephard, and A. W. Horne. 2011. Diagnosis and management of ectopic pregnancy. *The Journal of Family Planning and Reproductive Health Care*. 37(4):231–240.

Stedman, T. 2012. *Stedman's Medical Dictionary for the Health Professions and Nursing*, 7th ed. Philadelphia: Wolters Kluwer/Lippincott Williams & Wilkins.

Chapter 19

Certain Conditions Originating in the Perinatal Period (P00–P96)

Learning Objectives

At the conclusion of this chapter, you should be able to do the following:

- Describe the organization of the conditions and codes included in ICD-10-CM Chapter 16, Certain Conditions Originating in the Perinatal Period (P00–P96)

- Define the newborn or perinatal period

- Summarize the circumstances in which a code from Chapter 16 of ICD-10-CM can be assigned in terms of the age of the patient who has the condition

- Apply the newborn ICD-10-CM coding guidelines, including how to sequence the newborn and perinatal codes

- Identify the types of conditions classified in ICD-10-CM categories P00–P04, Newborn affected by maternal factors and by complications of pregnancy, labor, and delivery

- Describe the circumstances in which codes from ICD-10-CM categories P05–P08 are used on a newborn or perinatal record, including weeks of gestation and birth weight

- Explain the term *meconium* and describe the conditions associated with the passage of meconium

- Review the types of respiratory infections and cardiac dysrhythmias that can occur in newborn and perinatal infants

- Assign ICD-10-CM codes for certain conditions originating in the perinatal period

- Assign ICD-10-PCS procedure codes related to perinatal conditions

Key Terms

Bacterial sepsis of newborn
Exceptionally large baby
Extreme immaturity
Fetal growth retardation (FGR)

Gestational age
Heavy-for-dates
Large baby
Large-for-dates

Late newborn

Low birth weight

Meconium

Meconium aspiration syndrome

Meconium staining

Neonatal aspiration

Perinatal period

Postmaturity baby

Postterm newborn

Prematurity

Respiratory distress syndrome (RDS)

Short gestation

Overview of ICD-10-CM Chapter 16: Certain Conditions Originating in the Perinatal Period

Chapter 16 includes categories P00–P96 arranged in the following blocks:

P00–P04	Newborn affected by maternal factors and by complications of pregnancy, labor and delivery
P05–P08	Disorders of newborn related to length of gestation and fetal growth
P09	Abnormal findings on neonatal screening
P10–P15	Birth trauma
P19–P29	Respiratory and cardiovascular disorders specific to the perinatal period
P35–P39	Infections specific to the perinatal period
P50–P61	Hemorrhagic and hematological disorders of newborn
P70–P74	Transitory endocrine and metabolic disorders specific to newborn
P76–P78	Digestive system disorders of newborn
P80–P83	Conditions involving the integument and temperature regulation of newborn
P84	Other problems with newborn
P90–P96	Other disorders originating in the perinatal period

The codes in this chapter describe conditions that begin before birth or develop during the first 28 days of life, the **perinatal period**. These are not congenital conditions. Congenital condition codes are found in Chapter 17 of ICD-10-CM. The conditions that develop in the perinatal period may continue to exist past the first 28 days of life and can be coded regardless of the patient's age.

Codes P00–P04 are intended to describe newborns affected by maternal factors and by complications of pregnancy, labor, and delivery. The conditions have been confirmed to exist. An example of these codes is P00.3, Newborn affected by other maternal circulatory and respiratory diseases.

EXAMPLES: P00.3, Newborn affected by other maternal circulatory and respiratory diseases

P00.4, Newborn affected by maternal nutritional disorders

P00.5, Newborn affected by maternal injury

The block of codes for the perinatal conditions are organized by type; for example, disorders related to length of gestation and fetal growth versus conditions produced by birth trauma. Other blocks of codes are grouped by the type of condition or body system where the disease is present. For example, there are blocks of codes for infections versus respiratory and cardiovascular system disorders.

Coding Guidelines and Instructional Notes for ICD-10-CM Chapter 16

Codes from Chapter 16, Certain Conditions Originating in the Perinatal Period, are only for use on the newborn or infant record, never on the maternal record. This note appears at the beginning of Chapter 16. Codes from this chapter are also only applicable for liveborn infants.

Further, the following Includes note appears on the first page of Chapter 16, "Conditions that have their origin in the fetal or perinatal period (before birth through the first 28 days after birth) even if morbidity occurs later" (CDC 2018). This statement should be interpreted such that if a condition originated in the perinatal period and continued throughout the life of the child, the perinatal code should continue to be used regardless of the age of the patient.

Throughout Chapter 16 are notes that help to clarify how codes are to be sequenced. For example, the following note appears under P07: "When both birth weight and gestational age of the newborn are available, both should be coded with birth weight sequenced before gestational age" (CDC 2018).

The following note appears under P08.21 to define a **postterm newborn**: "Newborn with gestation period over 40 completed weeks to 42 completed weeks" (CDC 2018).

A note at block P00–P04, Newborn affected by maternal factors and by complications of pregnancy, labor, and delivery, also provides guidance:

> These codes are for use when the listed maternal conditions are specified as the cause of confirmed morbidity or potential morbidity which have their origin in the perinatal period (before birth through the first 28 days after birth) (CDC 2019).

The NCHS has published chapter-specific guidelines for Chapter 16 in the *ICD-10-CM Official Guidelines for Coding and Reporting*. The coding student should review all of the coding guidelines for Chapter 16 of ICD-10-CM, which appear in an ICD-10-CM code book or on the CDC website (CDC 2019) or in appendix E.

CG

Chapter 16: Certain Conditions Originating in the Perinatal Period (P00–P96): For coding and reporting purposes the perinatal period is defined as before birth through the 28th day following birth. The following guidelines are provided for reporting purposes.

Guideline I.C.16.a. General Perinatal Rules

Guideline I.C.16.a.1. Use of Chapter 16 Codes: Codes in this chapter are <u>never</u> for use on the maternal record. Codes from Chapter 15, the obstetric chapter, are never permitted on the newborn record. Chapter 16 codes may be used throughout the life of the patient if the condition is still present.

(Continued)

(Continued)

Guideline I.C.16.a.2. Principal Diagnosis for Birth Record: When coding the birth episode in a newborn record, assign a code from category Z38, Liveborn infants according to place of birth and type of delivery, as the principal diagnosis. A code from category Z38 is assigned only once, to a newborn at the time of birth. If a newborn is transferred to another institution, a code from category Z38 should not be used at the receiving hospital.

A code from category Z38 is used only on the newborn record, not on the mother's record.

Guideline I.C.16.a.3. Use of Codes from other Chapters with Codes from Chapter 16: Codes from other chapters may be used with codes from Chapter 16 if the codes from the other chapters provide more specific detail. Codes for signs and symptoms may be assigned when a definitive diagnosis has not been established. If the reason for the encounter is a perinatal condition, the code from Chapter 16 should be sequenced first.

Guideline I.C.16.a.4. Use of Chapter 16 Codes after the Perinatal Period: Should a condition originate in the perinatal period, and continue throughout the life of the patient, the perinatal code should continue to be used regardless of the patient's age.

Guideline I.C.16.a.5. Birth process or community acquired conditions: If a newborn has a condition that may be either due to the birth process or community acquired and the documentation does not indicate which it is, the default is due to the birth process and the code from Chapter 16 should be used. If the condition is community-acquired, a code from Chapter 16 should not be assigned.

Guideline I.C.16.a.6. Code all clinically significant conditions: All clinically significant conditions noted on routine newborn examination should be coded. A condition is clinically significant if it requires:

> clinical evaluation; or
>
> therapeutic treatment; or
>
> diagnostic procedures; or
>
> extended length of hospital stay; or
>
> increased nursing care and/or monitoring; or
>
> has implications for future health care needs

Note: The perinatal guidelines listed above are the same as the general coding guidelines for "additional diagnoses," except for the final point regarding implications for future health care needs. Codes should be assigned for conditions that have been specified by the provider as having implications for future health care needs.

Guideline I.C.16.b. Observation and Evaluation of Newborns for Suspected Conditions not Found:

1. Guideline I.C.16.b.1. Use of Z05 codes.

Assign a code from category Z05, Observation and evaluation of newborns and infants for suspected conditions ruled out, to identify those instances when a healthy newborn is evaluated for a suspected condition that is determined after study not to be present. Do not use a code from category Z05 when the patient has identified signs or symptoms of a suspected problem; in such cases code the sign or symptom.

2. Guideline I.C.16.b.2. Z05 on other than the birth record.

A code from category Z05 may also be assigned as a principal or first-listed code for readmissions or encounters when the code from category Z38 code no longer applies. Codes from category Z05 are for use only for healthy newborns and infants for which no condition after study is found to be present.

3. Guidelines I.C.16.b.3. Z05 on a birth record

A code from category Z05 is to be used as a secondary code after the code from category Z38, Liveborn infants according to place of birth and type of delivery.

Guideline I.C.16.c. Coding Additional Perinatal Diagnoses

Guideline I.C.16.c.1. Assigning codes for conditions that require treatment: Assign codes for conditions that require treatment or further investigation, prolong the length of stay, or require resource utilization.

Guideline I.C.16.c.2. Codes for conditions specified as having implications for future health care needs: Assign codes for conditions that have been specified by the provider as having implications for future health care needs. Note: This guideline should not be used for adult patients.

Guideline I.C.16.d. Prematurity and Fetal Growth Retardation: Providers utilize different criteria in determining prematurity. A code for prematurity should not be assigned unless it is documented. Assignment of codes in categories P05, Disorders of newborn related to slow fetal growth and fetal malnutrition, and P07, Disorders of newborn related to short gestation and low birth weight, not elsewhere classified, should be based on the recorded birth weight and estimated gestational age. Codes from category P05 should not be assigned with codes from category P07.

When both birth weight and gestational age are available, two codes from category P07 should be assigned, with the code for birth weight sequenced before the code for gestational age.

(Continued)

(Continued)

Guideline I.C.16.e. Low birth weight and immaturity status: Codes from category P07, Disorders of newborn related to short gestation and low birth weight, not elsewhere classified, are for use for a child or adult who was premature or had a low birth weight as a newborn and this is affecting the patient's current health status.

See Section I.C.21. Factors influencing health status and contact with health services, Status

Guideline I.C.16.f. Bacterial Sepsis of Newborn: Category P36, Bacterial sepsis of newborn, includes congenital sepsis. If a perinate is documented as having sepsis without documentation of congenital or community acquired, the default is congenital and a code from category P36 should be assigned. If the P36 code includes the causal organism, an additional code from category B95, Streptococcus, Staphylococcus, and Enterococcus as the cause of diseases classified elsewhere, or B96, Other bacterial agents as the cause of diseases classified elsewhere, should not be assigned. If the P36 code does not include the causal organism, assign an additional code from category B96. If applicable, use additional codes to identify severe sepsis (R65.2-) and any associated acute organ dysfunction.

Guideline I.C.16.g. Stillbirth: Code P95, Stillbirth, is only for use in institutions that maintain separate records for stillbirths. No other code should be used with P95. Code P95 should not be used on the mother's record.

Coding Certain Conditions Originating in the Perinatal Period in ICD-10-CM Chapter 16

The introductory notes at the beginning of the chapter provide clarification on how the codes from this chapter should be applied to health records. Codes from this chapter are for use on newborn records only, never on maternal records, and include conditions that have their origin in the fetal or perinatal period (before birth through the first 28 days after birth) even if morbidity occurs later. Coding Guideline I.C.16.a.1 further states that Chapter 16 codes may be used throughout the life of the patient if the condition is still present. Coding Guideline I.C.16.a.4 clarifies that conditions originating in the perinatal period, and continuing throughout the life of the patient, would have perinatal codes assigned regardless of the patient's age.

Although the perinatal period lasts through 28 days following birth, the codes within Chapter 15 may be assigned beyond that period when the condition still exists. However, the condition must have its origin in the perinatal period, even though it could continue to affect the patient beyond that time.

EXAMPLE: A six-month-old was admitted to the hospital with acute respiratory failure due to bronchopulmonary dysplasia: J96.00, Acute respiratory failure; P27.1, Bronchopulmonary dysplasia originating in the perinatal period.

In the above example, the patient developed bronchopulmonary dysplasia (BPD) during the perinatal period while receiving prolonged and high concentrations of inspired O_2. Although this patient is no longer in the perinatal period, the BPD is still present and, as such, should be coded. BPD occurs commonly in infants who had respiratory distress syndrome at birth, as well as in those who have required endotracheal intubation and a respirator for many days.

Codes in Chapter 16 identify newborns affected by maternal factors, disorders related to length of gestation and fetal growth, abnormal findings on neonatal screening, birth trauma, infections, and respiratory, cardiovascular, hemorrhagic, endocrine, and digestive conditions that originate in the perinatal period.

Newborn Affected by Maternal Factors and by Complications of Pregnancy, Labor, and Delivery (P00–P04)

These codes are used on the newborn or individual's record when a maternal condition is identified as the cause of the newborn or person's condition or possible condition and it originated in the perinatal period. On occasion, the newborn may be described as suspected of having a problem. The healthcare provider may describe the conditions as "suspected," and after an investigation, it may be determined that the condition does not exist or the physician may state that the condition is "ruled out." Codes for the "suspected" but ruled out conditions come from category Z05 instead of the P00-P04 codes.

A number of substances are known to have effects on the development of the fetus when the mother is exposed to the substance during pregnancy, also known as intrauterine exposure. Category P04, Newborn affected by noxious substances transmitted via placenta or breast milk, identifies through the use of the fourth or fifth character the substance found to have harmed the fetus or newborn. The substances include maternal anesthesia and analgesia, other maternal medication, maternal use of tobacco, maternal use of alcohol, maternal use of drugs of addiction, and maternal use of other chemical substances and noxious substances.

EXAMPLE: Live born infant (vaginal birth in hospital) to an alcohol-dependent mother; the physician determines the infant has the effects of the mother's use of alcohol during pregnancy: Z38.00, Single liveborn infant, delivered vaginally in hospital; P04.3, Newborn affected by maternal use of alcohol

EXAMPLE: Delivery of a normal and healthy infant (in hospital) to a mother who occasionally uses cocaine: Z38.00, Single liveborn, delivered vaginally in hospital

In the first example, the use of alcohol by the mother was manifested in the infant; therefore, a code for newborn affected by maternal use of alcohol.

In the second example, however, the infant was healthy and normal despite the mother's occasional use of cocaine; therefore, the code for newborn affected by maternal use of cocaine (P04.41) was not assigned. The P00–P04 codes are found in the Index under the main term "Newborn, affected by" with subterms for the maternal condition affecting the newborn.

Disorders of Newborn Related to Length of Gestation and Fetal Growth (P05–P08)

Categories P05, P07, and P08 are classified in this block of codes for disorders related to length of gestation and fetal growth. The specific categories are as follows:

P05	Disorders of newborn related to slow fetal growth and fetal malnutrition
P07	Disorders of newborn related to short gestation and low birth weight, not elsewhere classified
P08	Disorders of newborn related to long gestation and high birth weight

Disorders of Newborn Related to Slow Fetal Growth and Fetal Malnutrition (P05)

  Subcategories within P05 are used to classify an infant that the physician identifies as light-for-dates or light for gestational age. Other diagnoses written by the physician are small-for-dates or small for gestational age. Another subcategory is used when the physician diagnoses fetal (intrauterine) malnutrition. Other physicians may use an equivalent diagnosis of **fetal growth retardation (FGR),** or fetal growth restriction, that is a birth weight below the 10th percentile for infants in a given population (Dorland 2012, 1630). The coder must use the physician's terminology precisely and not substitute light-for-dates with small-for-dates and so on. These are infants who are born at a lighter weight or small size than expected at their full-term birth or at their gestational age. An infant's **gestational age** is the age of the infant expressed in elapsed time since the first day of the mother's last normal menstrual period (Stedman 2012, 694).

Most physicians and hospital staff indicate a newborn's weight in grams. However, weight may also be recorded in pounds and ounces. One pound equals approximately 454 grams. A 2-pound infant weighs about 907 grams, a 5-pound infant weighs about 2,268 grams, and a 10-pound infant weighs about 4,536 grams.

The following fifth characters are used with subcategories P05.0, Newborn light for gestational age, and P05.1, Newborn small for gestational age:

0   unspecified weight
1   less than 500 grams
2   500–749 grams
3   750–999 grams
4   1,000–1,249 grams
5   1,250–1,499 grams
6   1,500–1,749 grams
7   1,750–1,999 grams
8   2,000–2,499 grams
9   2,500 grams and over

These fifth digits are used to identify the weight of the infant at birth, not the weight at subsequent visits.

EXAMPLE: The newborn infant was described by the physician as "small-for-dates" weighing 1,800 grams: P05.17, Newborn small for gestational age, 1750–1999 grams. The Alphabetic Index to Diseases and Injuries using the main term of "small-for-dates" (infant) leads to code P05.17 for a weight of 1,800 grams.

Disorders of Newborn Related to Short Gestation and Low Birth Weight, Not Elsewhere Classified (P07)

The codes from category P07, Disorders of newborn related to **short gestation** and **low birth weight**, not elsewhere classified, are to be used for a child or an adult who was premature at birth or who had a low birth weight as a newborn and this condition is affecting the patient's current health status.

The first two subcategories in ICD-10-CM (CDC 2019) identify the low birth weight:

P07.0-, Extremely low birth weight newborn
         Codes describe birth weight of 999 grams or less
P07.1-, Other low birth weight newborn
         Codes describe birth weight of 1,000 to 2,499 grams

The last two subcategories in ICD-10-CM (CDC 2019) identify short gestational age:

P07.2-, Extreme immaturity of newborn
         Extreme immaturity is less than 28 completed weeks or less than 196 completed days of gestation
P07.3-, Preterm (premature) newborn
         Prematurity is 28 completed weeks or more but less than 37 completed weeks (or 196 completed days but less than 259 completed days) of gestation

Physicians must document a newborn's prematurity and estimated gestational age. A coder should not assign strictly based on the birth weight documented. A coder should not assign a code for prematurity unless the statement of prematurity has been made by the physician in the infant's health record. As is true in category P05, Disorders of newborn related to slow fetal growth and fetal malnutrition, the coder's assignment of codes from P07, Disorders of newborn related to short gestation and low birth weight, not elsewhere classified, should be based on the recorded birth weight and estimated gestational age. As the Excludes1 note under the category heading of P07 indicates, codes from category P05 should not be assigned with codes from category P07.

For a premature infant, the physician will likely document the baby's birth weight and estimated gestational age in the newborn's physical examination or other documentation. When both birth weight and gestational age are available, the coders should assign two codes from category P07, with the code for birth weight sequenced first. The code for gestational age is sequenced following the birth weight code. The code for the birth weight does not specify the gestational age and likewise for the gestational age codes. Both provide valuable information about the infant. Weeks of gestation may be predictive of the probability, but not a guarantee, of developmental problems for the infant in the future. The Alphabetic Index main terms are "low" for the newborn's birth weight and "preterm, newborn" for the newborn's gestational age.

> **EXAMPLE:**   The physician documented the preterm infant's birth weight as 1,690 grams with a gestational age of 34 completed weeks: P07.16, Low birth weight, 1500–1749 grams and P07.37, Preterm newborn, gestational age 34 completed weeks.

Disorders of Newborn Related to Long Gestation and High Birth Weight (P08)

Codes are also available for babies who have long gestational periods or have high birth weights. Physicians may describe the baby as a **large baby** or **exceptionally large baby**. Other phrases used by physicians are **heavy-for-dates** or **large-for-dates** to describe such a baby. The assignment of the code for the birth weight should take priority over the estimated gestational age code. Code P08.0, Exceptionally large newborn baby, is used for a baby who has a birth weight of 4,500 grams or more. The code P08.1 for heavy for gestational age is the code for a baby weighing between 4,000 and 4,499 grams (CDC 2019). The physician's documentation of a large baby or heavy-for-dates baby is critical to assigning the codes as the coder cannot assume the codes are appropriate for an infant strictly based on a weight listed in the newborn record.

Another subcategory code, P08.2, is titled **Late newborn**, not heavy for gestational age. The coder will find here a code for a postterm newborn, P08.21, which is defined as a gestation period over 40 completed weeks to 42 completed weeks. Code P08.22, Prolonged gestation of newborn, includes a definition of over 42 completed weeks of gestational age (CDC 2018). This code is the default code for the unspecified term of **postmaturity baby**. The physician's documentation of gestational age is required for coding.

The main terms used in the Index to locate the codes in the section P05–P08 include premature newborn, preterm newborn, immaturity, small-for-dates, light-for-dates, low birth weight, heavy-for-dates, and large baby.

> **EXAMPLE:** The physician documented the infant's diagnoses as postterm, exceptionally large newborn infant, 41 weeks of completed gestation with a birth weight of 4,600 grams: P08.0, Exceptionally large newborn baby and P08.21, Post-term newborn (newborn with gestation period over 30 completed weeks to 42 completed weeks).

Check Your Understanding 19.1

Assign diagnosis codes to the following conditions.

1. Newborn affected by prolapsed cord (Newborn transferred to Children's Hospital for treatment, code for the care at Children's Hospital)

2. Premature infant, 34 completed weeks, birth weight 2,100 grams, (Newborn transferred to Children's Hospital for treatment, code for care at Children's Hospital)

3. A 10-day-old infant seen in the physician's office to monitor the "large baby" with a birth weight of 4,100 grams

4. Newborn, light-for-dates, 37 completed week gestation, birth weight 1,700 grams

5. One-day-old infant transferred to Children's Hospital for evaluation of the newborn affected by maternal use of opiates. Code for care at Children's Hospital

Conditions Associated with Meconium

Meconium is present in the baby's first intestinal discharge and may be referred to as a newborn's first stool, although technically it is not stool. **Meconium** is a greenish intestinal discharge of the newborn infant consisting of epithelial cells, mucus, bile, and some amniotic fluid (Stedman 2012, 1028). However, a baby can pass meconium out of the bowel prior to birth, which excretes the meconium into the amniotic fluid. If this passage of meconium occurs *in utero*, the amniotic fluid will have **meconium staining** or a greenish tint that will be seen when the baby is delivered. If the meconium is present during labor and delivery, the infant will be watched more closely for signs of fetal distress. The concern is that when meconium is present in the amniotic fluid, the baby will aspirate the meconium in the throat and possibly into the lungs.

The passage of meconium before birth can be an indication of fetal distress. It is seen in infants small for gestational age, postterm infants, or those with cord complications or other factors compromising placental circulation. **Meconium aspiration syndrome** occurs when meconium from amniotic fluid in the upper airway is inhaled into the lungs by the newborn with his or her first breath (Stedman 2012, 1028). This invokes an inflammatory reaction in the lungs, which can be fatal. Meconium staining is not meconium aspiration. Meconium aspiration is not meconium aspiration syndrome. ICD-10-CM provides distinct codes for the different conditions involving meconium:

P03.82	Meconium passage during delivery
P24.00	Meconium aspiration without respiratory symptoms
P24.01	Meconium aspiration with respiratory symptoms (aspiration syndrome)
P76.0	Meconium ileus (plug syndrome)
P78.0	Peritoneal intestinal perforation and Meconium peritonitis
P96.83	Meconium staining (of amniotic fluid)

Respiratory and Cardiovascular Disorders Specific to the Perinatal Period (P19–P29)

Conditions classified to categories P19–P29, Respiratory and cardiovascular disorders specific to the perinatal period, are unfortunately present in many infants. An example of one of these conditions is **respiratory distress syndrome (RDS)** of newborn. This condition of inflamed lungs with pulmonary edema occurs in infants born prematurely. It is caused by pulmonary surfactant deficiency because surfactant is not produced in inadequate amounts until later in pregnancy, usually after 37 weeks of gestation. The diagnosis is made when the infant exhibits grunting respirations, nasal flaring, and the use of accessory muscles in the chest. The infant is treated with surfactant therapy and supportive oxygen replacement because the infant is hypoxemic (Balest 2018).

Category P22, Respiratory distress of newborn, contains subcategories such as the following:

P22.0,　Respiratory distress syndrome of newborn
This code would also be used for diagnoses of hyaline membrane disease, cardiorespiratory distress syndrome of newborns, and idiopathic RDS or RDS type I.

P22.1,　Transient tachypnea of newborn
This code would be used for RDS type II, idiopathic tachypnea of newborn or wet lung syndrome.

In addition to RDS, other codes are available for respiratory arrest of newborn (P28.81) and respiratory failure of newborn (P28.5).

Category P24, **Neonatal aspiration**, includes aspiration *in utero* and during delivery, of different substances, for example, meconium, clear amniotic fluid, blood, milk and regurgitated food, and other specified substances. Each of the subcategory codes P24.0–P24.8 has two options for the fifth character:

0—without respiratory symptoms
1—with respiratory symptoms

The respiratory symptoms are frequently pneumonia or pneumonitis. Each of the fifth-character codes has a "use additional code note" to identify any secondary pulmonary hypertension, I27.2, if applicable.

Category P29, Cardiovascular disorders originating in the perinatal period, contains neonatal cardiac conditions. Infants may have either bradycardia or tachycardia after birth that is unrelated to the stress of labor or delivery or other intrauterine complications. These symptoms are almost always a symptom of an underlying condition, but the cause may not be immediately known. Neonatal tachycardia is coded to P29.11 and neonatal bradycardia is coded to P29.12. Other codes for pulmonary hypertension of newborn (P29.30) and for other persistent fetal circulation, P29.39, are available for conditions described as delayed closure of ductus arteriosus or persistent pulmonary hypertension of newborn.

> **EXAMPLE:** The neonatologist documented that the infant in the neonatal intensive care unit was exhibiting neonatal bradycardia, with the cause undetermined: P29.12, Neonatal bradycardia.

Infections Specific to the Perinatal Period (P35–P39)

ICD-10-CM classifies perinatal infections to the block of codes from P35–P39, Infections specific to the perinatal period. According to the note that appears under the block heading of P35–P39, these infections can be acquired *in utero*, during birth via the umbilicus or during the first 28 days after birth (CDC 2018).

Therefore, an infant who develops a urinary tract infection at the age of 20 days would be assigned code P39.3, Neonatal urinary tract infection. Newborn, neonatal, and perinatal refer to the time period of birth through 28 days of life. If the infection is acquired within the first 28 days of life, the perinatal code is used.

According to Guideline I.C.16.a.5, the coder has discretion on how to code conditions that are community acquired or due to the birth process. If a newborn has a condition that may be either community acquired or due to the birth process and the documentation does not indicate which it is, the default code should be assigned to the code associated to the birth process. The code from Chapter 16 should be used. If the condition is community acquired, a code from Chapter 16 should not be assigned.

Category P36, **bacterial sepsis of newborn** or neonatal sepsis, contains codes used frequently to classify conditions in newborns with infections. Bacterial sepsis is the presence of bacteria in the blood of the infant. This produces an invasive infection, which is demonstrated in the infant having apnea, bradycardia, low temperature, respiratory distress, vomiting, diarrhea, abdominal distention, seizure, jaundice, and jitteriness. It is treated with intravenous antibiotics and is more common in low birth weight babies (Tesini 2018). Unique codes exist for septicemia or sepsis of newborn due to various organisms such as streptococcus group B, other streptococci, *Staphylococcus aureus*, as well as sepsis due to *Escherichia coli* and anaerobes. Because these codes include the causal organism, an additional code from categories B95–B96, Bacterial agents as the cause of diseases classified elsewhere, is not needed. However, if the P36 code does not include the causal organism, the coder should assign an additional code from category B96. If the infant has severe sepsis, the coder should use additional codes to identify severe sepsis (R65.2-) and any associated acute organ dysfunction.

According to Guideline I.C.16.f, congenital sepsis is included in category P36, Bacterial sepsis of newborn. If the documentation in the infant's record does not identify the sepsis as congenital or if it was community acquired, the coder should assume the condition is congenital and the default code of P36 is used.

EXAMPLE: A 5-day-old infant was readmitted to the hospital neonatal intensive care unit and diagnosed as having *Staphylococcus aureus* sepsis of newborn: P36.2, Sepsis of newborn due to Staphylococcus aureus. Explanation: If a perinate is documented as having sepsis without documentation of congenital or community acquired, the default is congenital and a code from category P36 should be assigned. If the P36 code includes the causal organism, an additional code from category B95, *Streptococcus, Staphylococcus,* and *Enterococcus* as the cause of diseases classified elsewhere, or B96, Other bacterial agents as the cause of diseases classified elsewhere, should not be assigned.

Check Your Understanding 19.2

Assign diagnosis codes to the following conditions.

1. Obstructive apnea of newborn

2. Facial palsy due to birth injury

3. Congenital Zika virus disease

4. Meconium aspiration pneumonia

5. Delayed closure of ductus arteriosus

Liveborn Infants According to Place of Birth and Type of Delivery (Z38)

The principal diagnosis for coding the birth episode of a newborn is not included in Chapter 16. The birth episode is coded with a code from category Z38, Liveborn infants according to place of birth and type of delivery, from Chapter 21, Factors influencing health status, and contact with health services. The Z38 category codes in ICD-10-CM identify the number of liveborn infants, where they are born (in hospital, outside hospital), and how they were delivered (vaginally or by cesarean). Other codes exist for twin, triplet, quadruplet, quintuplet, and other multiple liveborn infants. For example, the birth record for a single liveborn infant, born in the hospital, and delivered vaginally is code Z38.00. The birth record for a twin liveborn infant, born in the hospital, delivered by cesarean is code Z38.31. A code from category Z38 is assigned only once to a newborn at the time of birth. If the newborn is transferred to another institution or readmitted to the hospital, a code from category Z38 should not be used at the next hospital. The Z38 codes are located in the Index under the main term "newborn" with subterms of born in hospital, twin, triplet, quadruplet, and quintuplet.

EXAMPLE: The 5-day-old male newborn was discharged from the hospital following his birth by cesarean with his twin brother, also liveborn: Z38.31, Twin liveborn infant, delivered by cesarean

Check Your Understanding 19.3

Assign diagnosis codes to the following conditions.

1. Newborn male, born outside of hospital (vaginal delivery in private car while being driven to hospital)

2. Newborn twin female, born in hospital, by cesarean delivery

3. Newborn triplet male, born in hospital, by cesarean delivery

4. Newborn quadruplet female, born in hospital, by cesarean delivery

5. Newborn quintuplet male, born in hospital, by cesarean delivery

ICD-10-PCS Procedure Coding for Certain Conditions Originating in the Perinatal Period

There are no procedures unique to treating certain conditions originating in the perinatal period. Instead, the newborn or other patient may have procedures performed that relate to the Cardiovascular system, Respiratory system, Digestive systems, and others as appropriate. Other supportive procedures are coded for infants in the extracorporeal assistance and performance section of ICD-10-PCS for mechanical ventilation, continuous positive airway pressure breathing, or insertion of an intra-aortic balloon pump in seriously ill infants.

ICD-10-CM and ICD-10-PCS Review Exercises: Chapter 19

Assign the correct ICD-10-CM diagnosis codes or ICD-10-PCS procedure codes to the following exercises.

1. A 20-day-old infant was admitted with *Streptococcus* group B sepsis

2. Full-term newborn was delivered four days ago and discharged home. The infant was readmitted to the hospital and diagnosed with hyperbilirubinemia. Phototherapy was initiated, and the baby will continue to have phototherapy provided at home after discharge.

3. Newborn, full term, born in hospital, vaginal birth with ileus in the newborn due to meconium

4. Premature baby born in the hospital by cesarean section to a mother dependent on cocaine. The newborn affected by the mother's use of cocaine. Birth weight of 1,247 grams and 31 completed weeks of gestation. Dehydration was also diagnosed and treated.

ICD-10-CM and ICD-10-PCS Review Exercises: Chapter 19 (continued)

5. Full-term newborn, infant of diabetic mother syndrome. Baby was born by cesarean delivery in the hospital. Mother has pre-existing diabetes.

6. Newborn transferred to Children's Hospital after birth at local community hospital. Reasons for transfer are grade 1 intraventricular hemorrhage, birth weight of 1,800 grams and 32 weeks of gestation in a premature infant. Code for the Children's Hospital.

7. Full-term infant with omphalitis without hemorrhage, born in hospital by vaginal delivery

8. Premature infant, 35 weeks of gestation, birth weight 2,000 grams with stage 1 necrotizing enterocolitis, born in hospital by vaginal delivery

9. Single newborn, born in hospital, by cesarean delivery; birth injury of scalpel wound during cesarean delivery

10. Twin newborn, born in hospital, by cesarean delivery, full term; newborn with neonatal bradycardia

11. Full-term infant, born in hospital, vaginal delivery. Meconium staining was noted at the time of delivery. There were no complications in the infant as the result of it.

12. Full-term infant, born in hospital, vaginal delivery with respiratory distress syndrome, type II

13. Full-term infant, born in hospital, cesarean delivery, with hyponatremia of newborn

14. A 10-day-old infant readmitted for sepsis due to *E. coli* with severe sepsis

15. A 21-day-old infant readmitted with neonatal urinary tract infection due to *E. coli* bacteria

16. PROCEDURE: Mechanical ventilation, 18 consecutive hours following endotracheal intubation

17. PROCEDURE: Extracorporeal membrane oxygenation (ECMO) peripheral veno-arterial method

(Continued on next page)

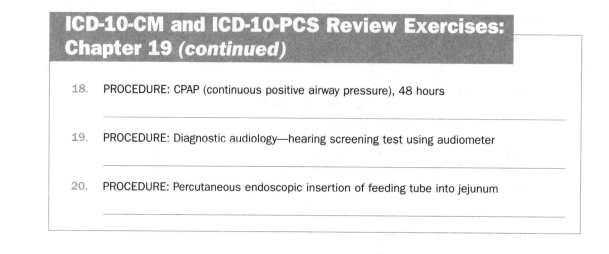

ICD-10-CM and ICD-10-PCS Review Exercises: Chapter 19 *(continued)*

18. PROCEDURE: CPAP (continuous positive airway pressure), 48 hours

19. PROCEDURE: Diagnostic audiology—hearing screening test using audiometer

20. PROCEDURE: Percutaneous endoscopic insertion of feeding tube into jejunum

References

Balest, Arcangela Lattari. 2018. *Merck Manual*. Respiratory Distress Syndrome in Neonates. http://www.merckmanuals.com/professional/pediatrics/perinatal-problems /respiratory-distress-syndrome-in-neonates.

Centers for Disease Control and Prevention (CDC), National Center for Health Statistics (NCHS). 2019. *ICD-10-CM Official Guidelines for Coding and Reporting*, 2020. http://www.cdc.gov/nchs/icd/icd10cm.htm or https://www.cdc.gov/nchs/data/ icd/10cmguidelines-FY2020_final.pdf.

Dorland, W.A.N., ed. 2012. *Dorland's Illustrated Medical Dictionary*, 32nd ed. Philadelphia: Elsevier Saunders.

Stedman, T. 2012. *Stedman's Medical Dictionary for the Health Professions and Nursing*, 7th ed. Philadelphia: Wolters Kluwer/Lippincott Williams & Wilkins.

Tesini, Brenda L. 2018. *Merck Manual*. Neonatal Sepsis. http://www.merckmanuals .com/professional/pediatrics/infections-in-neonates/neonatal-sepsis.

Chapter 20

Congenital Malformations, Deformations and Chromosomal Abnormalities (Q00–Q99)

Learning Objectives

At the conclusion of this chapter, you should be able to do the following:

- Summarize the organization of the conditions and codes included in ICD-10-CM Chapter 17, Congenital Malformations, Deformations and Chromosomal Abnormalities (Q00–Q99)

- Describe the types of common congenital anomalies classified in Chapter 17 of ICD-10-CM

- Identify the circumstances in which a code from Chapter 17 of ICD-10-CM can be assigned in terms of the age of the patient who has the condition

- Assign ICD-10-CM codes for congenital anomalies

- Assign ICD-10-PCS codes for procedures related to these conditions

Key Terms

Aortic valve stenosis (AS)
Atrial septal defect (ASD)
Bladder exstrophy
Chromosome
Chromosome abnormality
Cleft lip
Cleft palate
Clubfoot
Coarctation of aorta
Congenital anomaly

Cystic or polycystic kidney disease (PKD)
Down syndrome
Ebstein's anomaly
Edward's syndrome (trisomy 18)
Endocardial cushion defect
Epispadias
Hypoplastic left heart syndrome
Hypospadias
Lung hypoplasia (dysplasia)
Müllerian anomalies of the uterus

Obstructive genitourinary defect
Patau's syndrome
Patent ductus arteriosus (PDA)
Persistent/patent truncus
   arteriosus (PTA)
Pulmonary valve atresia
Pyloric stenosis
Renal agenesis or hypoplasia

Spina bifida
Stenosis
Tetralogy of Fallot (TOF)
Total anomalous pulmonary vein
   return (TAPVR)
Transposition of great vessels (TGV)
Tricuspid valve atresia (stenosis)
Ventricular septal defect (VSD)

Overview of ICD-10-CM Chapter 17: Congenital Malformations, Deformations and Chromosomal Abnormalities

Chapter 17 includes categories Q00–Q99 arranged in the following blocks:

Q00–Q07	Congenital malformations of the nervous system
Q10–Q18	Congenital malformations of eye, ear, face and neck
Q20–Q28	Congenital malformations of the circulatory system
Q30–Q34	Congenital malformations of the respiratory system
Q35–Q37	Cleft lip and cleft palate
Q38–Q45	Other congenital malformations of the digestive system
Q50–Q56	Congenital malformations of genital organs
Q60–Q64	Congenital malformations of the urinary system
Q65–Q79	Congenital malformations and deformations of the musculoskeletal system
Q80–Q89	Other congenital malformations
Q90–Q99	Chromosomal abnormalities, not elsewhere classified

A **congenital anomaly**, malformation, or deformation is an irregularity, abnormality, or a combination of abnormalities that are present at, and existing from, the time of birth (Dorland 2012, 95). In eukaryotic cells or cells with a true nucleus, a **chromosome** is the structure in the nucleus consisting of chromatin carrying the genetic information of the cell. A **chromosome abnormality** is an irregularity in the number or structure of chromosomes that may alter the course of the development of the embryo. The irregularity may be a duplicate of a chromosome, a deletion or loss of a chromosome, a translocation or exchange of a chromosome, or an alteration in the sequence of genetic material (Dorland 2012, 348).

Chapter 17 of ICD-10-CM is organized by body system, beginning with the Nervous system with a block of codes at the end of the chapter for chromosomal abnormalities. Because many conditions can be either congenital in origin or acquired, coders must carefully review the subterms in the Index to select the appropriate code to describe congenital conditions.

The congenital conditions are grouped into subcategories, or blocks, to make it easy to identify the type of condition included in Chapter 17. Updated terminology in the code descriptors in the chapter is specific as to the exact type of condition classified. An example of the ICD-10-CM codes for congenital conditions can be found in category Q61 with codes for specific forms of cystic kidney disease in addition to codes for less specified types of cystic kidney disease.

> **EXAMPLES:** Q61.00–Q61.02—Congenital renal cyst
> Q61.11–Q61.19—Polycystic kidney, infantile type
> Q61.2—Polycystic kidney, adult type
> Q61.3—Polycystic kidney, unspecified
> Q61.4—Renal dysplasia
> Q61.5—Medullary cystic kidney
> Q61.8—Other cystic kidney disease
> Q61.9—Cystic kidney disease

Chapter 17 includes classification that provides specificity according to the anatomic site and the combination of congenital conditions.

> **EXAMPLES:** Q35.1—Cleft hard palate
> Q35.3—Cleft soft palate
> Q35.5—Cleft hard palate with cleft soft palate
> Q35.7—Cleft uvula
> Q35.9—Cleft palate, unspecified

Coding Guidelines and Instructional Notes for ICD-10-CM Chapter 17

At the beginning of Chapter 17, a note states that codes from this chapter are not for use on maternal or fetal records. But this note should not be interpreted to state that the codes in this chapter cannot be used on infant or other records. When an infant is born with a congenital anomaly, an appropriate code from Chapter 17 should be used on the infant's record. During the admission when the infant is born, the appropriate code from category Z38 is sequenced first to identify the place of birth and the type of delivery. A secondary code is used to identify the congenital condition present at birth.

> **EXAMPLE:** Liveborn male infant, born in the hospital via vaginal birth with tetralogy of Fallot: Z38.00, Single liveborn, delivered in hospital without mention of cesarean delivery; Q21.3, Tetralogy of Fallot

However, if the patient was transferred on the day of birth to another hospital for care of the congenital anomaly, the principal diagnosis at the second hospital would be the congenital anomaly.

EXAMPLE: Liveborn male infant transferred to another hospital for care of thoracic spina bifida with hydrocephalus: Q05.1, Thoracic spina bifida with hydrocephalus

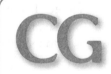
An important guideline states that codes for the congenital condition can be used throughout the entire life of the patient as long as it is still present. Congenital condition codes are not restricted for use at the time of birth or during the perinatal period. However, if a congenital condition has been corrected, the congenital condition should no longer be coded. Instead, the coder should indicate a personal history of a congenital condition, for example, from subcategory Z87.7, Personal history of (corrected) congenital malformation.

Instructions are included in Chapter 17 to direct the coder when additional codes are required. For example, a "use additional code for associated paraplegia, G82.2-" note appears with category Q05, Spina bifida. Another note appears with ICD-10-CM codes Q13.1 and Q13.81 to use an additional code for associated glaucoma, H42. Under section heading Q35–Q37, Cleft lip and cleft palate, a note appears to remind the coder to use an additional code to identify an associated malformation of the nose with code Q30.2. Another type of note appears under code Q55.3, Atresia of vas deferens, to code first any associated cystic fibrosis (E84.-). Coding guidelines also state that when a congenital condition does not have a unique code assignment, the coder should assign additional code(s) for any manifestations that may be present. For example, a malformation may be described as a syndrome with various conditions present. Under category Q87, Other specified congenital malformation syndromes affecting multiple systems, a directional note states "use additional code(s) to identify all associated manifestations." A similar type of instruction is also used with chromosomal abnormality codes. For example, under section Q90–Q99, Chromosomal abnormalities, not elsewhere classified, a note appears to remind the coder to use additional codes to identify any associated physical condition or the degree of intellectual disabilities that are present with the chromosomal abnormality (CDC 2019).

The NCHS has published chapter-specific guidelines for Chapter 17 in the *ICD-10-CM Official Guidelines for Coding and Reporting*. The coding student should review all of the coding guidelines for Chapter 17 of ICD-10-CM, which appear in an ICD-10-CM code book or on the CDC website (CDC 2019) or in appendix F.

CG **I.C.17. Chapter 17: Congenital malformations, deformations, and chromosomal abnormalities (Q00-Q99):** Assign an appropriate code(s) from categories Q00–Q99, Congenital Malformations, Deformations and Chromosomal Abnormalities when a malformation/deformation or chromosomal abnormality is documented. A malformation/deformation/or chromosomal abnormality may be the principal/first-listed diagnosis on a record or a secondary diagnosis.

When a malformation/deformation/or chromosomal abnormality does not have a unique code assignment, assign additional code(s) for any manifestations that may be present.

When the code assignment specifically identifies the malformation/deformation/or chromosomal abnormality, manifestations that are an inherent component of the anomaly should not be coded separately. Additional codes should be assigned for manifestations that are not an inherent component.

Codes from Chapter 17 may be used throughout the life of the patient. If a congenital malformation or deformity has been corrected, a personal history code should be used to identify the history of the malformation or deformity. Although present at birth, a malformation/deformation/or chromosomal abnormality may not be identified until later in life. Whenever the condition is diagnosed by the provider, it is appropriate to assign a code from codes Q00–Q99. For the birth admission, the appropriate code from category Z38, Liveborn infants, according to place of birth and type of delivery, should be sequenced as the principal diagnosis, followed by any congenital anomaly codes, Q00–Q99.

Coding Congenital Malformations, Deformations and Chromosomal Abnormalities in ICD-10-CM Chapter 17

Chapter 17 of ICD-10-CM, Congenital Malformations, Deformations and Chromosomal Abnormalities, contains codes in the range of Q00–Q99. Codes from Chapter 17 may be used throughout the life of the patient as long as the condition is present; the condition is not only coded at birth or when it is first diagnosed. If a congenital malformation or deformity has been corrected, a personal history code should be used to identify the history of the malformation or deformity.

Conditions included in Chapter 17 are organized by body system—for example, Q20–Q28, Congenital malformations of the circulatory system, and Q65–Q79, Congenital malformations and deformations of the musculoskeletal system—and include laterality for limbs and bones. Specific codes are included in ICD-10-CM to further describe the congenital condition. For example, there are four codes (Q90.0–Q90.9) to identify Down syndrome as trisomy 21, nonmosaicism, mosaicism, translocation, or unspecified. Updated terminology is also included. In place of Patau's syndrome and Edward's syndrome, the same conditions are coded with specific types of trisomy 18 and trisomy 13 codes in the range of Q91.0–Q91.7. The terminology of Patau's and Edward's syndrome does appear in the Alphabetic Index but directs the coder to the index entry for trisomy 18 or trisomy 13.

Many codes for congenital conditions and chromosomal abnormalities are included in ICD-10-CM. There are nine categories (Q90, Q91, Q92, Q93, Q95, Q96, Q97, Q98, and Q99) for chromosomal abnormalities, not elsewhere classified, to distinguish between the nonmosaicism, mosaicism, and translocation types of the abnormalities. As more has become known about these complex chromosomal abnormalities, the ICD-10-CM codes were included to report the different types of conditions.

Common Congenital Anomalies

A congenital anomaly, also known as a birth defect, has been the leading cause of infant mortality in the United States over the past several years. Birth defects substantially contribute to childhood morbidity and long-term disability. Congenital anomalies can affect almost every body system.

There are three major categories of known causes of congenital anomalies:

1. Chromosomal disorders (either hereditary or arising during conception)

2. Exposure to an environmental chemical (for example, medications, alcohol, cigarettes, solvents)

3. Mother's illness during pregnancy, exposing the infant to viral or bacterial infections

The stage of fetal development at the time of exposure to one of the two latter causes is critical. Fetal development is particularly vulnerable in the first trimester of pregnancy. The life expectancy and quality of life for individuals with many birth defects has improved greatly over the years. This is a result of pioneering surgery that can correct certain defects before the infant is born, as well as neonatal intensive care units that provide specialized care and advanced technology to treat the infant.

Congenital Defects of the Nervous System (Q00–Q07)

Central nervous system (CNS) defects involve the brain, spinal cord, and associated tissue. These include neural tube defects (anencephaly, spina bifida, and encephalocele), microcephalous, and hydrocephalus.

One of the more common CNS defects is spina bifida. **Spina bifida** is a defective closure of the vertebral column when a congenital neural tube defect occurs in which there is a developmental anomaly in the posterior vertebral arch (Mosby 2017, 1267). It ranges in severity from the occult type revealing few signs to a completely open spine (rachischisis). In spina bifida cystica, the protruding sac contains meninges (meningocele), the spinal cord (myelocele), or both (myelomeningocele). Commonly seen in the lumbar, low thoracic, or sacral region, spina bifida extends for three to six vertebral segments. Figure 20.1 shows the three most common types of spina bifida. Myelomeningocele is the most serious type of spina bifida. At birth, it is noted that a sac of fluid is coming through an opening in the child's back, and it contains damaged portions of the spinal cord and nerves. This condition causes many disabilities including urine and bowel elimination problems, loss of sensation in the feet and legs, and often the inability to move the legs (CDC 2018). Another type of spina bifida is a meningocele. When the baby is born, there is a sac of fluid coming through an opening in the back. It does not contain the spinal cord, and as a result, there is little to no nerve damage. Fortunately, the condition only causes minor disabilities. Spina bifida occulta may be referred to as a "hidden" spina bifida. When the child is born, there is no opening in the back. However, there is a small gap in the spine but hidden from view. The spinal cord and nerves are usually normal. The condition may not be discovered until later in life (CDC 2017a). This mildest form of spina bifida usually does not cause disabilities. When a baby is born with myelomeningocele, or open spina bifida with the spinal cord exposed, surgery is performed within the first few days of life to close the opening and repair of spinal cord as necessary. When the spinal cord or lumbosacral nerve roots are involved, as is usually the case, varying degrees of paralysis occur below the involved level. The paralysis also usually affects the sphincters of the bladder and rectum. In addition, an excessive accumulation of cerebrospinal fluid within the ventricles, called hydrocephalus, is associated with the lumbosacral type of spina bifida in at least 80 percent of affected patients. Health issues and treatments vary for people with different forms of spina bifida. Patients with open spina bifida unfortunately have more health issues and require more extensive treatment than do other spina bifida patients (CDC 2018).

Figure 20.1. Three most common types of spina bifida

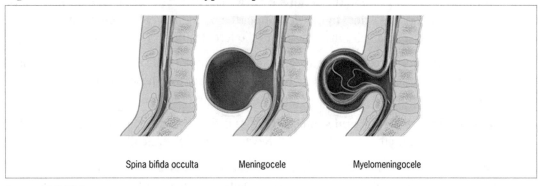

Spina bifida occulta   Meningocele   Myelomeningocele

Source: CDC 2018

In ICD-10-CM, most types of spina bifida, excluding spina bifida occulta, are assigned to category Q05. This category is further subdivided to fourth-digit subcategories that describe the sites, such as cervical, thoracic, lumbar, or sacral with presence or absence of hydrocephalus. As indicated by the Excludes1 note, Spina bifida occulta (Q76.0) would not be coded with the Q05 category codes, as it is mutually exclusive to those conditions.

> **EXAMPLE:** A newborn infant was transferred to the Children's Hospital after birth and was diagnosed with lumbosacral spina bifida, specifically myelomeningocele, without hydrocephalus: Q05.7, Lumbar spina bifida without hydrocephalus.

Cardiovascular System Defects (Q20–Q28)

Cardiovascular system defects involve the heart and circulatory system and are the most common group of birth defects in infants. Surgical procedures repair defects and restore circulation to as normal as possible. Some defects can be repaired before birth, whereas others may require multiple surgical procedures after birth. Smaller defects may be repaired in a cardiac catheterization laboratory instead of an operating room. Some of the more commonly occurring cardiovascular defects are patent ductus arteriosus, atrial septal defect, ventricular septal defect, and pulmonary artery anomalies.

Descriptions of cardiovascular system defects and their common abbreviations are as follows:

- **Hypoplastic left heart syndrome** (Q23.4) is a condition in which the entire left half of the heart is underdeveloped. This condition may be repaired in a series of three procedures over one year. If not treated, the condition can be fatal within one month.

- **Persistent/patent truncus arteriosus (PTA)** (Q25.0) is a failure of the fetal truncus arteriosus to divide into the aorta and pulmonary artery. It can be corrected surgically.

- **Pulmonary valve atresia** (Q22.0) and **stenosis** (Q22.1) are conditions that obstruct or narrow the pulmonary heart valve. Mild forms are relatively well tolerated and require no intervention. More severe forms are surgically corrected.

- **Tetralogy of Fallot (TOF)** (Q21.3) is a defect characterized by four anatomical abnormalities within the heart that results in poorly oxygenated blood being pumped to the body. It can be corrected surgically.

- **Total anomalous pulmonary venous return (TAPVR)** (Q26.2) is a malformation of all of the pulmonary veins. In this condition, the pulmonary veins empty into the right atrium, or a systemic vein, instead of into the left atrium.

- **Transposition of great vessels** or great arteries **(TGV)** (Q20.3) is a defect in which the positions of the aorta and the pulmonary artery are transposed. Immediate surgical correction is required.

- **Tricuspid valve atresia and stenosis** (Q22.4) is the absence or narrowing of the valve between the right atrium and ventricle. Severe cases are surgically corrected.

- **Aortic valve stenosis (AS)** (Q23.0) is the congenital narrowing or obstruction of the aortic heart valve. This can be surgically repaired in some cases.

- **Atrial septal defect (ASD)** (Q21.1) is a hole in the wall between the upper chambers of the heart (the atria). The openings may resolve without treatment or require surgical intervention. This condition may also be referred to as patent foramen ovale.

- **Coarctation of the aorta** (Q25.1) is a defect in which the aorta is narrowed somewhere along its length. Surgical correction is recommended even for mild defects.

- **Endocardial cushion defect** is a spectrum of septal defects arising from imperfect fusion of the endocardial cushions in the fetal heart (Q21.2). This diagnosis may also be specified as atrioventricular septal defect. This condition is repaired surgically.

- **Patent ductus arteriosus (PDA)** is a condition in which the channel between the pulmonary artery and the aorta fails to close at birth (Q25.0). Many of these close spontaneously and cause no consequences. The condition can also be surgically and medically repaired.

- **Ventricular septal defect (VSD)** (Q21.0) is a hole in the lower chambers of the heart, or the ventricles. The openings may resolve without treatment; however, the condition can be surgically corrected.

- **Ebstein's anomaly** (Q22.5) is a deformation or displacement of the tricuspid valve with the septal and posterior leaflets being attached to the wall of the right ventricle. Only severe cases are corrected surgically.

Respiratory System Defects (Q30–Q34)

Respiratory system congenital anomalies, mainly in the lungs, trachea, and nose, are life threatening, but less common than those involving other major organs. The major defect is **lung hypoplasia** or **dysplasia**, which is the underdevelopment or abnormal development of one or both lungs (Q33.6). Other unfortunate congenital malformations in the respiratory system are the underdevelopment or the lack or development of organs within the respiratory tract, such as the nose, trachea, bronchus, and lung. A web can be present in the larynx, and cystic lesions develop in the mediastinum. All of these respiratory anomalies require immediate medical and surgical care to correct the malformation so that the infant regains adequate respiratory function.

EXAMPLE: The newborn infant was transferred to the Children's Hospital for treatment of a subglottic web of the larynx: Q31.0, Web of larynx. The main term of "web" in the Alphabetic Index to Diseases and Injuries leads the reader to the correct code for glottis or subglottic web of the larynx.

Check Your Understanding 20.1

Assign diagnosis codes to the following conditions.

1. Arnold-Chiari syndrome with spina bifida
2. Glaucoma of newborn
3. Hypoplastic left heart syndrome
4. Dextrotransposition of aorta
5. Total anomalous pulmonary venous connection/return (TAPVR)
6. Congenital laryngomalacia
7. Congenital bronchomalacia
8. Congenital obstruction of the aqueduct of Sylvius
9. Coarctation of the aorta
10. Congenital supravalvular pulmonary artery stenosis

Digestive System and Orofacial Defects (Q35–Q37 and Q38–Q45)

Digestive system defects include orofacial defects (for example, choanal atresia, or cleft palate and lip) and gastrointestinal defects (for example, esophageal atresia, rectal and intestinal atresia and stenosis, and pyloric stenosis).

Cleft Lip and Cleft Palate (Q35–Q37)

Cleft lip, cleft palate, and combination of the two are the most common congenital anomalies of the head and neck. A cleft is a fissure or elongated opening of a specified site, usually occurring during the embryonic stage. A **cleft palate** is a split in the roof of the mouth (the palate), and a **cleft lip** is the presence of one or two splits in the upper lip. Figure 20.2 is an illustration of a cleft lip. Cleft lips and palates are classified as partial or complete and can occur either bilaterally or unilaterally. The most common clefts are left unilateral complete clefts of the primary and secondary palate, and partial midline clefts of the secondary palate involving the soft palate and part of the hard palate. The incisive foramen serves as the dividing point between the primary and the secondary palate (CDC 2017a).

Figure 20.2.   **Illustration of cleft lip**

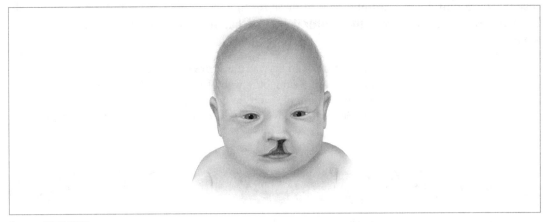

Source: CDC 2017

In ICD-10-CM, cleft palate is classified to Q35 and cleft lip is classified to category Q36. The category Q35 for cleft palate is subdivided to describe cleft hard palate (Q35.1), cleft soft palate (Q35.2), or when both conditions are present, cleft hard palate with cleft soft palate (Q35.3). Category Q36 for cleft lip is subdivided to identify bilateral, median, or unilateral forms of the cleft lip. When both conditions exist, cleft palate with cleft lip, the fourth character codes identify which palate is involved (hard or soft) and whether the cleft lip is a bilateral or unilateral type. As is true with all medical documentation, the physician should be queried when the documentation is unclear.

> **EXAMPLE:**   The infant was seen in the Orofacial Clinic for treatment of a cleft hard palate and left-sided cleft lip: Q37.1, Cleft hard palate with unilateral cleft lip.

Pyloric Stenosis (Q40.0)

Pyloric stenosis is the obstruction of the pyloric opening of the stomach (Dorland 2012, 1770). It results from hypertrophy of the circular and longitudinal muscularis of the pylorus and distal antrum of the stomach. Typically, the infant feeds well from birth until two or three weeks after birth, at which time occasional regurgitation of food, or spitting up, occurs, followed several days later by projectile vomiting. Dehydration due to the vomiting is common. ICD-10-CM assigns code Q40.0 for congenital hypertrophic pyloric stenosis.

> **EXAMPLE:**   The infant was seen in the Pediatric Surgery Clinic to be scheduled for surgery to repair his congenital hypertrophic pyloric stenosis: Q40.0, Congenital hypertrophic pyloric stenosis.

Genitourinary Tract Defects (Q50–Q56 and Q60–Q64)

Both male and female infants may be afflicted with defects of the reproductive organs and the urinary tract. Some are relatively minor and fairly common defects that can be repaired by surgery. Some of the genitourinary tract defects are as follows:

- Abnormalities of uterus codes (Q51.0–Q51.9) identify congenital anomalies such as agenesis and aplasia of uterus, doubling of uterus with doubling of cervix and vagina, septate uterus, unicornuate uterus, bicornuate uterus, arcuate uterus, and other anomalies of uterus. Collectively, these conditions may be referred to as **Müllerian anomalies of the uterus.** Women are likely to be diagnosed with these conditions after seeking medical attention for infertility or repeated pregnancy loss (Chandler et al. 2009).

- Different forms of **bladder exstrophy** (Q64.10–Q64.19) are conditions in which the bladder is turned inside out with portions of the abdominal and bladder walls missing. This must be surgically repaired (Dorland 2012, 662).

- Male or female **epispadias** (Q64.0) is a relatively rare defect in which the urethra opens on the top surface of the penis and surgical correction is needed (Dorland 2012, 635).

- Different forms of **hypospadias** (Q54.0–Q54.9) is a relatively common defect (1 in 250 male births) that appears as an abnormal urethral opening on the penis rather than at the end. The location of the abnormal condition is identified as anterior (balanic, glandular, coronal, or subcoronal) (Q54.0), middle (distal penile, midshaft, and proximal penile) (Q54.1), and posterior (penoscrotal or scrotal) (Q54.2). Another form of posterior hypospadias may be called perineal (Q54.3). A related condition also coded to this category is the condition known as congenital chordee or chordee without hypospadias. A chordee is a ventral curvature of the penis and may be present without hypospadias (Q54.4). Surgical correction may be needed for cosmetic, urologic, and reproductive reasons (CDC 2017b).

- **Obstructive genitourinary defect** is an obstruction of the ureter, renal pelvis, urethra, or bladder neck (Q62.0–Q62.8). Severity of the condition depends on the level of the obstruction. Urine accumulates behind the obstruction and produces organ damage. This condition can be corrected surgically while the fetus is in the uterus or after birth.

- **Renal agenesis or hypoplasia** (Q60.0–Q60.5) is the absence or underdevelopment of the kidneys and may be unilateral or bilateral. Newborns with bilateral renal agenesis often expire due to respiratory failure within a few hours of birth. Unilateral renal agenesis may not be detected for years (Dorland 2012, 37, 905).

- **Cystic or polycystic kidney disease (PKD)** is an inherited disorder characterized by multiple, bilateral, grapelike clusters of fluid-filled cysts that grossly enlarge the kidneys, compressing and eventually replacing functioning renal tissue. The infantile form of this condition reveals an infant with pronounced epicanthal folds, a pointed nose, a small chin, and floppy, low-set ears. Signs of respiratory distress and congestive heart failure also may be present. This condition eventually deteriorates into uremia and renal failure (NIDDK 2017). Figure 20.3 shows a comparison of a polycystic kidney and a normal kidney.

ICD-10-CM classifies cystic kidney disease to category Q61 with the following fourth-character subcategories:

Q61.00–Q61.02—Congenital renal cyst

Q61.11–Q61.19—Polycystic kidney, infantile type

Q61.2—Polycystic kidney, adult type

Q61.3—Polycystic kidney, unspecified

Q61.4—Renal dysplasia

Q61.5—Medullary cystic kidney

Q61.8—Other cystic kidney disease

Q61.9—Cystic kidney disease, unspecified

Figure 20.3. **A polycystic kidney and a normal kidney**

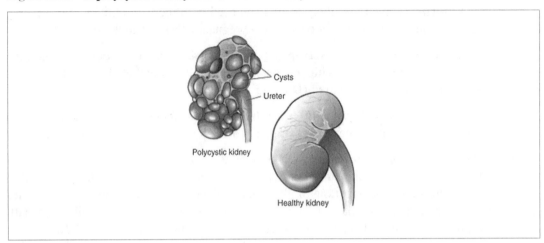

Source: HHS 2017

When there is no further specification as to type of polycystic kidney disease, assign code Q61.3. In addition, assign other complications that may be present, such as chronic kidney disease (N18.1–N18.9).

Musculoskeletal Defects (Q65–Q79)

Musculoskeletal defects are relatively common disorders and range from minor problems to more serious conditions. Clubfoot is the most common musculoskeletal congenital anomaly.

Clubfoot

Clubfoot, or talipes equinovarus, is a general term that is used to describe a variety of congenital structural foot deformities involving the lower leg, ankle, and foot joints, ligaments, and tendons (Stedman 2012, 1647). Clubfoot deformities include the following:

- Varus deformities, which are characterized by a turning inward of the feet (codes Q66.00–Q66.32)

- Valgus deformities, which are characterized by a turning outward of the feet (codes Q66.40-Q66.42, Q66.6)

- Talipes cavus, which is recognized by increased arch of the foot (code Q66.70-Q66.72)

- Talipes calcaneus or equinus, in which the entire foot exhibits an abnormal upward or downward misalignment (code Q66.89)

- The generic term clubfoot is classified as talipes, not otherwise specified (code Q66.90-Q66.92)

> **EXAMPLE:** A young male who was examined prior to acceptable into the Armed Forces was diagnosed with congenital flat feet: Q66.51 and Q66.52, Congenital pes planus, right foot and left foot.

Chromosomal Defects (Q90–Q99)

Chromosomal abnormalities are disorders that arise from abnormal numbers of chromosomes or from defects in specific fragments of the chromosomes. Each disorder is associated with a characteristic pattern of defects that arises as a consequence of the underlying chromosomal abnormality. Congenital heart defects, especially septal defects, are common among these infants and are a major cause of death. Specific forms of chromosomal abnormalities are classified with categories Q90–Q99.

The more common chromosomal conditions include the following:

- **Down syndrome (Q90.0–Q90.9)** is associated with the presence of a third number 21 chromosome. Another term for Down syndrome is trisomy 21. It results in mental retardation, distinctive malformations of the face and head, and other abnormalities. The severity of these problems varies widely among the affected individuals. Down syndrome is one of the more frequently occurring chromosomal abnormalities.

- **Edward's syndrome (Q91.0–Q91.3)** or trisomy 18 is associated with the presence of a third number 18 chromosome. It causes major physical abnormalities and severe mental retardation. Many children with this disorder expire in the first year of life due to the abnormalities of the lungs and diaphragm, heart defects, and blood vessel malformations.

- **Patau's syndrome (Q91.4–Q91.7)** or trisomy 13 is associated with the presence of a third number 13 chromosome. The infants have many internal and external abnormalities, including profound retardation. Death may occur in the first few days of life due to the respiratory difficulties, heart defects, and severe defects in other organ systems.

> **EXAMPLE:** The parents of a young child meet with the genetic counselor in the Genetics Center to review the findings of the testing done recently on their son. The parents learn that their son has abnormalities in his FMR-1 gene that has caused Fragile X syndrome that is the cause of the child's intellectual disability. The diagnosis code assigned for the visit is Q99.2, Fragile X syndrome.

Check Your Understanding 20.2

Assign diagnosis codes to the following conditions.

1. Congenital bile ducts atresia
2. Renal hypoplasia, left side
3. Craniosynostosis
4. High scrotal testis, bilateral
5. Osteogenesis imperfecta, primarily lower legs
6. Congenital sacral dimple
7. Velo-cardio-facial syndrome
8. Congenital hypertrophic pyloric stenosis
9. Partial septate uterus
10. Congenital metatarsus primus varus, right foot

ICD-10-PCS Procedure Coding to Correct Congenital Malformations and Deformations

The ICD-10-PCS procedure coding system does not have a specific group of procedure codes used to treat congenital malformations and deformities (CMS 2019). Instead, newborns or other patient may have procedures performed that relate to the cardiovascular system, respiratory system, digestive systems, and others as appropriate. Other congenital malformations and deformations are not treated surgically, for example, chromosomal abnormalities are treated with medical therapies instead.

Surgical procedures to correct congenital malformations, deformations, or congenital anomalies are coded based on the objective of the procedure. For example, if a hydrocephalus exists, the creation of a shunt may be necessary. The creation of a shunt is a Bypass within the Central Nervous system with the body part being the Cerebral Ventricle and the qualifier identifying the location where the bypass is directed to, for example, the peritoneal cavity for a ventriculo-peritoneal shunt.

Another example of a procedure to correct a congenital condition is a patient with spina bifida who requires surgical closure of the defect. The opening in the vertebral column is closed with the body part addressed as the spinal meninges. A closure as described in this type of procedure is Repair or the restoring, to the extent possible, a body part to its normal anatomic structure and function.

Surgical repair of cleft lip(s) or palate(s) may take place immediately after birth or delayed for several weeks after birth depending on the individual patient. The root operation Repair is used for procedures in the mouth and throat to restore the lip and palate to the correct anatomic position. Other possible root operations to be used depending on the procedure would be Supplement or Transfer for a palatoplasty. Each body part repaired is coded separately, for example, upper lip, hard palate, or soft palate.

Congenital pyloric stenosis is a narrowing of the outlet between the stomach and small intestine. It results from hypertrophy of the circular and longitudinal muscularis of the pylorus and distal antrum of the stomach. Surgery is the treatment of choice. It is usually an open procedure to cut into the pylorus. The condition is marked by a thickening of the pylorus, which is the muscular band of tissue in the stomach that controls the exit of food and gastric juices from the stomach into the small bowel. By making an incision into the pylorus to divide the muscular band, the stenosis is relieved. Based on the specific description of the procedure, the root operation is likely Division in Table 0D8 with the body part stomach, pylorus. Other possible root operations for a pyloroplasty would be Dilation, Supplement, or Repair.

ICD-10-CM and ICD-10-PCS Review Exercises: Chapter 20

Assign the correct ICD-10-CM diagnosis codes and ICD-10-PCS procedure codes to the following exercises.

1. Spina bifida, lumbar region, with hydrocephalus

    _____

2. Coloboma of right eye iris

    _____

ICD-10-CM and ICD-10-PCS Review Exercises: Chapter 20 (continued)

3. Full-term female infant was born in this hospital by vaginal delivery. Her mother has been an alcoholic for many years and would not stop drinking during her pregnancy. The baby was born with fetal alcohol syndrome and was placed in the NICU.

4. Fragile X syndrome

5. Occipital encephalocele with hydroencephalocele

6. Cleft palate involving both the soft and hard palate, with bilateral cleft lip

7. Penoscrotal hypospadias

8. Newborn was delivered by cesarean section. Congenital condition diagnosed was with infantile polycystic kidney disease with collecting duct dilatation, diagnosed at age 3 days old.

9. Karyotype 45, X (form of Turner's syndrome)

10. Arterial tortuosity syndrome

11. Duplication of uterine cervix

12. Tetralogy of Fallot congenital defect with ventricular septal defect, pulmonary stenosis, dextroposition of aorta with hypertrophy of right ventricle

13. Hirschsprung's congenital megacolon disease

14. Acoustic (Type 2) neurofibromatosis

15. Patent ductus arteriosus; primary pulmonary hypertension of newborn (age 2 day old infant transferred to Children's Hospital after birth at another hospital)

16. PROCEDURE: Open Blalock-Hanlon procedure with excision of the atrial septal opening for palliative treatment of transposition of great vessels

(Continued on next page)

ICD-10-CM and ICD-10-PCS Review Exercises: Chapter 20 (continued)

17. PROCEDURE: Laparoscopic Heller esophagomyotomy, which is described in the operative report as a complete myotomy of the esophagogastric junction to treat the patient's achalasia.

18. PROCEDURE: Reopening of chest wall to control bleeding after thoracic surgery to correct congenital pulmonary abnormality, bleeding controlled and incision closed

19. PROCEDURE: Frenulotomy to treat ankyloglossia and speech dysfunction

20. PROCEDURE: Repair of congenital cerebral artery aneurysm by restriction with intravascular coil

References

Centers for Disease Control and Prevention (CDC), National Center for Health Statistics (NCHS). 2019. *ICD-10-CM Official Guidelines for Coding and Reporting*, 2020. http://www.cdc.gov/nchs/icd/icd10cm.htm or https://www.cdc.gov/nchs/data/icd/10cmguidelines-FY2020_final.pdf.

Centers for Disease Control and Prevention (CDC), National Center on Birth Defects and Developmental Disabilities. 2018 Spina Bifida. http://www.cdc.gov/ncbddd/spinabifida/facts.html.

Centers for Disease Control and Prevention (CDC), National Center on Birth Defects and Developmental Disabilities. 2017a. Facts about Cleft Lip and Palate. https://www.cdc.gov/ncbddd/birthdefects/CleftLip.html.

Centers for Disease Control and Prevention (CDC), National Center on Birth Defects and Developmental Disabilities. 2017b. Facts about Hypospadias. http://www.cdc.gov/ncbddd/birthdefects/hypospadias.html.

Centers for Medicare and Medicaid Services (CMS). 2019. *ICD-10-PCS Official Guidelines for Coding and Reporting*, 2020. http://www.cms.gov/Medicare/Coding/ICD10/.

Chandler, T. M., L. S. Machan, P. L. Cooperberg, A. C. Harris, and S. D. Chang. 2009. Müllerian duct anomalies: from diagnosis to intervention. *British Journal of Radiology*. 82(984):1034–1042. http://www.birpublications.org/doi/abs/10.1259/bjr/99354802. Published online 2014.

Dorland, W. A. N., ed. 2012. *Dorland's Illustrated Medical Dictionary*, 32nd ed. Philadelphia: Elsevier Saunders.

Mosby. 2017. *Mosby's Pocket Dictionary of Medicine, Nursing, and Health Professions*, 8th ed. St. Louis: Mosby, Inc.

Stedman, T. 2012. *Stedman's Medical Dictionary for the Health Professions and Nursing*, 7th ed. Philadelphia: Wolters Kluwer/Lippincott Williams & Wilkins.

U.S. Department of Health and Human Services, National Institute of Diabetes and Digestive and Kidney Disease (NIDDK). 2017. Polycystic Kidney Disease. https://www.niddk.nih.gov/health-information/kidney-disease/polycystic-kidney-disease/what-is-pkd.

Chapter 21

Symptoms, Signs and Abnormal Clinical and Laboratory Findings, Not Elsewhere Classified (R00–R99)

Learning Objectives

At the conclusion of this chapter, you should be able to do the following:

- Describe the organization of the conditions and codes included in Chapter 18 of ICD-10-CM, Symptoms, Signs and Abnormal Clinical and Laboratory Findings, Not Elsewhere Classified (R00–R99)

- Identify the circumstances in which a coder should use a code from Chapter 18 of ICD-10-CM

- Apply the guidelines for the assignment of a symptom code with an established disease code

- Explain how symptom codes are organized in ICD-10-CM

- Identify the Alphabetic Index entries for locating nonspecific abnormal findings in order to code them

- Referring to the *ICD-10-CM Official Guidelines for Coding and Reporting*, briefly describe the use of sign and symptom codes for hospital inpatients as a principal or additional diagnosis

- Explain the differences in coding of qualified diagnosis, such as possible or probable, when the patient is an inpatient in the hospital as opposed to an outpatient in any healthcare setting

- Describe when the ICD-10-CM coma scale codes (R40.21–R40.24) are used

- Assign ICD-10-CM codes for symptoms, signs, and abnormal findings

- Assign ICD-10-PCS codes for procedures related to this chapter

Key Terms

Abnormal findings
Abnormal tumor markers
Altered mental status
Complex febrile seizure

Glasgow Coma Scale (GCS)
Sign
Simple febrile seizure
Symptom

Overview of ICD-10-CM Chapter 18: Symptoms, Signs and Abnormal Clinical and Laboratory Findings, Not Elsewhere Classified

Chapter 18 includes categories R00–R99 arranged in the following blocks:

R00–R09	Symptoms and signs involving the circulatory and respiratory systems
R10–R19	Symptoms and signs involving the digestive system and abdomen
R20–R23	Symptoms and signs involving the skin and subcutaneous tissue
R25–R29	Symptoms and signs involving the nervous and musculoskeletal systems
R30–R39	Symptoms and signs involving the genitourinary system
R40–R46	Symptoms and signs involving cognition, perception, emotional state and behavior
R47–R49	Symptoms and signs involving speech and voice
R50–R69	General symptoms and signs
R70–R79	Abnormal findings on examination of blood, without diagnosis
R80–R82	Abnormal findings on examination of urine, without diagnosis
R83–R89	Abnormal findings on examination of other body fluids, substances and tissues, without diagnosis
R90–R94	Abnormal findings on diagnostic imaging and in function studies, without diagnosis
R97	Abnormal tumor markers
R99	Ill-defined and unknown cause of mortality

A **symptom** is any subjective evidence of disease reported by the patient to the physician. A patient can describe the symptom of shortness of breath, chest pain, or abdominal pain. A **sign** is objective evidence of a disease observed by the physician as the result of a physical examination or test result such as an abnormal result of a laboratory test or imaging study.

Some symptoms, such as hives or urticaria (L50.9), gastrointestinal hemorrhage (K92.2), menstrual pain (N94.6), and low back pain (M54.5), have been classified elsewhere in ICD-10-CM. Such symptoms are associated with a given organ system and thus are assigned to the chapter in ICD-10-CM that deals with the corresponding organ system.

Other symptoms and signs are associated with different body systems or are of unknown cause; these are classified to Chapter 18. Examples of these types of symptoms and signs include tachycardia, epistaxis, dyspnea, chest pain, abdominal pain, nausea, vomiting, rash, dysuria, coma, fever, fatigue, syncope, anorexia, and dry mouth.

As opposed to subjective symptoms, objective signs are a measurement or observation confirmed by diagnostic testing. **Abnormal findings** include objective measurements documented in laboratory reports that are reported after examination of blood, urine, or other body fluids taken from the patient. ICD-10-CM provides codes for abnormal findings on examination of blood, urine, other body fluids, diagnostic imaging, and function studies (CDC 2018). Abnormal findings of imaging studies are the conclusions written by radiologists based on review of images collected during diagnostic x-rays, ultrasound, computed axial tomography, magnetic resonance imaging, positron emission tomography, and thermography studies of the various parts of the patient's body. Abnormal findings also include conclusions written by physicians in reports produced after the examination of body function with radioisotope studies or scans, electroencephalogram, electromyogram, electrocardiogram, and other function studies.

Abnormal tumor markers are objective measurements of biochemical substances that are indicative of the presence of tumors. A tumor marker is a substance released into the circulation by tumor tissue, and its detection in the serum indicates the presence and type of tumor (Stedman 2012, 1731). Tumor markers are used to screen, diagnose, assess prognosis, follow response to treatment, and monitor for recurrence of neoplasia. Usually the measurement is an elevation in tumor-associated antigens (TAA) or tumor-specific antigens (TSA) such as carcinoembryonic antigen (CEA) or prostate-specific antigen (PSA).

One category, R99, is provided to describe ill-defined and unknown cause of mortality; it is only for use in the situation when a patient arrives at the emergency department or other facility as dead on arrival (DOA) and pronounced dead by the examining physicians. It does not represent the discharge disposition of death and would not be used on every patient who has expired.

Coding Guidelines and Instructional Notes for ICD-10-CM Chapter 18

The following note appears at the beginning of Chapter 18 outlining the conditions classified to this chapter: "This chapter includes symptoms, signs, abnormal results of clinical or other investigative procedures, and ill-defined conditions regarding which no diagnosis classifiable elsewhere is recorded" (CDC 2019).

Signs and symptoms that point rather definitely to a given diagnosis have been assigned to a category in other chapters of the classification. In general, categories in this chapter include the less well-defined conditions and symptoms that, without the necessary study of the case to establish a final diagnosis, point perhaps equally to two or more diseases or to two or more systems of the body. Practically all categories in the chapter could be designated not otherwise specified, unknown etiology, or transient. The Alphabetic Index should be consulted to determine which symptoms and signs are to be allocated here and which to other chapters.

The conditions, signs, and symptoms included in Chapter 18 consist of the following:

- Cases for which no more specific diagnosis can be made even after all the facts bearing on the case have been investigated

- Signs or symptoms existing at the time of the initial encounter that proved to be transient and whose causes could not be determined

- Provisional diagnosis in a patient who failed to return for further investigation or care

- Cases referred elsewhere for investigation or treatment before the diagnosis was made

- Cases in which a more precise diagnosis was not available for any other reason

- Certain symptoms, for which supplementary information is provided, that represent important problems in medical care in their own right (CDC 2019)

Additionally, notes for code usage appear at the subchapter level. Many of the blocks and categories in Chapter 18 have Excludes1 notes such as the one found under R09, Other symptoms and signs involving the circulatory and respiratory system, that directs the coder to locate diagnosis codes that appear in other chapters of ICD-10-CM. Guidelines that clarify code usage are also found under specific codes. Code R52, Pain unspecified, includes inclusive terms and Excludes1 notes (CDC 2019).

The NCHS has published chapter-specific guidelines for Chapter 18 in the *ICD-10-CM Official Guidelines for Coding and Reporting*. The coding student should review all of the coding guidelines for Chapter 18 of ICD-10-CM that appear in an ICD-10-CM code book or on the CDC website (CDC 2019) or in appendix F.

CG

I.C.18. Chapter 18: Symptoms, signs, and abnormal clinical and laboratory findings, not elsewhere classified (R00–R99): Chapter 18 includes symptoms, signs, abnormal results of clinical or other investigative procedures, and ill-defined conditions regarding which no diagnosis classifiable elsewhere is recorded. Signs and symptoms that point to a specific diagnosis have been assigned to a category in other chapters of the classification.

I.C.18.a. Use of symptom codes: Codes that describe symptoms and signs are acceptable for reporting purposes when a related definitive diagnosis has not been established (confirmed) by the provider.

I.C.18.b. Use of a symptom code with a definitive diagnosis code: Codes for signs and symptoms may be reported in addition to a related definitive diagnosis when the sign or symptom is not routinely associated with that diagnosis, such as the various signs and symptoms associated with complex syndromes. The definitive diagnosis code should be sequenced before the symptom code.

Signs or symptoms that are associated routinely with a disease process should not be assigned as additional codes, unless otherwise instructed by the classification.

I.C.18.c. Combination codes that include symptoms: ICD-10-CM contains a number of combination codes that identify both the definitive diagnosis and common symptoms of that diagnosis. When using one of these combination codes, an additional code should not be assigned for the symptom.

I.C.18.d. Repeated falls: Code R29.6, Repeated falls, is for use for encounters when a patient has recently fallen and the reason for the fall is being investigated.

Code Z91.81, History of falling, is for use when a patient has fallen in the past and is at risk for future falls. When appropriate, both codes R29.6 and Z91.81 may be assigned together.

I.C.18.e. Coma scale: The coma scale codes (R40.2-) can be used in conjunction with traumatic brain injury codes, acute cerebrovascular disease or sequelae of cerebrovascular disease codes. These codes are primarily for use by trauma registries, but they may be used in any setting where this information is collected. The coma scale may also be used to assess the status of the central nervous system for other non-trauma conditions, such as monitoring patients in the intensive care unit regardless of medical condition. The coma scale codes should be sequenced after the diagnosis code(s).

These codes, one from each subcategory, are needed to complete the scale. The 7th character indicates when the scale was recorded. The 7th character should match for all three codes.

At a minimum, report the initial score documented on presentation at your facility. This may be a score from the emergency medicine technician (EMT) or in the emergency department. If desired, a facility may choose to capture multiple coma scale scores.

Assign code R40.24, Glasgow coma scale, total score, when only the total score is documented in the medical record and not the individual score(s).

Do not report codes for individual or total Glasgow coma scale scores for a patient with a medically induced coma or a sedated patient.

See Section I.B.14 for coma scale documentation by clinicians other than patient's provider

I.C.18.f. Functional quadriplegia: Guideline has been deleted effective October 1, 2017.

I.C.18.g. SIRS due to Non-Infectious Process: The systemic inflammatory response syndrome (SIRS) can develop as a result of certain non-infectious disease processes, such as trauma, malignant neoplasm, or pancreatitis. When SIRS is documented with a noninfectious condition, and no subsequent infection is documented, the code for the underlying condition, such as an injury, should be assigned, followed by code R65.10, Systemic inflammatory response syndrome (SIRS) of non-infectious origin without acute organ dysfunction, or code R65.11, Systemic inflammatory response syndrome (SIRS) of non-infectious origin with acute organ dysfunction. If an associated acute organ dysfunction is documented, the appropriate code(s) for the specific type of organ dysfunction(s) should be assigned in addition to code R65.11. If acute organ dysfunction is documented, but it cannot be determined if the acute organ dysfunction is associated

(Continued)

(Continued)

with SIRS or due to another condition (e.g., directly due to the trauma), the provider should be queried.

I.C.18.h. Death NOS: Code R99, Ill-defined and unknown cause of mortality, is only for use in the very limited circumstance when a patient who has already died is brought into an emergency department or other healthcare facility and is pronounced dead upon arrival. It does not represent the discharge disposition of death.

I.C.18.i. NIHSS Stroke Scale: The NIH stroke scale (NIHSS) codes (R29.7–) can be used in conjunction with acute stroke codes (I63) to identify the patient's neurological status and the severity of the stroke. The stroke scale codes should be sequenced after the acute stroke diagnosis code(s).

At a minimum, report the initial score documented. If desired, the facility may choose to capture multiple stroke scale scores.

See Section I.B.14. for information concerning the medical record documentation that may be used for assignment of the NIHSS codes.

Coding Symptoms, Signs and Abnormal Clinical and Laboratory Findings in ICD-10-CM Chapter 18

Chapter 18 of ICD-10-CM, Symptoms, Signs and Abnormal Clinical and Laboratory Findings, Not Elsewhere Classified (R00–R99), includes symptoms, signs, and abnormal findings that relate to conditions in multiple body systems. Many of these codes are used for patients evaluated and treated in the outpatient settings, for example, in the physician's office, clinic, or emergency department. That does not mean a patient with a symptom could not be admitted to the hospital. It is possible to use a Chapter 18 code as a principal or secondary diagnosis for an inpatient if the reason for the symptom, sign, or finding could not be explained after inpatient studies were completed.

To help the coder locate the symptoms and signs without an established diagnosis, the ICD-10-CM Alphabetic Index to Diseases and Injuries contains such entries as abnormal, abnormalities, elevated, elevation, findings, abnormal, inconclusive, without diagnosis, and positive.

Symptoms and Signs by Body System (R00–R69)

Chapter 18 includes codes for a variety of symptoms. In some cases, symptom codes may be assigned in addition to a related definitive diagnosis when the symptoms or signs are not routinely associated with that diagnosis. The following discussion should be of assistance in determining when to assign a symptom as an additional diagnosis:

- Conditions that are routinely associated with a disease process: Symptoms and signs that are routinely associated with the disease process should not be assigned as additional codes unless otherwise instructed by the classification.

> **EXAMPLE:** Nausea and vomiting with gastroenteritis: K52.9, Noninfectious gastroenteritis and colitis, unspecified
> Only the code for gastroenteritis (K52.9) is assigned. The code for nausea and vomiting (R11.2) is not assigned because these are symptoms of gastroenteritis.

- Conditions that are not routinely associated with a disease process: Additional signs and symptoms that are not routinely associated with a disease process should be coded when present.

> **EXAMPLE:** Patient with metastases to brain admitted in comatose state: C79.31, Secondary malignant neoplasm of brain and spinal cord; R40.20, Coma
>
> The code for coma (R40.20) should be added as an additional diagnosis; coma is a significant condition that is not routinely associated with brain metastases.

Symptoms and signs are used frequently to describe reasons for service in outpatient settings. Outpatient visits do not always allow for the type of study that is needed to determine a diagnosis. Often the purpose of the outpatient visit is to relieve the symptom rather than to determine or treat the underlying condition. Coders must code the outpatient's condition to the highest level of certainty. The highest level of certainty is often an abnormal sign or symptom code that is assigned as the reason for the outpatient visit.

Most of the categories in the blocks of codes for symptoms and signs (R00–R69) are grouped by body systems, such as categories R00–R09, Symptoms and signs involving the circulatory and respiratory systems, and categories R10–R19, Symptoms and signs involving the digestive system and abdomen.

Coma Scale (R40.2)

According to the *ICD-10-CM Official Guidelines for Coding and Reporting*, subcategory R40.2, Coma, incorporates what may be documented in the health record as the **Glasgow Coma Scale (GCS)** (R40.211–R40.236). The GCS is a way to describe and communicate about the level of consciousness of patients with an acute brain injury that could be the result of trauma, neurologic disease, or other etiologies. The findings of the physician's examination of the patient's eyes, verbal responses, and motor responses are intended to help the physician decide what medical or surgical treatment is necessary to improve the patient's condition (GCS 2014, 2019). Figure 21.1 shows a GCS scoring tool that correlates the patient's responses with the scale numbers assigned for each response that can be reported as individual scores for eyes open, best verbal response, or best motor response.

Figure 21.1.   **Glasgow Coma Scale scoring tool**

Physical Factor	Patient's Response	Score
Eyes Opening	Opens eyes spontaneously	4
	Opens eyes when spoken to or in reaction to a sound	3
	Opens eyes in response to physical pressure or pain applied to body part	2
	Does not open eyes in response to any factor	1
	Eyes have been closed by medical factor, non-testable	NT
Verbal Speech	Normal conversation, oriented to name, place and date	5
	Speaks coherently but is confused, disoriented	4
	Speaks single coherent words, may use inappropriate words, no sentences	3
	Speech is incomprehensible or only moans or groans	2
	No audible responses, makes no sounds spontaneously or to stimuli	1
	Cannot speak due to medical intervention, non-testable	NT
Motor Response	Obeys commands or requests to do something	6
	Localizes painful stimuli, reaches to painful area	5
	Normal flexion of limb to withdraw from painful stimuli	4
	Abnormal flexion of limb in response to pain	3
	Extension of limb to painful stimuli	2
	No movement, no motor response	1
	Paralyzed or other limiting medical factor, non-testable	NT
Score may be documented as "GCS 10 = Eyes 3, Verbal 3, Motor 4" or a single total score is reported		
Minimum/worst score = 3 that usually indicates patient is in deep unconsciousness		
Maximum/best score = 15 that usually indicates patient is fully alert		

Adapted from GlasgowComaScale.org.

Although the GCS codes are commonly used to assess patients, including children, with traumatic brain injury. The GCS can be used to evaluate patients with a stroke such as a spontaneous subarachnoid hemorrhage, spontaneous intracerebral hemorrhage, or ischemic stroke. Other conditions that can be evaluated with the GCS to determine the patient's clinical neurologic status are intracerebral infections, brain abscess, nontraumatic coma, and poisonings. Each code includes the response from a child under the age of 2 years and from a child between 2 and 5 years of age as a child's response at that age is different from that of an older child or adult. For example, under code R40.222, Coma scale, best verbal response, incomprehensive words, would include incomprehensible sounds from a 2- to 5-year-old child. The best score available for a patient is 15 and the worse score is a 3. The score is a way of communicating the severity of the patient's condition (GCS 2014, 2019). The GCS scores are collected by trauma registries and research databases, but they may be used in any setting where this information is collected. The ICD-10-CM coma scale codes are sequenced after the diagnosis code(s). These codes, one from each subcategory (R40.21, R40.22, R40.23), are needed to complete the scale. The seventh character indicates when the scale was recorded, and it should match for all three codes:

0—unspecified time
1—in the field [EMT or ambulance]
2—at arrival to emergency department
3—at hospital admission
4—24 hours or more after hospital admission

At a minimum, report the initial score documented on presentation at the facility. This may be a score from the emergency medicine technician (EMT) or in the emergency department. If desired, a facility may choose to capture multiple GCS scores during the course of the patient's hospitalization.

Some physicians and emergency department personnel may document only one total Glasgow score. According to the coding guidelines, one ICD-10-CM code from the range of codes R40.241–R40.244, Glasgow coma scale, total score, may be the only coma scale code assigned instead of individual codes when only the total score is documented.

Example of GCS scoring

The emergency department physician determined the patient had a moderate traumatic brain injury based on his examination of the patient who demonstrated:

a. The patient opened his eyes in response to painful stimuli (score of 2)

b. The patient's verbal response to questions was confused and he was disoriented (score of 4)

c. The patient had abnormal flexion as his motor response (score of 3)

d. Total score was 9

For this patient, the GCS codes would be (a) R40.212, Coma scale, eyes open, to pain; (b) R40.224, Coma scale, best verbal response, confused conversation; and (c) R40.233, Coma scale, best motor response, abnormal.

Altered Mental Status, Unspecified (R41.82)

Code R41.82, **Altered mental status**, unspecified, identifies a frequent clinical state that requires investigation. This condition is a general change in brain function, such as confusion, amnesia, loss of alertness, loss of orientation, unusual or strange behavior, and other abnormalities of perception (Stöppler 2018).

Altered mental status or a change in mental status can be a symptom of many different illnesses. Underlying etiologies may include trauma, infection, neoplasm, or alcohol and drug use, as well as endocrine disorders, neurological disorders, psychiatric disorders, and diseases of the kidney. Altered mental status is not to be confused with altered level of consciousness (R40.-) or delirium (R41.0). Altered level of consciousness is difficult to define as this condition can vary widely from confusion to stupor to coma. Sometimes, the patient will be described as sleeping a lot and remaining drowsy and confused when awake. Delirium is a serious condition that exhibits a sudden state of severe confusion and rapid decline in brain function, sometimes associated with hallucinations and hyperactivity, during which the patient is not in contact with reality (MedicineNet 2016). It is important that the coder codes the diagnosis or condition as documented by the physician, that is, altered mental status, altered level of consciousness or delirium, and not consider the terminology as equivalent as the physician will apply the description of the patient considering each particular patient and his or her medical situation.

After workup, if a specific cause of the altered mental status is known, that condition should be coded, and the symptom code should not be used. An Excludes1 note appears under code R41.82 that states if the altered mental status is due to a known condition, the coder should code to that condition and not use this code.

> **EXAMPLE:** The patient is an 80-year-old female who was brought to the physician's office by her husband who explains to the physician that his wife "hasn't been herself" the past two days as she originally stated she had painful urination but then became confused and seemingly less alert. The physician ordered a urinalysis and complete blood count and advised the patient and husband that she would call them at home when the results of the lab work were completed in the event that medications should be prescribed. The physician documented the diagnosis of altered mental status and possible urinary tract infection in the patient's record: R41.82, Altered mental status, unspecified. The possible urinary tract infection was not coded as qualified diagnoses are not coded as if it exists for an outpatient visit.

General Symptoms and Signs (R50–R69)

The block of codes for general symptoms and signs (R50–R69) classifies general symptoms that are not related to one specific body system. Category R56, Convulsions, not elsewhere classified, is subdivided to recognize different forms of seizures or convulsions not identified as epileptic. Two codes exist for febrile seizures. A **complex febrile seizure** (code R56.01) is defined as a fever-associated seizure that is focal, prolonged (lasting more than 15 minutes), or recurs within 24 hours, or seizures in which only one side of the body is affected. These may also be described as "atypical" or "complicated" febrile seizures. Simple febrile seizures are ones that last less than 15 minutes and are without recurrence within the next 24 hours (or within the same febrile illness) (Holmes 2019).

Any other fever-associated seizure that does not meet this definition is defined as a **simple febrile seizure** (code R56.00). A febrile seizure that is not specified as simple or complex will also be coded to the R56.00 code. Another code is included for posttraumatic seizures (code R56.1). The last code under this category, R56.9, includes other or recurrent convulsions that are not related to fever and may also be described as "convulsive seizure or fit" in the diagnostic statement.

Category R52, Pain, unspecified, is a symptom code for generalized pain or pain without specificity of site. This code would not be used if the pain is described as acute or chronic or if the patient has localized pain that would be coded to pain by anatomic site. This is a three-character code with no subdivisions.

Category R68, Other general symptoms and signs, is subdivided to include conditions that do not fit in other body system categories. Examples of conditions in this category are codes R68.12, Fussy infant (baby); R68.11, Excessive crying of infant (baby); R68.81, Early satiety; and R68.83, chills (without fever).

Other categories in this chapter include codes for symptoms involving different body systems:

R00	Abnormalities of heart beat
R06	Abnormalities of breathing
R10	Abdominal and pelvic pain
R11	Nausea and vomiting
R21	Rash and other nonspecific skin eruption
R26	Abnormalities of gait and mobility
R31	Hematuria
R40	Somnolence, stupor and coma
R42	Dizziness and giddiness
R50	Fever of other and unknown origin
R55	Syncope and collapse
R57	Shock, not elsewhere classified
R63	Symptoms and signs concerning food and fluid intake

As stated previously, symptom and sign categories are frequently used in outpatient settings to indicate that the patient has a physical complaint for which a definitive diagnosis has not been established. It is possible that a symptom code might be used for an inpatient diagnosis when a reason for the complaint cannot be determined. In addition, symptom codes may be used as additional codes with an established diagnosis to describe the complete story of the patient's illness if the symptom is not an integral or usual part of the disease.

EXAMPLE: The patient is a 25-year-old female who comes to the urgent care center complaining of abdominal pain that she described as occurring in her right upper quadrant with nausea and vomiting and syncope. The patient was transferred by ambulance to the hospital emergency department with the following diagnoses of right upper quadrant abdominal pain, nausea and vomiting, and syncope and possible acute appendicitis. The diagnoses for the urgent care visit are R10.11, Right upper quadrant (abdominal) pain; R11.2, nausea with vomiting; and R55, Syncope. The acute appendicitis described as a possible condition is not coded in the outpatient setting.

Check Your Understanding 21.1

Assign diagnosis codes to the following diagnostic statements.

1. Change in bowel habits, diarrhea, and bright red blood per rectum
2. Fainting, malaise, and weakness
3. Chills with fever, cough, and acute respiratory distress
4. Nervousness, restlessness, and agitation
5. Palpitations, dizziness, and rapid heartbeat
6. Lower Abdominal pain, periumbilical; nausea with vomiting
7. Dysuria, gross hematuria, and chronic bladder pain
8. Altered mental status, painful urination
9. Facial pain, jaw pain, and chest pain
10. Epistaxis and headache and facial pain

Abnormal Findings (R70–R94)

Abnormal findings codes contain descriptors for nonspecific abnormal findings from laboratory, x-ray, pathologic, and other diagnostic tests. These nonspecific findings may be referred to as signs or clinical signs. Codes for nonspecific abnormal test results or findings may be found in the Alphabetic Index under such entries as the name of the test or one of the following:

abnormal, abnormality, abnormalities
findings, abnormal, without diagnosis
elevated, elevation
high
low
positive

Abnormal findings from laboratory, x-ray, pathologic, and other diagnostic results are not coded and reported unless the physician indicates their clinical significance. If the findings are outside the normal range and the physician has ordered other tests to evaluate the condition or has prescribed treatment, it is appropriate to ask the physician whether the diagnosis code(s) for the abnormal findings should be added.

Often abnormal findings are the reason for additional testing to be performed on patients in the outpatient setting. For example, elevated prostate specific antigen (PSA) (code R97.20) may be a reason for continued testing or monitoring of a patient. The code does not provide a specific diagnosis but indicates an abnormal finding for a specific organ. Abnormal findings recorded in the record may or may not be appropriate to code. If the coder notes an abnormal laboratory finding that appears to have triggered additional testing or therapy, the coder should ask the physician whether the abnormal finding is a clinically significant condition.

On other occasions, the coder will notice abnormal findings on radiologic studies that may well be incidental to the patient's current condition. For example, an elderly patient with congestive heart failure is given a chest x-ray. A finding of degenerative arthritis is noted in the radiologist's conclusion, but no apparent treatment or further evaluation has occurred. It is unlikely that the arthritis should be coded as it is considered an incidental finding.

The radiologist's findings can be used to identify the specific site of a fracture when the attending or ordering physician's diagnosis statement is nonspecific. For example, the attending physician writes, "Fracture, left tibia." However, the radiologist describes the injury as a fracture of the shaft of the tibia. The coder may code S82.20-, Fracture, tibia, shaft, based on the specific findings of the radiologist.

The radiologist's findings may also be used to clarify an outpatient's diagnosis or reason for services. For example, a patient comes to the hospital for an outpatient x-ray. The physician's order for the x-ray is "possible kidney stones." The radiologist's statement on the radiology report is "bilateral nephrolithiasis." Based on the fact that the radiologist is a physician, it is appropriate to code the calculus of the kidney as the patient's diagnosis.

The title of category R92, Abnormal and inconclusive findings on diagnostic imaging of breast, includes the term "inconclusive." This category includes findings that are considered inconclusive and not necessarily abnormal. For example, a routine mammogram may be considered inconclusive due to what is termed "dense breasts." This is not an abnormal condition but a condition that may require further testing—for example, an ultrasound—to conclude that no malignant condition exists that cannot be found on the mammogram. The diagnosis of dense breast or inconclusive mammography is assigned code R92.2, Inconclusive mammogram.

Coding of Papanicolaou Test (Pap Smear) Findings (R87)

The coding of Papanicolaou tests (Pap smears) often involves the coding of nonspecific abnormal findings. Because the classification of abnormal Pap smears has become more specific in recent years, ICD-10-CM includes code options under subcategories R87.6–R87.9, Abnormal cytological, histological and other abnormal findings in specimens from female genital organs.

The Bethesda System of Cytologic Examination is used by most of the laboratories in the United States and has been endorsed by national and international societies as the preferred method of reporting the results of abnormal Pap smears (Apgar et al. 2003). In ICD-10-CM, code R87.612 describes Pap smear of the cervix with low-grade squamous intraepithelial lesion and code R87.613 describes Pap smear of the cervix with high-grade squamous intraepithelial lesion. Other codes describe Pap smear with cervical high-risk human papillomavirus (HPV) DNA test positive (R87.810), Pap smear of the cervix with cytologic evidence of malignancy (R87.614), and Pap smear with cervical low-risk HPV DNA test positive (R87.820). Another code describes an unsatisfactory cytologic smear of the cervix or an inadequate sample from the cervix (R87.615).

The Excludes note for subcategory R87.61 refers the coder to other subcategories for confirmed dysplasia, CIN I–III, or carcinoma *in situ* conditions.

EXAMPLE: The patient is a 40-year-old female who returns to her gynecologist's office to review the results of her recent Pap smear. The physician stated the cytology report included the diagnosis of low-grade squamous intraepithelial lesion based on examination of cervical specimen submitted for study. The physician recommended that a colposcopy be performed in the following month to further investigate the abnormal findings of the Pap smear. The diagnosis code is R87.612, Low grade squamous intraepithelial lesion on cytologic smear of cervix.

Abnormal Tumor Markers (R97)

Testing has become common practice for elevations in TAA, antigens that are relatively restricted to tumor cells; in TSA, antigens unique to tumor cells; and in the diagnosis of and the follow-up care for many malignancies. A unique code for elevated PSA was created when this test became routine in the monitoring of prostate cancer. Many other TAA and TSA tests have become standard practice, and other elevated TAA codes are available for use: R97.0, Elevated carcinoembryonic antigen (CEA); R97.1, Elevated cancer antigen 125 (CA 125); R97.20, Elevated prostate specific antigen (PSA); R97.21, Rising PSA following treatment for malignant neoplasm of prostate.

EXAMPLE: The 75-year-old male brought his physician's order to the outpatient laboratory department of the hospital to complete a prostate-specific antigen (PSA) laboratory test. The laboratory used the diagnosis of "elevated PSA" as written by the doctor on the laboratory test order form to complete the claim for the lab test service: R97.20, Elevated prostate specific antigen (PSA).

Ill-Defined and Unknown Causes of Mortality (R99)

The ill-defined and unknown causes of mortality section of Chapter 18 include death or unexplained death and other conditions that are unspecified causes of mortality. These codes should not be used when a more definitive diagnosis is available. Code R99 is likely to be used for the patient who is brought to the hospital emergency department or other facility but has appeared to die prior to arrival. There may or may not be resuscitation efforts depending on the individual circumstances. The reason for the death may not be known. The diagnosis in the record for this patient may be written as "dead on arrival" (DOA). The physician will pronounce the patient dead and document the date and time in the health record.

Otherwise, the terminology of "death" is not a diagnosis. It is considered the healthcare outcome or the discharge disposition. The code R99 is not to be used on every health record when a patient expires. Instead, the cause of death and the underlying illness are coded on the health record. Code R99 is only used when the death is unexplained and there is no cause of death documented.

Check Your Understanding 21.2

Assign diagnosis codes to the following diagnostic statements.

1. Bacteremia in an otherwise healthy appearing child with bacteriuria

2. Positive tuberculin skin test; solitary lung nodule

3. Atypical squamous cells of undetermined significance on cytologic smear of the cervix (ASC-US)

4. Cervical high-risk human papillomavirus (HPV) DNA test positive

5. Abnormal electroencephalogram findings; post-traumatic seizures

6. Abnormal cardiac stress test findings, prediabetes, and elevated blood pressure readings

7. Abnormal liver function studies and abnormal radiology liver scan

8. Abnormal/prolonged prothrombin (PT) and partial thromboplastin times (PTT) lab results

9. Low-grade squamous Intraepithelial lesion on cytologic smear of vagina (LGSIL)

10. Positive blood drug screen for heroin and cocaine

ICD-10-PCS Procedure Coding to Investigate Symptoms, Signs and Abnormal Clinical and Laboratory Findings

Diagnostic procedures may be performed to investigate symptoms, signs, and abnormal test findings. In the Medical and Surgical section, procedures falling under the root operations Excision or Drainage may be performed as diagnostic studies or biopsies. The seventh character for these procedures would be X to distinguish this procedure as diagnostic when the procedure is identified as a biopsy. Other diagnostic procedures from the Medical and Surgical section are also possible tests that can be performed to investigate symptoms and signs, for example, inspection procedures such as bronchoscopy, cystoscopy, and colonoscopy that may be performed without a companion procedure such as a biopsy.

Diagnostic procedures also appear in other sections of the ICD-10-PCS classification system, for example, procedures in the Administration, Measurement and Monitoring, Imaging, and Nuclear Medicine sections. It would be up to the institution or provider to decide what procedures outside the Medical and Surgical section would be coded; just because there is a code for a procedure does not mean it requires coding.

Administration

The codes in the Administration section identify procedures for putting in or on a therapeutic, prophylactic, protective, diagnostic, nutritional, or physiological substance. This section includes transfusions, infusions, and injections. The seven characters for the administration procedures are shown in table 21.1.

Table 21.1.   **Administration procedures**

Character 1—Section	Administration procedure codes have the first-character value of 3
Character 2—Body System	Three values: Circulatory, Indwelling Device, Physiological Systems and Anatomical Regions
Character 3—Root Operation	Three values: Transfusion, Irrigation and Introduction
Character 4—Body/System Region	Identifies the site where the substance is administered, not the site where the substance administered takes effect
Character 5—Approach	Approaches are Open, Percutaneous, Via Natural or Artificial Opening, Via Natural or Artificial Opening Endoscopic and External
Character 6—Substance	Specifies the substance being introduced such as blood products, stem cells, irrigating substances, antineoplastic, thrombolytic, Anesthetic, Contrast, Dialysate, and Immunotherapeutic, and so on
Character 7—Qualifier	Indicates whether the substance is Autologous or Nonautologous, high-dose or low-dose Interleukin, Recombinant human-activated protein C, and so on

Source: CMS 2018

The main terms for procedures in the Administration section include such procedures as "Transfusion" and "Introduction of substance in or on." For example, the transfusion of nonautologous blood platelets through a peripheral vein is coded as 30233R1. The infusion of an electrolyte substance through a peripheral vein is coded as 3E0337Z.

Measurement and Monitoring

 The codes in the Measurement and Monitoring section identify and describe procedures for determining the level of a physiological or physical function. A measurement is defined as determining the level of a physiological or physical function at a point in time. Monitoring is defined as determining the level of a physiological or physical function over a period of time. The seven characters for measurement and monitoring procedures are shown in table 21.2.

Examples of procedures coded to this section are electrocardiograms (EKG), electroencephalograms (EEG), and cardiac catheterization. An EKG is a measurement of cardiac electrical activity (4A02X4Z). An EEG is a measurement of the electrical activity of the central nervous system (4A00X4Z). A cardiac catheterization is a measurement of the sampling and pressures in the heart performed through a percutaneous approach. A left heart diagnostic cardiac catheterization is coded 4A023N7. The main terms used to locate the procedure codes are "measurement" and "monitoring" or the title of the procedure; for example, stress test is 4A12XM4.

Table 21.2. **Measurement and monitoring procedures**

Character 1—Section	Measurement and Monitoring procedure codes have the first-character value of 4
Character 2—Body System	Two values: Physiological Systems and Physiological Devices
Character 3—Root Operation	Two values: Measurement and Monitoring
Character 4—Body/System Region	Specifies the specific body system measured or monitored
Character 5—Approach	Approaches are Open, Percutaneous, Via Natural or Artificial Opening, Via Natural or Artificial Opening Endoscopic, and External
Character 6—Function/Device	Specifies the physiological or physical function being measured or monitored, for example, Conductivity, Metabolism, Pulse, Temperature, and Volume. If a device is required and left in place, the insertion of the device is coded as a separate Medical and Surgical procedure
Character 7—Qualifier	Specific values to further identify the body part or the variation of the procedure performed

Source: CMS 2018

Imaging Section

The codes in the Imaging section include procedures such as plain radiography, fluoroscopy, CT, MRI, and ultrasound. The seven characters for the procedures in the Imaging section are shown in table 21.3.

Table 21.3. **Imaging procedures**

Character 1—Section	Imaging procedure codes have the first-character value of letter B
Character 2—Body System	Defines the body system such as Central Nervous System, Heart, Upper Arteries, Respiratory System, Digestive System, and such
Character 3—Root Operation	Five values: Plain Radiology, Fluoroscopy, Computerized Tomography, Magnetic Resonance Imaging, and Ultrasonography

Character 4—Body Part	Defines the body part with different values for each of the body systems identified with character 2
Character 5—Contrast	Identifies whether the contrast material used in the imaging procedure is high or low osmolar or other contrast when applicable
Character 6—Qualifier	Provides further details about the nature of the substance used or the technology involved
Character 7—Qualifier	Specifies the circumstances of the imaging performed, for example, Intraoperative, Intravascular, or Transesophageal

Source: CMS 2017

Examples of procedures coded to this section are the fluoroscopy performed on a single coronary artery using low-osmolar contrast during a cardiac catheterization (B2101ZZ), CT of the abdomen (BW201ZZ), ultrasound of the bilateral breasts (BH42ZZZ), and plain x-ray of the right hip (BQ00ZZZ). The main terms used to locate the procedure codes are the root operations Computerized Tomography, Fluoroscopy, Magnetic Resonance Imaging, Plain Radiology, and Ultrasonography.

ICD-10-CM and ICD-10-PCS Review Exercises: Chapter 21

Assign the correct ICD-10-CM diagnosis codes or ICD-10-PCS procedure codes to the following exercises.

1. Right upper quadrant rebound abdominal tenderness, asymptomatic microscopic hematuria

   _____

2. Assign the Glasgow Coma Scale code(s) when the patient had the following documented by the EMT: eyes do not open, no verbal response, with no motor response. The neurologist documented the following on day 2 of the hospital admission: eyes open to sound, verbal response produced inappropriate words, and motor response with flexion withdrawal.

   _____

3. Microcalcification found on breast mammography, dense breasts producing an inconclusive mammogram

   _____

4. The patient comes to the physician's office for an annual physical, and two readings of elevated blood pressure are found. The physician requests the patient to return to the office in two weeks after the patient follows certain dietary and exercise instructions. The diagnosis recorded for the office visit is high blood pressure readings, rule out hypertension and systolic murmur.

   _____

5. Malignant ascites due to carcinoma of the ovary, right side (primary site neoplasm)

   _____

(Continued on next page)

ICD-10-CM and ICD-10-PCS Review Exercises: Chapter 21 (continued)

6. A 2-year-old child seen in emergency department (ED) with diarrhea, fever, and chills with a witnessed febrile seizure in the ED

7. The 65-year-old female patient was seen in the physician's office complaining of chest pain, back pain, and jaw pain with shortness of breath and excessive sweating. An ambulance was summoned and the patient was taken to the hospital emergency room with the diagnosis of rule out acute myocardial infarction.

8. Dyspnea, fatigue, and syncope

9. Elevated PSA in a patient currently under treatment for carcinoma of the prostate

10. At the conclusion of the physician office visit, the doctor wrote the final diagnosis in the record as "Rule out diabetes." Patient complained of weight loss and polydipsia with polyuria for several weeks

11. At the conclusion of the physician office visit, the physician documented "Postnasal drip, headache, cough, and localized lymphadenopathy, possible seasonal allergies."

12. Elevated glucose tolerance test

13. Elevated CEA and abnormal radiology imaging study of gastrointestinal tract

14. Physician office visit conclusion: Radiology study finding of nonvisualization of gallbladder; possible chronic cholecystitis

15. Physician office visit conclusion: Radiology study of coin lesion of lung and chronic cough

16. PROCEDURE: Bronchoscopy with biopsy of left main bronchus

17. PROCEDURE: Destruction of lesion in nasal mucosa by electrocautery

18. PROCEDURE: EGD with mid-esophageal biopsy

ICD-10-CM and ICD-10-PCS Review Exercises: Chapter 21 (continued)

19. PROCEDURE: Maxillary sinusoscopy

   _____

20. PROCEDURE: Cystoscopy with bladder biopsy

   _____

References

Apgar, B. S., L. Zoschnick, and T. C. Wright. 2003. The 2001 Bethesda System Terminology. *American Family Physician*. 68(10):1992–1998. http://www.aafp.org/afp/2003/1115/p1992.html.

Centers for Disease Control and Prevention (CDC), National Center for Health Statistics (NCHS). 2019. *ICD-10-CM Official Guidelines for Coding and Reporting*, 2020. http://www.cdc.gov/nchs/icd/icd10cm.htm or https://www.cdc.gov/nchs/data/icd/10cmguidelines-FY2020_final.pdf.

Centers for Medicare and Medicaid Services (CMS). 2019. *ICD-10-PCS Official Guidelines for Coding and Reporting*, 2020. http://www.cms.gov/Medicare/Coding/ICD10/.

Glasgow Coma Scale. 2014. What Is the Glasgow Coma Scale? http://www.glasgowcomascale.org/. (Accessed 07/2019)

Holmes, G. L. 2019. Epilepsy Foundation. Febrile Seizures. http://www.epilepsy.com/learn/types-seizures/febrile-seizures.

MedicineNet. 2018. Definition of Delirium. http://www.medicinenet.com/script/main/art.asp?articlekey=23364.

Stedman, T. 2012. *Stedman's Medical Dictionary for the Health Professions and Nursing*, 7th ed. Philadelphia: Wolters Kluwer/Lippincott Williams & Wilkins.

Stöppler, M. C. 2018. Altered Mental Status. MedicineNet. http://www.medicinenet.com/altered_mental_status/symptoms.htm.

Chapter 22A

Injury (S00–T34)

Learning Objectives

At the conclusion of this chapter, you should be able to do the following:

- Describe the organization of the conditions and codes included in Chapter 19 of ICD-10-CM, with a focus on injuries, categories S00–T34

- Identify the correct seventh character required for reporting certain injury codes in ICD-10-CM

- Apply the ICD-10-CM coding guidelines to the coding and reporting of injuries

- Assign ICD-10-CM diagnosis codes for injuries

- Assign ICD-10-PCS codes for procedures related to injuries

Key Terms

Burn
Closed fracture
Comminuted fracture
Contusion
Corrosion
Crush injury
Dislocation
Displaced fracture
First-degree burn
Frostbite
Greenstick fracture
Iatrogenic injuries
Immobilization
Impacted fracture
Initial encounter
Insertion
Malunion
Nondisplaced fracture
Nonunion

Oblique fracture
Open fracture
Open wound
Pathological fracture
Placeholder character
Repair
Reposition
Second-degree burn
Sequela
Sprain
Strain
Stress fracture
Subluxation
Subsequent encounter
Superficial injuries
Third-degree burn
Transverse fracture
Traumatic amputation
Traumatic fracture

Overview of the Injury Portion of ICD-10-CM Chapter 19

The Injury portion of Chapter 19 includes categories S00–T34 arranged in the following blocks:

S00–S09	Injuries to the head
S10–S19	Injuries to the neck
S20–S29	Injuries to the thorax
S30–S39	Injuries to the abdomen, lower back, lumbar spine, pelvis and external genitals
S40–S49	Injuries to the shoulder and upper arm
S50–S59	Injuries to the elbow and forearm
S60–S69	Injuries to the wrist, hand and fingers
S70–S79	Injuries to the hip and thigh
S80–S89	Injuries to the knee and lower leg
S90–S99	Injuries to the ankle and foot
T07	Injuries involving multiple body regions
T14	Injury of unspecified body region
T15–T19	Effects of foreign body entering through natural orifice
T20–T25	Burns and corrosions of external body surface, specified by site
T26–T28	Burns and corrosions confined to eye and internal organs
T30–T32	Burns and corrosions of multiple and unspecified body regions
T33–T34	Frostbite

This chapter focuses on the ICD-10-CM coding of injuries (S00-T34). The coding of drug-related illnesses (T35 T88) such as poisoning, adverse effects, and underdosing of drugs is addressed in Chapter 22B of this text.

Specific types of injuries found in categories S00–S99 of Chapter 19 of ICD-10-CM are arranged by body region beginning with the head and concluding with the ankle and foot. This results in the grouping of injury types together under the site where it occurred.

In addition, generally the listings of conditions that follow the anatomic site are as follows:

- Superficial injury

- Open wound

- Fracture

- Dislocation and sprain

- Injury of nerves

- Injury of blood vessels

- Injury of muscle and tendon

- Crushing injury

- Traumatic amputation

- Other and unspecified injuries

ICD-10-CM uses the terms "displaced" and "nondisplaced" in the code descriptor for fracture. Codes from blocks T20–T32 classify burns and corrosions. The burn codes identify thermal burns, except for sunburns, that come from a heat source. The burn codes are also for burns resulting from electricity and radiation. Corrosions are burns due to chemicals.

Coding Guidelines and Instructional Notes for the Injury Portion of ICD-10-CM Chapter 19

The following guideline appears at the beginning of ICD-10-CM Chapter 19: "Use secondary code(s) from ICD-10-CM Chapter 20: External Causes of Morbidity, to indicate cause of injury. Codes within the T code section that include the external cause do not require an additional external cause code" (CDC 2019).

Instructions for coding open wounds are included in ICD-10-CM. ICD-10-CM contains a note under the different categories for open wounds and directs the coding professional to code also any associated injuries or wound infection.

Most categories in ICD-10-CM Chapter 19 have seventh characters that identify the encounter:

A—Initial encounter
D—Subsequent encounter
S—Sequela

The fracture categories in Chapter 19 have different seventh characters that identify the fracture-care encounter:

A—Initial encounter for closed fracture
B—Initial encounter for open fracture or open fracture type I or II
C—Initial encounter for open fracture type IIIA, IIIB, or IIIC
D—Subsequent encounter for fracture with routine healing
E—Subsequent encounter for open fracture type I or II with routine healing
F—Subsequent encounter for open fracture type IIIA, IIIB, or IIIC with routine healing
G—Subsequent encounter for fracture with delayed healing
H—Subsequent encounter for open fracture type I or II with delayed healing
J—Subsequent encounter for open fracture type IIIA, IIIB, or IIIC with delayed healing
K—Subsequent encounter for fracture with nonunion
M—Subsequent encounter for open fracture type I or II with nonunion
N—Subsequent encounter for open fracture type IIIA, IIIB, or IIIC with nonunion
P—Subsequent encounter for fracture with malunion
Q—Subsequent encounter for open fracture type I or II with malunion
R—Subsequent encounter for open fracture type IIIA, IIIB, or IIIC with malunion
S—Sequela

The seventh characters for fractures are unique to each type of bone and type of fracture. Not all of these seventh characters are used with every fracture. It is necessary to review the fracture carefully before assigning a seventh character.

The NCHS has published chapter-specific guidelines for Chapter 19 in the *ICD-10-CM Official Guidelines for Coding and Reporting*. The coding student should review all of the coding guidelines for Chapter 19 of ICD-10-CM that appear in an ICD-10-CM code book or on the CDC website (CDC 2019) or in appendix F.

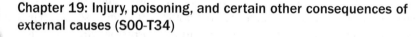

Chapter 19: Injury, poisoning, and certain other consequences of external causes (S00-T34)

I.C.19.a. Application of 7th Characters in Chapter 19: Most categories in chapter 19 have a 7th character requirement for each applicable code. Most categories in this chapter have three 7th character values (with the exception of fractures): A, initial encounter, D, subsequent encounter and S, sequela. Categories for traumatic fractures have additional 7th character values. While the patient may be seen by a new or different provider over the course of treatment for an injury, assignment of the 7th character is based on whether the patient is undergoing active treatment and not whether the provider is seeing the patient for the first time.

For complication codes, active treatment refers to treatment for the condition described by the code, even though it may be related to an earlier precipitating problem. For example, code T84.50XA, Infection and inflammatory reaction due to unspecified internal joint prosthesis, initial encounter, is used when active treatment is provided for the infection, even though the condition related to the prosthetic device, implant or graft that was placed at a previous encounter.

7th character "A", initial encounter is used for each encounter where the patient is receiving active treatment for the condition.

7th character "D" subsequent encounter is used for encounters after the patient has completed active treatment of the condition and is receiving routine care for the condition during the healing or recovery phase.

The aftercare Z codes should not be used for aftercare for conditions such as injuries or poisonings, where 7th characters are provided to identify subsequent care. For example, for aftercare of an injury, assign the acute injury code with the 7th character "D" (subsequent encounter).

7th character "S", sequela, is for use for complications or conditions that arise as a direct result of a condition, such as scar formation after a burn. The scars are sequelae of the burn. When using 7th character "S", it is necessary to use both the injury code that precipitated the sequela and the code for the sequela itself. The "S" is added only to the injury code, not the sequela code. The 7th character "S" identifies the injury responsible for the sequela. The specific type of sequela (e.g. scar) is sequenced first, followed by the injury code.

See Section I.B.10 Sequelae, (Late Effects)

I.C.19.b. Coding of Injuries: When coding injuries, assign separate codes for each injury unless a combination code is provided, in which case the combination code is assigned. Codes from category T07, Unspecified multiple injuries should not be assigned in the inpatient setting unless information for a more specific code is not available. Traumatic injury codes (S00-T14.9) are not to be used for normal, healing surgical wounds or to identify complications of surgical wounds.

The code for the most serious injury, as determined by the provider and the focus of treatment, is sequenced first.

I.C.19.b.1. Superficial injuries: Superficial injuries such as abrasions or contusions are not coded when associated with more severe injuries of the same site.

I.C.19.b.2. Primary injury with damage to nerves/blood vessels: When a primary injury results in minor damage to peripheral nerves or blood vessels, the primary injury is sequenced first with additional code(s) for injuries to nerves and spinal cord (such as category S04), and/or injury to blood vessels (such as category S15). When the primary injury is to the blood vessels or nerves, that injury should be sequenced first.

I.C.19.b.3. Iatrogenic injuries: Injury codes from Chapter 19 should not be assigned for injuries that occur during, or as a result of, a medical intervention. Assign the appropriate complication code(s).

IC.19.c. Coding of Traumatic Fractures: The principles of multiple coding of injuries should be followed in coding fractures. Fractures of specified sites are coded individually by site in accordance with both the provisions within categories S02, S12, S22, S32, S42, S49, S52, S59, S62, S72, S79, S82, S89, S92 and the level of detail furnished by medical record content.

A fracture not indicated as open or closed should be coded to closed. A fracture not indicated whether displaced or not displaced should be coded to displaced.

More specific guidelines are as follows:

I.C.19.c.1. Initial vs. subsequent encounter for fractures: Traumatic fractures are coded using the appropriate 7th character for initial encounter (A, B, C) for each encounter where the patient is receiving active treatment for the fracture. The appropriate 7th character for initial encounter should also be assigned for a patient who delayed seeking treatment for the fracture or nonunion.

Fractures are coded using the appropriate 7th character for subsequent care for encounters after the patient has completed active treatment of the fracture and is receiving routine care for the fracture during the healing or recovery phase.

(Continued)

(Continued)

Care for complications of surgical treatment for fracture repairs during the healing or recovery phase should be coded with the appropriate complication codes.

Care of complications of fractures, such as malunion and non-union, should be reported with the appropriate 7th character for subsequent care with nonunion (K, M, N,) or subsequent care with malunion (P, Q, R).

Malunion/nonunion: The appropriate 7th character for initial encounter should also be assigned for a patient who delayed seeking treatment for the fracture or nonunion.

The open fracture designations in the assignment of the 7th character for fractures of the forearm, femur and lower leg, including the ankle are based on the Gustilo open fracture classification. When the Gustilo classification type is not specified for an open fracture, the 7th character for open fracture type I or II should be assigned (B, E, H, M, Q.)

A code from category M80, not a traumatic fracture code, should be used for any patient with known osteoporosis who suffers a fracture, even if the patient had a minor fall or trauma, if that fall or trauma would not usually break a normal, healthy bone.

See Section I.C.13. Osteoporosis.

The aftercare Z codes should not be used for aftercare for traumatic fractures. For aftercare of a traumatic fracture, assign the acute fracture code with the appropriate 7th character.

I.C.19.c.2. Multiple fractures sequencing: Multiple fractures are sequenced in accordance with the severity of the fracture.

I.C.19.c.3. Physeal fractures: For physeal fractures, assign only the code identifying the type of physeal fracture. Do not assign a separate code to identify the specific bone that is fractured.

I.C.19.d. Coding of Burns and Corrosions: The ICD-10-CM makes a distinction between burns and corrosions. The burn codes are for thermal burns, except sunburns, that come from a heat source, such as a fire or hot appliance. The burn codes are also for burns resulting from electricity and radiation. Corrosions are burns due to chemicals. The guidelines are the same for burns and corrosions.

Current burns (T20–T25) are classified by depth, extent and by agent (X code). Burns are classified by depth as first degree (erythema), second degree (blistering), and third degree (full-thickness involvement). Burns of the eye and internal organs (T26–T28) are classified by site, but not by degree.

I.C.19.d.1. Sequencing of burn and related condition codes: Sequence first the code that reflects the highest degree of burn when more than one burn is present.

I.C.19.d.1.a. When the reason for the admission or encounter is for treatment of external multiple burns, sequence first the code that reflects the burn of the highest degree.

I.C.19.d.1.b. When a patient has both internal and external burns, the circumstances of admission govern the selection of the principal diagnosis or first-listed diagnosis.

I.C.19.d.1.c. When a patient is admitted for burn injuries and other related conditions such as smoke inhalation and/or respiratory failure, the circumstances of admission govern the selection of the principal or first-listed diagnosis.

I.C.19.d.2. Burns of the same anatomic site: Classify burns of the same anatomic site and on the same side but of different degrees to the subcategory identifying the highest degree recorded in the diagnosis (e.g., for second and third degree burns of right thigh, assign only code T24.311-).

I.C.19.d.3. Non-healing burns: Non-healing burns are coded as acute burns.

Necrosis of burned skin should be coded as a non-healed burn.

I.C.19.d.4. Infected burn: For any documented infected burn site, use an additional code for the infection.

I.C.19.d.5. Assign separate codes for each burn site: When coding burns, assign separate codes for each burn site. Category T30, Burn and corrosion, body region unspecified is extremely vague and should rarely be used. Codes for burns of "multiple sites" should only be assigned when the medical record documentation does not specify the individual sites.

I.C.19.d.6. Burns and corrosions classified according to extent of body surface involved: Assign codes from category T31, Burns classified according to extent of body surface involved, or T32, Corrosions classified according to extent of body surface involved, when the site of the burn is not specified or when there is a need for additional data. It is advisable to use category T31 as additional coding when needed to provide data for evaluating burn mortality, such as that needed by burn units. It is also advisable to use category T31 as an additional code for reporting purposes when there is mention of a third-degree burn involving 20 percent or more of the body surface.

Categories T31 and T32 are based on the classic "rule of nines" in estimating body surface involved: head and neck are assigned nine percent, each arm nine percent, each leg 18 percent, the anterior trunk 18 percent, posterior trunk 18 percent, and genitalia one percent. Providers may change these percentage assignments where necessary to accommodate infants and children who have proportionately larger heads than adults, and patients who have large buttocks, thighs, or abdomen that involve burns.

(Continued)

(Continued)

I.C.19.d.7. Encounters for treatment of sequela of burns: Encounters for the treatment of the late effects of burns or corrosions (i.e., scars or joint contractures) should be coded with a burn or corrosion code with the 7th character "S" for sequela.

I.C.19.d.8. Sequelae with a late effect code and current burn: When appropriate, both a code for a current burn or corrosion with 7th character "A" or "D" and a burn or corrosion code with 7th character "S" may be assigned on the same record (when both a current burn and sequelae of an old burn exist). Burns and corrosions do not heal at the same rate and a current healing wound may still exist with sequela of a healed burn or corrosion.

See Section I.B.10 Sequela (Late Effects)

I.C.19.d.9. Use of an external cause code with burns and corrosions: An external cause code should be used with burns and corrosions to identify the source and intent of the burn, as well as the place where it occurred.

Coding of Injuries in Chapter 19 of ICD-10-CM

The Alphabetic Index to Diseases in ICD-10-CM classifies injuries according to their general type, such as a burn, dislocation, fracture, or wound. The subterms under the general type of injury identify the anatomical site:

Burn (electricity)(flame)(hot gas, liquid or hot object)(radiation)(steam)(thermal)
    abdomen, abdominal (muscle)(wall) T21.02
        first degree T21.12-
        second degree T21.22-
        third degree T21.32-

Dislocation (articular)
    with fracture—see Fracture
    acromioclavicular (joint) S43.10-
        with displacement
        100%–200% S43.12-
        more than 200% S43.13-

Fracture, traumatic (abduction)(adduction)(separation)(see also Fracture, pathological)
    acetabulum S32.40-
    column
        anterior (displaced) (iliopubic) S32.43-
            nondisplaced S32.436

Wound, open
    abdomen, abdominal

wall S31.109-
    with penetration into peritoneal cavity S31.609-
    bite—see Bite, abdomen, wall
    epigastric region S31.102-
        with penetration into peritoneal cavity S31.602-

In ICD-10-CM, injuries are grouped by body parts rather than by categories of injury, so that all injuries of the specific site (such as head and neck) are grouped together rather than groupings of all fractures or all open wounds. For example, categories are grouped by site, such as injuries to the head (S00–S09), injuries to the neck (S10–S19), injuries to the thorax (S20–S29), and so on.

Chapter 19 encompasses two alpha characters. The S section provides codes for the various types of injuries related to single body regions; the T section covers injuries to unspecified body regions as well as poisonings and certain other consequences of external causes. For example, the codes in the ranges of S00–S99 are specific injuries to specific anatomical sites, such as the head, neck, thorax, abdomen, lower back, lumbar spine, and so on. Injury codes using the first character of T identify other and unspecified injuries sites such as T07, Unspecified multiple injuries, and T14.8, Other injury of unspecified body region.

The codes to classify traumatic fractures start with the first character of S. The fracture codes include detailed specificity in ICD-10-CM. For example, some of the information that may be found in fracture codes includes the type of fracture, specific anatomical site, whether the fracture is displaced or not, laterality, routine versus delayed healing, nonunions, and malunions. Laterality and identification of type of encounter (initial, subsequent, sequela) are a significant component of the code expansion. A seventh character is required for many of the injury codes to identify the encounter of care.

Because some of the injury codes are less than seven characters in length, ICD-10-CM uses a **placeholder character** X for certain codes. The X is used as a placeholder at certain codes to allow for future expansion. For example, S01.01XA for an initial encounter for care of a laceration without foreign body of scalp requires the sixth character to have a placeholder X to allow the addition of the seventh character to indicate the initial encounter of care.

It is common for patients to have multiple injuries as a result of an accident. Separate ICD-10-CM codes are assigned for each injury unless there is a combination code available. However, some combination codes should not be assigned. For example, code T07, Unspecified multiple injuries, should not be assigned in an inpatient setting if at all possible. The only time a code like T07 should be used is when no more specific information is available from the provider, for example, in a brief physician office visit note when the patient is transferred to an acute-care setting for care.

When patients have multiple injuries that can be coded, the code for the most serious injury is sequenced first. The physician determines the most serious injury in a patient with multiple injuries. It is common for a patient to have both significant and superficial injuries on the same site. For example, if a patient suffers a fractured distal radius (wrist) in a fall, it is likely the patient would also have contusions and abrasions at the site of the distal radius fracture. When a patient has superficial injuries associated with a more serious injury at the same site, the code for the superficial injuries such as contusions and abrasions are not coded as the superficial injuries are expected to be present with a more serious injury.

Injury codes from ICD-10-CM Chapter 19 should not be assigned for iatrogenic injuries, that is, injuries that occur during, or as a result of, a medical intervention. The coder should assign the appropriate complication code(s) instead.

Seventh Characters

Most categories in Chapter 19 of ICD-10-CM have a seventh character required for each applicable code. Most categories have three applicable codes. Three seventh character values are used for most of the categories except for fractures, which have a most extensive list of seventh characters. The characters are as follows:

- The seventh character A for **initial encounter** is used for each encounter where the patient is receiving active treatment for the injury.

- The seventh character D for **subsequent encounter** is used for encounters after the patient has received completed active treatment of the injury and is receiving routine care for the injury during the healing or recovery phase.

- The seventh character S for **sequela** is used for complications or conditions that arise as a direct result of an injury, such as scar formation after a burn. When using the seventh character S, it is necessary to use both the injury code that precipitated the sequela and the code for the sequela itself. The S is added only to the injury code, not the sequela code. The seventh character S identifies the injury responsible for the sequela. The specific type of sequela (for example, contracture) is sequenced first, followed by the injury code (CDC 2019).

The aftercare Z codes should not be used for aftercare for injuries according to the *ICD-10-CM Official Guidelines for Coding and Reporting*. For aftercare of an injury, the coder should assign the acute injury code with the seventh character D for subsequent encounter.

Fractures

A **traumatic fracture** is a break in the bone or rupture in a bone due to a traumatic injury (Dorland 2012, 740). Tenderness and swelling develop at the site of the break, with a visible or palpable deformity, pain, and weakness. X-rays show a partial or an incomplete break at the site of the fracture.

In ICD-10-CM, traumatic fractures are coded to the specific sites of the fracture within categories S02, S12, S22, S32, S42, S49, S52, S59, S62, S72, S79, S82, S89, and S92. A fracture that is not indicated as an open fracture or a closed fracture is coded as a closed fracture. A fracture that is not indicated as a displaced fracture or a nondisplaced fracture is coded to a displaced fracture.

There are different types of fractures that may be described by physicians: closed, open, displaced, and nondisplaced. A **closed fracture** is when the bone breaks but there is no puncture or open wound in the skin. An **open fracture** is one in which the bone breaks through the skin even though it may fall back into the wound and may or may not be visible through the wound. A **displaced fracture** is described for a bone that breaks into two or more parts and the two ends of the bone are out of place and need to be realigned. This may also be called a comminuted fracture. In a **nondisplaced fracture**, the fracture of the bone occurs with a crack either part way or all the way through the bone but the bone remains in alignment. Some fractures are more severe than others based on fracture location and damage done to the bone and surrounding tissue. Fractures can damage blood vessels and nerves around the bone. A fractured bone can become infected or develop osteomyelitis. Healing time varies depending on the type of bone as well as the age and the overall health of a patient.

Figure 22A.1 shows three types of fractures. The stable, closed, or simple fractures show the fractured ends of the bone barely out of position. The oblique fracture has an angled pattern where the break in the bone has occurred. The comminuted fracture occurs when the bone breaks into several pieces that require realignment for fracture healing (AAOS 2013b).

Figure 22A.1. **Types of fractures**

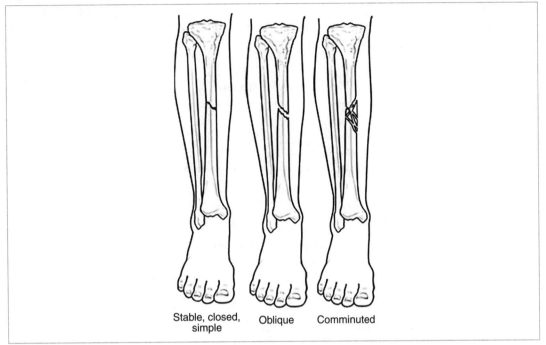

Reproduced with permission from *OrthoInfo*. ©American Academy of Orthopaedic Surgeons. http://orthoinfo.aaos.org.

Figure 22A.2 illustrates an open fracture. In this example of an open fracture of the tibia, the fractured end of the bone has torn through the soft tissue and may protrude through the skin or may be visible through an open wound at the site (AAOS 2017a).

Figure 22A.2. **Open fracture of the tibia**

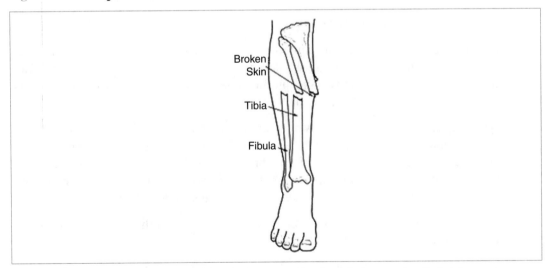

Reproduced with permission from *OrthoInfo*. ©American Academy of Orthopaedic Surgeons. http://orthoinfo.aaos.org.

Figure 22A.3 are images of extra-articular and intra-articular fractures of the forearm, the radius or ulna. Illustrations of both displaced and nondisplaced fractures appear here to demonstrate how the bone is separated as a displaced fracture and how the bone remains in alignment as a nondisplaced fracture (AAOS 2013a).

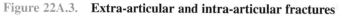

Figure 22A.3. **Extra-articular and intra-articular fractures**

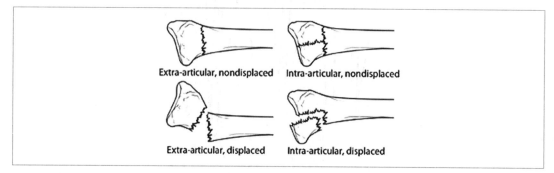

Reproduced with permission from JF Sarwark, ed: *Essentials of Musculoskeletal Care*, ed 4. Rosemont, IL, American Academy of Orthopaedic Surgeons, 2010.

Physicians may use other terminology to describe a fracture:

- A **comminuted fracture** occurs when a bone breaks into several pieces or splintered.

- A **greenstick fracture** is an incomplete fracture in which one side of the bone is broken and the other side of the bone is bent.

- An **impacted fracture** occurs when the bone breaks and the ends of the bone are pushed into each other or one end of the bone impacted into the other end of the bone at the site of the break. This type of fracture may also be referred to as a buckle fracture.

- An **oblique fracture** occurs when the bone breaks in a curved or sloped shape.

- A **pathological fracture** is one caused by disease that weakens the bone and breaks with minor trauma that otherwise would not break a healthy bone. Pathological fractures may occur in patients with neoplastic bone disease, osteoporosis, osteomalacia, osteomyelitis, and other diseases.

- **Stress fractures** are caused by overuse or repetitive force applied to a limb or bone, most commonly occurring in the bones of the lower leg and foot of athletes who run and jump in their sport. A stress fracture appears as small cracks in a bone that does not always appear on the first imaging or x-ray. Stress fractures can also occur with normal use of a bone when the bone is weakened by disease such as osteoporosis.

- A **transverse fracture** is one that breaks at a right angle to the bone's axis (Dorland 2012, 741–743).

Traumatic fractures are coded with the appropriate seventh characters to identify the episode of care: initial treatment, subsequent treatment, or to identify an injury that is the cause of a sequela. Fracture seventh characters are expanded to include options for the initial care for a closed versus open fracture, subsequent care that includes routine and delayed healing, complications of nonunion and malunion, and identification of a sequela situation:

A—Initial encounter for closed fracture
B—Initial encounter for open fracture
D—Subsequent encounter for fracture with routine healing
G—Subsequent encounter for fracture with delayed healing
K—Subsequent encounter for fracture with nonunion
P—Subsequent encounter for fracture with malunion
S—Sequela

Some fracture categories provide for seventh characters to designate the specific type of open fracture. These seventh character designations are based on the Gustilo open fracture classification:

B—Initial encounter for open fracture type I or II (open NOS or not otherwise specified)
C—Initial encounter for open fracture type IIIA, IIIB, or IIIC
E—Subsequent encounter for open fracture type I or II with routine healing
F—Subsequent encounter for open fracture type IIIA, IIIB, or IIIC with routine healing
H—Subsequent encounter for open fracture type I or II with delayed healing
J—Subsequent encounter for open fracture type IIIA, IIIB, or IIIC with delayed healing
M—Subsequent encounter for open fracture type I or II with nonunion
N—Subsequent encounter for open fracture type IIIA, IIIB, or IIIC with nonunion
Q—Subsequent encounter for open fracture type I or II with malunion
R—Subsequent encounter for open fracture type IIIA, IIIB, or IIIC with malunion

There may be complications of fracture injuries, and the care for these complications should be coded with the appropriate complication codes, such as postoperative wound infections. If there is a complication of the fracture healing such as malunion or nonunion, the code for the fracture should be reported with the seventh character for subsequent encounter for fracture with nonunion or malunion. A **malunion** fracture (Stedman 2012, 1011) is a fractured bone that has healed in a poor alignment and may cause the bone to be shorter than it was before the break. A **nonunion** is a fracture (Stedman 2012, 1167) that has failed to heal after several months of recovery. Both conditions cause significant impairment in the patient and usually require additional treatment including surgery.

Remember that pathologic fractures due to underlying bone disease are not considered traumatic and, as such, are not classified to Chapter 19 of ICD-10-CM with the traumatic fracture codes. A code from category M80, Age related osteoporosis with pathologic fracture, should be assigned when a patient with known osteoporosis acquires a fracture from a minor injury that normally would not cause a bone to break in a person without osteoporosis.

> **EXAMPLE:** Two patients with a fracture of the right distal (lower end) radius, subsequent treatment for normal healing
>
> a. Patient with no known bone disease with a traumatic fracture of right distal radius, S52.501D
>
> b. Patient with age related osteoporosis with pathologic fracture of right distal radius, M80.031D

Multiple Fractures

When coding fractures, the coder should assign separate codes for each fracture unless a complication code is provided in the Alphabetic Index, in which case the combination code is assigned.

EXAMPLE: Initial encounter for a patient who has a closed fracture of the distal radius and the first metacarpal bone of the right upper limb. This patient has multiple fractures, one in the distal radius or wrist and one in the first metacarpal bone of the hand. The Alphabetic Index to Diseases and Injuries has an entry for "Fracture, traumatic, multiple, hand (and wrist) NEC—see Fracture by site." This directs the coder to use two codes, one for each fracture site, as a combination code is not available.

Closed fracture of the distal radius (radius, lower end): S52.501A, Unspecified fracture of the lower end of the right radius

Closed fracture of the first metacarpal bone, right hand: S62.201A, Unspecified fracture of first metacarpal bone, right hand

Combination categories for multiple fractures are provided for use when the health record contains a description of multiple fractures at one site but without specific details.

EXAMPLE: Initial encounter for multiple fractures of ribs right side is the only information provided in the health record: S22.41XA, Multiple fractures of ribs, right side. The Alphabetic Index to Diseases and Injuries has an entry for "Fracture, traumatic, multiple, ribs—see Fracture, rib, multiple." For this reason, one code can be used to classify multiple rib fractures.

EXAMPLE: Initial encounter for multiple pelvic fractures without disruption of the pelvic ring: S32.82XA, Multiple fractures of pelvic without disruption of pelvic ring. The Alphabetic Index to Diseases and Injuries has an entry for "Fracture, traumatic, pelvis (pelvic bone), multiple, without disruption of pelvic ring (circle)." For this reason, one code can be used to classify the multiple pelvic fractures.

Dislocation and Subluxation

Dislocation is the displacement of a bone from its joint, specifically a disarrangement of the normal relation of the bones that form the joint. A dislocation may also be called a luxation (Stedman 2012, 491). The joints most commonly affected are in the fingers, thumbs, and shoulders. Pain and swelling occur, as well as the loss of use of the injured part. To promote healing, the dislocation can be reduced and the joint immobilized by applying a cast. A dislocation that occurs with a fracture is included in the fracture code. The reduction of the dislocation is included in the code for the fracture reduction. Figure 22A.4 illustrates the anatomy of the shoulder joint. The human shoulder is one of the most active joints in the body. The shoulder can be rotated forward, backward, or raised upward or sideways. Because of its mobility, a shoulder can be easily dislocated when a trauma occurs. A shoulder can dislocate partially and completely. A partial dislocation occurs when the humeral head comes partially out of its socket or the glenoid process. A complete dislocation occurs then the humeral head is completely out of the glenoid socket (AAOS 2017b).

Figure 22A.4. **Shoulder anatomy**

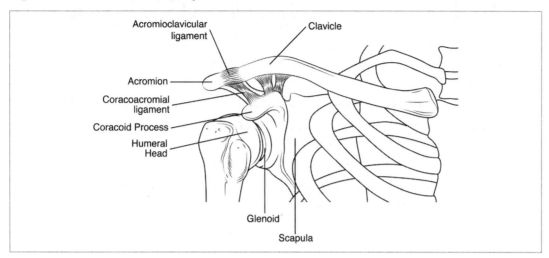

©AHIMA

A **subluxation** is an incomplete dislocation with the contact between the joint surfaces remaining in place (Stedman 2012, 1610). A subluxation commonly seen in children under the age of five is "nursemaid's elbow." This injury occurs when a small child is lifted, yanked, or swung by the hand or wrist or falls on an outstretched arm. The injury is a subluxation of the radial head from the annular ligament. The ligament is trapped in the elbow joint and causes acute pain. By manipulating the elbow joint to release the trapped tissue, the subluxation can be corrected, and the pain is immediately relieved.

In ICD-10-CM, traumatic dislocations and subluxations are coded to the specific sites of the dislocation within categories S03, S13, S23, S33, S43, S53, S63, S73, S83, and S93 with specific fourth characters to identify the dislocation and subluxation. The main term for dislocation and subluxation is "Dislocation" by site and "Subluxation" by site. Each of these codes requires a seventh character to identify whether the encounter of care for the condition is the initial (A) or a subsequent (D) encounter, or is for a sequela (S).

Dislocations may also be described as pathological or recurrent. These are not the same as traumatic dislocations. Codes for these conditions are contained in Chapter 13: Diseases of the Musculoskeletal System and Connective Tissue, in subcategories M24.3-, Pathological dislocation of joint, not elsewhere classified, and M24.4-, Recurrent dislocation of joint. The main term is dislocation, pathological or dislocation, recurrent, by site.

Once a dislocation of a joint has occurred, it takes less effort to produce another dislocation. Only the initial occurrence of the joint dislocation is coded to the injury code. All subsequent dislocations of the same joint are coded as recurrent dislocation.

> **EXAMPLE:**   A college athlete was brought to the ED with a dislocation of the right shoulder that occurred while he was wrestling at a sporting event. The athlete stated he has had a dislocated shoulder previously. The physician describes the dislocation as "recurrent." This would be accessed in the Alphabetic Index as Dislocation, recurrent, shoulder, M24.41-

The patient's condition for this episode of care is coded: M24.411, Recurrent dislocation of joint, right shoulder. The M is from the ICD-10-CM chapter on musculoskeletal diseases. It is not coded as a traumatic injury with an acute dislocation code for the shoulder, S43.005A.

Check Your Understanding 22A.1

Assign diagnosis codes to the following injuries.

1. Acute fracture, left distal tibia, physeal, Salter-Harris Type III, emergency department (ED) visit

2. Greater trochanteric traumatic fracture of the hip/femur, right side, surgical episode of care

3. Nondisplaced traumatic torus fracture of the left ulna, lower end, follow-up visit in physician's office, normal healing phase

4. Dislocation of left clavicle with displacement 100 percent, ED visit

5. Subluxation, radial head, right (nursemaid's elbow), physician office visit for initial care

Sprains

A **sprain** is a traumatic injury of the tendons, muscles, or supporting ligaments around a joint that may be the result of a turning or twisting of a body part. Sprains are extremely painful and are accompanied by pain, swelling, and discoloration of the skin over the joint. Treatment includes support, rest, and alternating heat and cold packs for the injury to heal (Mosby 2017, 1273). Whiplash is a specific type of sprain, usually due to a sudden throwing of the head forward and then backward. It is an injury to the supporting structure, ligaments and tendons, of the cervical vertebrae and results in pain and tenderness in the neck (Mosby 2017, 1451). An illustration of the ligaments in the ankle is shown in figure 22A.5a. When an ankle sprain occurs, one or more ligaments in the joint are torn away from the joint structures as illustration in figure 22A.5b.

Figure 22A.5. **Ankle sprain**

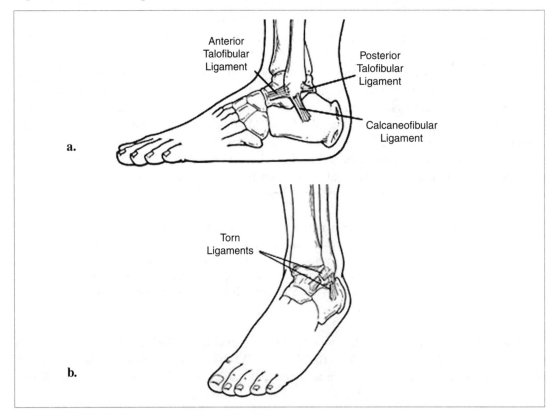

Reprinted with permission from American College of Foot and Ankle Surgeons.

A **strain** is an overstretching or overexertion of some part of the musculature. Strains usually respond to rest. Strains commonly occur in the musculature of the spine, especially in the neck (cervical strain) and in the low back (lumbar). A strain can be a partial tear in the muscle attached to a bone. The injury usually occurs when there is an unusual force applied to the muscle, for example, in an accident or during an athletic exercise or sport activity. The treatment is usually rest of the site, application of ice, and compression of the area with a wrap or supportive device (Mosby 2017, 1286).

In ICD-10-CM, traumatic sprains are coded to the specific site within categories S03, S13, S23, S33, S43, S53, S63, S73, S83, and S93 with specific fourth characters to identify the sprain. The main term is "Sprain" by site. Each of these codes requires a seventh character to identify whether the encounter for care of the condition is the initial (A) or a subsequent (D) encounter, or is for a sequela (S).

A strain may also be a traumatic injury. The Alphabetic Index contains the main term "Strain" with subterms for a limited number of sites that direct the coder to the injury chapter for codes such as:

Strain
  back S39.012
  cervical S16.1
  low back S39.012
  muscle—see Injury, muscle, by site, strain
  neck S16.1
  tendon—see Injury, muscle, by site, strain

Injuries to muscles and tendons are coded to the specific site within categories S09, S16, S29, S29, S39, S46, S56, S66, S76, S86, and S96 with specific fourth characters to identify the strain. The main term is "Injury, muscle (and tendon)" or "Injury, tendon (see also Injury, muscle)" by site. Each of these codes requires a seventh character to identify whether the encounter for care for the condition is the initial (A) or a subsequent encounter (D), or is for a sequela (S).

> **EXAMPLE:** The patient is brought to the ED after being in a car accident complaining of neck and low back pain. After examination and treatment, the ED physician documented the final diagnosis for the ED visit as "Whiplash injury of the neck" and "Lumbosacral sprain"
>
> S13.4, Sprain of ligaments of cervical spine (Whiplash injury of cervical spine)
> S33.9, Sprain of unspecified parts of lumbar spine and pelvis

Intracranial Injury, Excluding Those with Skull Fracture (S06)

Category S06, Intracranial injury, is used for various forms of traumatic brain injury excluding these injuries that occur with a skull fracture. The fourth-character subterms identify the specific intracranial injuries of concussion (S06.0), traumatic cerebral edema (S06.1), diffuse traumatic brain injury (S06.2), focal traumatic brain injury (S06.3), epidural hemorrhage (S06.4), traumatic subdural hemorrhage (S06.5), traumatic subarachnoid hemorrhage (S06.6), other specific intracranial injuries (S06.8), which includes injuries to carotid arteries, and unspecified intracranial injury (S06.9).

The sixth characters for the codes in subcategories S06.1–S06.9 identify whether the patient did or did not have a loss of consciousness:

0—without loss of consciousness
1—with loss of consciousness of 30 minutes or less
2—with loss of consciousness of 31 to 59 minutes
3—with loss of consciousness 1 hour to 5 hours 59 minutes
4—with loss of consciousness of 6 hours to 24 hours
5—with loss of consciousness of greater than 24 hours with return to preexisting conscious level
6—with loss of consciousness of greater than 24 hours without return to preexisting conscious level with patient surviving
7—with loss of consciousness of any duration with death due to brain injury prior to regaining consciousness
8—with loss of consciousness of any duration with death due to other cause prior to regaining consciousness
9—with loss of consciousness of unspecified duration

There are only three codes in subcategory S06.0X Concussion:

- S06.0X0, Concussion without loss of consciousness

- S06.0X1, Concussion with loss of consciousness of 30 minutes or less

- S06.0X9, Concussion with loss of consciousness of unspecified duration

Category S06, Intracranial injury, includes two instructional notes so that the coder will recognize that a patient with both an intracranial injury with an open wound or with a skull fracture will require two codes:

Code also any associated:
  Open wound of head (S01.1-)
  Skull fracture (S02.-)

An Excludes1 note appears under category S06: "head injury NOS (S09.90)." If the coder finds the diagnosis of "head injury" without the specificity of an intracranial injury, the coder should access the Alphabetic Index under the main term of "injury, head." The entry of "injury, head" directs the coder to code S09.90. In addition, the Index entry of injury, head, with loss of consciousness provides the code S06.9-. This code identifies the condition as one classified to the intracranial injury category. A loss of consciousness is an indication that an intracranial injury has occurred.

Another Index entry for "injury, head, specified type NEC" directs the coder to code S09.8. The diagnosis of "head injury" is a nonspecific description and should only be used if no further detail is provided in the health record documentation. Under code S09.90, Unspecified injury of head, an inclusion term of head injury NOS is provided to explain this is the code to use for the diagnosis of head injury when no further information is provided. The coder is reminded with an Excludes1 note that other specified descriptions of a head injury are coded elsewhere, for example, brain injury (S06.9-), head injury with loss of consciousness (S06.9-), and intracranial injury (S06.9-). The Excludes1 note means that category S06 codes are not used with code S09.90 for unspecified head injury.

EXAMPLE: The patient is admitted to the hospital from the ED after suffering trauma to his head that the physician documented as an intracranial injury with loss of consciousness of less than five minutes and a laceration of his scalp:
S06.9X1A, Unspecified intracranial injury with loss of consciousness of 30 minutes or less, initial encounter
S01.01XA, Laceration without foreign body of scalp, initial encounter

Injury to Internal Organs

ICD-10-CM classifies injuries to internal organs as well. The main term to use in the Alphabetic Index is Injury with the subterms for the organ site or a region, for example, "Injury, internal" with subterms for the anatomic sites of the aorta, bladder, bronchus, cecum, intestine, intrathoracic, ureter, uterus, and such. Other entries in the Index are Injury, internal, intra-abdominal, intracranial, or intrathoracic for injuries to internal organs within the cavity. The following are examples of categories for injuries to internal organs with their instructional notes:

S26, Injury of heart
  Code also any associated:
    Open wound of thorax (S21.-)
    Traumatic hemopneumothorax (S27.2)
    Traumatic hemothorax (S27.1)
    Traumatic pneumothorax (S27.0)
  S36, Injury of intra-abdominal organs
  Code also any associated open wound (S31.-)
  S37, Injury to urinary and pelvic organs
  Code also any associated open wound (S31.-)

Again, these codes require the use of the seventh characters A, D, or S to identify the encounter of care or the sequela of an injury.

EXAMPLE: The patient is brought to the ED by ambulance after suffering a gunshot wound to the stomach:
S36.33XA, Gunshot wound/laceration, internal organ, see Injury by site, stomach, laceration, initial encounter

---

Check Your Understanding 22A.2

Assign diagnosis codes to the following injuries.

1. Sprain of medial collateral ligament of the right knee, emergency department (ED) visit

2. Neck strain, cervical spine, subsequent visit, physician's office

3. Gunshot wound, intrathoracic, left lung, major laceration, ED visit with admission to ICU

4. Concussion with minimal loss of consciousness (5 minutes), ED visit

5. Stab wound with internal injury (laceration) to descending colon, with puncture wound of abdominal wall with penetration into peritoneal cavity, ED visit

Open Wound and Crush Injury

A traumatic **open wound** is an injury of the soft tissue parts associated with a break or a rupture of the skin (Mosby 2017, 954). Open wounds may be animal bites, avulsions, cuts, lacerations, puncture wounds, and traumatic amputation. In addition, an open wound may be a penetrating wound, which involves the passage of an object through tissue that leaves an entrance and exit, as in the case of a knife or gunshot wound.

The seriousness of an open wound depends on its site and extent. If a major vessel or organ is involved, a wound may be life threatening. For example, the rupture of a large artery or vein may cause blood to accumulate in one of the body cavities, which is referred to as hemothorax, hemopericardium, hemoperitoneum, or hemarthrosis, depending on the body cavity involved. The significance of the hemorrhage rests on the volume of the blood loss, the rate of loss, and the site of hemorrhage. Large losses may induce hemorrhagic shock.

Open wounds in ICD-10-CM include such diagnoses as laceration, with and without foreign body; puncture wounds, with or without foreign body; and open bites as well as codes for unspecified open wounds. Animals or humans can cause the bites. The open wounds are classified by site, for example:

S01	Open wound of head
S11	Open wound of neck
S21	Open wound of thorax
S31	Open wound of abdomen, lower back, pelvis and external genitals
S41	Open wound of shoulder and upper arm
S51	Open wound of elbow and forearm
S61	Open wound of wrist, hand and fingers
S71	Open wound of hip and thigh
S81	Open wound of knee and lower leg
S91	Open wound of ankle, foot and toes

Instructional notes appear with the open wound categories to code also any associated injury to nerve, injury to muscle and tendon, intracranial injury, spinal cord injury, or associated wound infection. In addition, there are notes to code any associated injury, such as injury to the heart, intrathoracic organs, rib fractures, and such.

A **crush injury** or crushing wound occurs when a body part is caught or squeezed between two heavy objects usually by a high degree of pressure or force (Mosby 2017, 346). Crushing injuries cause bruising, bleeding, compartment syndrome, fractures, lacerations, nerve injuries, and wound infections. Crushing syndrome is a serious condition caused by extensive crushing trauma, characterized by destruction of muscle and bone with hemorrhage and fluid loss resulting in hypovolemic shock, hematuria, renal failure, and coma (Mosby 2017, 346). Less traumatic crush injuries occur in motor vehicle accidents when a body part is caught for a short period of time. For instance, a finger smashed in a car door or legs being trapped for a period of time between metal or heavy objects before the patient can be extricated from a vehicle. Crushing injuries can occur when part or all of an extremity is pulled into and compressed by rollers in a machine, such as those found in industrial plants. Avulsion of the skin and fat or a friction burn of the tissues may result. Abrasion burns are often severe, including third degree. Vessels, nerves, and muscles may be avulsed, and bones may be dislocated or fractured. A common complication is secondary congestion, which can lead to paralysis and to severe muscle fibrosis and joint stiffness. Muscle compartments may need decompression, and muscles and ligaments may need to be sectioned. Often, the overall circulation of the extremity is of greater concern than definitive management of specific structures. These types of injuries may also be called wringer or compression injuries in addition to crush, crushed, or crushing injuries.

Crushing wounds are classified to the following categories in Chapter 19 of ICD-10-CM:

S07	Crushing injury of head
S17	Crushing injury of neck
S28	Crushing injury of thorax, and traumatic amputation of part of thorax
S38	Crushing injury and traumatic amputation of abdomen, lower back, pelvis and external genitals
S47	Crushing injury of shoulder and upper arm
S57	Crushing injury of elbow and forearm
S67	Crushing injury of wrist, hand, and fingers
S77	Crushing injury of hip and thigh
S87	Crushing injury of lower leg
S97	Crushing injury of ankle and foot

Instructional notes with the categories for crushing injuries remind the coder to use additional codes for all associated injuries such as intracranial or spinal cord injuries, fractures, injury to blood vessels, and open wounds as applicable.

The main terms to be used in the Alphabetic Index are "Crush, crushed, crushing," by site or injury, crushing—see Crush. These codes require the use of the seventh characters of A, D, or S to identify the encounter of care or the fact that the crushing injury is the sequel of an injury.

EXAMPLE: The patient was brought to the ED for initial treatment of an injury to his right foot that was trapped under the dashboard of his car as the result of an auto accident. The surgeon took the patient to surgery immediately to repair the crushing injury to the right foot: S97.81XA, Crushing injury of right foot

Burns and Corrosions

ICD-10-CM contains codes for burns and corrosions. **Burns** are caused by a heat source such as fire, electricity, radiation, or a hot appliance. **Corrosions** are burns due to a chemical (CDC 2019). The same ICD-10-CM coding guidelines apply to both burns and corrosions. Current burns are coded to categories T20–T25 and classified by depth, extent, and by agent or external cause code. Burns of the eye and internal organs are coded by site, T26–T28, but are not classified by degree (CDC 2019).

The burns coded by depth are classified as first degree (erythema), second degree (blistering), and third degree (full thickness) described as follows:

- A **first-degree burn** is the least severe and includes damage to the epidermis or outer layer of skin alone. The burn may also be described as superficial. The skin appears pink to red and painful. There is some edema, but no blisters or eschar. Dead skin may peel away two to three days after the burn (Dorland 2012, 261).

- A **second-degree burn** involves the epidermis and dermis. There is mild to moderate edema, and the burn will blister, but there is no eschar. The burn may also be described as either superficial partial thickness or deep partial thickness. Superficial partial-thickness burns extend into the upper dermal layer and leave the skin pink to red. Because the nerve endings are exposed, any stimulation causes extreme pain. Deep partial-thickness burns extend into the deeper layers of derma, leaving the skin red to pale with moderate edema. Blisters are infrequent, but there will be soft, dry eschar. The patient will experience pain but not as severe as in a superficial partial-thickness burn because some of the nerve endings have been destroyed (Dorland 2012, 262).

- A **third-degree burn** is the most severe and includes all three layers of skin: epidermis, dermis, and subcutaneous. A third-degree burn is also known as a full-thickness burn. The skin may appear black, brown, yellow, white, or red. Edema is severe. The burn penetrates the derma and may reach the subcutaneous fat. Pain is minimal because nerve endings are almost completely destroyed. There are no blisters, but there is hard eschar (Dorland 2012, 262).

Burns often exist with other injuries from the same accident. When the reason for the encounter is for treatment of multiple external burns, the site of the burn with the highest degree is coded and sequenced first. Additional codes are used for additional sites with lesser degree burns. When a patient has both an external and internal burn, either type of burn could be coded and sequenced first depending on the circumstances of the admission or encounter. When the patient is admitted with burns and related injuries such as smoke inhalation or organ failure such as respiratory or renal failure, the circumstances of the admission will determine the sequencing of the principal diagnosis.

When a patient has burns of varying degrees on one site (a single category between T20–T28), one code is assigned for the highest degree for that site. If burns exist on multiple sites, multiple separate codes are assigned. The category code T30, Burn and corrosion, body region unspecified, should rarely be used as it is too vague and only appropriate if there is no possibility of getting more information to further specify the burn site.

Complications can exist with burns. If a burn is not healing, it is coded as an acute burn for each encounter in which it is treated. If the condition is described as necrosis of burned skin, it is equivalent to a nonhealing burn. Burns can also become infected. If a burn site is documented as infection, an additional code for the infection is also assigned.

Category T31, Burns classified according to extent of body surface involved, is used as the primary code when the site of the burn is unspecified. This category is used as an additional code with categories T20–T25 when the site is specified. The same rule applies for category T32, Corrosions classified according to extent of body surface involved, which is to be used as an additional code with categories T20–T25 when the site is specified. The use of category T31 can provide valuable data for evaluating burn care and the mortality that unfortunately results from burn injuries. Category T31 will be used as an additional code to report what extent of the body surface is covered and what percent of that body surface is a third-degree burn. For example, a patient who has 20 percent of the body surface burned with 10 percent of that surface covered with a third-degree burn would be coded with T31.21. The main term to locate these codes is "burn" or "corrosion," extent (percentage of body surface) followed by the percentage of third-degree burn (CDC 2019).

Burns can cause long-term problems for patients. A patient may have a condition as the result of a healed burn that requires treatment. The condition the patient has for the long term is called the late effect of the sequela of the burn. The burn is healed, but the secondary condition remains. Common sequelae of burns are scars on the skin or joint contractures. The current condition is coded, such as the scar or contracture, as well as the code for the original burn with the seventh character of S to identify the burn as causing the sequela condition. It is possible for a patient with multiple burns to have a healed burn and a current healing burn existing at the same time, as burns do not heal at the same rate.

An external cause of morbidity code should be used with burns or corrosions to identify the cause of the accident as well as the place where it occurred, information about what the patient was doing at the time of the accident, and their work or nonwork status.

EXAMPLE: Two patients were being treated in the ED at the same time for burn injuries that occurred within the hour before being brought to the ED. Patient 1 had a second- and third-degree burn of multiple sites on her right hand and wrist as well as a first-degree burn on her right forearm as a result of a kitchen fire at home. Patient 2 had second-degree burns on his right and left forearms as a result of a chemical burn from fire at the factory where he worked.

Patient 1: T23.391A, Burn of third degree of multiple sites of right wrist and hand, initial encounter; T22.111A, Burn of first degree of right forearm. Only the third-degree burn of the multiple sites on the right wrist and hand are coded per coding guidelines when both second- and third-degree burns are present at the same site. The forearm is coded separately as it is a different site than the hand and wrist and is listed second as it is a less severe (first-degree) burn.

Patient 2: T22.611A, Corrosion of second degree of right forearm, initial encounter; T22.612A, Corrosion of second degree of left forearm, initial encounter

Both sites are coded as laterality is included in the codes: right and left. The Alphabetic Index to Diseases and Injuries includes an entry for burns, chemical—see—Corrosion by site.

Check Your Understanding 22A.3

Assign diagnosis codes to the following injuries.

1. Dog bite, right index finger, first care in emergency department visit

2. Laceration of right foot with foreign body removed, urgent care clinic visit

3. Crushing injury of right index finger, physician office visit for wound healing evaluation

4. Second degree burns of left foot and third-degree burns of right foot, ED visit

5. Normal healing burn, multiple sites on face and neck, subsequent physician office visit

Superficial Injury

Superficial injuries such as abrasions or contusions are not coded when associated with more severe injuries (for example, fracture or open wound) of the same site. The following subsections describe the conditions for coding superficial injuries.

Contusion

Contusions are injuries of the soft tissue. Although the skin is not broken, the small vessels or capillaries are ruptured, and the result is bleeding into the tissue. It may also be referred to as a bruise. When blood becomes trapped in the interstitial spaces, the result is a hematoma (Stedman 2012, 251, 392). ICD-10-CM classifies contusions according to the body site with laterality for right, left, and unspecified site.

> **EXAMPLE:** The patient went to the urgent care center after falling off a ladder at home and landing on her knees. After x-rays were taken, the physician concluded that there were no fractures in either leg, and the diagnoses documented were contusions of both knees: S80.01XA, Contusion of right knee and S80.02XA, Contusion of left knee

Superficial Injury

Superficial injuries include a variety of less serious conditions such as abrasion, blister, external constriction, superficial foreign body, insect bite, and other superficial bite of a specific location. These injuries are coded according to the body site where they exist and according to the specified laterality of the site with codes for right, left, and unspecified side.

The main terms to be used in the Alphabetic Index to locate these injuries are either "Injury, superficial" followed by the body part or by the word for the injury, such as abrasion, contusion, or bite, by site and superficial (CDC 2019). The appropriate seventh character is used with the superficial injury codes to identify whether the episode of care is the initial encounter (A) or a subsequent encounter (D), or for a sequela (S).

> **EXAMPLE:** The patient was seen in the physician's office complaining of a painful right foot that was scraped when a board fell on her foot. Upon direction of the physician, the medical assistant cleaned the scrapes and denuded skin on the patient's foot and applied a soft dressing to protect the injured skin. The physician documented the reason for the visit as severe abrasions of the right foot: S90.811A, Abrasion, right foot.

Injury to Blood Vessels, Nerves, and Spinal Cord

This subsection describes the conditions for coding injury to blood vessels and the nerves and spinal cord.

When a primary injury results in minor damage to peripheral nerves or blood vessels, the coder must assign a code for the primary injury that is sequenced first with additional code(s) for injuries to nerves, spinal cord, or blood vessels. When the primary or major injury is to the blood vessel or nerve (for example, represented by codes from category S15 or category S04), the code for that injury to the blood vessel or nerve is sequenced first.

Injuries to blood vessels can be a minor laceration that may also be described as an incomplete transection of a vessel or a superficial laceration of a blood vessel. A blood vessel may also have a major laceration that would be a complete transection or traumatic rupture of the blood vessel. Injuries to regions of the spinal cord are classified as to the type of injury, such as complete lesion, central cord syndrome, anterior cord syndrome, Brown-Séquard syndrome, or other incomplete lesions. Injuries to nerves are classified by the specific nerve involved.

Some examples of Alphabetic Index entries for locating injuries to blood vessels, nerves, and spinal cord are as follows:

- Injury, blood vessel, by site, such as abdomen, laceration (S35.91)

- Injury, aorta, abdominal (S35.00)

- Injury, blood vessel, uterine, vein (S35.53-)

- Injury, nerve (by site) such as abducens, followed by the type of injury—contusion, laceration or specified type (S04.4-)

- Injury, nerve, cranial, fifth (trigeminal)—see Injury, nerve, trigeminal (S04.3-)

- Injury, spinal cord, by spinal region and then by level, for example,

  ○ Injury, spinal (cord), cervical, anterior cord syndrome, C1 level (S14.131)

  ○ Injury, spinal (cord), lumbar, complete lesion, L1 level (S34.111)

Each of these injuries requires a seventh character to identify the initial encounter of care (A), subsequent encounter of care (D), or sequel episode (S). Instructional notes appear throughout the chapter with categories for injuries to blood vessels, nerves, and spinal cord. Examples of notes include the following:

- Code first any associated intracranial injury

- Code any associated open wound

- Code any associated fracture

- Code any associated transient paralysis

Codes for injuries of the cranial nerves are coded with the selection of the side or laterality based on the side of the body being affected. Codes for spinal cord injuries are coded to the highest level of spinal cord injury.

Check Your Understanding 22A.4

Assign diagnosis codes to the following injuries.

1. Spinal cord injury, incomplete lesion, L3 with transient paralysis, emergency department visit

2. Injury to the seventh cranial nerve (facial nerve), left side affected, follow up visit to physician office during recovery/healing phase

3. Superficial human bite to left external ear and left side of neck, first visit to urgent care center

4. Contusion of right shoulder and right upper arm, follow-up visit to physician's office for routine care during healing phase

5. Abrasions of both knees and to right forearm, first visit to urgent care center

Traumatic Amputation

A traumatic amputation is another type of injury classified to codes within Chapter 19 of ICD-10-CM. A **traumatic amputation** is the loss of a body part as the result of an accident or injury (Stedman 2012, 80). The most common sites of a traumatic removal of a limb or part of a limb are the finger, hand, toe, and foot. An amputation not identified as partial or complete is coded as a complete amputation. The categories for amputations of upper and lower extremities are as follows:

S48	Traumatic amputation of shoulder and upper arm
S58	Traumatic amputation of elbow and forearm
S68	Traumatic amputation of wrist, hand and fingers
S78	Traumatic amputation of hip and thigh
S88	Traumatic amputation of lower leg
S98	Traumatic amputation of ankle and foot

Each category requires the use of the appropriate seventh character to identify whether the treatment for the traumatic amputation is the initial encounter (A), a subsequent encounter (D), or is a sequela of the amputation (S). The codes for the traumatic amputations identify whether the right or left extremity is affected with other specificity as to the level of the amputation, such as between hip and knee, at knee level, between knee and ankle, and such.

> **EXAMPLE:** The patient was brought to the ED by ambulance from the factory where he works after he suffered a partial amputation of his right index and middle fingers when his hand was caught in a machine. The patient was taken to surgery for repair of his two fingers and discharged from the hospital in two days. The final diagnosis for the patient was partial metacarpophalangeal amputation of index and middle fingers of right hand: S68.120A, Partial traumatic metacarpophalangeal amputation of right index finger; S68.122A, Partial traumatic metacarpophalangeal amputation of right middle finger.

Effects of Foreign Body Entering through Natural Orifice (T15–T19)

The condition created in the body as a result of a foreign body entering through a natural orifice is coded with categories T15–T19. These codes do not include foreign body accidentally left in operative wound (T81.5-), foreign body in penetrating wound (see open wound by body region), residual foreign body in soft tissue (M79.5), or splinter without open wound (see foreign body, superficial by site such as finger, foot, knee, and so on).

Categories for the coding of foreign body are body systems, for example, respiratory tract, with fourth, fifth, and sixth character codes to identify the specific body part when the foreign body was located. The sixth character identifies a complication of the presence of the foreign body, for example, causing asphyxiation, compression, or other injury when this can occur based on the anatomic site.

Foreign objects often are found in various body openings in the pediatric population. Children sometimes put small items in their nose or ears or swallow small items, such as coins or marbles. Foreign bodies also can lodge in the larynx, bronchi, or esophagus, usually during eating. Foreign bodies in the larynx may produce hoarseness, coughing, and gagging, and partially obstruct the airway, causing stridor. A grasping forceps through a direct laryngoscope can remove foreign bodies from the larynx.

Foreign bodies in the bronchi usually produce an initial episode of coughing, followed by an asymptomatic period before obstructive and inflammatory symptoms occur. Foreign bodies are removed from the bronchi through a bronchoscope. Foreign bodies in the esophagus produce the immediate symptoms of coughing and gagging, with the sensation of something being "stuck in the throat," as well as causing difficulty in swallowing. Foreign bodies in the esophagus can be removed through an esophagoscope. Intraocular foreign bodies require removal by an ophthalmic surgeon.

These codes can be found in the Alphabetic Index by referencing the main term "Foreign body" and the various subterms such as by site or "entering through orifice." When the foreign body is associated with a laceration, this is located in the Index under "foreign body, in, laceration—see Laceration, by site, with foreign body." A foreign body accidentally left following a procedure is coded according to the type of procedure that was performed. The codes in categories T15–T19 require an appropriate seventh character to be added to indicate whether the episode of care was the initial encounter (A) or a subsequent encounter (D), or a sequela of the foreign body event (S).

EXAMPLE: A 55-year-old male patient came to the ED complaining of "food stuck in his throat." The patient was eating at a restaurant with family members and took a big bite of steak and felt it stick in his "throat." He tried to dislodge the meat himself in the restroom by forcing himself to vomit but the object did not move. The patient stated he could not even swallow water after this occurred. The ED physician called the gastroenterologist to examine the patient who decided the patient needed an esophagogastroduodenoscopy (EGD) to remove the substance. The gastroenterologist documented in his EGD report that the patient had an abrasion injury in his esophagus due to lodged meat. The physician could push the substance into the patient's stomach where it would be eliminated from the body naturally. The diagnosis for this patient would be coded as T18.128A, Food in esophagus causing other injury, initial encounter.

Frostbite

Frostbite damages skin and subcutaneous tissue when the skin is exposed to low environmental temperatures (Dorland 2012, 746). The damage can occur when body parts are exposed to cold temperatures for a prolonged period of time or extreme cold for a short period of time. Patients with peripheral vascular disease and diabetes are more likely to develop frostbite when exposed to the cold. Symptoms of frostbite include varying sensations at the site, including the feeling of pins and needles followed by numbness, as well as a lack of sensation when the area is touched. The skin may appear hard and pale, and after the area thaws, the body surface becomes red and painful. Severe cases of frostbite will have blisters and damage to tendons, muscles, nerves, and bone. If frostbite affects blood vessels, the damage is likely to be permanent with possible gangrene developing that requires amputation of the affected site. If the blood vessels are not involved, the patient most likely will have a complete recovery. While frostbite can occur when any part of the body is exposed to cold temperatures, the most common sites of frostbite are the hands, fingers, feet, toes, nose, and ears.

The injury of frostbite is classified in ICD-10-CM according to whether it is superficial frostbite (T33) or frostbite with tissue necrosis (T34). A superficial frostbite involves only the epidermis and upper epidermis with partial-thickness skin loss (Dorland 2012, 746). The severe type of frostbite involves tissue necrosis (may be documented as fourth-degree frostbite) that extends through a part of the body where the frostbite occurred and where gangrene develops and the site must be amputated (Dorland 2012, 746). Sites include parts of the body that are more likely to be exposed to low environmental temperatures, for example, head and face, ear, nose, neck, thorax, abdominal wall, arm, wrist, hand, finger, hip, thigh, knee, ankle, foot, and toe. The codes include the laterality of the site as well as an unspecified side. The categories for frostbite require the appropriate seventh character for the initial encounter (A) or a subsequent encounter (D), or for a sequela (S).

EXAMPLE: A 60-year-old male patient was brought to the ED by fire ambulance called by homeless shelter workers who found the homeless man exposed to very cold temperatures that night and noticed his fingers looked "frozen." The ED physician determined the patient had superficial frostbite of both hands and placed the patient in observation overnight and requested a social work consultation to help the patient find appropriate lodging. The diagnoses for the patient would be coded: T33.521A, Superficial frostbite of right hand, initial encounter, and T33.522A, Superficial frostbite of left hand, initial encounter.

Check Your Understanding 22A.5

Assign diagnosis codes to the following diagnostic statements.

1. Foreign body removed from cornea, right eye, in physician's office, initial care

2. Foreign body, external ear, left, removed in urgent care clinic

3. Foreign body in larynx (food and bone) causing injury to larynx, removed in emergency department (ED)

4. Superficial frostbite, right foot and frostbite with tissue necrosis, left foot, first treatment at urgent care center

5. Traumatic amputation, left lower leg, between knee and ankle, partial, treated in ED of hospital, transferred to inpatient status for definitive surgery

---

ICD-10-PCS Coding for Procedures Related to the Treatment of Injuries

Two of the more commonly coded procedures related to the injuries is the coding of fracture treatment and the repair of skin lacerations. The following sections describe the root operations that are used for these types of injuries. Fracture treatment depends on the type of fracture and surgical and non-surgical treatment that is appropriate depending on the type of fracture. The repair of the skin lacerations will depend on the location and the depth of the injury.

Coding Fracture Treatment

The root operations typically used for coding fracture treatment are Reposition, Insertion, and Immobilization.

The definition of **Reposition** is moving to its normal location or other suitable location all or a portion of a body part (CMS 2019). The body part is moved from an abnormal location or from a normal location where it is not functioning properly. The object of the procedure is to restore or establish normal function. The most common use of the root operation Reposition is to code a fracture or dislocation reduction. In a fracture reduction, the physician moves the bone or bone fragments back into their proper location. For a dislocation reposition, the physician moves a dislocation joint back into the correct position for articulation or movement of the joint. The terminology used by the physician will likely be "reduction," and the coder needs to translate that term to the ICD-10-PCS root operation Reposition. The approach for a Reposition procedure may be External or Closed, Percutaneous, Percutaneous Endoscopic, or Open.

The definition of **Insertion** is putting in a nonbiological device that monitors, assists, performs, or prevents a physiological function but does not physically take the place of a body part (CMS 2019). In this procedure, the sole objective is to put in a device without performing any other procedure. If the insertion of a device is a component of another procedure, the device is included in the device character for that procedure. Examples of an insertion procedure is putting in a pin to hold a nondisplaced fracture to allow it to heal properly or putting in a bone growth stimulator to promote healing of a fracture that is slow to heal.

The definition of **Immobilization** is limiting or preventing motion of a body region (CMS 2019). An example of an immobilization procedure is the placement of cast or splint to promote healing of a nondisplaced fracture or a dislocation. The body region for an immobilization procedure for musculoskeletal procedures includes upper and lower extremity, upper and lower arm, upper and lower leg, hand, thumb, finger, foot, and toe. The approach is always External. The device used for an immobilization may be a Splint, Cast, Brace, or another device. These devices are premade, out of the box items, and do not require extensive adjustment or fitting. There is no qualifier used for immobilization procedures.

The reduction or manipulation of a displaced fracture is coded in ICD-10-PCS to the root operation Reposition. The application of a cast or splint with a fracture reduction is not coded separately. A nondisplaced fracture does not require a repositioning. Any treatment of a nondisplaced fracture is coded to the procedure performed. For example, if a nondisplaced fracture is treated by putting in a fixation pin, the root operation is Insertion. If the nondisplaced fracture only requires the application of a cast or splint, the root operation is Immobilization.

Coding Repair of Lacerations

Repair is defined in ICD-10-PCS as a root operation to restore, to the extent possible, a body part to its normal anatomical structure and function. Repair is the root operation that is used if no other root operation applies. Repair is essentially the not elsewhere classifiable (NEC) root operation (CMS 2019). Repair procedures include a variety of procedures such as suturing lacerations of the skin or internal organs and herniorrhaphy that does not include mesh. If a fixation device is used to repair a bone or joint, it is included in the Repair root operation. If a Repair is performed on overlapping layers of the musculoskeletal system, the body part specifying the deepest layer is coded. The repair of skin lacerations is coded to 0HQ with the body part being skin of a specific location, such as skin of the scalp, face, right upper arm, left lower arm, right upper leg, left lower leg, right foot, and such. The approach is always external as the site can be accessed directly. There is no device included in the ICD-10-PCS code for repairs even though sutures remain in the body after the procedure but do not meet the definition of a device.

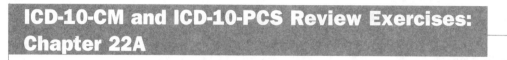

ICD-10-CM and ICD-10-PCS Review Exercises: Chapter 22A

Assign the correct ICD-10-CM diagnosis codes or ICD-10-PCS procedure to the following exercises.

Chapter 22A will provide practice coding ICD-10-CM Chapter 19 codes. External cause codes will be discussed and coded in Chapter 23. For Chapter 22A, assign only diagnosis and procedure codes, not the external cause of morbidity (V–Y) codes.

1. Superficial foreign body, right middle finger, initial encounter in emergency department

   _____

2. This patient is seen for increased pain in her ankle. She has a displaced trimalleolar fracture of the left ankle. During this subsequent evaluation for her fracture care, she was found to have a nonunion of her left trimalleolar fracture.

   _____

3. Fracture of left tibia, lower end, physeal, Salter-Harris, type II, initial fracture care

   _____

4. The patient is a complete paraplegic due to a traumatic L2 vertebral fracture five years ago. At this time, she is experiencing no new problems.

   _____

5. This is a follow-up visit for the healing of the patient's partial amputation of the right index finger through the metacarpophalangeal joint.

   _____

6. Crushing injury of the left hand sustained in an industrial accident when the patient's hand was caught in a piece of machinery. The crushing injury also produced an open fracture of the base of the first metacarpal bone of the left hand at the same time. This is the emergency department initial encounter for care of the injury.

   _____

7. The patient was seen in the emergency department for the initial encounter. The patient was playing a high school football game and received a hard tackle by an opponent and complained of acute severe pain in his right side. Examination and imaging prove there was a moderate laceration of the right kidney.

   _____

8. The patient is seen in her physician's office complaining of acute ankle pain. Based on her history of twisting her ankle while going down stairs during a recent move from one apartment to another and the physical examination performed, the physician diagnosed the patient with an acute sprain of the talofibular ligament of the right ankle.

   _____

9. The patient came to the physician's office for follow-up during the healing phase of the injury to the left index finger, specifically a laceration of the left index finger that was cut with a knife when the patient was preparing dinner one week ago. The physician also diagnosed a laceration to a digital nerve of the left index finger that occurred at the same time as the skin laceration. Both injuries are healing satisfactorily.

   _____

ICD-10-CM and ICD-10-PCS Review Exercises: Chapter 22A *(continued)*

10. Laceration of the scalp with foreign body, initial encounter for care in emergency department

   _____

11. The patient is seen in the emergency department for initial treatment of a dislocation of the right patella.

   _____

12. The patient is seen in the physician's office for a follow-up examination or subsequent visit during the recovery phrase for a sprain of the radial collateral ligaments of the right elbow.

   _____

13. The patient is seen in the emergency department for the first time for a first- and second-degree burn of the right shoulder.

   _____

14. The patient was brought to the emergency department and treated prior to transfer to a trauma center hospital with burns to multiple sites of the right leg (lower limb) above the ankle and foot. The burns were diagnosed as first- and second-degree burns.

   _____

15. Gunshot injury, right upper arm producing an open wound with laceration injury to brachial artery and retained foreign body in wound. Initial encounter in emergency department prior to transfer to trauma center hospital.

   _____

16. PROCEDURE: Closed reduction, fracture distal ulna, right with cast application

   _____

17. PROCEDURE: Open reduction with internal fixation, right femur shaft

   _____

18. PROCEDURE: Application of right lower leg brace for severe sprain

   _____

19. PROCEDURE: Suture laceration repair, skin laceration of forehead

   _____

20. PROCEDURE: Removal of foreign body, bullet from open wound, right neck muscle by incision

   _____

References

American Academy of Orthopaedic Surgeons (AAOS). 2017a. Open Fractures. http://www.orthoinfo.org/topic.cfm?topic=A00582.

American Academy of Orthopedic Surgeons (AAOS). 2017b. Dislocated Shoulder. http://orthoinfo.aaos.org/topic.cfm?topic=A00035.

American Academy of Orthopaedic Surgeons (AAOS). 2013a. Distal Radius Fractures (Broken Wrist). http://orthoinfo.aaos.org/topic.cfm?topic=A00412.

American Academy of Orthopaedic Surgeons (AAOS). 2013b. Fractures (Broken Bones). http://www.orthoinfo.org/topic.cfm?topic=A00139.

American College of Foot and Ankle Surgeons. 2019. Ankle Sprain. http://www.acfas.org/footankleinfo/ankle-sprain.htm.

Centers for Disease Control and Prevention (CDC), National Center for Health Statistics (NCHS). 2019. *ICD-10-CM Official Guidelines for Coding and Reporting*, 2020. http://www.cdc.gov/nchs/icd/icd10cm.htm or https://www.cdc.gov/nchs/data/icd/10cmguidelines-FY2020_final.pdf.

Centers for Medicare and Medicaid Services (CMS). 2019. *ICD-10-PCS Official Guidelines for Coding and Reporting*, 2020. http://www.cms.gov/Medicare/Coding/ICD10/.

Dorland, W.A.N., ed. 2012. *Dorland's Illustrated Medical Dictionary*, 32nd ed. Philadelphia: Elsevier Saunders.

Mosby. 2017. *Mosby's Pocket Dictionary of Medicine, Nursing, and Health Professions*, 8th ed. St. Louis: Mosby, Inc.

Stedman, T. 2012. *Stedman's Medical Dictionary for the Health Professions and Nursing*, 7th ed. Philadelphia: Wolters Kluwer/Lippincott Williams & Wilkins.

Chapter 22B

Poisoning and Certain Other Consequences of External Causes (T36–T88)

Learning Objectives

At the conclusion of this chapter, you should be able to do the following:

- Describe the organization of the conditions and codes included in Chapter 19 of ICD-10-CM, Injury, Poisoning, and Certain Other Categories of External Causes, with a focus on poisoning and certain other consequences of external causes, categories T36–T88

- Explain the organization of the ICD-10-CM Table of Drugs and Chemicals and identify which codes are used for which of the following circumstances: poisoning, adverse effect, and underdosing

- Identify the correct seventh characters required for reporting codes in Chapter 19 of ICD-10-CM

- Assign ICD-10-CM codes for adverse effects, poisonings, underdosing, and complications of surgical and medical care

- Assign ICD-10-PCS codes for procedures for adverse effects, poisonings, underdosing, and complications of surgical and medical care

Key Terms

Adverse effect
Complications
Dilation
Extirpation
Infection or inflammatory
   reaction
Insertion
Mechanical complications

Poisoning
Removal
Replacement
Revision
Toxic effect
Transplant complications
Transplantation
Underdosing

Overview of Poisoning and Certain Other Consequences of External Causes in ICD-10-CM Chapter 19

Chapter 19 includes categories T36–T88 arranged in the following blocks for poisoning, adverse effect, underdosing, toxic effects, other consequences of external causes, and complications of surgical and medical care, not elsewhere classified:

T36–T50	Poisoning by, adverse effect of and underdosing of drugs, medicaments and biological substances
T51–T65	Toxic effects of substances chiefly nonmedicinal as to source
T66–T78	Other and unspecified effects of external causes
T79	Certain early complications of trauma, not elsewhere classified
T80–T88	Complications of surgical and medical care, not elsewhere classified

This chapter's discussion of Chapter 19 focuses on the poisoning and certain other consequences of external cause codes.

ICD-10-CM does not provide different category codes to identify poisonings versus adverse effect. Instead, under a single category for a specific drug, there is one code for each drug to identify poisoning, adverse effects, and underdosing by the drug (T36–T50). The sixth character of the code generally identifies the condition resulting from the use of the drug. The poisoning codes include the intent of the poisoning, if known, such as accidental, intentional self-harm, or assault as well as a code for undetermined when the facts are not known.

Underdosing is a term in ICD-10-CM defined as taking less of a medication than is prescribed by a provider or the manufacturer's instructions with a resulting negative health consequence. As a consequence, the patient suffers a negative health consequence, such as a worsening of the condition intended to be treated by the medication (CDC 2019).

> **EXAMPLE:** T46.1, Poisoning by, adverse effect of, and underdosing of calcium-channel blockers
> T46.1X1-, Poisoning by calcium-channel blocker, accidental (unintentional)
> T46.1X2-, Poisoning by calcium-channel blocker, intentional self-harm
> T46.1X3-, Poisoning by calcium-channel blocker, assault
> T46.1X4-, Poisoning by calcium-channel blocker, undetermined
> T46.1X5-, Adverse effect of calcium-channel blocker
> T46.1X6-, Underdosing of calcium-channel blocker

Coding Guidelines and Instructional Notes for Chapter 19

A note at the beginning of the chapter states "Use secondary code(s) from Chapter 20: External Causes of Morbidity, to indicate cause of injury. Codes within the T section that include the external cause do not require an additional external cause code" (CDC 2019).

Under the block of codes T36–T50, Poisoning by, adverse effects of and underdosing of drugs, medicaments and biological substances, there is an Includes note that states the block of codes includes

- Adverse effect of correct substance properly administered
- Poisoning by overdose of substance
- Poisoning by wrong substance given or taken in error
- Underdosing by (inadvertently)(deliberately) taking less substance than prescribed or instructed

Other instructions appear under the section heading for T36–T50 such as code first notes, directions, and use additional code notes.

1. Code first, for adverse effects, the nature of the adverse effect, such as:

    Adverse effect NOS (T88.7)
    Aspirin gastritis (K29-)
    Blood disorders (D56-D76)
    Contact dermatitis (L23–L25)
    Dermatitis due to substance taken internally (L27-)
    Nephropathy (N14.0–N14.2)

2. Note: The drug giving rise to the adverse effect should be identified by use of codes from categories T36–T50 with fifth or sixth character 5.

3. Use additional code(s) to specify:

    Manifestations of poisoning
    Underdosing or failure in dosage during medical and surgical care (Y63.6, Y63.8–Y63.9)
    Underdosing of medication regimen (Z91.12-, Z91.13-)

In ICD-10-CM, a note is included stating to use an additional code (Y62–Y82) to identify devices involved and details of circumstances.

The NCHS has published chapter-specific guidelines for Chapter 19 in the *ICD-10-CM Official Guidelines for Coding and Reporting*. The coding student should review all of the coding guidelines for Chapter 19 of ICD-10-CM, that appear in an ICD-10-CM code book or on the CDC website (CDC 2019) or in appendix F.

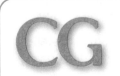

Chapter 19: Injury, poisoning, and certain other consequences of external causes (T36-T88)

Guideline I.C.19.e. Adverse Effects, Poisoning, Underdosing and Toxic Effects: Codes in categories T36–T65 are combination codes that include the substance that was taken as well as the intent. No additional external cause code is required for poisonings, toxic effects, adverse effects and underdosing codes.

Guideline I.C.19.e.1. Do not code directly from the Table of Drugs: Do not code directly from the Table of Drugs and Chemicals. Always refer back to the Tabular List.

(Continued)

(Continued)

Guideline I.C.19.e.2. Use as many codes as necessary to describe: Use as many codes as necessary to describe completely all drugs, medicinal or biological substances.

Guideline I.C.19.e.3. If the same code would describe the causative agent: If the same code would describe the causative agent for more than one adverse reaction, poisoning, toxic effect or underdosing, assign the code only once.

Guideline I.C.19.e.4. If two or more drugs, medicinal or biological substances: If two or more drugs, medicinal or biological substances are taken, code each individually unless a combination code is listed in the Table of Drugs and Chemicals.

If multiple unspecified drugs, medicinal or biological substances were taken, assign the appropriate code from subcategory T50.91, Poisoning by, adverse effect of and underdosing of multiple unspecified drugs, medicaments and biological substances.

Guideline I.C.19.e.5. The occurrence of drug toxicity is classified in ICD-10-CM as follows:

Guideline I.C.19.e.5(a). Adverse Effect: When coding an adverse effect of a drug that has been correctly prescribed and properly administered, assign the appropriate code for the nature of the adverse effect followed by the appropriate code for the adverse effect of the drug (T36–T50). The code for the drug should have a 5th or 6th character "5" (for example T36.0X5-) Examples of the nature of an adverse effect are tachycardia, delirium, gastrointestinal hemorrhaging, vomiting, hypokalemia, hepatitis, renal failure, or respiratory failure.

Guideline I.C.19.e.5(b). Poisoning: When coding a poisoning or reaction to the improper use of a medication (e.g., overdose, wrong substance given or taken in error, wrong route of administration), first assign the appropriate code from categories T36–T50. The poisoning codes have an associated intent as their 5th or 6th character (accidental, intentional self-harm, assault and undetermined). If the intent of the poisoning is unknown or unspecified, code the intent as accidental intent. The undetermined intent is only for use if the documentation in the record specified that the intent cannot be determined. Use additional code(s) for all manifestations of poisonings.

If there is also a diagnosis of abuse or dependence of the substance, the abuse or dependence is assigned as an additional code.

Examples of poisoning include:

i. Error was made in drug prescription

    Errors made in drug prescription or in the administration of the drug by provider, nurse, patient, or other person.

ii.   Overdose of a drug intentionally taken

If an overdose of a drug was intentionally taken or administered and resulted in drug toxicity, it would be coded as a poisoning.

iii.   Nonprescribed drug taken with correctly prescribed and properly administered drug

If a nonprescribed drug or medicinal agent was taken in combination with a correctly prescribed and properly administered drug, any drug toxicity or other reaction resulting from the interaction of the two drugs would be classified as a poisoning.

iv.   Interaction of drug(s) and alcohol

When a reaction results from the interaction of a drug(s) and alcohol, this would be classified as poisoning.

See Section I.C.4. if poisoning is the result of insulin pump malfunctions.

Guideline I.C.19.e.5(c). Underdosing: Underdosing refers to taking less of a medication than is prescribed by a provider or a manufacturer's instruction. Discontinuing the use of a prescribed medication on the patient's own initiative (not directed by the patient's provider) is also classified as an underdosing. For underdosing, assign the code from categories T36–T50 (fifth or sixth character "6").

Codes for underdosing should never be assigned as principal or first-listed codes. If a patient has a relapse or exacerbation of the medical condition for which the drug is prescribed because of the reduction in dose, then the medical condition itself should be coded.

Noncompliance (Z91.12-, Z91.13- and Z91.14-) or complication of care (Y63.8–Y63.9) codes are to be used with an underdosing code to indicate intent, if known.

Guideline I.C.19.e.5 (d). Toxic Effects: When a harmful substance is ingested or comes in contact with a person, this is classified as a toxic effect. The toxic effect codes are in categories T51–T65.

Toxic effect codes have an associated intent: accidental, intentional self-harm, assault and undetermined.

I.C.19.f. Adult and child abuse, neglect and other maltreatment: Sequence first the appropriate code from categories T74.- (Adult and child abuse, neglect and other maltreatment, confirmed) or T76.- (Adult and child abuse, neglect and other maltreatment, suspected) for abuse, neglect and other maltreatment, followed by any accompanying mental health or injury code(s).

If the documentation in the medical record states abuse or neglect it is coded as confirmed (T74.-). It is coded as suspected if it is documented as suspected (T76.-).

(Continued)

(Continued)

For cases of confirmed abuse or neglect an external cause code from the assault section (X92–Y09) should be added to identify the cause of any physical injuries. A perpetrator code (Y07) should be added when the perpetrator of the abuse is known. For suspected cases of abuse or neglect, do not report external cause or perpetrator code.

If a suspected case of abuse, neglect or mistreatment is ruled out during an encounter code Z04.71, Encounter for examination and observation following alleged physical adult abuse, ruled out, or code Z04.72, Encounter for examination and observation following alleged child physical abuse, ruled out, should be used, not a code from T76.

If a suspected case of alleged rape or sexual abuse is ruled out during an encounter code Z04.41, Encounter for examination and observation following alleged physical adult abuse, ruled out, or code Z04.42, Encounter for examination and observation following alleged rape or sexual abuse, ruled out, should be used, not a code from T76.

If a suspected case of forced sexual exploitation or forced labor exploitation is ruled out during an encounter, code Z04.81, Encounter for examination and observation of victim following forced sexual exploitation, or code Z04.82, Encounter for examination and observation of victim following forced labor exploitation, should be used, not a code from T76.

See Section I.C.15. Abuse in a pregnant patient.

Guideline I.C.19.g. Complications of care

Guideline I.C.19.g.1. General guidelines for complications of care

a. **Documentation of complications of care**

See Section I.B.16. for information on documentation of complications of care.

Guideline I.C.19.g.2. Pain due to medical devices: Pain associated with devices, implants or grafts left in a surgical site (for example painful hip prosthesis) is assigned to the appropriate code(s) found in Chapter 19, Injury, poisoning, and certain other consequences of external causes. Specific codes for pain due to medical devices are found in the T code section of the ICD-10-CM. Use additional code(s) from category G89 to identify acute or chronic pain due to presence of the device, implant or graft (G89.18 or G89.28).

Guideline I.C.19.g.3. Transplant complications

Guideline I.C.19.g.3c (a). Transplant complications other than kidney: Codes under category T86, Complications of transplanted organs and tissues, are for use for both complications and rejection of transplanted organs. A transplant complication code is only assigned if the complication affects the function of the transplanted organ. Two codes are required to fully describe a transplant complication: the appropriate code from category T86 and a secondary code that identifies the complication.

Pre-existing conditions or conditions that develop after the transplant are not coded as complications unless they affect the function of the transplanted organs.

See I.C.21. for transplant organ removal status

See I.C.2. for malignant neoplasm associated with transplanted organ.

Guideline I.C.19.g.3 (b). Kidney transplant complications: Patients who have undergone kidney transplant may still have some form of chronic kidney disease (CKD) because the kidney transplant may not fully restore kidney function. Code T86.1- should be assigned for documented complications of a kidney transplant, such as transplant failure or rejection or other transplant complication. Code T86.1- should not be assigned for post kidney transplant patients who have chronic kidney (CKD) unless a transplant complication such as transplant failure or rejection is documented. If the documentation is unclear as to whether the patient has a complication of the transplant, query the provider.

Conditions that affect the function of the transplanted kidney, other than CKD, should be assigned a code from subcategory T86.1, Complications of transplanted organ, Kidney, and a secondary code that identifies the complication.

For patients with CKD following a kidney transplant, but who do not have a complication such as failure or rejection, *see section I.C.14. Chronic kidney disease and kidney transplant status.*

Guideline I.C.19.g.4. Complication codes that include the external cause: As with certain other T codes, some of the complications of care codes have the external cause included in the code. The code includes the nature of the complication as well as the type of procedure that caused the complication. No external cause code indicating the type of procedure is necessary for these codes.

Guideline I.C.19.g.5. Complications of care codes within the body system chapters: Intraoperative and postprocedural complication codes are found within the body system chapters with codes specific to the organs and structures of that body system. These codes should be sequenced first, followed by a code(s) for the specific complication, if applicable.

Complication codes from the body system chapters should be assigned for intraoperative and postprocedural complications (e.g., the appropriate complication code from chapter 9 would be assigned for a vascular intraoperative or postprocedural complication) unless the complication is specifically indexed to a T code in chapter 19.

Coding Poisoning, Adverse Effects, Underdosing, and Certain Consequences of External Causes in ICD-10-CM Chapter 19

The coding of poisoning, adverse effect, and underdosing of drugs is discussed in this section.

Alphabetic Index

The ICD-10-CM Alphabetic Index provides direction on how to code medical conditions caused by drugs used appropriately and inappropriately by a patient and causing a medical condition. Using the main term "Adverse effect," the coder is directed to see Table of Drugs and Chemicals, categories T36–T50, with the sixth character of S. The main term "Poisoning" or "Poisoning, drug" in the Index directs the coder to see also Table of Drugs and Chemicals. The third entry for underdosing states "see also Table of Drugs and Chemicals, categories T36–T50, with final character of 6" (CDC 2019). The Table of Drugs and Chemicals follows the ICD-10-CM Neoplasm Table that appears after the ICD-10-CM Index to Diseases and Injuries.

Table of Drugs and Chemicals

The ICD-10-CM Table of Drugs and Chemicals is organized into seven columns with rows for the substances involved. The first, left-most column contains the name of the drug, chemical, or biologic substance. The next six columns contain ICD-10-CM codes for the following:

- Poisoning, accidental (nonintentional)

- Poisoning, intentional self-harm

- Poisoning, assault

- Poisoning, undetermined

- Adverse effect

- Underdosing

 Not every row with a chemical name has a code in each of the six columns. This is because certain chemicals cannot produce an adverse effect or an underdosing because the substance is never used for therapeutic purposes. Codes that are found on the Table of Drugs and Chemicals are in the range of codes from T36–T50. These are combination codes that include the substance that was taken by the patient, appropriately or inappropriately, and describe the intent as well. There is a subcategory code if multiple, unspecified drugs, medicinal or biological substances are taken. For example, the codes differentiate between poisonings that are accidental, intentional, assault, or are of an undetermined nature. For this reason, there is no need for an additional external cause of morbidity code for poisonings, adverse effects, and underdosing codes.

Adverse Effects of Drugs

An **adverse effect** or adverse drug effect (Mosby 2017, 37) is an unintended reaction to a drug administered at normal dosage. An adverse effect can occur in situations in which medication is prescribed correctly and administered properly in both therapeutic and diagnostic procedures. An adverse effect can occur when everything is done right—right drug, right dose, right patient receiving it, right route of administration—but a physical reaction is experienced. Common causes of adverse effects are as follows:

- Cumulative effects result when the inactivation or excretion of the drug is slower than the rate at which the drug is being administered. This is often documented as drug toxicity of a prescribed drug in the health record.

- Hypersensitivity or allergic reaction is a qualitatively different response to a drug acquired only after re-exposure to the drug.

- Synergistic reaction is enhancing the effect of a prior or concurrent administration of another drug.

- The effectiveness of a drug may change as the result of interaction with another prescribed medication.

- Side effects are the unwanted predictable pharmacologic effects that occur within therapeutic code ranges.

Instructions for Coding Adverse Effects

The following instructions apply when coding adverse effects:

1. Code first the manifestation or the nature of the adverse effects, such as urticaria, vertigo, gastritis, and so forth.

2. Locate the drug responsible for the adverse effect in the Substance column of the Table of Drugs and Chemicals in the Alphabetic Index to Diseases.

3. Assign the appropriate seventh character to the drug or chemical code to identify whether the healthcare was provided during the initial encounter, a subsequent encounter, or for a sequela.

4. If more than one drug or chemical is involved, the coder should use as many codes as necessary from the Table of Drugs and Chemicals to completely describe all the drugs or chemicals involved.

5. If the same drug produced more than one manifestation or adverse effect, the coder should assign the drug code only once.

6. If two or more drugs or chemicals are involved, each drug or chemical should be coded separately unless there is a combination code included in the Table of Drugs and Chemicals.

> **EXAMPLE:** Initial encounter to treat atrial tachycardia due to digitalis glycosides: I47.1, Supraventricular tachycardia; T46.0X5A, Adverse effect of cardiac-stimulant glycosides and drugs of similar action

7. If the patient has a current condition that is the late effect or sequela of an adverse effect of a correct substance properly administered, it is coded as follows:

   - First code the residual or late effect, such as blindness or deafness.

• Assign the code for the drug that produced the adverse effect with the seventh character of S for sequela.

> **EXAMPLE:** Deafness in the right ear occurring as a result of previously administered streptomycin therapy: H91.91, Unspecified hearing loss, right ear; T36.5X5S, Adverse effect of aminoglycosides, sequela

See table 22B.1 for assistance in coding adverse reactions to correct substances properly administered. If the patient has a present condition when the patient is experiencing a physical condition as the result of reacting to a drug, the current condition is coded first with an additional code describing the drug causing the reaction by accessing the Table of Drugs and Chemicals to locate drug name and using the code from the column identified as "adverse effect" that will have the fifth or sixth character of 5. The same process is followed when the patient has a sequela or a long-term effect of once having a reaction to a properly administered drug. First a diagnosis code should be assigned for the condition that the patient is experiencing as a result of the adverse effect of a drug. An additional code is assigned to identify the drug that caused the original reaction. The additional code for the drug is located by accessing the drug name on the Table of Drugs and Chemicals and selecting the code from the "adverse effect" column of the table.

Table 22B.1. **Coding adverse reactions to correct substances properly administered**

Current Condition		Sequela
Code effect: Coma, vertigo, and such	← Principal or First-Listed Diagnosis →	Code effect: Deafness, blindness, and such
And		**And**
Adverse effect of drug code from Table of Drugs and Chemicals with the fifth or sixth character of 5 with the seventh character of A or D for initial or subsequent encounter	← Other Diagnosis →	Adverse effect of drug code from Table of Drugs and Chemicals with the fifth or sixth character of 5 with the seventh character of S for sequela

Check Your Understanding 22B.1

Assign diagnosis codes to the following conditions.

1. The patient came to the physician's office complaining of nausea, vomiting, and diarrhea within 24 hours of taking her prescription as directed for acyclovir for her herpes zoster neuralgia.

2. The patient was being treated in the emergency department for severe low back pain with the medication Demerol and shortly thereafter was found to have shortness of breath and a slow heartbeat that were attributed to a side effect of the Demerol properly administered.

3. The patient had been prescribed famotidine for GERD and was taking it for three days as prescribed, but the drug was discontinued during this office visit as the patient required treatment for drug-induced diarrhea.

4. The patient returned to her oncologist's office for further evaluation of her severe hot flashes that were thought to be due to her prescribed tamoxifen for her history of breast cancer in remission. The patient had been seen in the office three days ago when the drug was discontinued and received a follow-up visit today to address her continuing side effect from the drug.

(Continued)

(Continued)

5. The patient was examined for visual blurring, bilateral conjunctival hyperemia and bilateral eye pain at the urgent care center. The urgent care center physician determined the patient's eye complaints were an adverse reaction to the gentamicin sulfate ophthalmic solution prescribed by her eye doctor. The patient did not know the name of the eye disease she had.

Poisonings

Poisoning is a reaction to the improper use of a medication (CDC 2019). A poisoning is a condition caused by drugs, medicinal substances, and other biological substances when the substance involved is not used according to a physician's instructions. A poisoning occurs when something is done wrong—wrong drug, wrong dose, wrong route of administration, wrong person receiving the drug, or the drug should not have been used. A poisoning can occur with prescription drugs, over-the-counter purchased medications, illegal drugs, or when drugs are taken with alcohol beverages. Poisonings can occur in the following ways:

- There is an error made in the drug prescription. This includes errors made in drug prescription or in the administration of the drug by the provider, the nurse, the patient, or another person.

- An overdose of a drug is intentionally taken. If an overdose of a drug was intentionally taken or administered and resulted in drug toxicity, the situation would be classified as a poisoning.

- A nonprescribed drug is taken with a correctly prescribed and properly administered drug. If the nonprescribed drug or medicinal agent was taken in combination with a correctly prescribed and properly administered drug, any drug toxicity or other reaction resulting from the interaction of these two drugs would be classified as a poisoning.

- A drug is taken with alcohol. When a patient has a medical condition or reaction produced from the interaction of a drug or drugs and alcohol, the condition would be classified as a poisoning.

Instructions for Coding Poisonings

The following instructions apply when coding poisonings (Note the difference in coding and sequencing of poisonings from the coding and sequencing of adverse effects):

1. Use the Table of Drugs and Chemicals in the Alphabetic Index to Diseases to locate the drug or other agent.

2. Code first the code from the "Poisoning" column depending on the associated intent with the fifth or sixth character identifying it as accidental, intentional self-harm, assault, and undetermined.

3. Next code all the specified manifestation or effect of the poisoning, such as coma, vertigo, drowsiness, that might be experienced.

4. If there is also a diagnosis of drug abuse or dependence to the drug, the abuse or dependence is coded as an additional diagnosis.

> **EXAMPLE:** Overdosed on aspirin, suicide attempt, initial episode of care:
> T39.012A, Poisoning by aspirin, intentional self-harm, initial episode of care

5. If the patient has a current condition that is the late effect or sequela of an adverse effect of a poisoning or overdose, it is coded as follows:

   • First code the residual condition or late effect, such as organ or nerve damage.

   • Assign the code for the drug that produced the poisoning with the seventh character of S for sequela.

> **EXAMPLE:** Anoxic brain damage as a result of previously narcotic intentional overdose: G93.1, Anoxic brain damage, not elsewhere classified; T40.602S, Poisoning by unspecified narcotics, intentional self-harm, sequela

See table 22B.2 for assistance in coding poisonings. When the patient has a current poisoning event, the first code is taken from the Table of Drugs and Chemicals by locating the drug involved and using the code from the columns 1–4 depending on the intent of the poisoning (accidental, intentional, assault, or undetermined). A second code is assigned to identify the specified effect of the poisoning, that is, what physical or other condition the poisoning produced. When a patient has a sequela of a poisoning that occurred in the past, the first code is the condition the patient continues to experience. The second code is assigned to identify the drug that poisoned the patient in the past using a code from the Table of Drugs and Chemicals from columns 1–4 depending on the original intent of the poisoning (accidental, intentional, assault, or undetermined).

Table 22B.2. **Coding poisonings**

Current Poisoning Event		Sequela
Code from T36–T50 with fifth or sixth character for the associated intent (accidental, intentional self-harm, assault, or undetermined) from the Table of Drugs and Chemicals with the seventh character for initial or subsequent encounter	← Principal or First-Listed Diagnosis →	Code for the residual condition first that is currently present
Plus		*Plus*
Specified effect—tachycardia, coma	← Other Diagnosis →	Code from T36–T50 with fifth or sixth character for the associated intent, accidental, intentional self-harm, assault, or undetermined with the seventh character for sequela

Check Your Understanding 22B.2

Assign diagnosis codes to the following conditions.

1. The patient was treated in the emergency department (ED) for an accidental overdose of heroin and fentanyl (patient purchased illegally) with respiratory arrest.

(Continued)

(Continued)

2. Accidental overdose of ecstasy treated in the ED in a patient with secondary symptoms of shortness of breath, excessive sweating, and tachycardia.

3. The patient came to the ED stating that he was having a heart attack because he had developed chest pain and found to have elevated blood pressure readings that were attributed to the patient's admitted excessive use of crack (cocaine).

4. The patient was brought to the ED by ambulance after being found at home by her parents having seizures. Once stabilized, the patient admitted to taking an overdose of her antidepressant medication (Sinequan) as a suicide attempt. She had been prescribed the medication for persistent anxiety and depression.

5. The patient was brought to the emergency department by family after it was determined that the patient took a second dose of insulin by mistake and then did not eat breakfast. The patient was found to have severe hypoglycemia due to (accidental poisoning of?) insulin.

Underdosing

The concept of underdosing in ICD-10-CM refers to the situation when a patient takes less of a medication than is prescribed by the provider or a manufacturer's instruction. When the patient decides to discontinue the use of a prescription medication without being told by the patient's provider to discontinue the drug, that is also classified as an underdosing. For this situation, the code from T36–T50 specifying the drug is assigned with the fifth or sixth character of 6. The code for the drug that was underdosed is never listed first or as the principal diagnosis. When underdosing occurs, most likely the patient returns to the healthcare provider because the patient has a worsening of the medical condition that is being treated by the drug. In this situation, the medical condition is coded first. Noncompliance codes (Z91.12- or Z91.13- or Z91.14-) or complication of care (Y63.6, Y63.8–Y63.9) codes are used with the underdosing code to identify the intent if it is known.

> **EXAMPLE:** Hyperglycemia with type 2 diabetes as a result of the patient not taking his oral antidiabetic agents. The patient stated he cannot afford his prescriptions so he has not been taking his medications every day in order to make his prescription last longer: E11.65, Type 2 diabetes with hyperglycemia; T38.3X6A, Underdosing of insulin or oral hypoglycemic [antidiabetic] drugs, initial encounter; Z91.120, Patient's intentional underdosing of medication regimen due to financial hardship

Toxic Effects

A patient may come in contact with or ingest, accidentally or otherwise, a harmful substance that would be classified in ICD-10-CM as a **toxic effect** (CDC 2019). The toxic effect code is included in categories T51–T65 and include the associated intent of accidental, intentional self-harm, assault, or undetermined. A note appears under the block of codes T51–T65 for toxic effects of substances chiefly nonmedicinal as to source that a code for accidental intent should be used if no intent is indicated. The undetermined intent is only for use when there is specific documentation in the record that the intent of the toxic effect cannot be determined.

> **EXAMPLE:** The patient came in contact with chloroform in the industrial plant where he worked and was brought to the emergency department with severe shortness of breath. This was the initial episode of care. T53.1X1A, Toxic effect of chloroform, accidental, initial encounter; R06.02, Shortness of breath.

Other and Unspecified Effects of External Cause (T66–T78)

The diagnoses represented by this block of codes represent injuries and conditions that are caused by an external agent, such as radiation, heat, light, cold, air, and water pressure as an example. The codes require the use of the appropriate seventh character to identify the episode of care, that is, the initial encounter (A), a subsequent encounter (D), or if the event represents a sequela (S).

Asphyxiation (T71)

Asphyxiation is also called suffocation. Asphyxiation is a physiological change in the body cause by a lack of oxygen in respired air, resulting in a lack of oxygen and an increased amount of carbon dioxide in the blood (Dorland 2012, 166). Specific codes are provided to identify when a condition of asphyxiation is being treated. The diagnosis for this situation may also be described by the provider as a traumatic or mechanical suffocation. These are ICD-10-CM combination codes that identify the state of asphyxiation as well as the cause of it. For example, asphyxiation could be caused by smothering under a pillow, a plastic bag placed over the head, being trapped in bed linens, or smothering by being face down or trapped in furniture. Other external events that can cause asphyxiation are accidental or intentional hanging, being trapped in a car trunk, a cave-in, or otherwise being caught in a low-oxygen environment. The codes in this category require a seventh character to identify whether the care is provided in the initial encounter, a subsequent encounter, or as a sequela.

EXAMPLE: The 20-year-old male patient was brought to the emergency department (ED) by fire ambulance after being found unconscious by his father in the family's garage hanging from the rafters with a rope around his neck. The family found a suicide note written by the patient indicating his intent to end his life. ED physician and staff were unable to resuscitate the patient, and he was pronounced dead. The ED physician documented the final diagnosis as "asphyxiation by mechanical means by hanging by the patient's own hands": T71.162, Asphyxiation due to hanging, intentional self harm.

Adult and Child Abuse, Neglect and Other Maltreatment, Confirmed (T74) and Suspected (T76)

When an adult or child is treated for confirmed or suspected abuse, neglect, or other maltreatment, the appropriate code from categories T74 (Adult and child abuse, neglect and other maltreatment, confirmed) or T76 (Adult and child abuse, neglect and other maltreatment, suspected) is assigned as the principal or first-listed diagnosis code. Any injury or mental health condition that occurs as a result of the abuse, neglect, or maltreatment is coded as an additional diagnosis. The coder must examine the record for the provider's conclusion as to whether the abuse has been confirmed at the end of the encounter or is still suspected and unconfirmed. If the provider documents the patient's situation as abuse or neglect, it is coded as confirmed with category T74. If the documentation states the abuse or neglect is suspected, it is coded as suspected with category T76. A perpetrator code from category Y07 is added when the perpetrator of the abuse or neglect is known. If the patient's abuse or neglect is suspected, no code is assigned for the perpetrator identification.

EXAMPLE: A 90-year-old lady was brought to the emergency department (ED) by fire ambulance and police after being called by neighbors who had not seen the patient's daughter around the house for several days, and the neighbors feared the patient was inside the house alone. The ED physician found the patient to have dehydration and suffering from dementia as she was unable to communicate with the hospital staff as to who she was, where she was, or what physical complaints that she had. The police later found the patient's daughter at her job and took her to the police station for questioning. The ED physician contacted a family physician to admit the patient to the hospital. When she was discharged three days later to be cared for in a long-term care facility, the final diagnoses were suspected adult neglect, dehydration, and dementia: T76.01XA, Adult neglect or abandonment, suspected, initial encounter; E86.0, Dehydration and F03.90, Unspecified dementia without behavioral disturbance.

Check Your Understanding 22B.3

Assign diagnosis codes to the following conditions.

1. The patient was brought to the emergency department at the hospital by ambulance after becoming overcome by fumes from the toxic effects of liquid hydrochloric acid at the factory where he works. The patient was revived with intravenous fluids and had no further ill effects.

2. The patient returned to the pain clinic complaining of worsening cervicobrachial syndrome pain and was found to be taking less of the nonsteroidal anti-inflammatory medication that she was prescribed because she did not want to become "addicted" to the medication.

3. The patient was brought to the ER by police for evaluation and treatment as a suspected adult rape victim, female, with facial contusions and bilateral knee contusions.

4. The patient was brought to the ER by ambulance after being found by family members unresponsive in the patient's garage as a result of asphyxia by mechanical hanging. The patient left a note that indicated he intended to commit suicide by hanging. The patient was unable to be resuscitated and expired.

5. The police were asked to perform a well-being check on an elderly patient and found her unresponsive in her bed in a very hot apartment with windows closed and no air conditioning or fans running. She was able to be resuscitated and was taken to the hospital. The patient was treated in the hospital for heat stroke and systemic inflammatory response syndrome (SIRS) of non-infectious origin but was unable to recover and died three days later.

Complications of Surgical and Medical Care, Not Elsewhere Classified (T80–T88)

Codes for intraoperative and postprocedural complications and disorders are provided in specific body system chapters throughout ICD-10-CM, for example, code N99.0, Postprocedural (acute)(chronic) kidney failure. These chapter-specific codes are sequenced first when coding the condition, but an additional code should be assigned for the specific complication, if applicable. Complication codes from the body system chapters should be assigned for intraoperative and postprocedural complications. For example, the appropriate complication code from chapter 9, the circulatory system, would be assigned for a vascular intraoperative or postprocedural complication unless the complication is specifically indexed to a T code in chapter 19 described here.

Specific **complications** are identified in this block of codes to represent all types of conditions that are unwanted but may not be entirely unavoidable in medical care. The coding guidelines direct the coder that the documentation of complications of care must be specific. The assignment of a complications code must be based on the provider's documentation, and the fact that the provider has made a connection between the condition and the medical care or procedure that apparently caused it. As stated in the guidelines, not every condition that develops following medical care or a surgical procedure should be coded as a complication. The provider must indicate the condition is a complication and was caused by the care provided. It is the coder's responsibility to query the physician for this relationship if the documentation is not specific as to the cause of the condition the patient exhibits after medical care or a procedure has been provided.

Some of the complication codes in this chapter have the external cause as well as the condition included in the code. No external cause code is required when the code includes the nature of the complication as well as the type of procedure that caused the complication.

> **EXAMPLES:** 1. The patient had a central line infection due to the presence of the central venous catheter
>   T80.211A, Bloodstream infection due to central venous catheter, initial encounter
> 2. The patient had a cystostomy catheter following bladder surgery and it was found to be leaking urine.
>   T83.030A, Leakage of cystostomy catheter, initial encounter
> 3. The patient was found to have an infected internal fixation device in his right femur
>   T84.620A, Infection and inflammatory reaction due to internal fixation device of right femur, initial encounter

The conditions identified in this block of codes, T80–T88, identify complications of surgical and medical care that are not specific to a particular body system. A seventh character is required for these category codes to identify if the condition was treated in an initial encounter, subsequent encounter, or represents a sequela.

Three directional notes appear under the heading for these codes to remind the coder of the following:

1. Use additional code for adverse effect, if applicable, to identify drug (T36–T50) with fifth or sixth character of five (5).

2. Use additional code(s) to identify the specified condition resulting from the complication.

3. Use additional code to identify devices involved and details of circumstances (Y62–Y83).

Complications of Procedures, Not Elsewhere Classified (T81)

Codes within this category include postprocedural shock, disruption of operative or surgical wound, infection following a procedure, complications of a foreign body accidentally left in the body following a procedure, acute reaction to foreign substance accidentally left during a procedure, and not elsewhere classified vascular complications.

Directional notes remind the coder to use an additional code for an adverse effect, if applicable, to identify a responsible drug from categories T36–T50 with a fifth or sixth character of 5. When a patient is diagnosed with an infection following a procedure, the coder should use an additional code to identify the infection by type or organism as well as use an additional code if the infection advances to severe sepsis. If the code is not specific, a use additional code note appears to remind the coder to specify the complication with an additional code.

> **EXAMPLE:** The patient was readmitted from a hip replacement procedure and was found to have methicillin-susceptible *Staphylococcus aureus* that was apparently introduced into the patient's body during the orthopedic surgery
> T81.44XA, Sepsis following a procedure, caused by Staphylococcus aureus, Methicillin susceptible, initial encounter
> B95.61, Methicillin susceptible Staphylococcus aureus infection as the cause of diseases classified elsewhere

Complications of Prosthetic Devices, Implants and Grafts (T82–T85)

Subcategory codes T82.0- to T82.5- identify **mechanical complications** of specific cardiac and vascular prosthetic devices, implants, and grafts. Complications include the mechanical breakdown, displacement, leakage, or other mechanical complication of the device, implant, or graft. The types of devices identified in these codes are heart valves, cardiac electronic devices, coronary artery bypass grafts, other vascular grafts, vascular dialysis catheters, and surgically created arteriovenous fistula.

Subcategory codes T82.6–T82.7 identify an **infection or inflammatory reaction** to a specific cardiac and vascular prosthetic device, implant, or graft. Both of these subcategory codes would have an additional code to identify the infection if the documentation is provided. Subcategory codes T82.8–T82.9 identify other specified complications due to the presence of these devices. These complications include embolism, fibrosis, hemorrhage, pain, stenosis, thrombosis, or other specified condition that is due to the cardiac or vascular prosthetic device, implant, or graft.

Similar codes appear for complications of prosthetic devices, implants, and grafts in other body systems, for example, in category T83 for genitourinary devices, T84 for orthopedic devices, and T85 for other internal prosthetic devices, implants, and grafts. These codes also have subcategories including mechanical complications, infections, and inflammations as a result of the device and other specific conditions such as embolism, fibrosis, hemorrhage, pain, and such. All the codes in categories T82–T85 require the use of the seventh character to identify the initial or subsequent encounter or the sequela situation.

> **EXAMPLE:**
> 1. The patient's cardiac pacemaker was found to be in mechanical failure and needed to be replaced.
>   T82.111A, Breakdown (mechanical) of cardiac pulse generator (battery), initial encounter
> 2. Following an endoscopic retrograde cholangiopancreatography, it was determined that a chip from a catheter used during the procedure was obstructing a bile duct and had to be removed and treated.
>   T81.524A, Obstruction due to foreign body accidentally left in body following endoscopic examination, initial encounter
> 3. A thrombosis was found in the patient's popliteal artery following bypass surgery.
>   T82.868A, Thrombosis of vascular prosthetic device, implants and grafts, initial encounter
> 4. The patient was taken back to surgery to remove and replace an intraocular lens that was found to be displaced.
>   T85.22XA, Displacement of intraocular lens, initial encounter

Complications of Transplanted Organs and Tissues (T86)

Three "use additional code" notes appear under the category heading for complications of transplanted organs and tissues. The notes remind the coder to use an additional code to identify other **transplant complications** such as graft versus host disease, malignancy associated with organ transplant, and posttransplant lymphoproliferative disorders.

It is important to note that patients may still have some form of chronic kidney disease after they have had a kidney transplant. The kidney transplant may not restore the kidney function completely. Code T86.1- should be assigned for a documented complication of a kidney transplant such as transplant failure or rejection. Chronic kidney disease in a kidney transplant patient is not assigned as a complication code unless the condition is documented as a complication. If the documentation is not clearly stated, the coder is obligated to ask the provider for clarification. Patients may have another condition that affects the function of the transplanted kidney. When a provider documents that another condition affects the transplanted kidney, a code from subcategory T86.1, Complications of kidney transplant, is assigned with an additional code for the specific complication. Complications of renal transplantation can occur both during the medical and surgical treatments related to the procedure. Table 22B.3 shows examples of the types of complications that can occur in renal transplant patients as a result of the surgical and medical treatments related to the disease and transplant procedure.

Table 22B.3. **Complications during renal transplantation**

Surgical/Mechanical	Medical
• Obstruction	• Acute rejection/acute renal failure
• Hematuria	• Delayed graft function
• Urinoma	• Acute cyclosporine/tacrolimus nephrotoxicity
• Arterial stenosis	• Prerenal azotemia
• Arterial thrombosis	• Drug toxicity
• Renal vein thrombosis	• Infection
• Postoperative hemorrhage	• Recurrent disease
• Lymphocele	

Reproduced with permission Singapuri MS, Subramanian RM. Renal Transplant: Procedures and Complications. *Crit Connections.* 2011; 10(1):14–15. Copyright © 2011 the Society of Critical Care Medicine.

Specific codes exist in category T86 for transplant rejection, failure, or infection for various types of organs and tissues that have been transplanted, for example, bone marrow, heart, lung, liver, skin, bone, corneal, intestine, and other transplanted tissue.

EXAMPLE: The patient was taken to surgery to remove what remained from a failed skin graft that was the result of an allograft skin rejection following a skin graft replacement procedure, initial encounter
T86.820, Skin graft (allograft) rejection

Complications Peculiar to Reattachment and Amputation (T87)

Specific codes are provided in this category to identify when there are complications related to a reattached (part of the) upper extremity, lower extremity, or other body part specified as right, left, or unspecified side. Other subcategory codes identify when there is a complication of an amputation stump, specifically a neuroma, infection, necrosis, or other specified and unspecified complication.

> **EXAMPLE:** The patient was readmitted to the hospital for treatment of an infection of the below-knee amputation stump on the right lower leg that was amputated the prior week because of gangrene and peripheral vascular disease.
>
> T87.43, Infection of amputation stump, right lower extremity

Other Complications of Surgical and Medical Care, Not Elsewhere Classified (T88)

The final category in Chapter 19 of ICD-10-CM contains less frequently occurring complications of surgical and medical care. Codes related to complications of anesthesia, such as shock, malignant hyperthermia, and other complications require the use of an additional code for the drug responsible for an adverse effect if it was applicable to this patient. The serious emergency of an anaphylactic reaction or shock due to an adverse effect of a drug is classified with code T88.6XX with the seventh character identifying the episode of care. The drug responsible for the adverse effect is identified with an additional code. If the specific adverse effect of a drug cannot be identified, the subcategory code T88.7XX is used with the seventh character to identify the episode of care. This code is used when the provider can only identify the condition as a "drug reaction" or "drug hypersensitivity."

> **EXAMPLE:** The patient was transferred to the emergency department to be treated for an anaphylactic reaction due to adverse effect of penicillin given by injection for a respiratory infection. The correct dose of penicillin was given in the physician's office according to the usual protocol for the condition the patient had.
>
> 1. T88.6XXA, Anaphylactic reaction due to adverse effect of correct drug or medicament properly administered, initial encounter
> 2. T36.0X5A, Penicillin drug causing the adverse effect (Table of Drugs and Chemicals, fifth column)

Check Your Understanding 22B.4

Assign diagnosis codes to the following conditions.

1. Dehiscence of closure of sternum (sternotomy) wound, following aortocoronary bypass surgery 2 weeks ago, subsequent cardiovascular surgery clinic visit

2. Mechanical loosening of internal left hip joint prosthesis, postoperative wound check post repair, normal healing

3. Kidney transplant rejection, left kidney. Concurrent chronic kidney disease, right kidney, stage 4

4. Thrombosis complication within intraperitoneal dialysis catheter, initial encounter

5. Mechanical leakage of insulin pump, initial evaluation in the physician's office

ICD-10-PCS Coding for Procedures Related to Poisoning and Certain Other Consequences of External Causes

There is no particular group of procedures that relate to coding of conditions addressed in this chapter. Surgical procedures are more commonly performed to treat complications of medical and surgical care. While any of the 31 root operations could be the objective of a procedure, there are a few root operations that should be addressed in this chapter.

One of the four root operations that involve procedures to alter the diameter or route of a tubular body part is **Dilation**. Solids, liquids, or gases pass through tubular body parts. These body parts are part of the circulatory system, digestive system, genitourinary, and respiratory system. Sometimes, these tubular body parts become narrow or stenotic and can create problems as the solids, liquids, or gases cannot pass through it. The root operation Dilation is to expand the orifice or the lumen of the tubular body part to open it or make it larger. The dilation can be accomplished by stretching a tubular body part using intraluminal pressure or by cutting part of the orifice or wall of the tubular body part. It is also possible that dilation may be an approach for another procedure to achieve its objective, for example, dilation and curettage where the objective is to remove the lining of the uterus, that is, an extraction procedure. An example of a Dilation procedure is an angioplasty of a coronary or noncoronary vessel. A device can be used to perform the Dilation, such as a balloon catheter, and other devices can be left in place in the vessel to maintain the opening of the vessel, such as a stent or intraluminal device. Only a device left in place at the end of the procedure is considered in the sixth character of an ICD-10-PCS code (CMS 2019).

An **Extirpation** procedure takes out or cuts out a solid matter from a body part (CMS 2019). The solid matter may be a foreign body, such as piece of metal, or it may be a by-product of a biological function, for example, a blood clot or a plaque deposit in a blood vessel. The medical term of "extirpation" is not commonly used in health record documentation. Instead, the coder should trust the Alphabetic Index of ICD-10-PCS when the title of an operation, such as thrombectomy, directs the coder to the code tables for Extirpation. The removal of foreign objects from the body will also be coded as Extirpation procedures. The coder must realize that the likely procedure title of "removal" of a foreign body would not be the root operation when the objective of the procedure is to take a solid matter like a foreign body. A Removal procedure in ICD-10-PCS always involves removing a device, and a foreign body is not a device.

Other procedures that are often required to treat complications of disease all involve devices. These root operations are Insertion, Replacement, Removal, Revision, Supplement, and Change. Each of these procedures put in a device, remove a device, correct a device, or exchange a device. The root operation **Insertion** has the objective of putting in a nonbiological device that monitors, assists, performs, or prevents a physiological function but does not physically take the place of a body part (CMS 2019). Commonly inserted devices include a central venous catheter for infusion or a cardiac pacemaker or cardioverter defibrillator.

In a **Replacement** procedure, the original body part may be taken out before the Replacement is performed (CMS 2019). The removal of the original body part is included in the Replacement procedure. However, if the Replacement is a repeat of a previous procedure, removing the device placed during the previous procedure is coded separately as a Removal. Examples of musculoskeletal Replacement procedures are joint replacements such as hips, knees, or shoulders.

A **Removal** procedure takes out or off a device from any body part and does not involve putting in another device (CMS 2019). Usually, the patient's condition no longer requires the device to remain in place for therapy when a Removal procedure is performed. The removal of an infusion device, drainage device, internal fixation, or joint prosthetic device is an example of this root operation.

A **Revision** procedure is the correction of a malfunctioning or displace device to the extent possible (CMS 2019). The objective of a Revision procedure is to fix a device that remains in place at the end of the procedure. If the device is removed during the procedure, it is not a Revision. However, a part of the device may be taken out or put back in as part of a Revision procedure. Examples of Revision procedures are adjustment to catheters, cardiac devices, joint prostheses, or internal fixator.

A transplant procedure may be performed to treat complications of diseases. A **Transplantation** is putting in the body a portion or all of a living body part (CMS 2019). The body part may be taken from another human or from an animal. The transplanted organ takes the place and function of the entire body part or a portion of the body part that is being replaced. The commonly replaced body parts are kidney, liver, heart, and lung. The seventh character for the root operation Transplantation identifies the type of transplant that is performed, that is, allogeneic, syngeneic, or zooplastic.

- An allogeneic transplant is an organ taken from different individuals of the same species or another human.

- A syngeneic transplant is an organ taken from an individual that has identical genetic composition as the recipient, such as an identical twin.

- A zooplastic transplant is an organ or tissue taken from an animal and place in a human.

Some procedures that are commonly referred to as transplants are not coded with this root operation. For example, there is no code available for a corneal transplant, because the procedure performed in a corneal transplant does not involve a body part by ICD-10-PCS definition. In a corneal transplant, a layer of tissue is placed in a body part. For that reason, a corneal transplant is classified as a Replacement procedure by ICD-10-PCS definition. Other procedures also called transplants are bone marrow, stem cell, and pancreatic islet cell transplantations. These procedures are not coded to transplant either. Instead, these procedures are coded to the root operation Administration because these procedures involve putting in autologous or nonautologous cells instead of organs or body parts.

Hemodialysis and renal replacement therapy may be performed for patients with conditions that produce renal failure that may be coded from this chapter. The amount of time the dialysis is performed is not the important factor. The type of dialysis is what should be coded. Intermittent hemodialysis is the conventional treatment usually performed for ESRD, three times a week, for less than six hours per session. Two other forms of hemodialysis are referred to as renal replacement therapy (RRT). These are performed on patients with acute kidney injury or acute renal failure and delivered to critically ill patients. Prolonged intermittent renal replacement therapy (PIRRT), also called SLED or EDD, is performed for 6–18 hours per day and is a gentler form of dialysis on very ill patients. The second type is continuous renal replacement therapy (CRRT), also called CVVH or CCVHD or CVVHDF, is performed for at least 18 hours a day and is the slowest and gentlest hemodialysis for patients who have acute kidney injury that has resulted in hemodynamic instability. They would not be able to tolerate the other forms of dialysis. The hemodialysis and renal replacement therapy codes are included in the Extracorporeal or Systemic Assistance and Performance tables for the Urinary body system with the 5th character identifying the duration or type of filtration, that is dialysis or renal replacement therapy:

5A1D70Z for intermittent hemodialysis
5A1D80Z for prolonged intermittent renal replacement therapy
5A1D90Z for continuous renal replacement therapy

Generally, the hospital can decide how often to code the procedures on a hospitalized patient. Usually the practice is to code the intermittent hemodialysis one time for each patient receiving it, no matter how many days it is done. The practice may be coded one time per admission for each type of dialysis or renal replacement therapy instead of coding when it is performed, for example, every day during a hospital stay.

ICD-10-CM and ICD-10-PCS Coding Exercises: Chapter 22B

Assign the correct ICD-10-CM diagnosis codes or ICD-10-PCS procedure to the following exercises.

Chapter 22B will provide practice coding ICD-10-CM Chapter 19 codes. External cause codes will be discussed and coded in Chapter 23. For Chapter 22B, assign only diagnosis and procedure codes, not external cause of morbidity (V–Y) codes.

1. A child is seen emergently for an accidental overdose of vitamins. He inadvertently ate several gummy vitamins when he found an open bottle at home.

2. A patient has been taking digoxin and is experiencing nausea and vomiting and profound fatigue. The patient indicates that he has been taking the drug appropriately. The evaluation and treatment was focused on adjustment of medication dosage only.

3. This patient is seen in the hospital with a diagnosis of congestive heart failure due to hypertensive heart disease. The patient also has stage 5 chronic kidney failure. The patient had been prescribed Lasix previously but admits that he forgets to take his medication every day. This is due to his advanced age. What are the correct diagnosis codes?

4. The patient was in the Cardiac Cath Lab for insertion of a dual chamber pacemaker to treat his sick sinus syndrome. During the procedure, the pacemaker electrode broke upon insertion. The procedure was abandoned and will be rescheduled.

5. The patient was seen in the emergency department complaining of right hip pain after falling at home. She stated that she had her right hip replaced six weeks ago and was walking fine before this fall. X-rays show the right hip prosthesis was dislocated. The patient was admitted for care by her orthopedic surgeon.

6. A college-age male was brought to the emergency department by ambulance called by his friends after they were unable to wake him this morning. The patient now responds to commands but is very drowsy. Based on the history provided by friends the patient was drinking heavily last night and was seen taking a handful of pills that were later determined to be Naproxen (Naprosyn) because the patient said he had a headache. After receiving IV fluids and being placed on telemetry, the patient became more alert and confirmed the history told by his friends. The ER physician discharged the patient with the final diagnosis of drowsiness due to the interaction of alcohol and naproxen.

7. The patient is seen in his internal medicine physician's office for the second time complaining of fatigue. This is a follow-up visit for both the patient's hypertension that was recently diagnosed and the fatigue he is experiencing. The patient stated that he feels even more tired than his last visit and the dizziness started after he started taking his new antihypertensive medication, metoprolol. The physician orders a new antihypertensive medication to hopefully relieve the patient's side effect from the metoprolol.

8. The patient is a two-year-old female who had a heart transplant in the past year and was admitted to the hospital and diagnosed with a viral pericarditis due to parvovirus, which is a complication of her heart transplant status.

9. The patient is a 27-year-old male who was prescribed 14 days of amoxicillin for acute suppurative right otitis media. The patient felt better after taking the drug for seven days and discontinued taking the pills that he then threw in the trash. However, the right ear pain returned and the patient came back to the physician's office for another prescription. (This is the initial episode of care for the underdosing condition.)

10. Accidental overdose of PCP (phencyclidine), initial encounter, emergency department treatment

11. Allergic reaction to contrast medium for radiology study exams. The patient experienced flushing of the face and neck and generalized itching.

12. The 65-year-old male is an ESRD patient on renal dialysis. The patient's arteriovenous dialysis catheter is clogged with a thrombosis. The patient will have a revision of the dialysis catheter the next day in the outpatient surgery department.

13. The patient is a 45-year-old female who attempted suicide (message left with a friend) by ingesting a large amount of alcohol with a dozen tricyclic antidepressant pills; she was found disoriented and confused by her family, brought to the emergency department for treatment.

(Continued on next page)

ICD-10-CM and ICD-10-PCS Coding Exercises: Chapter 22B *(continued)*

14. The patient is a 30-year-old male who works in a local zoo and was bitten by a venomous rattlesnake on his left arm while attempting to move the snake to a transportation container. A small open wound was treated on his left forearm that did not need sutures.

15. The patient was seen in the Pediatric Clinic of University Hospital as a follow-up or subsequent visit for a recent emergency department visit for suspected child abuse. The patient's Colles' fracture of the right arm is healing normally according to an x-ray exam taken during the clinic visit.

16. PROCEDURE: Open thrombectomy, left brachial artery

17. PROCEDURE: Right kidney transplant from living donor

18. PROCEDURE: Hemodialysis, performed as intermittent convention dialysis for 3 hours every other day during the inpatient hospital stay

19. PROCEDURE: Percutaneous insertion of a peripherally inserted central catheter (PICC) venous catheter into the superior vena cava from upper arm access

20. PROCEDURE: Angioplasty of left renal artery with insertion of a vascular stent

References

Centers for Disease Control and Prevention (CDC), National Center for Health Statistics (NCHS). 2019. *ICD-10-CM Official Guidelines for Coding and Reporting*, 2020. http://www.cdc.gov/nchs/icd/icd10cm.htm or https://www.cdc.gov/nchs/data/icd/10cmguidelines-FY2020_final.pdf.

Centers for Medicare and Medicaid Services (CMS). 2019. *ICD-10-PCS Official Guidelines for Coding and Reporting*, 2020. http://www.cms.gov/Medicare/Coding/ICD10/.

Dorland, W.A.N., ed. 2012. *Dorland's Illustrated Medical Dictionary*, 32nd ed. Philadelphia: Elsevier Saunders.

Mosby. 2017. *Mosby's Pocket Dictionary of Medicine, Nursing, and Health Profession*s, 8th ed. St. Louis: Mosby, Inc.

Singapuri, M.S. and R.M. Subramanian. 2011. Renal Transplant–Procedures and Complications. *Critical Connections* 10(1).

Chapter 23

External Causes of Morbidity (V00–Y99)

Learning Objectives

At the conclusion of this chapter, you should be able to do the following:

- Describe the organization of the codes included in Chapter 20 of ICD-10-CM, External Causes of Morbidity (V00–Y99)

- Identify the types of entries found in the ICD-10-CM Index to External Causes that are used to locate the code for the external cause

- Identify the correct seventh character required for reporting certain External Causes of Morbidity codes in ICD-10-CM

- Explain the sequencing of ICD-10-CM external cause in comparison with diagnosis codes

- Summarize how the ICD-10-CM external cause codes can be used to describe the late effect of an illness or injury

- Assign ICD-10-CM codes for external causes of morbidity

Key Terms

Activity codes
External cause status
External causes
ICD-10-CM External Cause of
   Injuries Index

Intent of the event
Never events
Place of occurrence
Sequela
Seventh (7th) character

Overview of ICD-10-CM Chapter 20: External Cause of Morbidity

Chapter 20 includes categories V00–Y99 arranged in the following blocks:

V00–X58	Accidents
V00–V99	Transport accidents
V00–V09	Pedestrian injured in transport accident
V10–V19	Pedal cycle rider injured in transport accident
V20–V29	Motorcycle rider injured in transport accident
V30–V39	Occupant of three-wheeled motor vehicle injured in transport accident
V40–V49	Car occupant injured in transport accident
V50–V59	Occupant of pick-up truck or van injured in transport accident
V60–V69	Occupant of heavy transport vehicle injured in transport accident
V70–V79	Bus occupant injured in transport accident
V80–V89	Other land transport accidents
V90–V94	Water transport accidents
V95–V97	Air and space transport accidents
V98–V99	Other and unspecified transport accidents
W00–X58	Other external causes of accidental injury
W00–W19	Slipping, tripping, stumbling and falls
W20–W49	Exposure to inanimate mechanical forces
W50–W64	Exposure to animate mechanical forces
W65–W74	Accidental non-transport drowning and submersion
W85–W99	Exposure to electric current, radiation and extreme ambient air temperature and pressure
X00–X08	Exposure to smoke, fire and flames
X10–X19	Contact with heat and hot substances
X30–X39	Exposure to forces of nature
X50	Overexertion and strenuous or repetitive movements
X52–X58	Accidental exposure to other specified forces
X71–X83	Intentional self-harm
X92–Y09	Assault
Y21–Y33	Event of undetermined intent
Y35–Y38	Legal intervention, operations of war, military operations and terrorism

Y62–Y84	Complications of medical and surgical care
Y62–Y69	Misadventures to patients during surgical and medical care
Y70–Y82	Medical devices associated with adverse incidents in diagnostic and therapeutic use
Y83–Y84	Surgical and other medical procedures as the cause of abnormal reaction of the patient, or of later complication, without mention of misadventure at the time of the procedure
Y90–Y99	Supplementary factors related to causes of morbidity classified elsewhere

Chapter 20: External Causes of Morbidity (V00–Y99), contains codes that have the first character of V, W, X, and Y. It is helpful to review the Tabular List and read all the instructional notes to gain an understanding of the possible codes available.

This chapter permits the classification of **external causes** that are intended to provide data for injury research and evaluation of injury prevention strategies. External cause codes in Chapter 20 of ICD-10-CM capture the cause of the injury or health condition, the **intent of the event** (accidental or incidental), the place where the event occurred, the activity of the patient at the time of the event, and the patient's status (such as civilian or military). Coding external causes of injuries and other conditions provides valuable data for research and evaluation of injury prevention strategies (CDC 2019). External cause codes provide information that is extremely useful to public health agencies and may assist healthcare planners in determining the kind of accidents a particular facility or physician treats.

No external cause code can be assigned as the principal, first-listed, or only listed diagnosis code. When a code from this section is applicable, it is intended that it will be used secondary to a code from another chapter of the classification indicating the nature of the condition. Most often, the condition will be classifiable to ICD-10-CM Chapter 19: Injury, Poisoning, and Certain Other Consequences of External Causes (S00–T88). Other conditions that may be stated to be due to external causes are classified in Chapters 1 to 18. For these conditions, the external cause codes from ICD-10-CM Chapter 20 should be used to provide additional information as to the cause of the condition.

The use of external cause codes is optional for physicians and healthcare facilities unless there is state-based mandatory reporting. Each provider or facility must decide whether it needs the information the external cause codes provide. Today, the information about accidents and other external causes of patients' injuries and illnesses may be of great value to hospital planning and to public health agencies. Because of the value of this information, many state governments have mandated the use of some or all of the types of external causes that can be reported. For example, some states have required the external cause of the injury and the place of occurrence. Other states have required reporting of external cause codes by certain providers, such as hospitals that are regional trauma centers. Each physician or hospital must consider the requirements of their state agencies to decide what reporting is mandated.

Coding Guidelines and Instructional Notes for ICD-10-CM Chapter 20

There are many notes in Chapter 20 to show which categories require the seventh character to indicate whether the episode of care being identified was the initial, subsequent, or a secondary encounter, or if the condition is a result of a past event (sequela). The category codes that require a seventh character include a note box that lists the instruction to it.

In addition to the external cause code that identifies the event that cause the illness or injury, three other external cause codes identify other factors concerning the event. The additional facts that are available to be reported are as follows:

Y92, Place of occurrence of the external cause
Y93, Activity codes
Y99, External cause status

The *ICD-10-CM Guidelines for Coding and Reporting* and the instructional note in the code book with category Y92, **Place of occurrence** of the external cause, states to use Y92 in conjunction with the activity code. A note under category Y92 states "The following category is for use, when relevant, to identify the place of occurrence of the external cause. Use in conjunction with an activity code. Generally, the place of occurrence should be recorded only at the initial encounter for treatment. However, in the rare instance that a new injury occurs during hospitalization, an additional place of occurrence code may be assigned" (CDC 2019).

The guidelines and the instructional note with category Y93, **Activity codes**, states, "Category Y93 is provided for use to indicate the activity of the person seeking healthcare for an injury or health condition, such as a heart attack while shoveling snow, which resulted from, or was contributed to, by the activity." The activity code should be recorded only once at the initial encounter for treatment (CDC 2019).

The third category used to provide additional facts about the event is category Y99, **External cause status.** The note that appears in the ICD-10-CM code book under category Y99 states "A single code from category Y99 should be used in conjunction with the external cause code(s) assigned to a record to indicate the status of the person at the time the event occurred" (CDC 2019). The external cause status code indicates the work status of the person at the time the event occurred. The external cause status code is used only once at the initial encounter for treatment.

The NCHS has published chapter-specific guidelines for Chapter 20 in the *ICD-10-CM Official Guidelines for Coding and Reporting*. The coding student should review all of the coding guidelines for Chapter 20 of ICD-10-CM, which appear in an ICD-10-CM code book or on the CDC website (CDC 2019) or in appendix F.

CG **Guidelines for Chapter 20: External Causes of Morbidity (V01–Y99):** The external causes of morbidity codes should never be sequenced as the first-listed or principal diagnosis.

External cause codes are intended to provide data for injury research and evaluation of injury prevention strategies. These codes capture how the injury or health condition happened (cause), the intent (unintentional or accidental; or intentional, such as suicide or assault), the place where the event occurred, the activity of the patient at the time of the event, and the person's status (e.g., civilian, military).

There is no national requirement for mandatory ICD-10-CM external cause code reporting. Unless a provider is subject to a state-based external code reporting mandate or these codes are required by a particular payer, reporting of ICD-10-CM codes in Chapter 20, External Causes of Morbidity, is not required. In the absence of a mandatory reporting requirement, providers are encouraged to voluntarily report external cause codes, as they provide valuable data for injury research and evaluation of injury prevention strategies.

Guideline I.C.20.a. General External Cause Coding Guidelines

Guideline I.C.20.a.1. Used with any code in the range of A00.0–T88.9, Z00–Z99: An external cause code may be used with any code in the range of A00.0–T88.9, Z00–Z99, classification that represents a health condition due to an external cause. Though they are most applicable to injuries, they are also valid for use with such things as infections or diseases due to an external source, and other health conditions, such as a heart attack that occurs during strenuous physical activity.

Guideline I.C.20.a.2. External cause code used for length of treatment: Assign the external cause code, with the appropriate 7th character (initial encounter, subsequent encounter or sequela) for each encounter for which the injury or condition is being treated.

Most categories in chapter 20 have a 7th character requirement for each applicable code. Most categories in this chapter have three 7th character values: A, initial encounter, D, subsequent encounter, and S, sequela. While the patient may be seen by a new or different provider over the course of treatment for an injury or condition, assignment of the 7th character for external cause should match the 7th character of the code assigned for the associated injury or condition for the encounter.

Guideline I.C.20.a.3. Use the full range of external cause codes: Use the full range of external cause codes to completely describe the cause, the intent, the place of occurrence, and if applicable, the activity of the patient at the time of the event, and the patient's status, for all injuries, and other health conditions due to an external cause.

Guideline I.C.20.a.4. Assign as many external cause codes as necessary: Assign as many external cause codes as necessary to fully explain each cause. If only one external code can be recorded, assign the code most related to the principal diagnosis.

Guideline I.C.20.a.5. The selection of the appropriate external cause code: The selection of the appropriate external cause code is guided by the Alphabetic Index of External Causes and by Inclusion and Exclusion notes in the Tabular List.

Guideline I.C.20.a.6. External cause code can never be a principal diagnosis: An external cause code can never be a principal (first-listed) diagnosis.

(Continued)

(Continued)

Guideline I.C.20.a.7. Combination external cause codes: Certain of the external cause codes are combination codes that identify sequential events that result in an injury, such as a fall which results in striking against an object. The injury may be due to either event or both. The combination external cause code used should correspond to the sequence of events regardless of which caused the most serious injury.

Guideline I.C.20.a.8. No external cause code needed in certain circumstances: No external cause code from Chapter 20 is needed if the external cause and intent are included in a code from another chapter (e.g. T36.0X1- Poisoning by penicillins, accidental (unintentional)).

Guideline I.C.20.b. Place of Occurrence Guideline: Codes from category Y92, Place of occurrence of the external cause, are secondary codes for use after other external cause codes to identify the location of the patient at the time of injury or other condition.

Generally, a place of occurrence code is used only once, at the initial encounter for treatment. However, in the rare instance that a new injury occurs during the hospitalization, an additional place of occurrence code may be assigned. No 7th characters are used for Y92. Do not use place of occurrence code Y92.9 if the place is not stated or is not applicable.

Guideline I.C.20.c. Activity Code: Assign a code from category Y93, Activity code, to describe the activity of the patient at the time the injury or other health condition occurred.

An activity code is used only once, at the initial encounter for treatment. Only one code from Y93 should be recorded on a medical record. The activity codes are not applicable to poisonings, adverse effects, misadventures or sequela.

Do not assign Y93.9, Unspecified activity, if the activity is not stated.

A code from category Y93 is appropriate for use with external cause and intent codes if identifying the activity provides additional information about the event.

Guideline I.C.20.d. Place of Occurrence, Activity, and Status Codes Used with other External Cause Code: When applicable, place of occurrence, activity, and external cause status codes are sequenced after the main external cause code(s). Regardless of the number of external cause codes assigned, there should be only one place of occurrence code, one activity code, and one external cause status code assigned to an encounter. However, in the rare instances when a new injury occurs during hospitalization, an additional place of occurrence code may be assigned.

Guideline I.C.20.e. If the Reporting Format Limits the Number of External Cause Codes: If the reporting format limits the number of external cause codes that can be used in reporting clinical data, report the code for the cause/intent most related to the principal diagnosis. If the format permits capture of additional external cause codes, the cause/intent, including medical misadventures, of the additional events should be reported rather than the codes for place, activity, or external status.

Guideline I.C.20.f. Multiple External Cause Coding Guidelines: More than one external cause code is required to fully describe the external cause of an illness or injury. The assignment of external cause codes should be sequenced in the following priority:

If two or more events cause separate injuries, an external cause code should be assigned for each cause. The first-listed external cause code will be selected in the following order:

External codes for child and adult abuse take priority over all other external cause codes.

See Section I.C.19. Child and Adult abuse guidelines.

External cause codes for terrorism events take priority over all other external cause codes except child and adult abuse.

External cause codes for cataclysmic events take priority over all other external cause codes except child and adult abuse and terrorism.

External cause codes for transport accidents take priority over all other external cause codes except cataclysmic events, child and adult abuse and terrorism.

Activity and external cause status codes are assigned following all causal (intent) external cause codes.

The first-listed external cause code should correspond to the cause of the most serious diagnosis due to an assault, accident, or self-harm, following the order of hierarchy listed above.

Guideline I.C.20.g. Child and Adult Abuse Guideline: Adult and child abuse, neglect and maltreatment are classified as assault. Any of the assault codes may be used to indicate the external cause of any injury resulting from the confirmed abuse.

For confirmed cases of abuse, neglect and maltreatment, when the perpetrator is known, a code from Y07, Perpetrator of maltreatment and neglect, should accompany any other assault codes.

See Section I.C.19. Adult and child abuse, neglect and other maltreatment

(Continued)

(Continued)

Guideline I.C.20.h. Unknown or Undetermined Intent Guideline: If the intent (accident, self-harm, assault) of the cause of an injury or other condition is unknown or unspecified, code the intent as accidental intent. All transport accident categories assume accidental intent.

Guideline I.C.20.h.1. Use of undetermined intent: External cause codes for events of undetermined intent are only for use if the documentation in the record specifies that the intent cannot be determined.

Guideline I.C.20.i. Sequelae (Late Effects) of External Cause Guidelines

Guideline I.C.20.i.1. *Sequelae* **external cause codes:** Sequela are reported using the external cause code with the 7th character "S" for sequela. These codes should be used with any report of a late effect or sequela resulting from a previous injury.

See Section I.B.10 Sequela (Late Effects)

Guideline I.C.20.i.2. *Sequela* **external cause code with a related current injury:** A sequela external cause code should never be used with a related current nature of injury code.

Guideline I.C.20.i.3. Use of *sequela* **external cause codes for subsequent visits:** Use a late effect external cause code for subsequent visits when a late effect of the initial injury is being treated. Do not use a late effect external cause code for subsequent visits for follow-up care (e.g., to assess healing, to receive rehabilitative therapy) of the injury when no late effect of the injury has been documented.

Guideline I.C.20.j. Terrorism Guidelines

Guideline I.C.20.j.1. Cause of injury identified by the Federal Government (FBI) as terrorism: When the cause of an injury is identified by the Federal Government (FBI) as terrorism, the first-listed external cause code should be a code from category Y38, Terrorism. The definition of terrorism employed by the FBI is found at the inclusion note at the beginning of category Y38. Use additional code for place of occurrence (Y92.-). More than one Y38 code may be assigned if the injury is the result of more than one mechanism of terrorism.

Guideline I.C.20.j.2. Cause of an injury is suspected to be the result of terrorism: When the cause of an injury is suspected to be the result of terrorism a code from category Y38 should not be assigned. Suspected cases should be classified as assault.

Guideline I.C.20.j.3. Code Y38.9, Terrorism, secondary effects: Assign code Y38.9, Terrorism, secondary effects, for conditions occurring subsequent to the terrorist event. This code should not be assigned for conditions that are due to the initial terrorist act.

It is acceptable to assign code Y38.9 with another code from Y38 if there is an injury due to the initial terrorist event and an injury that is a subsequent result of the terrorist event.

Guideline I.C.20.k. External Cause Status: A code from category Y99, External cause status, should be assigned whenever any other external cause code is assigned for an encounter, including an Activity code, except for the events noted below. Assign a code from category Y99, External cause status, to indicate the work status of the person at the time the event occurred. The status code indicates whether the event occurred during military activity, whether a non-military person was at work, whether an individual including a student or volunteer was involved in a non-work activity at the time of the causal event.

A code from Y99, External cause status, should be assigned, when applicable, with other external cause codes, such as transport accidents and falls. The external cause status codes are not applicable to poisonings, adverse effects, misadventures or late effects.

Do not assign a code from category Y99 if no other external cause codes (cause, activity) are applicable for the encounter.

An external cause status code is used only once, at the initial encounter for treatment. Only one code from Y99 should be recorded on a medical record.

Do not assign code Y99.9, Unspecified external cause status, if the status is not stated.

Coding External Cause of Morbidity in ICD-10-CM Chapter 20

As stated previously, an external cause code can never be a principal, first-listed, or only diagnosis code reported. An external cause code, with the appropriate seventh character (initial encounter, subsequent encounter, or sequela), is assigned for each encounter for which the injury or condition is being treated. This includes the initial encounter and all subsequent encounters when the condition being treated was caused by an external cause. Some of these healthcare encounters can be years later when the patient continues to suffer from the consequences of the original problem that was caused by an external event.

When it is applicable, an external cause code is used as an additional code with another code from other chapters in ICD-10-CM in the range of A00.0–T88.9, Z00–Z99 to identify when a health condition or injury is due to an external cause. External cause codes are used most commonly with codes for injuries. However, there may also be an external cause to be reported as the cause of other conditions such as infections or diseases, for example, when a musculoskeletal condition is produced as the result of overuse or repetitive motions.

The coder may use the full range of external cause codes to completely describe the cause, the intent, the place of occurrence, and if applicable, the activity of the patient at the time of the event, and the patient's status, for all injuries, and other health conditions due to an external cause. The coder may assign as many external cause codes as necessary to fully explain each cause. If only one external code can be recorded, the coder should assign the code most related to the principal diagnosis.

The coder must recognize that no external cause code from Chapter 20 is needed if the external cause and intent are included in a code from another chapter. For example, an external cause code is not used with a code for a poisoning. The code T36.0X1, Poisoning by penicillins, accidental (unintentional), includes the intent and therefore would not require the use of an external cause code.

Certain external cause codes are combination codes that identify sequential events that result in an injury, such as a fall that results in striking against an object. The injury may be due to either event or both. The combination external cause code used should correspond to the sequence of events regardless of which event caused the most serious injury.

If the reporting format limits the number of external cause codes that can be used in reporting clinical data, the coder should report the code for the cause or intent most relative to the principal diagnosis. If additional external cause codes are allowed, the cause or intent, including medical misadventures, of the additional events should be reported rather than the codes for place, activity, or external status (CDC 2019).

Seventh Character to Identify the Encounter

ICD-10-CM indicates when one of the external cause codes in the range of V00–Y99 codes require a seventh character to indicate whether the healthcare encounter was the

A—Initial encounter,
D—Subsequent encounter, or
S—Sequela.

Because an external cause code is assigned for each encounter for which the injury or condition is being treated, the **seventh character** identifies the timing of the care for the condition. The encounter could be the first time the patient is treated, it could be a follow-up visit or subsequent encounter, or it could be a much later encounter. When the external cause is recognized as the cause of a **sequela**, or condition that the patient has today, and continues to receive treatment, the external cause is reported with the seventh character S for sequela. These later encounters identify when the long-term effect of an injury is being treated.

Certain external causes are only used once, at the initial encounter for treatment, such as the place of occurrence codes, the activity code, and the external status code(s). The actual external cause, such as a fall or transportation accident, continues to be reported with the appropriate seventh character for as long as the patient receives treatment.

The seventh character of an external cause code must always be the seventh character in the data field. If a code that requires a seventh character is not six characters, a placeholder X must be used to fill in the empty characters.

ICD-10-CM External Cause of Injuries Index

The selection of the appropriate external cause code is guided by the **ICD-10-CM External Cause of Injuries** (alphabetic) **Index** and by inclusion and exclusion notes in the Tabular List. In the ICD-10-CM External Cause of Injuries Index, the entries use main terms identifying the event with such entries as accident, drowning, exposure, the force of nature, falling, slipping, and other events that can cause an injury. Other entries exist for assignment of the activity of the person, place of occurrence, and status of external cause, such as civilian activity, leisure activity, student activity, and such.

The external cause code is organized by the main term describing the accident, circumstance, event, or specific agent that caused the injury or illness, such as a motor vehicle crash earthquake, or dog bite:

Fall, falling (accidental) W19
building W20.1
  burning (uncontrolled fire) X00.3
down
  embankment W17.81
  escalator W10.0
  hill W17.81
  ladder W11
  ramp W10.2
  stairs, steps W10.9

EXAMPLES

1. Patient was injured when he was kicked by another person in a fight and brought to the emergency department (ED) for treatment
Main term: Kicked by
Subterm: person
Subterm: in, fight
Code: Y04.0XXA

2. Patient was assaulted by another person who shot the patient with a handgun and the patient was brought to the ED for treatment
Main term: Assault
Subterm: firearm
Subterm: handgun
Code: X93.XXXA

3. Patient was diving into a swimming pool and got injured when he struck the bottom and was brought to the ED for treatment
Main term: Diving—see Accident, diving
Main term: Accident, diving—see Fall, into, water
Main term: Fall, into, water, in, swimming pool, striking, bottom (W16.022)
However, the direct cause of the patient's injury is the "striking the bottom." If he had not struck bottom of pool he probably would not have been injured, so using the direct cause:
Main term: Striking against, bottom when, diving or jumping into water (in)
Subterm: swimming pool (W16.022)
Code: W16.022A

Check Your Understanding 23.1

Using the ICD-10-CM External Cause of Injuries Index and Tabular List, assign the external cause codes only for the following events, consider all initial encounters.

1. Fall off balcony

2. Knocked down by another person in a brawl

3. Drowning in a lake

4. Bumped into sports equipment

5. Injured during a hurricane

6. Injured by contact with a powered bench saw as industrial accident

---

Sequence of Place of Occurrence (Y92), Activity (Y93), and Status Codes (Y99)

The place of occurrence, activity, and external cause status codes are sequenced after the main external cause code(s). Regardless of the number of external cause codes assigned, there should be only one place of occurrence code except an additional place of occurrence code can be assigned when an accident occurs during a hospital stay for a patient, one activity code, and one external cause status code assigned to the initial encounter. For example, if a patient was treated during an initial encounter for two injuries from two external causes that occurred at the same time, such as a burn from hot stove (X15.0XXA) and a fracture from a fall (W18.30XA), there is only one place of occurrence code used, for example, the kitchen in a single family residence (Y92.000), only one activity code, for example, baking and cooking (Y93.G3), and only one external cause status code, for example, this was a leisure activity for the patient (Y99.8). When the patient is treated during subsequent healthcare visits, only the main external cause code will be assigned with the seventh character D, but no additional external cause codes will be assigned for the place of occurrence, activity, or external cause status.

Multiple External Cause Codes

The first-listed external cause code should correspond to the cause of the most serious diagnosis due to an assault, accident, or self-harm, following an established hierarchy. If two or more events cause separate injuries, an external cause code should be assigned for each cause. The first-listed external cause code will be selected in the following order (CDC 2019):

1. External codes for child and adult abuse take priority over all other external cause codes.

2. External cause codes for terrorism events take priority over all other external cause codes except child and adult abuse.

3. External cause codes for cataclysmic events take priority over all other external cause codes except child and adult abuse and terrorism.

4. External cause codes for transport accidents take priority over all other external cause codes except cataclysmic events, child and adult abuse, and terrorism.

5. Activity and external cause status codes are assigned following all causal (intent) external cause codes.

External Cause Codes for Child and Adult Abuse (X92–Y09)

Adult and child abuse, neglect, and maltreatment are classified as assault. For cases of confirmed abuse or neglect is documented in the record, an external cause code from the assault section (X92–Y09) should be added to identify the cause of any physical injuries.

For confirmed cases of abuse, neglect, and maltreatment, when the perpetrator is known, a code from Y07, Perpetrator of maltreatment and neglect, should accompany any other assault codes. The relationship between the perpetrator and victim is identified with the Y07 code, for example, spouse or partner, parent, or sibling; the perpetrator may also be a nonfamily member, such as a daycare provider or teacher.

For suspected cases of abuse or neglect, the coder does not report an external cause of injury or perpetrator code for the encounter (CDC 2019).

> **EXAMPLE:** The mother of the two-year-old male child brought the patient to the emergency department (ED) for an evaluation of the contusions on his legs that the mother found after the child had been at a day care center. The mother feared the child had been abused. The day care worker who came with the mother said the child fell on playground equipment. The child could not tell what happened. The ED physician wrote the final diagnosis as child and family referred to State Agency for investigation of "Suspected physical abuse of a child:" T76.12XA, Child abuse suspected. No external cause code for child abuse, such as X58 or the perpetrator of maltreatment (Y07), is assigned as the case is still under investigation and a perpetrator has not been identified.

Identifying the Intent for External Cause Codes

All transport accident categories are assumed to be accidental and reported as having an accidental intent. In addition, if the intent of an event is unknown or unspecified, that is, it is not stated to be an accident, self-harm, or an assault, the coder can assume the intent of the event is accidental. The only time the coder uses the event codes that state there is an undetermined intent is when the documentation in the record specifically states the intent of the event cannot be determined.

Sequelae or Late Effect External Cause Codes

To identify that a patient's condition being treated today is from an event that occurred in the past, the external cause code is reported with the seventh character S for sequela. These external cause codes should be used with any report of a late effect or sequela resulting from a previous injury. A sequela external cause code should never be used with a related current nature of injury code. Typically, a patient with a sequela of a past injury or illness is coded as follows (CDC 2019):

1. Residual effect or the condition the patient has at present, which is found in the Alphabetic Index to Diseases and Injuries

2. Sequela or late effect or the condition the patient originally had that produced the residual effect found in the Alphabetic Index to Disease and Injuries under the term "sequelae."

3. External cause code for the original accident or event, found in the Index to External Causes with the seventh character of "S" for sequelae.

EXAMPLE: The 30-year-old male patient was seen in the physician's office for ongoing evaluation of his sensorineural deafness in his left ear only that was the result of a snow skiing accident when he fell off a ski lift and suffered a skull fracture. The coding for this example of a sequela of an injury with a sequela external cause code is as follows:

H90.42, Sensorineural hearing loss, unilateral, left ear, with unrestricted hearing on the contralateral side
S02.91XS, Unspecified fracture, skull, sequela
V98.3XXS, Accident, ski(ing)—see Accident, transport, ski lift, sequela

Transport Accidents (V00–V99)

The transport accidents section (V00–V99) is structured in 12 groups:

Accidents	V00–X58
Transport accidents	V00–V99
Pedestrian injured in transport accident	V00–V09
Pedal cycle rider injured in transport accident	V10–V19
Motorcycle rider injured in transport accident	V20–V29
Occupant of three-wheeled motor vehicle injured in transport accident	V30–V39
Car occupant injured in transport accident	V40–V49
Occupant of pick-up truck or van injured in transport accident	V50–V59
Occupant of heavy transport vehicle injured in transport accident	V60–V69
Bus occupant injured in transport accident	V70–V79
Other land transport accidents	V80–V89
Water transport accidents	V90–V94
Air and space transport accidents	V95–V97
Other and unspecified transport accidents	V98–V99

Those relating to land transport accidents (V00–V89) reflect the victim's mode of transport and are subdivided to identify the victim's counterpart or the type of event. The vehicle of which the injured person is an occupant is identified in the first two characters since it is seen as the most important factor to identify for prevention purposes. A transport accident is one in which the vehicle involved must be moving or running or in use for transport purposes at the time of the accident. The definitions of transport vehicles are provided at the beginning of Chapter 20. A "use additional code" note appears under the heading for transport accidents (V00–V99) to use another code for airbag injury (W22.1-), type of street or road (Y92.4-), and use of cellular telephone or other electronic equipment at the time of the transport accident (Y93.C-).

EXAMPLE: The patient was brought to the emergency department for treatment of injuries suffered in a motor vehicle crash when the patient was the driver of a vehicle involved in a collision with another vehicle (assign external cause code only):

Main term: Accident
Sub term: transport

Sub term: car occupant
Sub term: driver
Sub term: collision (with)
Sub term: car (traffic)

Code: V43.52XA, Car driver injured in collision with other type of car in traffic accident, initial encounter

Check Your Understanding 23.2

Assign the transport accident external cause codes for the following events, consider all as initial encounter.

1. Patient was driver occupant of a bus involved in a transport accident, collision with a vehicle in traffic

2. Patient was passenger of a vehicle in a collision with sport utility vehicle in traffic

3. Patient was driver of motorcycle in collision with vehicle in traffic

4. Patient was a passenger occupant in a pickup truck in collision with a bus in traffic

5. Patient was a heavy truck driver in collision with another heavy truck in traffic

6. Patient was pedal cyclist (alone driving/riding a bicycle) in collision with bus in traffic

Never Events or Serious Reportable Events

ICD-10-CM contains external cause codes to identify and track the occurrence of wrong site surgery, wrong surgery, and wrong patient having surgery to support the collection of data related to the National Quality Forum's **never events**. The federal government's Institute of Medicine (IOM) developed a comprehensive approach to improving patient safety in American healthcare organizations by identifying certain healthcare errors and particular events that were reported in a systemic manner. To accomplish this, the IOM worked with the National Quality Forum to identify a list of "serious reportable events" in healthcare that should never occur. This list of events has become known as "never events" as a result of the National Quality Forum's report "Serious Reportable Events in Healthcare: A Consensus Report" (Kizer and Stegun 2005). A complete list of the never events and the work of the Department of Health and Human Services' Agency for Healthcare Research and Quality (AHRQ) can be found in table 23.1.

The wrong site, wrong surgery, and wrong patient never events or serious reportable events are among the list of adverse medical events that are serious, largely preventable, and of concern to patients and healthcare providers. The Joint Commission, the federal government, and state governments use the never events list as the basis for quality indicators and state-based reporting systems. The following are examples of external cause codes that can be used to describe the external cause of several of these factors:

Y65.51	Performance of wrong procedure (operation) on correct patient
Y65.52	Performance of procedure (operation) on patient not scheduled for surgery
Y65.53	Performance of correct procedure (operation) on wrong side or body part

Some of these events—such as stage 3 and 4 pressure ulcers acquired after admission to the healthcare facility and intravascular air embolisms that occur while being cared for in a healthcare facility—can be captured by ICD-10-CM diagnosis codes and present-on-admission indicators. Other events in this area cannot be captured using ICD-10-CM codes because the event is beyond the scope of the classification system. An example of a never event that cannot be coded is an infant discharged to the wrong patient or the abduction of a patient of any age. The main terms used in the External Cause of Injuries Index may be misadventure(s) to patient(s) during surgical or medical care, wrong, or the problem itself.

Table 23.1.   **List of serious reportable events or never events**

Event	Additional specifications
1. Surgical events	
A. Surgery performed on the wrong body part	Defined as any surgery performed on a body part that is not consistent with the documented informed consent for that patient. Excludes emergent situations that occur in the course of surgery and/or whose exigency precludes obtaining informed consent.
B. Surgery performed on the wrong patient	Defined as any surgery on a patient that is not consistent with the documented informed consent for that patient.
C. Wrong surgical procedure performed on a patient	Defined as any procedure performed on a patient that is not consistent with the documented informed consent for that patient. Excludes emergent situations that occur in the course of surgery and/or whose exigency precludes obtaining informed consent. Surgery includes endoscopies and other invasive procedures.
D. Retention of a foreign object in a patient after surgery or other procedure	Excludes objects intentionally implanted as part of a planned intervention and objects present prior to surgery that were intentionally retained.
E. Intraoperative or immediately postoperative death in an ASA Class I patient	Includes all ASA Class I patient deaths in situations where anesthesia was administered; the planned surgical procedure may or may not have been carried out. Immediately postoperative means within 24 hours after induction of anesthesia (if surgery not completed), surgery, or other invasive procedure was completed.
2. Product or device events	
A. Patient death or serious disability associated with the use of contaminated drugs, devices, or biologics provided by the healthcare facility	Includes generally detectable contaminants in drugs, devices, or biologics regardless of the source of contamination and/or product.
B. Patient death or serious disability associated with the use or function of a device in patient care, in which the device is used for functions other than as intended	Includes, but is not limited to, catheters, drains, and other specialized tubes, infusion pumps, and ventilators.
C. Patient death or serious disability associated with intravascular air embolism that occurs while being cared for in a healthcare facility	Excludes deaths associated with neurosurgical procedures known to be a high risk of intravascular air embolism.

Event	Additional specifications
3. Patient protection events	
A. Infant discharged to the wrong person	
B. Patient death or serious disability associated with patient elopement (disappearance) for more than four hours	Excludes events involving competent adults.
C. Patient suicide, or attempted suicide resulting in serious disability, while being cared for in a healthcare facility	Defined as events that result from patient actions after admission to a healthcare facility. Excludes deaths resulting from self-inflicted injuries that were the reason for admission to the healthcare facility.
4. Care management events	
A. Patient death or serious disability associated with a medication error (e.g., errors involving the wrong drug, wrong dose, wrong patient, wrong time, wrong rate, wrong preparation, or wrong route of administration).	Excludes reasonable differences in clinical judgment on drug selection and dose
B. Patient death or serious disability associated with a hemolytic reaction due to the administration of ABO-incompatible blood or blood products	
C. Maternal death or serious disability associated with labor or delivery in a low-risk pregnancy while being cared for in a healthcare facility	Includes events that occur within 42 days postdelivery. Excludes deaths from pulmonary or amniotic fluid embolism, acute fatty liver of pregnancy, or cardiomyopathy.
D. Patient death or serious disability associated with hypoglycemia, the onset of which occurs while the patient is being cared for in a healthcare facility	
E. Death or serious disability (kernicterus) associated with failure to identify and treat hyperbilirubinemia in neonates	Hyperbilirubinemia is defined as bilirubin levels >30 mg/dL. Neonates refers to the first 28 days of life.
F. Stage 3 or 4 pressure ulcers acquired after admission to a healthcare facility	Excludes progression from Stage 2 to Stage 3 if Stage 2 was recognized upon admission.
G. Patient death or serious disability due to spinal manipulative therapy	
5. Environmental events	
A. Patient death or serious disability associated with an electric shock while being cared for in a healthcare facility	Excludes events involving planned treatments such as electric countershock
B. Any incident in which a line designated for oxygen or other gas to be delivered to a patient contains the wrong gas or is contaminated by toxic substances	
C. Patient death or serious disability associated with a burn incurred from any source while being cared for in a healthcare facility	

(Continued)

Event	Additional specifications
D. Patient death associated with a fall while being cared for in a healthcare facility	
E. Patient death or serious disability associated with the use of restraints or bedrails while being cared for in a healthcare facility	
6. Criminal events	
A. Any instance of care ordered by or provided by someone impersonating a physician, nurse, pharmacist, or other licensed healthcare provider	
B. Abduction of a patient of any age	
C. Sexual assault on a patient within or on the grounds of the healthcare facility	
D. Death or significant injury of a patient or staff member resulting from a physical assault (i.e., battery) that occurs within or on the grounds of the healthcare facility	

Source: Kizer and Stegun 2005

Military Operations

The US Department of Defense initiated the addition and expansion of external cause codes for the identification of the causes of injuries among the military population to assist with the prevention of such injuries. Two categories of ICD-10-CM external cause codes are available to report the cause of an injury or illness.

Operations of War (Y36)

The Includes note under category Y36 states these codes describe the cause of injuries to military personnel and civilians caused by war, civil insurrections, and peacekeeping missions. The Excludes1 note states this category is not to be used with category Y37, Military operations, which identify the cause of injuries to military personnel occurring during peacetime operations.

> **EXAMPLE:** The patient is an active military member of the US Army who lost his right arm due to explosion of an improvised explosive device (IED) during military operations (external cause code only):
>
> Y36.230, Explosion, war operations—see War operations, explosion, improvised explosive device, military personnel

Military Operations (Y37)

The Includes note under category Y37 states these codes describe the cause of injuries to military personnel and civilians occurring during peacetime on military property and during routine military exercises and operations. The Excludes1 note states that military aircraft accidents, military vehicles transport accidents, and military watercraft transport accidents with civilian aircraft, vehicles, or watercrafts are coded to other categories. In addition, war operations that caused an injury are not reported with these external cause codes in category Y37. Examples of external cause codes to identify injuries from military operations are as follows:

Y37.010-	Military operations involving explosion of depth-charge, military personnel
Y37.210-	Military operations involving explosion of aerial bomb, military personnel
Y37.320-	Military operations involving incendiary bullet, military personnel
Y37.421-	Military operations involving firearms pellets, civilian
Y37.6X1-	Military operations involving biological weapons, civilian
Y37.92X-	Military operations involving friendly fire

Terrorism External Cause Codes

When the cause of an injury is identified by the Federal Bureau of Investigation (FBI) as terrorism, the first-listed external cause code should be a code from category Y38, Terrorism. The definition of terrorism employed by the FBI is found at the inclusion note at the beginning of category Y38. The note reads, "These codes are for use to identify injuries resulting from the unlawful use of force or violence against persons or property to intimidate or coerce a government, the civilian population, or any segment thereof, in furtherance of a political or social objective" (CDC 2019). Use an additional code for place of occurrence (Y92.-). More than one Y38 code may be assigned if the injury is the result of more than one mechanism of terrorism. When the cause of an injury is suspected to be the result of terrorism, a code from category Y38 should not be assigned. Suspected cases should be classified as assault. Assign code Y38.9, Terrorism, secondary effects, for conditions occurring subsequent to the terrorist event. This code should not be assigned for conditions that are due to the initial terrorist act. It is acceptable to assign code Y38.9 with another code from Y38 if there is an injury due to the initial terrorist event and an injury that is a subsequent result of the terrorist event. The main term to be used in the External Cause of Injuries Index would be "terrorism."

EXAMPLE: The patient was a civilian injured when a bomb was exploded that was determined to be an act of terrorism (external cause code only).

Y38.2X2A, Terrorism, explosion, civilian injured, initial encounter

Check Your Understanding 23.3

Assign an external cause code for the following descriptions of never events, military operations, and terrorism, do not code place of occurrence, status or activity codes.

1. The patient was taken to surgery and the lung biopsy was performed on the wrong patient.

2. The patient was treated for an intra-abdominal infection after it was determined there was a failure in sterile precautions during a surgical operation.

3. The patient was an active member of the US Army involved in war operations when he was injured in a "friendly fire" incident, initial encounter for care.

4. The patient was an active member of the US Air Force involved in military operations and was injured when the aircraft he was piloting had an onboard fire and was destroyed. This visit is a follow-up or subsequent visit for treatment of burns on the patient.

5. The patient is a city fireman who was injured while fighting a fire in a building that was determined to have been set on first as an act of terrorism, initial encounter.

6. Wrong fluids were administered to patient in intravenous fluids that caused a patient reaction or misadventure

Place of Occurrence

The code for the place of occurrence is used to identify, when documented, where the event occurred. Category Y92 codes, Place of occurrence of the external cause, are used in conjunction with an activity code if the activity is stated by the healthcare provider. Place of occurrence should be recorded only at the initial encounter for treatment to identify the location of the patient at the time when the injury or other condition occurred. Only one code from Y92 should be recorded on a medical record. According to official ICD-10-CM coding guidelines, the coder should not use the unspecified place of occurrence code Y92.9 if the place is not stated in the record or is not applicable. The main term to be used in the External Cause of Injuries Index is "Place of occurrence."

Check Your Understanding 23.4

Assign a place of occurrence external cause code for the following descriptions.

1. Campsite area

2. Same day surgery center

3. Residence, apartment, kitchen

4. Residence, single family house, garage

5. Golf course

6. Public high school

Activity Code

A code from category Y93, Activity code, is used to describe the activity of the patient at the time the injury or other health condition occurred. An activity code is used only once, at the initial encounter for treatment. Only one code from Y93 should be recorded on a medical record. An activity code should be used in conjunction with a place of occurrence code, Y92. The activity codes are not applicable to poisonings, adverse effects, misadventures, or sequela. According to the official ICD-10-CM coding guidelines, the coder should not assign code Y93.9 for an unspecified activity if the activity is not stated.

A code from category Y93 is appropriate for use with external cause and intent codes if identifying the activity provides additional information about the event. A note at the beginning of category Y93 in the Tabular states the activity code is provided to indicate the activity of the person seeking healthcare for an injury or health condition that resulted from the activity or was contributed to by the activity, such as a heart attack while shoveling snow. These codes are appropriate for use for both acute injuries, such as those from Chapter 19 and conditions that are due to the long-term, cumulative effects of an activity, such as those from Chapter 13. They are also appropriate for use with external cause codes for cause and intent if identifying the activity provides additional information on the event. These codes should be used in conjunction with codes for external cause status (Y99) and place of occurrence (Y92). The activity code is used only once, at the initial encounter for treatment. The main term to be used in the External Cause of Injuries Index is "Activity."

This section contains the following broad activity categories:

Y93.0	Activities involving walking and running
Y93.1	Activities involving water and water craft
Y93.2	Activities involving ice and snow

Y93.3	Activities involving climbing, rappelling, and jumping off
Y93.4	Activities involving dancing and other rhythmic movement
Y93.5	Activities involving other sports and athletics played individually
Y93.6	Activities involving other sports and athletics played as a team or group
Y93.7	Activities involving other specified sports and athletics
Y93.a	Activities involving other cardiorespiratory exercise
Y93.b	Activities involving other muscle strengthening exercises
Y93.c	Activities involving computer technology and electronic devices
Y93.d	Activities involving arts and handcrafts
Y93.e	Activities involving personal hygiene and interior property and clothing maintenance
Y93.f	Activities involving caregiving
Y93.g	Activities involving food preparation, cooking, and grilling
Y93.h	Activities involving exterior property and land maintenance, building and construction
Y93.i	Activities involving roller coasters and other types of external motion
Y93.j	Activities involving playing musical instrument
Y93.k	Activities involving animal care
Y93.8	Activities, other specified
Y93.9	Activity, unspecified

Check Your Understanding 23.5

Assign an activity external cause code for the following descriptions.

1. Patient's activity at time of accident: Nordic skiing

2. Patient's activity at time of accident: running on treadmill

3. Patient's activity at time of accident: wall climbing

4. Patient's activity at time of accident: skateboarding

5. Patient's activity at time of accident: cheerleading

6. Patient's activity at time of accident: packing up for residential relocation to new home

External Cause Status Codes

A code from category Y99, External cause status, should be assigned whenever any other external cause code is assigned for an encounter, including an activity code, except for the events noted below. A code from category Y99, External cause status, should be assigned to indicate the work status of the person at the time the event occurred. The status code indicates whether the event occurred during military activity, whether a nonmilitary person was at work, or whether an individual including a student or volunteer was involved in a nonwork activity at the time of the causal event.

A code from Y99, External cause status, should be assigned, when applicable, with other external cause codes, such as transport accidents and falls. The external cause status codes are not applicable to poisonings, adverse effects, misadventures, or late effects. The coder should not assign a code from category Y99 if no other external cause codes (cause, activity) are applicable for the encounter.

An external cause status code is used only once, at the initial encounter for treatment. Only one code from Y99 should be recorded on a medical record. According to the official ICD-10-CM coding guidelines, the coder should not assign code Y99.9, Unspecified external cause status, if the status is not stated in the record. The main terms to be used in the External Cause of Injuries Index may be "External cause status" or "Status of external cause."

Check Your Understanding 23.6

Assign a status of external cause code for the following descriptions.

1. Civilian activity done for financial compensation
2. Leisure activity
3. Military activity
4. Volunteer activity
5. Civilian activity working in factory for income
6. Student activity at school

ICD-10-CM Review Exercises: Chapter 23

Assign the appropriate external cause codes only and not the injury or illness codes.

1. Assign external cause codes for this case: An 18-year-old driver of a vehicle that collided with a truck on the interstate highway. The driver confessed to using his cell phone to send a text message to his girlfriend.

2. Assign external cause only codes for this case: An army officer was injured while on patrol on the military base in Afghanistan by an explosion of an IED. This was not a result of war operations.

3. Assign external cause only codes for this case: The patient was bitten by a horse while attempting to rescue it from a barn while performing his job at animal control.

4. Assign initial encounter for this case: The patient was burned on his face by a fireworks accident that occurred in the neighborhood park. The patient is a high school student and was at the park as part of a student outing from his school.

5. Assign initial encounter for this case: The patient was injured while playing in an American football game at a football field. He was injured when he was tackled by an opposing team player.

ICD-10-CM Review Exercises: Chapter 23 (continued)

6. Assign initial encounter for this case: The patient was injured when he was burned by hot food spilled on him while he was eating at a hospital cafeteria during a business lunch. The patient is employed as a company salesman.

   _____

7. Assign initial encounter for this case: The patient was hit by a falling tree and debris while hiking in a forest when a tornado suddenly occurred. The patient was on vacation at the time.

   _____

8. Assign initial encounter for this case: The patient was injured when he was thrown off a horse as a student at a riding school; there was no collision with another object. The patient is a student in college.

   _____

9. Assign initial encounter for this case: The patient was hit by a water ski while waterskiing but boat was unpowered at the time. The patient was on vacation at a lake.

   _____

10. Assign late effect or sequela encounter for this case: The patient was treated for a deviated septum that developed after a nose fracture. He had been hit in the face by a football while playing a football game with his high school team when he was a student.

    _____

11. Assign initial encounter for this case: The patient had a back injury after she fell into a hole while she was gardening in her single-family residence backyard. The patient is unemployed and gardening is her hobby.

    _____

12. Assign late effect or sequela encounter for this case: The patient was treated for hearing loss after years of noise damage from playing loud music with his professional rock band. He was paid for his band's appearances at concerts. He quit playing in his band several years ago and has been treated for hearing losses on several past visits.

    _____

13. Assign initial encounter for this case: The patient was in the hospital when he had the cataract removed from his right eye when he was supposed to have a cataract extraction on his left eye. The procedure was performed in a hospital operating room.

    _____

14. Assign initial encounter for this case: The patient was injured when she was hit by a car while walking across a local residential street in her neighborhood. The patient was a retired woman.

    _____

15. Assign initial encounter for this case: The patient was stabbed in the back with a knife during a fight at a basketball court while playing basketball with a group of people.

    _____

(Continued on next page)

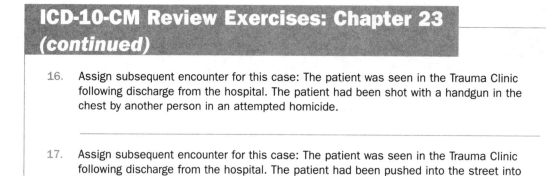

ICD-10-CM Review Exercises: Chapter 23 (continued)

16. Assign subsequent encounter for this case: The patient was seen in the Trauma Clinic following discharge from the hospital. The patient had been shot with a handgun in the chest by another person in an attempted homicide.

   _____

17. Assign subsequent encounter for this case: The patient was seen in the Trauma Clinic following discharge from the hospital. The patient had been pushed into the street into the path of a moving car by another person who was assaulting the patient.

   _____

18. Assign subsequent encounter for this case: The patient was seen in the Occupational Health Clinic following discharge from the hospital. The patient works for the local power company and came in contact with the electrical current while working on electric transmission lines.

   _____

19. Assign external cause code to describe the original event for the sequela the patient has: The patient is seen in the Dermatology Clinic for evaluation of scars on her skin from years of radiation damage from ultraviolet light from tanning beds.

   _____

20. Assign initial encounter for this case: The patient, a 20-year-old college student, fell down stairs while rough housing with friends in the school dormitory at his college and injured his face when he hit his head on the wall.

   _____

References

Centers for Disease Control and Prevention (CDC), National Center for Health Statistics (NCHS). 2019. *ICD-10-CM Official Guidelines for Coding and Reporting*, 2020. http://www.cdc.gov/nchs/icd/icd10cm.htm or https://www.cdc.gov/nchs/data/icd/10cmguidelines-FY2020_final.pdf.

Kizer, K. W. and M. B. Stegun. 2005. Serious Reportable Adverse Events in Health Care. In: Henriksen K., J. B. Battles, E. S. Marks, et al., eds. *Advances in Patient Safety: From Research to Implementation (Volume 4: Programs, Tools, and Products)*. Rockville: Agency for Healthcare Research and Quality (US). https://www.ahrq.gov/downloads/pub/advances/vol4/Kizer2.pdf.

Chapter 24

Factors Influencing Health Status and Contact with Health Services (Z00–Z99)

Learning Objectives

At the conclusion of this chapter, you should be able to do the following:

- Describe the organization of the codes included in Chapter 21 of ICD-10-CM, Factors Influencing Health Status and Contact with Health Services (Z00–Z99)

- Identify the healthcare settings and scenarios when Z code classifications are available for use

- Explain the intent of the codes in Chapter 21 and assign ICD-10-CM codes for factors influencing health status and contact with health services

- Assign ICD-10-CM diagnosis codes for factors influencing health status and contact with health services

Key Terms

Aftercare
Antenatal screening
Body mass index (BMI)
Do not resuscitate (DNR)
Family history
Follow-up codes
Genetic carrier
Genetic susceptibility

Noncompliance
Outcome of delivery
Personal history
Resistance
Ruled out
Screening
Underimmunization

Overview of ICD-10-CM Chapter 21: Factors Influencing Health Status and Contact with Health Services

Chapter 21 includes categories Z00–Z99 arranged in the following blocks:

Z00–Z13	Persons encountering health services for examinations
Z14–Z15	Genetic carrier and genetic susceptibility to disease
Z16	Resistance to antimicrobial drugs
Z17	Estrogen receptor status
Z18	Retained foreign body fragment
Z19	Hormone sensitivity malignancy status
Z20–Z29	Persons with potential health hazards related to communicable diseases
Z30–Z39	Persons encountering health services in circumstances related to reproduction
Z40–Z53	Encounters for other specific health care
Z55–Z65	Persons with potential health hazards related to socioeconomic and psychosocial circumstances
Z66	Do not resuscitate status
Z67	Blood type
Z68	Body mass index (BMI)
Z69–Z76	Persons encountering health services in other circumstances
Z77–Z99	Persons with potential health hazards related to family and personal history and certain conditions influencing health status

Codes included in Chapter 21: Factors Influencing Health Status and Contact with Health Services (Z00–Z99), represent reasons for encounters. Z codes are diagnosis codes. If a procedure is performed, a corresponding procedure code must be used with the Z code that identifies the reason for the encounter. Z codes are provided for encounters when circumstances other than a disease or injury are recorded in the health record as the diagnosis—the problem or reason for the encounter.

EXAMPLE: The patient is a 50-year-old female who was admitted to the hospital for chemotherapy for carcinoma of the lower-outer quadrant of her right breast. The intravenous chemotherapy was given through a central vein by percutaneous approach. The patient was discharged the second day. The codes for this admission are as follows:

Z51.11, Encounter for antineoplastic chemotherapy
C50.511, Malignant neoplasm of lower-outer quadrant of right female breast
3E04305, Administration through central vein, percutaneous approach, antineoplastic, other antineoplastic (Introduction of substance, vein, central, antineoplastic)

Some categories in Chapter 21 have titles to clearly describe the situations the code will classify. For example, the description for Z08 is "Encounter for follow-up examination after completed treatment for malignant neoplasm" to identify the reason for the visit for the patient who is being seen after having completed treatment for cancer. Another example of a clear description of the reason for the patient's examination is subcategory Z00.0, Encounter for general adult medical examination. Code Z00.00 identifies a general adult medical examination without abnormal findings, and code Z00.01 identifies a general adult medical examination with abnormal findings. These codes distinguish between the encounter when a patient is found to be completely healthy and when an abnormal finding has been identified in the patient who presented for a medical examination. Under code Z00.01 is a "use additional code" note to identify the abnormal finding so that the patient's situation can be fully described.

However, some conditions are not specifically identified. In ICD-10-CM there is a category, Z16, to represent infection with antimicrobial drug–resistant microorganisms. For example, if a patient had an infection that did not respond to treatment by the usual penicillin medication, code Z16.11 would identify the resistance of the condition to this antimicrobial drug. Another example of a nonspecific situation is code Z23, Encounter for immunization. This code does not identify the types of immunizations that were administered.

Coding Guidelines and Instructional Notes for ICD-10-CM Chapter 21

Instructional notes are available in the different categories to explain how codes should be assigned. For example, under category Z01, Encounter for other special examination without complaint, suspected or reported diagnosis, is the following note: "Codes from category Z01 represent the reason for the encounter. A separate procedure code is required to identify any examination or procedure performed" (CDC 2019). Also, under category Z85, Personal history of malignant neoplasm, is the following note: "Code first any follow-up examination after treatment of malignant neoplasm (Z08)" (CDC 2019).

The NCHS has published chapter-specific guidelines for Chapter 21 in the *ICD-10-CM Official Guidelines for Coding and Reporting*. The coding student should review all of the coding guidelines for Chapter 21 of ICD-10-CM that appear in an ICD-10-CM code book or on the CDC website (CDC 2019) or in appendix F.

CG **Chapter 21: Factors influencing health status and contact with health services (Z00–Z99):** Note: The chapter specific guidelines provide additional information about the use of Z codes for specified encounters.

Guideline I.C.21.a. Use of Z Codes in Any Healthcare Setting: Z codes are for use in any healthcare setting. Z codes may be used as either a first-listed (principal diagnosis code in the inpatient setting) or secondary code, depending on the circumstances of the encounter. Certain Z codes may only be used as first-listed or principal diagnosis.

Guideline I.C.21.b. Z Codes Indicate a Reason for an Encounter: Z codes are not procedure codes. A corresponding procedure code must accompany a Z code to describe any procedure performed.

Guideline I.C.21.c. Categories of Z Codes

Guideline I.C.21.c.1. Contact/Exposure: Category Z20 indicates contact with, and suspected exposure to, communicable diseases. These codes are for patients who do not show

(Continued)

(Continued)

any sign or symptom of a disease but are suspected to have been exposed to it by close personal contact with an infected individual or are in an area where a disease is epidemic.

Category Z77, Other contact with and (suspected) exposures hazardous to health, indicates contact with and suspected exposures hazardous to health.

Contact/exposure codes may be used as a first-listed code to explain an encounter for testing, or, more commonly, as a secondary code to identify a potential risk.

Guideline I.C.21.c.2. Inoculations and vaccinations: Code Z23 is for encounters for inoculations and vaccinations. It indicates that a patient is being seen to receive a prophylactic inoculation against a disease. Procedure codes are required to identify the actual administration of the injection and the type(s) of immunizations given. Code Z23 may be used as a secondary code if the inoculation is given as a routine part of preventive health care, such as a well-baby visit.

Guideline I.C.21.c.3. Status: Status codes indicate that a patient is either a carrier of a disease or has the sequelae or residual of a past disease or condition. This includes such things as the presence of prosthetic or mechanical devices resulting from past treatment. A status code is informative, because the status may affect the course of treatment and its outcome. A status code is distinct from a history code. The history code indicates that the patient no longer has the condition.

A status code should not be used with a diagnosis code from one of the body system chapters, if the diagnosis code includes the information provided by the status code. For example, code Z94.1, Heart transplant status, should not be used with a code from subcategory T86.2, Complications of heart transplant. The status code does not provide additional information. The complication code indicates that the patient is a heart transplant patient.

For encounters for weaning from a mechanical ventilator, assign a code from subcategory J96.1, Chronic respiratory failure, followed by code Z99.11, Dependence on respirator [ventilator] status.

The status Z codes/categories are:

Z14, Genetic carrier

Genetic carrier status indicates that a person carries a gene, associated with a particular disease, which may be passed to offspring who may develop that disease. The person does not have the disease and is not at risk of developing the disease.

Z15, Genetic susceptibility to disease

Genetic susceptibility indicates that a person has a gene that increases the risk of that person developing the disease.

Codes from category Z15 should not be used as principal or first-listed codes. If the patient has the condition to which he/she is susceptible, and that condition is the reason for the encounter, the code for the current condition should be sequenced first.

If the patient is being seen for follow-up after completed treatment for this condition, and the condition no longer exists, a follow-up code should be sequenced first, followed by the appropriate personal history and genetic susceptibility codes. If the purpose of the encounter is genetic counseling associated with procreative management, code Z31.5, Encounter for genetic counseling, should be assigned as the first-listed code, followed by a code from category Z15. Additional codes should be assigned for any applicable family or personal history.

Z16, Resistance to antimicrobial drugs

This code indicates that a patient has a condition that is resistant to antimicrobial drug treatment. Sequence the infection code first.

Z17, Estrogen receptor status

Z18, Retained foreign body fragments

Z19, Hormone sensitivity malignancy status

Z21, Asymptomatic HIV infection status

This code indicates that a patient has tested positive for HIV but has manifested no signs or symptoms of the disease.

Z22, Carrier of infectious disease

Carrier status indicates that a person harbors the specific organisms of a disease without manifest symptoms and is capable of transmitting the infection.

Z28.3, Underimmunization status

Z33.1, Pregnant state, incidental

This code is a secondary code only for use when the pregnancy is in no way complicating the reason for visit. Otherwise, a code from the obstetric chapter is required.

Z66, Do not resuscitate

This code may be used when it is documented by the provider that a patient is on do not resuscitate status at any time during the stay.

Z67, Blood type

Z68, Body mass index (BMI)

BMI codes should only be assigned when there is an associated, reportable diagnosis (such as obesity). Do not assign BMI codes during pregnancy.

(Continued)

(Continued)

See Section I.B.14 for BMI documentation by clinicians other than the patient's provider.

Z74.01, Bed confinement status

Z76.82, Awaiting organ transplant status

Z78, Other specified health status

Code Z78.1, Physical restraint status, may be used when it is documented by the provider that a patient has been put in restraints during the current encounter. Please note that this code should not be reported when it is documented by the provider that a patient is temporarily restrained during a procedure.

Z79, Long-term (current) drug therapy

Codes from this category indicate a patient's continuous use of a prescribed drug (including such things as aspirin therapy) for the long-term treatment of a condition or for prophylactic use. It is not for use for patients who have addictions to drugs. This subcategory is not for use of medications for detoxification or maintenance programs to prevent withdrawal symptoms in patients with drug dependence (e.g., methadone maintenance for opiate dependence). Assign the appropriate code for the drug dependence instead.

Assign a code from Z79 if the patient is receiving a medication for an extended period as a prophylactic measure (such as for the prevention of deep vein thrombosis) or as treatment of a chronic condition (such as arthritis) or a disease requiring a lengthy course of treatment (such as cancer). Do not assign a code from category Z79 for medication being administered for a brief period of time to treat an acute illness or injury (such as a course of antibiotics to treat acute bronchitis).

Z88, Allergy status to drugs, medicaments and biological substances

Except: Z88.9, Allergy status to unspecified drugs, medicaments and biological substances status

Z89, Acquired absence of limb

Z90, Acquired absence of organs, not elsewhere classified

Z91.0-, Allergy status, other than to drugs and biological substances

Z92.82, Status post administration of tPA (rtPA) in a different facility within the last 24 hours prior to admission to a current facility

Assign code Z92.82, Status post administration of tPA (rtPA) in a different facility within the last 24 hours prior to admission to current facility, as a secondary diagnosis when a patient is received by transfer into a facility and documentation indicates they were administered tissue plasminogen activator (tPA) within the last 24 hours prior to admission to the current facility.

This guideline applies even if the patient is still receiving the tPA at the time they are received into the current facility.

The appropriate code for the condition for which the tPA was administered (such as cerebrovascular disease or myocardial infarction) should be assigned first.

Code Z92.82 is only applicable to the receiving facility record and not to the transferring facility record.

Z93, Artificial opening status

Z94, Transplanted organ and tissue status

Z95, Presence of cardiac and vascular implants and grafts

Z96, Presence of other functional implants

Z97, Presence of other devices

Z98, Other postprocedural states

Assign code Z98.85, Transplanted organ removal status, to indicate that a transplanted organ has been previously removed. This code should not be assigned for the encounter in which the transplanted organ is removed. The complication necessitating removal of the transplant organ should be assigned for that encounter.

See Section I.C19. for information on the coding of organ transplant complications.

Z99, Dependence on enabling machines and devices, not elsewhere classified

Note: Categories Z89–Z90 and Z93–Z99 are for use only if there are no complications or malfunctions of the organ or tissue replaced, the amputation site or the equipment on which the patient is dependent.

Guideline I.C.21.c.4. History (of): There are two types of history Z codes, personal and family. Personal history codes explain a patient's past medical condition that no longer exists and is not receiving any treatment, but that has the potential for recurrence, and therefore may require continued monitoring.

Family history codes are for use when a patient has a family member(s) who has had a particular disease that causes the patient to be at higher risk of also contracting the disease.

Personal history codes may be used in conjunction with follow-up codes and family history codes may be used in conjunction with screening codes to explain the need for a test or procedure. History codes are also acceptable on any medical record

(Continued)

(Continued)

regardless of the reason for visit. A history of an illness, even if no longer present, is important information that may alter the type of treatment ordered.

The history Z code categories are:

Z80, Family history of primary malignant neoplasm

Z81, Family history of mental and behavioral disorders

Z82, Family history of certain disabilities and chronic diseases (leading to disablement)

Z83, Family history of other specific disorders

Z84, Family history of other conditions

Z85, Personal history of malignant neoplasm

Z86, Personal history of certain other diseases

Z87, Personal history of other diseases and conditions

Z91.4-, Personal history of psychological trauma, not elsewhere classified

Z91.5, Personal history of self-harm

Z91.81, History of falling

Z91.82, Personal history of military deployment

Z92, Personal history of medical treatment

Except: Z92.0, Personal history of contraception

Except: Z92.82, Status post administration of tPA (rtPA) in a different facility within the last 24 hours prior to admission to a current facility

Guideline I.C.21.c.5. Screening: Screening is the testing for disease or disease precursors in seemingly well individuals so that early detection and treatment can be provided for those who test positive for the disease (e.g., screening mammogram).

The testing of a person to rule out or confirm a suspected diagnosis because the patient has some sign or symptom is a diagnostic examination, not a screening. In these cases, the sign or symptom is used to explain the reason for the test.

A screening code may be a first-listed code if the reason for the visit is specifically the screening exam. It may also be used as an additional code if the screening is done during an office visit for other health problems. A screening code is not necessary if the screening is inherent to a routine examination, such as a pap smear done during a routine pelvic examination.

Should a condition be discovered during the screening then the code for the condition may be assigned as an additional diagnosis.

The Z code indicates that a screening exam is planned. A procedure code is required to confirm that the screening was performed.

The screening Z codes/categories:

Z11, Encounter for screening for infectious and parasitic diseases

Z12, Encounter for screening for malignant neoplasms

Z13, Encounter for screening for other diseases and disorders

Except: Z13.9, Encounter for screening, unspecified

Z36, Encounter for antenatal screening for mother

Guideline I.C.21.c.6. Observation: There are two observation Z code categories. They are for use in very limited circumstances when a person is being observed for a suspected condition that is ruled out. The observation codes are not for use if an injury or illness or any signs or symptoms related to the suspected condition are present. In such cases the diagnosis/symptom code is used with the corresponding external cause code.

The observation codes are to be used as principal diagnosis only. The only exception to this is when the principal diagnosis is required to be a code from category Z38, Liveborn infants according to place of birth and type of delivery. Then the code from category Z05, Encounter for observation and evaluation of newborn for suspected diseases and conditions ruled out, is sequenced after the Z38. code. Additional codes may be used in addition to the observation code but only if they are unrelated to the suspected condition being observed.

Codes from subcategory Z03.7, Encounter for suspected maternal and fetal conditions ruled out, may either be used as a first-listed or as an additional code assignment depending on the case. They are for use in very limited circumstances on a maternal record when an encounter is for a suspected maternal or fetal condition that is ruled out during that encounter (for example, a maternal or fetal condition may be suspected due to an abnormal test result). These codes should not be used when the condition is confirmed. In those cases, the confirmed condition should be coded. In addition, these codes are not for use if an illness or any signs or symptoms related to the suspected condition or problem are present. In such cases the diagnosis/symptom code is used.

Additional codes may be used in addition to the code from subcategory Z03.7, but only if they are unrelated to the suspected condition being evaluated.

Codes from subcategory Z03.7 may not be used for encounters for antenatal screening of mother. *See Section I.C.21. Screening.*

(Continued)

(Continued)

For encounters for suspected fetal condition that are inconclusive following testing and evaluation, assign the appropriate code from category O35, O36, O40 or O41.

The observation Z code categories:

Z03, Encounter for medical observation for suspected diseases and conditions ruled out

Z04, Encounter for examination and observation for other reasons

Except: Z04.9, Encounter for examination and observation for unspecified reason

Z05, Encounter for observation and evaluation of newborn for suspected diseases and conditions ruled out

Guideline I.C.21.c.7. Aftercare: Aftercare visit codes cover situations when the initial treatment of a disease has been performed and the patient requires continued care during the healing or recovery phase, or for the long-term consequences of the disease. The aftercare Z code should not be used if treatment is directed at a current, acute disease. The diagnosis code is to be used in these cases. Exceptions to this rule are codes Z51.0, Encounter for antineoplastic radiation therapy, and codes from subcategory Z51.1, Encounter for antineoplastic chemotherapy and immunotherapy. These codes are to be first-listed, followed by the diagnosis code when a patient's encounter is solely to receive radiation therapy, chemotherapy, or immunotherapy for the treatment of a neoplasm. If the reason for the encounter is more than one type of antineoplastic therapy, code Z51.0 and a code from subcategory Z51.1 may be assigned together, in which case one of these codes would be reported as a secondary diagnosis.

The aftercare Z codes should also not be used for aftercare for injuries. For aftercare of an injury, assign the acute injury code with the appropriate 7th character (for subsequent encounter).

The aftercare codes are generally first-listed to explain the specific reason for the encounter. An aftercare code may be used as an additional code when some type of aftercare is provided in addition to the reason for admission and no diagnosis code is applicable. An example of this would be the closure of a colostomy during an encounter for treatment of another condition.

Aftercare codes should be used in conjunction with other aftercare codes or diagnosis codes to provide better detail on the specifics of an aftercare encounter visit, unless otherwise directed by the classification. Should a patient receive multiple types of antineoplastic therapy during the same encounter, code Z51.0, Encounter for antineoplastic radiation therapy, and codes from subcategory Z51.1, Encounter for antineoplastic chemotherapy and immunotherapy, may be used together on a record. The sequencing of multiple aftercare codes depends on the circumstances of the encounter.

Certain aftercare Z code categories need a secondary diagnosis code to describe the resolving condition or sequelae. For others, the condition is included in the code title.

Additional Z code aftercare category terms include fitting and adjustment, and attention to artificial openings.

Status Z codes may be used with aftercare Z codes to indicate the nature of the aftercare. For example code Z95.1, Presence of aortocoronary bypass graft, may be used with code Z48.812, Encounter for surgical aftercare following surgery on the circulatory system, to indicate the surgery for which the aftercare is being performed. A status code should not be used when the aftercare code indicates the type of status, such as using Z43.0, Encounter for attention to tracheostomy, with Z93.0, Tracheostomy status.

The aftercare Z category/codes:

Z42, Encounter for plastic and reconstructive surgery following medical procedure or healed injury

Z43, Encounter for attention to artificial openings

Z44, Encounter for fitting and adjustment of external prosthetic device

Z45, Encounter for adjustment and management of implanted device

Z46, Encounter for fitting and adjustment of other devices

Z47, Orthopedic aftercare

Z48, Encounter for other postprocedural aftercare

Z49, Encounter for care involving renal dialysis

Z51, Encounter for other aftercare

Guideline I.C.21.c.8. Follow-up: The follow-up codes are used to explain continuing surveillance following completed treatment of a disease, condition, or injury. They imply that the condition has been fully treated and no longer exists. They should not be confused with aftercare codes, or injury codes with a 7th character for subsequent encounter, that explain ongoing care of a healing condition or its sequelae. Follow-up codes may be used in conjunction with history codes to provide the full picture of the healed condition and its treatment. The follow-up code is sequenced first, followed by the history code.

A follow-up code may be used to explain multiple visits. Should a condition be found to have recurred on the follow-up visit,

(Continued)

(Continued)

then the diagnosis code for the condition should be assigned in place of the follow-up code.

The follow-up Z code categories:

Z08, Encounter for follow-up examination after completed treatment for malignant neoplasm

Z09, Encounter for follow-up examination after completed treatment for conditions other than malignant neoplasm

Z39, Encounter for maternal postpartum care and examination

Guideline I.C.21.c.9. Donor: Codes in category Z52, Donors of organs and tissues, are used for living individuals who are donating blood or other body tissue. These codes are only for individuals donating for others, not for self-donations. They are not used to identify cadaveric donations.

Guideline I.C.21.c.10. Counseling: Counseling Z codes are used when a patient or family member receives assistance in the aftermath of an illness or injury, or when support is required in coping with family or social problems. They are not used in conjunction with a diagnosis code when the counseling component of care is considered integral to standard treatment.

The counseling Z codes/categories:

Z30.0-, Encounter for general counseling and advice on contraception

Z31.5, Encounter for procreative genetic counseling

Z31.6-, Encounter for general counseling and advice on procreation

Z32.2, Encounter for childbirth instruction

Z32.3, Encounter for childcare instruction

Z69, Encounter for mental health services for victim and perpetrator of abuse

Z70, Counseling related to sexual attitude, behavior and orientation

Z71, Persons encountering health services for other counseling and medical advice, not elsewhere classified

Note: Code Z71.84, Encounter for health counseling related to travel, is to be used for health risk and safety counseling for future travel purposes.

Z76.81, Expectant mother prebirth pediatrician visit

Guideline I.C.21.c.11. Encounters for Obstetrical and Reproductive Services: *See Section I.C.15. Pregnancy, Childbirth, and the Puerperium, for further instruction on the use of these codes.*

Z codes for pregnancy are for use in those circumstances when none of the problems or complications included in the codes from the Obstetrics chapter exist (a routine prenatal visit or postpartum care). Codes in category Z34, Encounter for supervision of normal pregnancy, are always first-listed and are not to be used with any other code from the OB chapter.

Codes in category Z3A, Weeks of gestation, may be assigned to provide additional information about the pregnancy. Category Z3A codes should not be assigned for pregnancies with abortive outcomes (categories O00–O08), elective termination of pregnancy (Z33.2), nor for postpartum conditions, as category Z3A is not applicable to these conditions. The date of admission should be used to determine weeks of gestation for inpatient admissions that encompass more than one gestational week.

The outcome of delivery, category Z37, should be included on all maternal delivery records. It is always a secondary code. Codes in category Z37 should not be used on the newborn record.

Z codes for family planning (contraceptive) or procreative management and counseling should be included on an obstetric record either during the pregnancy or the postpartum stage, if applicable.

Z codes/categories for obstetrical and reproductive services:

Z30, Encounter for contraceptive management

Z31, Encounter for procreative management

Z32.2, Encounter for childbirth instruction

Z32.3, Encounter for childcare instruction

Z33, Pregnant state

Z34, Encounter for supervision of normal pregnancy

Z36, Encounter for antenatal screening of mother

Z3A, Weeks of gestation

Z37, Outcome of delivery

Z39, Encounter for maternal postpartum care and examination

Z76.81, Expectant mother prebirth pediatrician visit

Guideline. I.C.21.c.12. Newborns and Infants: *See Section I.C.16. Newborn (Perinatal) Guidelines, for further instruction on the use of these codes.*

Newborn Z codes/categories:

Z76.1, Encounter for health supervision and care of foundling

Z00.1-, Encounter for routine child health examination

(Continued)

(Continued)

Z38, Liveborn infants according to place of birth and type of delivery

Guideline I.C.21.c.13. Routine and Administrative Examinations: The Z codes allow for the description of encounters for routine examinations, such as, a general check-up, or, examinations for administrative purposes, such as, a pre-employment physical. The codes are not to be used if the examination is for diagnosis of a suspected condition or for treatment purposes. In such cases the diagnosis code is used. During a routine exam, should a diagnosis or condition be discovered, it should be coded as an additional code. Pre-existing and chronic conditions and history codes may also be included as additional codes as long as the examination is for administrative purposes and not focused on any particular condition.

Some of the codes for routine health examinations distinguish between "with" and "without" abnormal findings. Code assignment depends on the information that is known at the time the encounter is being coded. For example, if no abnormal findings were found during the examination, but the encounter is being coded before test results are back, it is acceptable to assign the code for "without abnormal findings." When assigning a code for "with abnormal findings," additional code(s) should be assigned to identify the specific abnormal finding(s).

Pre-operative examination and pre-procedural laboratory examination Z codes are for use only in those situations when a patient is being cleared for a procedure or surgery and no treatment is given.

The Z codes/categories for routine and administrative examinations:

Z00, Encounter for general examination without complaint, suspected or reported diagnosis

Z01, Encounter for other special examination without complaint, suspected or reported diagnosis

Z02, Encounter for administrative examination

Except: Z02.9, Encounter for administrative examinations, unspecified

Z32.0-, Encounter for pregnancy test

Guideline I.C.21.c.14. Miscellaneous Z Codes: The miscellaneous Z codes capture a number of other health care encounters that do not fall into one of the other categories. Certain of these codes identify the reason for the encounter; others are for use as additional codes that provide useful information on circumstances that may affect a patient's care and treatment.

Prophylactic Organ Removal: For encounters specifically for prophylactic removal of an organ (such as prophylactic removal of breasts due to a genetic susceptibility to cancer or a family history of cancer), the principal or first-listed code should be a code from category Z40, Encounter for prophylactic surgery, followed by the appropriate codes to identify the associated risk factor (such as genetic susceptibility or family history).

If the patient has a malignancy of one site and is having prophylactic removal at another site to prevent either a new primary malignancy or metastatic disease, a code for the malignancy should also be assigned in addition to a code from subcategory Z40.0, Encounter for prophylactic surgery for risk factors related to malignant neoplasms. A Z40.0 code should not be assigned if the patient is having organ removal for treatment of a malignancy, such as the removal of the testes for the treatment of prostate cancer.

Miscellaneous Z codes/categories:

Z28, Immunization not carried out

Except: Z28.3, Underimmunization status

Z29, Encounter for other prophylactic measures

Z40, Encounter for prophylactic surgery

Z41, Encounter for procedures for purposes other than remedying health state

Except: Z41.9, Encounter for procedure for purposes other than remedying health state, unspecified

Z53, Persons encountering health services for specific procedures and treatment, not carried out

Z55, Problems related to education and literacy

Z56, Problems related to employment and unemployment

Z57, Occupational exposure to risk factors

Z58, Problems related to physical environment

Z59, Problems related to housing and economic circumstances

Z60, Problems related to social environment

Z62, Problems related to upbringing

Z63, Other problems related to primary support group, including family circumstances

Z64, Problems related to certain psychosocial circumstances

Z65, Problems related to other psychosocial circumstances

Z72, Problems related to lifestyle

Note: These codes should be assigned only when the documentation specifies that the patient has an associated problem.

Z73, Problems related to life management difficulty

(Continued)

(Continued)

Z74, Problems related to care provider dependency

Except: Z74.01, Bed confinement status

Z75, Problems related to medical facilities and other health care

Z76.0, Encounter for issue of repeat prescription

Z76.3, Healthy person accompanying sick person

Z76.4, Other boarder to healthcare facility

Z76.5, Malingerer [conscious simulation]

Z91.1-, Patient's noncompliance with medical treatment and regimen

Z91.83, Wandering in diseases classified elsewhere

Z91.84-, Oral health risk factors

Z91.89, Other specified personal risk factors, not elsewhere classified

See Section I.B.14 for Z55–Z65, Persons with potential health hazards related to socioeconomic and psychosocial circumstances, documentation by clinicians other than the patient's provider

Guideline I.C.21.c.15. Nonspecific Z Codes: Certain Z codes are so non-specific, or potentially redundant with other codes in the classification, that there can be little justification for their use in the inpatient setting. Their use in the outpatient setting should be limited to those instances when there is no further documentation to permit more precise coding. Otherwise, any sign or symptom or any other reason for visit that is captured in another code should be used.

Nonspecific Z codes/categories:

Z02.9, Encounter for administrative examinations, unspecified

Z04.9, Encounter for examination and observation for unspecified reason

Z13.9, Encounter for screening, unspecified

Z41.9, Encounter for procedure for purposes other than remedying health state, unspecified

Z52.9, Donor of unspecified organ or tissue

Z86.59, Personal history of other mental and behavioral disorders

Z88.9, Allergy status to unspecified drugs, medicaments and biological substances status

Z92.0, Personal history of contraception

Guideline I.C.21.c.16. Z Codes That May Only be Principal/First-Listed Diagnosis: The following Z codes/categories may only be reported as the principal/first-listed diagnosis, except when there are multiple encounters on the same day and the medical records for the encounters are combined:

Z00, Encounter for general examination without complaint, suspected or reported diagnosis

Except: Z00.6

Z01, Encounter for other special examination without complaint, suspected or reported diagnosis

Z02, Encounter for administrative examination

Z03, Encounter for medical observation for suspected diseases and conditions ruled out

Z04, Encounter for examination and observation for other reasons

Z33.2, Encounter for elective termination of pregnancy

Z31.81, Encounter for male factor infertility in female patient

Z31.82, Encounter for Rh incompatibility status

Z31.83, Encounter for assisted reproductive fertility procedure cycle

Z31.84, Encounter for fertility preservation procedure

Z34, Encounter for supervision of normal pregnancy

Z38, Liveborn infants according to place of birth and type of delivery

Z39, Encounter for maternal postpartum care and examination

Z40, Encounter for prophylactic surgery

Z42, Encounter for plastic and reconstructive surgery following medical procedure or healed injury

Z51.0, Encounter for antineoplastic radiation therapy

Z51.1-, Encounter for antineoplastic chemotherapy and immunotherapy

Z52, Donors of organs and tissues

Except: Z52.9, Donor of unspecified organ or tissue

Z76.1, Encounter for health supervision and care of foundling

Z76.2, Encounter for health supervision and care of other healthy infant and child

Z99.12, Encounter for respirator [ventilator] dependence during power failure

Coding Factors Influencing Health Status and Contact with Health Services in ICD-10-CM Chapter 21

The Z codes are intended to provide reasons for healthcare encounters in different types of settings: ambulatory, inpatient, and postacute care. Z codes are diagnosis codes. If a procedure is performed during the encounter, a procedure code is required. The Z code for the reason for the visit does not state that a procedure was performed. Z codes are used for patients who may or may not be sick but need healthcare services for a particular reason. Patients may need care for a current condition. The patient may be receiving prophylactic vaccination or immunization. An organ or tissue donor is identified with a Z code. A patient may need counseling or other services to address a problem that is not a disease or illness. The patient may be at risk for a disease that is identified with a Z code. Many times a coder will use a Z code to describe a condition or problem that has an impact on the patient's health status and need for health services, but the situation described by the Z code is not a current illness or injury. An outline of the Z codes is as follows:

Z00–Z13, Persons encountering health services for examinations

    EXAMPLES: Z00.00, Encounter for general adult medical examination without abnormal findings

                Z00.01, Encounter for general adult medical examination with abnormal findings

Z14–Z15, Genetic carrier and genetic susceptibility to disease

    EXAMPLES: Z14.01, Asymptomatic hemophilia A carrier

                Z15.01, Genetic susceptibility to malignant neoplasm of breast

Z16, Resistance to antimicrobial drugs

    EXAMPLE: Z16.11, Resistance to penicillins

Z17, Estrogen receptor status

    EXAMPLE: Z17.0, Estrogen receptor positive status [ER+]

Z20–Z28, Persons with potential health hazards related to communicable diseases

    EXAMPLES: Z21, Asymptomatic human immunodeficiency virus (HIV) infection

                Z23, Encounter for immunization

Z30–Z39, Persons encountering health services in circumstances related to reproduction

    EXAMPLES: Z30.011, Encounter for initial prescription of contraceptive pills

                Z34.81, Encounter for supervision of other normal pregnancy, first trimester

> Z37.-, Outcome of delivery
> Z38.-, Liveborn infants according to place of birth and type of delivery
> Z3A.-, Weeks of gestation

Z40–Z53, Encounters for other specific health care

> **EXAMPLES:** Z48.22, Encounter for aftercare following kidney transplant
> Z51.11, Encounter for antineoplastic chemotherapy

Z55–Z65, Persons with potential health hazards related to socioeconomic and psychosocial circumstances

> **EXAMPLES:** Z59.5, Extreme poverty
> Z62.0, Inadequate parental supervision and control
> Z66, Do not resuscitate (DNR) status
> Z67.10, Type A blood, Rh positive
> Z67.41, Type O blood, Rh negative
> Z68.41, Body mass index (BMI) 40.0–40.9, adult

Z69–Z76, Persons encountering health services in other circumstances

> **EXAMPLES:** Z71.42, Counseling for family member of alcoholic
> Z72.0, Tobacco use

Z77–Z99, Persons with potential health hazards related to family and personal history and certain conditions influencing health status

> **EXAMPLES:** Z79.4, Long term (current) use of insulin
> Z85.3, Personal history of malignant neoplasm of breast

There is an explanation of the use of the codes with a note at the beginning of Chapter 21: Factors Influencing Health Status and Contact with Health Services (Z00–Z99) that states:

Z codes represent reasons for encounters. A corresponding procedure code must accompany a Z code if a procedure is performed. Categories Z00–Z99 are provided for occasions when circumstances other than a disease, injury or external cause classifiable to categories A00–Y89 are recorded as "diagnoses" or "problems." This can arise in two main ways:

(a) When a person who may or may not be sick encounters the health services for some specific purpose, such as to receive limited care or service for a current condition, to donate an organ or tissue, to receive prophylactic vaccination (immunization), or to discuss a problem which is in itself not a disease or injury.

(b) When some circumstance or problem is present which influences the person's health status but is not in itself a current illness or injury (CDC 2019).

Z code classifications are available for the following situations:

- When a person who is currently not sick uses health services for some purpose, such as acting as a donor, receiving prophylactic care such as an inoculation or vaccination, or receiving counseling on health-related issues.

> **EXAMPLE:** The patient was admitted to donate bone marrow for another patient: Z52.3, Bone marrow donor

- When a person with a resolving disease or injury or one with a chronic long-term condition requiring continuous care encounters the healthcare system for specific aftercare of that disease or injury (for example, chemotherapy for malignancy). A diagnosis or symptom code should be used whenever a current, acute diagnosis is being treated or a sign or symptom is being studied.

> **EXAMPLE:** The patient is admitted for antineoplastic radiation therapy, Z51.0

- When circumstances or problems influence a person's health status but are not in themselves a current illness or injury.

> **EXAMPLE:** Patient visits physician's office with a complaint of chest pain with an undetermined cause; patient is status post open-heart surgery for mitral valve replacement, six months ago: R07.9, Chest pain, unspecified; Z95.2, Presence of prosthetic heart valve

- For newborns, to indicate birth status.

> **EXAMPLE:** Single newborn delivered via cesarean section: Z38.01, Single liveborn delivered by cesarean delivery

Z codes are assigned more frequently in hospital ambulatory care departments and other primary care sites, such as physicians' offices, than in acute inpatient facilities. Z codes may be used as either a first-listed (principal diagnosis code in the inpatient setting) or secondary code depending on the circumstances of the encounter. Certain Z codes may only be used as first listed, others only as secondary codes.

Main Terms

Z codes are indexed in the ICD-10-CM Index to Diseases and Injuries (Alphabetic Index) along with codes for diseases, conditions, and symptoms. It is necessary, however, to become familiar with the main terms in the Alphabetic Index that are related to Z codes. First, the coder should look for main terms in the Alphabetic Index that describe the reason for the encounter or admission. The terms documented in the health record will often not lead to the appropriate code. Then, the coder should ask why the patient is receiving services and what the reason is for the visit.

> **EXAMPLE:** The health record states closure of colostomy: Z43.3, Encounter for attention to colostomy

The statement in the preceding example requires a Z code (Z43.3) because the patient was admitted for attention to an artificial opening. In addition, a procedure code must be assigned for the actual surgical closure.

Figure 24.1 shows how the main terms in the Alphabetic Index to Diseases lead to Z codes. These are examples of words that indicate the reason for an encounter for healthcare services, that is, the patient is at the healthcare provider today to receive "attention to" an artificial opening such as a colostomy or to receive renal or peritoneal "dialysis."

Figure 24.1. **Examples of main terms to use in the Alphabetic Index to locate Z codes**

Admission (encounter)	Donor	Pregnancy
Aftercare	Encounter for	Problem
Attention to	Examination	Prophylactic
Boarder	Exposure	Replacement by artificial or
Care (of)	Fitting (of)	mechanical device or prosthesis of
Carrier (suspected) of	Follow-up	Resistance, resistant
Checking	Healthy	Screening
Chemotherapy	History (personal) of	Status (post)
Contact	Maintenance	Supervision (of)
Contraception, contraceptives	Maladjustment	Test(s)
Counseling	Newborn	Therapy
Dependence	Observation	Transplant(ed)
Dialysis	Outcome of delivery	Unavailability of medical facilities
		Vaccination

Persons Encountering Health Services for Examination (Z00–Z13)

The codes from this section are used for patients who may not be acutely ill but require or request an examination by a healthcare provider for routine physical examinations and other administrative purposes such as examinations for pre-employment, entrance into the military, sports participation, and insurance reasons. Other codes here identify patients who must be observed for suspected conditions that later were proven not to exist or for follow-up examinations following the completed treatment of malignant neoplasms and other health conditions.

Category Z00, Encounter for General Examination without Complaint, Suspected or Reported Diagnosis

The codes in category Z00 describe reasonably healthy adults and children who seek healthcare services for routine examinations, such as a general physical examination. Generally, the codes are only used as first-listed diagnoses. If a diagnosis or condition is identified during the course of the general medical examination, it should be reported as an additional diagnosis code. Pre-existing or chronic conditions, as well as history codes, may also be used as additional diagnoses as long as the examination was for an administrative purpose and not focused on treatment of the medical condition. Nonspecific abnormal findings found at the time of these examinations are classified to categories R70–R94. These codes are indexed in the Alphabetic Index under Admission, Encounter, Evaluation, Examination and Test.

In subcategory Z00.0, Encounter for general adult medical examination, there are two specific codes to distinguish between the examination without abnormal findings and an examination when abnormal findings are identified. In this case, the coder would use an additional code to identify the abnormal finding or disease.

> **EXAMPLE:** A 55-year-old male has an appointment at his primary care physician's office for his annual physical examination. The patient has mild

eczema that is treated with over-the-counter lotions, and he had an inguinal hernia repaired during the past year.

Z00.01, Encounter for general adult medical examination with abnormal findings; Eczema, L30.9. The hernia is not coded because it no longer exists.

Subcategory Z00.1, Encounter for newborn, infant and child health examination, identifies outpatient clinic or doctor office encounters with newborns and young children. Z00.12, Encounter for routine infant or child health examination, identifies a child over 28 days old who the physician may identify as a "well baby" or "well child" visit in the office or clinic when the infant or child does not have an illness but is seen for developmental testing, immunizations, or routine health checkups. Two specific codes, Z00.110, Health examination for newborn under eight days old and Z00.111, Health examination for newborn 8 to 28 days old, were created for specific posthospital newborn care visits in the doctor's office or clinic. Most healthy newborns are discharged from the hospital less than 48 hours after birth. Pediatric care standards recommend an examination by the physician within two days of that discharge or no later than 28 days after birth. During this encounter, the infant is evaluated for feeding, jaundice, hydration, and elimination problems; the clinician also assesses how well mother and infant are interacting, reviews the newborn's laboratory and screening tests, and communicates the plan for healthcare maintenance, future immunizations, and periodic examinations.

Other subcategory codes under Z00 identify examinations for a period of rapid growth in childhood, for adolescent development state, for a potential donor of organ and tissue, and for normal comparison and control in a clinical research program, along with examinations during periods of delayed growth in childhood. Finally, one code, Z00.8, Encounter for other general examination, is used for a health examination in a population survey, for example, a public health study.

Category Z01, Encounter for Other Special Examination without Complaint, Suspected or Reported Condition

Category Z01, Encounter for other special examination without complaint, suspected or reported condition, is used to identify the reason for another type of encounter. A separate procedure code is used to identify the examination or procedure actually performed. Subcategory codes under Z01 are used to code visits for eye and vision examinations, ear and hearing examinations, dental examinations and cleanings, and blood pressure examinations. There are specific codes under subcategory Z01 that state whether or not an abnormal finding was identified during the examination. If there was an abnormal finding, a note reminds the coder to use an additional code to identify the abnormal finding. An example of this is code Z01.411, encounter for gynecological examination with abnormal findings. The coder is reminded with a "use additional code" note to add a code for screening for human papillomavirus, if applicable (Z11.51); for screening vaginal Pap smear, if applicable (Z12.72); and to identify acquired absence of uterus, if applicable (Z90.71-). Again, there are options to report the routine gynecological examination with and without abnormal findings. Codes in this category are indexed Admission for, Encounter for, or Examination, follow-up in the Alphabetic Index.

Another subcategory code, Encounter for other specified special examination, Z01.8-, will be used for preprocedural cardiovascular and respiratory examinations provided to the patient, which include physical examinations as well as visits specifically for radiological examinations, laboratory examinations, and preoperative examinations. Coding guidelines state when coding encounters for routine laboratory or radiology testing in the absence of any signs, symptoms, or associated diagnosis, the coder should assign a code from subcategory Z01. If routine testing is performed during the same encounter as a test to evaluate a sign, symptom, or diagnosis, it is appropriate to assign both the Z code and the codes describing the reason for the nonroutine test. For patients receiving preoperative evaluations only, the coder should sequence first a code from subcategory Z01.81 to describe the pre-op consultation. Then, the coder should assign a code for the condition to describe the reason for the surgery as an additional diagnosis. The coder would also assign an additional code for any diagnosis or problem for which the service is being performed.

> **EXAMPLE:** The patient is examined in the cardiologist's office for a preprocedural cardiovascular examination prior to scheduled surgery for a right hip replacement for osteoarthritis of the right hip. The patient is known to have essential hypertension as well. The codes to be assigned are as follows:
>
> Z01.810, Encounter for preprocedural cardiovascular examination
> M16.11, Osteoarthritis of right hip
> I10, Essential hypertension

The codes in category Z01 are not used for examinations for administrative purposes (Z02.-), for suspected conditions proven not to exist (Z03.-), for laboratory or radiology examinations as a component of general medical examinations (Z00.0-), or for encounters for laboratory, radiology, and imaging examinations for signs and symptoms. In those circumstances when a sign or symptom exists, the code for the sign or symptom should be used instead of the Z01 category codes.

Category Z03, Encounter for Medical Observation for Suspected Diseases and Conditions Ruled Out

Category Z03, Encounter for medical observation for suspected diseases and conditions ruled out, is used when a person without a diagnosis is suspected of having an abnormal condition. The patient does not have any signs or symptoms. However, the patient requires study for the suspected condition. However, test results and examinations prove the condition does not exist or is **ruled out**. Again, if the patient has signs and symptoms of a suspected disease, the coder should assign a code for the sign or symptom instead of the Z03 category codes. Conditions that were ruled out and reported with the Z03 category codes include toxic effect from ingested substance, problem with amniotic fluids in the pregnant female, suspected fetal anomaly, and suspected exposure to biological agents. Codes in this category are indexed "Observation; Suspected condition ruled out" in the Alphabetic Index.

> **EXAMPLE:** The patient was seen in the physician's office with vague complaints that the patient thought was due to new prescription medication she was taking. After examination, the physician ruled out suspected adverse effect from the drug, essential hypertension as well. The codes to be assigned are as follows:
>
> Z03.6, Encounter for observation for suspected toxic effect from ingested substance ruled out

Category Z04, Encounter for Examination and Observation for Other Reasons

Category Z04, Encounter for examination and observation for other reasons, includes encounters primarily for medical legal reasons. This category is used when a person is suspected of having an abnormal condition but does not have signs or symptoms of the condition. The patient is examined and tests may be done, and after study, it is proven that the condition does not exist or it is ruled out. Codes from this category would be assigned to patients who were seen for examination and observation following various events, such as a work accident, other accident, alleged rape, or requested psychiatric examination by authority (usually a court system) and following alleged physical abuse. Codes in this category are indexed Admission, Evaluation, Examination, Observation, or Test in the Alphabetic Index.

> **EXAMPLE:** The male patient is a construction worker who fell on the job at a work site but declared himself unhurt. However, the company sent the patient to the emergency department (ED) to be examined. The ED physician could not find any injuries on the patient and documented that the patient was examined and observed after a work accident, no injuries found.
>
> Z04.2, Encounter for examination and observation following work accident

Category Z05, Encounter for Observation and Evaluation of Newborn for Suspected Diseases and Conditions

Category Z05 codes are used for newborns within the first 28 days of life or during the perinatal period. These codes are used when the newborn is suspected of having an abnormal condition. These infants do not have signs or symptoms of the disease. But the newborn's condition is found not to exist, that is, it is ruled out after examination and observation (CDC 2019).

> **EXAMPLE**: The newborn infant was investigated for a genetic condition that was present in the newborn infant's two older siblings. After study, the genetic condition was not found to exist.
>
> Z05.41, Observation and evaluation of newborn for suspected genetic condition ruled out

Encounter for Follow-up Examination after Completed Treatment for Malignant Neoplasm (Z08) and Encounter for Follow-up Examination after Completed Treatment for Conditions Other Than Malignant Neoplasm (Z09)

Together, Z08 and Z09 category codes are called follow-up codes. The **follow-up codes** are used to explain medical surveillance following completed treatment of a disease, condition, or injury. The code means the patient has been fully treated for the condition that no longer exists. These codes are not the same as the aftercare codes in ICD-10-CM or the injury codes with a seventh character for subsequent encounter, which explain ongoing care of a healing condition or its sequelae. Follow-up codes may be used in conjunction with history codes to provide the full picture of the healed condition and its treatment. The follow-up code is sequenced first, followed by the history code.

A patient may have multiple visits for follow-up for these conditions, and the codes may be used each time. If a condition is found to have recurred during the follow-up visit, a diagnosis code for the condition would be assigned instead of the Z08 or Z09 follow-up code. Two notes appear under category code Z08 to remind the coder to use an additional code for any acquired absence of organ (Z90.-) and an additional code for a personal history of malignant neoplasm (Z85.-). Under category code Z09, a "use additional code" note appears to remind the coder to assign any applicable history of disease code (Z86.-, Z87.-) (CDC 2019). The coder must be aware that these codes are intended to represent the visit of a patient who has completed treatment for a condition and is being "followed" to assure the patient remains disease free. The coder must also be aware the term follow-up as it is intended in ICD-10-CM can be different from what a physician intends to describe when he uses the same phrase. When a physician documents follow-up, the physician may be describing ongoing medical treatment or a recovery phase of the illness or recent surgery.

Categories Z08 and Z09 are to be used only to describe an encounter where the treatment of the condition is completed, and the patient is undergoing surveillance or a checkup to determine if his or her disease-free status continues. When a physician states "follow-up" for hypertension that remains under treatment or follow-up after recent cardiac surgery, the Z09 category is unlikely to be the appropriate set of codes to use. In these circumstances described by the physician, the hypertension under treatment is likely to be coded or a surgical aftercare code may be more appropriate to describe the healing or recovery phase after surgery. Codes in this category are indexed "Examination, follow-up" in the Alphabetic Index.

EXAMPLE: Patient was admitted for follow-up cystoscopy to rule out recurrence of malignant neoplasm of the urinary bladder; patient had a transurethral resection of the bladder one year ago and has been cancer-free to date; cystoscopy revealed no recurrence: Z08, Follow-up examination after completed treatment for malignant neoplasm; Z85.51, History of malignant neoplasm of the urinary bladder. A procedure code would be assigned for the cystoscopy.

Encounter for Screening for Malignant Neoplasms, Z12

Category Z12 is used to describe when a patient is being examined by a screening examination. **Screening** is defined in ICD-10-CM coding guidelines as testing for disease or disease precursors in seemingly well individuals so that early detection and treatment can be provided to those who test positive for the disease (CDC 2019, I.21.C.5). These patients do not have signs of symptoms of a disease. Instead, the screening is intended to detect an unidentified condition so that it can be treated promptly. A note appears with category Z12 codes to use an additional code to identify any family history of malignant neoplasm (Z80.-) as patients with a family history of malignancy puts the patient at higher risk of having the same or related condition (CDC 2019).

Codes in this category that will be used frequently are Z12.11, Encounter for screening for malignant neoplasm of colon or otherwise described as an encounter for a screening colonoscopy, and Z12.31, Encounter for screening mammogram for malignant neoplasm of breast. Two other commonly used codes are Z12.4, Encounter for screening for malignant neoplasm of cervix when the physician performs a screening Pap smear on an asymptomatic female patient, and Z12.72, Encounter for screening for malignant neoplasm of vagina when the physician performs a vaginal Pap smear on a patient who has had a hysterectomy that included the removal of the cervix. If the patient had any signs or symptoms, category codes from Z12 would not be used but rather the diagnosis codes for the signs or symptoms are assigned for the encounter. Codes in this category are indexed Admission, Encounter, Mammogram, Papanicolaou, or Screening in the Alphabetic Index.

EXAMPLE: The 70-year-old male patient visited the outpatient laboratory department with an order from his physician for a screening prostate-specific antigen test with the diagnosis written on the order as "screening for malignant neoplasm of prostate."

Z12.5, Encounter for screening for malignant neoplasm of cervix

Encounter for Screening for Other Diseases and Disorders, Z13

Category Z13 is used to describe a screening procedure on an asymptomatic patient for a condition other than malignant neoplasms. If a patient had signs or symptoms, these conditions would be coded instead of using a Z13 category code. A screening procedure is performed on an asymptomatic patient. The commonly used codes in this category are encounter for screening for certain developmental disorders in childhood (Z13.4-), encounter for screening for osteoporosis (Z13.820), and encounter for screening of traumatic brain injury (Z13.850). Codes in this category are indexed Screening in the Alphabetic Index.

EXAMPLE: The patient is a four-year-old female with an appointment in the Pediatric Assessment center with her mother for screening of global developmental handicaps in childhood.

Z13.42, Encounter for screening for global developmental delays (milestones)

Genetic Carrier and Genetic Susceptibility to Disease (Z14–Z15)

Codes in category Z14, **Genetic carrier**, are intended to describe a patient who is known to carry a particular gene that could cause a disease to be passed on to his or her children. The code does not mean the patient has this particular disease. It also does not mean there is 100 percent certainty that the disease would be passed on genetically to the next generation. The code could be used to explain why a patient is receiving additional monitoring or testing. The codes in this category identify patients who are asymptomatic and symptomatic hemophilia A carriers, cystic fibrosis carriers, and genetic carriers of another disease. Codes in this category are indexed Carrier and Genetic in the Alphabetic Index.

Codes in category Z15, **Genetic susceptibility** to disease, are intended to describe a patient who has a confirmed abnormal gene that makes the patient more susceptible to a particular disease. Subcategory Z15.0, Genetic susceptibility to malignant neoplasm, is used with an additional code for any personal history of malignant neoplasm (Z85.-) if applicable. If the patient has a current malignant neoplasm (C00–C75, C81–C96), the code for the current neoplasm is sequenced first before the genetic susceptibility code. Genetic susceptibility to malignant neoplasms of the breast, ovary, prostate, endometrium, and other specified sites are reported with these subcategory codes. Codes in this category are indexed Genetic; Susceptibility to disease in the Alphabetic Index.

EXAMPLE: The female patient has an appointment with the genetic counselor to review her recent diagnostic studies that confirmed she has genetic susceptibility to a malignant neoplasm of the breast and what further studies or therapies may be appropriate.

Z15.01, Genetic susceptibility to malignant neoplasm of breast

Resistance to Antimicrobial Drugs (Z16)

Category Z16, Resistance to antimicrobial drugs, should be used as an additional code to indicate the **resistance** and nonresponsiveness of a condition to an antimicrobial drug. An important note, "Code first the infection," appears here to identify the type and site of the current infection present in the patient who is known to be resistant to these drugs. If the patient has a methicillin-resistant *Staphylococcus* infection, other codes in ICD-10-CM should be used in place of the Z16 codes, for example, A49.02, Methicillin resistant *Staphylococcus aureus* infection, unspecified site; J15.212, Pneumonia due to Methicillin resistant *Staphylococcus aureus*; and A41.02, Sepsis due to Methicillin resistant *Staphylococcus aureus*. The coder should sequence the infection code first and then the Z16 code. Z16 codes are to be used when the documentation in the health record indicates that a patient's infection has a known causative bacteria or other organism that is resistant to the medication therapy administered. Subcategory Z16.1 is used to identify patients with resistance to beta-lactam antibiotics, such as penicillins and cephalosporins. Subcategory Z16.2 is used to identify patients with resistance to other antibiotics, such as vancomycins, vancomycin-related antibiotics, quinolones, or other multiple or single specified antibiotics. Subcategory Z16.3 is used to identify resistance in a patient to such drugs as antiparasitic, antifungal, or antimycobacterial preparations. The organism resistance codes are indexed under the main term "Resistance, resistant, organism (to) drug, followed by the drug" type or name.

> **EXAMPLE:** The patient was hospitalized and treated for vancomycin-resistant sepsis that required treatment with other specific antibiotics. The diagnosis codes to be used for this patient are as follows:
>
> A41.9, Sepsis
> Z16.21, Resistant to vancomycin

Estrogen Receptor Status (Z17)

The status codes Z17.0, Estrogen receptor positive status [ER+], or Z17.1, Estrogen receptor negative status [ER–], are used as an additional code for patients who have been diagnosed with breast cancer, both females and males, and have had their estrogen receptor status determined. About two-thirds of breast cancer patients have an estrogen receptor–positive [ER+] tumor (ACS 2017). The incidence is greater among postmenopausal women. These patients are more likely to benefit from endocrine therapies, so knowledge of their receptor status is important in the selection of adjuvant or palliative therapy. Oral hormones, such as tamoxifen, and estrogen ablation by oophorectomy have proven effective to prolong the duration of disease-free survival, as well as for palliation in the patient with advanced disease when the patient's tumor was estrogen receptor positive. Codes in this category are indexed "Status" in the Alphabetic Index.

> **EXAMPLE:** The patient is a 70-year-old female who was diagnosed with carcinoma of the right breast, upper-inner quadrant and was found to have estrogen receptor–positive status. The diagnosis codes for the patient are as follows:
>
> C50.211, Malignant neoplasm of upper-inner quadrant of right female breast
> Z17.0, Estrogen receptor positive status [ER+]

Retained Foreign Body Fragment (Z18)

Category Z18 contains codes created for embedded foreign body fragment status to identify the type of embedded material. The codes were requested primarily to identify military personnel who have had an injury, most likely from an explosion that resulted in embedded fragments remaining in the body because the location of the fragment makes it too difficult to remove. Any embedded object has the potential to cause infection due to the object itself or any organism present on it when it entered the body. An embedded magnetic object is a contraindication to certain imaging studies and can pose long-term toxicological hazards. Codes in the range of Z18.0–Z18.9 identify radioactive, metal, plastic, organic, and other types of foreign body fragments. Another code, Z87.821, identifies the personal history of a retained foreign body having been removed. An Excludes1 note appears under category Z18 to direct the coder to other ICD-10-CM diagnosis codes that describe other types of foreign body that may be present in the patient. Codes in this category are indexed Retained in the Alphabetic Index.

EXAMPLE: The 26-year-old male patient was seen in the physician's office for a pre-employment physical. The patient told the physician that he had bullet fragments near his spine from a gunshot wound 10 years ago. The physician confirms the presence of nonmagnetic fragments in the patient's lower back. The diagnosis codes for this visit are as follows:

Z02.1, Encounter for pre-employment examination
Z18.12, Retained nonmagnetic metal fragments

Check Your Understanding 24.1

Assign diagnosis codes for the following conditions.

1. Emergency department visit for examination and observation following an alleged adult rape

2. Outpatient visit for screening routine mammogram for malignant neoplasm of the breast

3. Office visit for screening for depression

4. Office visit for general adult medical annual physical examination with elevated blood pressure readings

5. Specialty center visit for screening for autism in a 5-year-old child

---

Persons with Potential Health Hazards Related to Communicable Diseases (Z20–Z28)

Codes from categories Z20–Z28 are assigned when a patient has come in contact with, or has been exposed to, a communicable disease. The person does not show any signs or symptoms of the disease he or she was exposed to or came in contact with.

Category Z20, Contact with and (Suspected) Exposure to Communicable Diseases

The Z20 category codes for contact and exposure or suspected exposure to communicable disease may be used as the first-listed code to explain an encounter for testing. However, these

codes may be used more commonly as secondary codes to identify a potential health risk. The types of communicable disease that the patient may have come in contact with include *Escherichia coli* intestinal disease, tuberculosis, sexually transmitted disease, rabies, rubella, viral hepatitis, HIV, anthrax, varicella, and other and unspecified communicable diseases. Codes in this category are indexed Contact and Exposure in the Alphabetic Index.

> **EXAMPLE:** The patient was seen in his physician's office to be evaluated for pulmonary tuberculosis. His brother recently visited, and after the brother returned home, he was diagnosed with pulmonary tuberculosis, so the patient was concerned that he may have contract the disease from his brother. The physician ordered diagnostic tests and recommended the patient stay at home until his follow-up visit with the physician in five days. The physician documented the diagnosis for this visit as "contact and suspected exposure to tuberculosis."
>
> Z20.1, Contact with and (suspected) exposure to tuberculosis

Category Z21, Asymptomatic Human Immunodeficiency Virus (HIV) Infection Status

The Z21 code indicates that the patient has tested positive for the HIV virus but has not manifested symptoms of HIV or AIDS. The health record documentation may include "HIV positive." This code should not be confused with code B20, human immunodeficiency virus [HIV] disease or AIDS, which means that the patient has the consequences of human immunodeficiency virus in the blood that causes the patient to have certain neoplasms or infections as a result of the patient's immune-compromised condition. A "code first" note appears under code Z21 to code HIV disease complicating pregnancy, childbirth, and the puerperium, if applicable, with O98.7-. Codes in this category are indexed HIV, Human, Status, or Test in the Alphabetic Index.

> **EXAMPLE:** The patient was seen in his primary care physician's office to discuss his recent laboratory result showing the presence of the HIV virus in his blood. The patient has no signs or symptoms of the disease or other infections. The physician documented "HIV positive" as the patient's visit diagnosis.
>
> Z21, Asymptomatic human immunodeficiency virus [HIV] infection status.

Category Z22, Carrier of Infectious Disease

The Z22 category codes describe colonization status or the presence on or in the body of a particular organism without it causing an illness in the patient. Codes within this category recognize carrier status for typhoid, diphtheria, specific bacterial diseases, sexually transmitted disease, viral hepatitis, and other viral and infectious diseases. Some of the commonly used codes in this category are Z22.330, Carrier of group B streptococcus; Z22.321, Carrier or suspected carrier of Methicillin susceptible *Staphylococcus aureus* (MSSA); Z22.322, Carrier or suspected carrier Methicillin resistant *Staphylococcus aureus* (MRSA); and Z22.52, Carrier of viral hepatitis C. Many hospitals test patients routinely for MRSA colonization by performing a nasal swab test upon admission that can identify positive or negative MRSA colonization in the patient.

The category Z22 codes indicate that the patient is either a carrier or a suspected carrier of an infectious disease but currently does not exhibit the symptoms of the disease. Status codes in the Z code classification are informational because the conditions they describe may affect the course of treatment. Remember, "status" is different from "history" in ICD-10-CM. The history codes indicate the patient no longer has the disease. Codes in this category are indexed Carrier, and Colonization in the Alphabetic Index.

> **EXAMPLE:** The patient was seen in her primary care physician's office to follow-up on recent laboratory testing that determined she was a carrier of Methicillin resistant *Staphylococcus aureus (MRSA)* or has MRSA colonization
>
> Z22.322, Carrier or suspected carrier of Methicillin resistant *Staphylococcus aureus*

Categories Z23, Encounter for Immunization and Z28, Immunization Not Carried Out and Underimmunization Status

These codes are located in the Alphabetic Index under the main terms Admissions, Immunization, Prophylactic, and Vaccination.

> **EXAMPLE:** The child was brought to the pediatrician's office for the regularly scheduled infant immunizations. The physician documented the visit for immunization.
>
> Z23, Encounter for immunization

Category Z23, Encounter for immunization, is a three-character code that is used for any encounter when the purpose of the visit is to receive any prophylactic inoculation against a disease. A procedure code must also be used to show the inoculation occurred. Vaccinations and inoculation codes may be used as secondary codes during well-baby or well-child care visits if the service was given as part of routine preventive healthcare. The type of vaccine administered is not identified by diagnosis code Z23. Under category code Z23 is a "code first" note to code any routine child examination.

Category Z28, Immunization Not Carried Out and Underimmunization Status

Codes Z28.01 through Z28.9 describe specific reasons why an immunization or vaccination was not given. The reasons an immunization may not be given are medical contraindications, for example, the patient has an acute or chronic illness or an allergy, or the patient is immune compromised, which are all reasons not to receive vaccinations. Other reasons are patient's decisions not to become immunized for reasons of belief or group pressure or simply because the patient refuses the vaccination. Other reasons identified with the codes are the fact that the patient has already had the illness the vaccine is intended to prevent or the immunization was not carried out because of the caregiver's, parent's, or guardian's refusal to have it done or due to the unavailability of the vaccine. Tracking why an immunization was not given can be as important as tracking those that are given, according to the American Academy of Pediatrics. These codes identify the multiple reasons why a patient did not receive a routine immunization. Another important health status that can be identified with these codes is the fact that the person or child is "underimmunized." Code Z28.3, **Underimmunization** status, identifies the patient who has not received the vaccinations that are appropriate for the person's age. It is a level of immunization that is suboptimal for a person or population (AHA 2009, 115). The doctor may describe this status in the record as "delinquent immunization status" or "lapsed immunization scheduled status." These codes are located in the Alphabetic Index under the main terms Delayed, Delinquent immunization status, Immunization, Lapsed immunization status, Status, Underimmunization status, or Vaccination.

> **EXAMPLE:** The child was brought to the pediatrician's office by her mother to ask the physician what vaccinations did her child need to catch up with as the family had moved to the city but had not been to a physician's office until this date. The physician documented that the child's reason for the visit was her status as being underimmunized or unvaccinated.
>
> Z28.3, Underimmunization status

Persons Encountering Health Services in Circumstances Related to Reproduction (Z30–Z39)

The codes from this section are used to describe healthcare services related to contraceptive and procreative management. Examples of codes in this section are codes that describe the status of the newborn at the time of the birth including the place where the infant was born and the type of delivery the mother experienced with this newborn. Other codes in this section identify how many infants were born to a mother, such as a single live birth, twins, triplets, and other types of multiple births. Codes in this section are also used to describe the supervision of pregnancy care provided to the pregnant woman during an uncomplicated, normal pregnancy.

Category Z30, Encounter for Contraceptive Management

Category Z30 includes codes for contraceptive management, such as initial prescription of contraceptives, counseling and instruction for natural family planning, and other general contraceptive counseling and advice. Codes from this category are indexed under Contraception, contraceptive, Intrauterine contraceptive device, Planning, family, and Prescription of contraceptives in the Alphabetic Index.

> **EXAMPLE:** Visit to physician for prescription of initial prescription of birth control pills: Z30.011, Encounter for initial prescription of contraceptive pills

Code Z30.2, Encounter for sterilization, is often assigned as an additional diagnosis when a sterilization procedure is performed during the same admission as a delivery. It may also be assigned as a principal diagnosis when the admission is solely for sterilization.

> **EXAMPLE:** Spontaneous delivery of full-term live infant with tubal ligation performed the day after delivery: O80, Encounter for full-term uncomplicated delivery; Z37.0, Outcome of delivery, single live birth; Z30.2, Encounter for sterilization with a procedure code to describe the specific delivery and sterilization procedure

> **EXAMPLE:** Patient desires permanent sterilization:
>
> Z30.2 with a procedure code for the specific sterilization procedure performed

Subcategory codes Z30.4 are used to report encounters for surveillance of contraceptives, which include encounters for repeat prescription for contraceptive pills as well as surveillance of injectable contraceptive. These subcategory codes are frequently used for office visits when the encounter is for the insertion of an intrauterine device (IUD) (Z30.430), for removal of an IUD (Z30.432), and for removal and reinsertion of an IUD (Z30.433). An encounter for routine checking of an IUD would be reported with code Z30.431, Encounter for routine checking of intrauterine contraceptive device.

Category Z31, Encounter for Procreative Management

Procreative management describes healthcare services related to providing reproductive fertility services. Services related to genetic testing and infertility services can be described with these codes. Screening for genetic carrier status is becoming more commonplace to identify individuals for certain serious genetic disease. For example, a couple may be screened either preconception or early in pregnancy to determine carrier status. If both partners are carriers, different pregnancy management may be instituted. Because most of the individuals are noncarriers, it is inappropriate to use disease codes to describe the screening encounter; instead, subcategory codes Z31.43- is used to identify an encounter for genetic testing of female for procreative management and/or Z31.4- is used to identify the testing of the male partner for genetic disease carrier status. Other codes within category Z31 identify encounters for genetic counseling and advice on procreation as well as such specific codes as Z31.83 for an encounter for assisted reproductive fertility procedure cycle. Healthcare encounters for reversal of a previous tubal ligation or vasectomy, artificial insemination, procreative investigation and testing, and genetic counseling are also coded within this category. Codes from this category are indexed under Admission, Counseling, Encounter, Test, Tuboplasty, and Vasoplasty in the Alphabetic Index.

EXAMPLE: The female patient was seen today to have genetic testing with her husband prior to discontinuing birth control and attempting to get pregnant. The patient is concerned because she has relatives with sickle cell disease and does not know if she is a carrier of the disease. Her husband will also be tested as he is unaware of his status as well, and there is a history of sickle cell disease in his family too. The diagnosis code for the female patient's visit is:

Z31.430, Encounter of female for testing for genetic disease carrier status for procreative management.

Category Z32, Encounter for Pregnancy Test and Childbirth and Childcare Instruction

Subcategory code Z32.0, Encounter for pregnancy test, contains codes to identify an encounter when the result of a pregnancy test is positive, negative, or unknown. Other codes in this category describe encounters for childbirth and childcare instructions. Codes from this category are indexed under "encounter" in the Alphabetic Index.

Code Z33.1, Pregnant State, Incidental

Code Z33.1, Pregnant state, incidental, is used to identify the fact that a patient is pregnant. This code is used when the provider documents that the pregnancy is incidental or unrelated to the encounter, such as an injury sustained during an accident. In that event, code Z33.1 is used in place of an obstetric code from Chapter 15. It is the provider's responsibility to state that the patient's condition being treated is not affecting the pregnancy. Codes are indexed under the main terms of Abortion, Pregnancy, Status, and Termination in the Alphabetic Index.

Code Z33.2, Encounter for Elective Termination of Pregnancy

Category Z33.2 is used to code the healthcare encounter when a patient has requested an elective abortion for personal reasons or has been recommended to have an elective termination of pregnancy for medical reasons. A procedure code would be used to identify the abortion procedure performed. This code would not be used if the encounter was for the purpose of completing a procedure to terminate the pregnancy because of an early fetal death with retention of the dead fetus, for example, a missed abortion that would be coded O02.1, Missed Abortion. It is also not applicable to the treatment of a patient with a spontaneous incomplete abortion that would be coded with category O03, Spontaneous abortion codes depending on the patient's clinical status. The Alphabetic Index entry for the encounter for elective termination of pregnancy would be "abortion, induced (encounter for)" for an uncomplicated patient.

Category Z34, Encounter for Supervision of Normal Pregnancy

Codes in category Z34 are assigned for supervision of a normal pregnancy. Codes Z34.0, Encounter for supervision of normal first pregnancy, and Z34.8, Encounter for supervision of other normal pregnancy, are generally used in outpatient settings and for routine prenatal visits. The fifth character with these codes identifies whether the patient is in her first, second, or third trimester of pregnancy or unspecified trimester. When a complication of the pregnancy is present, the code for that condition is assigned rather than a code from category Z34. These codes are not used with any other pregnancy code in Chapter 15 of ICD-10-CM because the Z34 code indicates the patient is pregnant and healthy, whereas the Chapter 15 codes indicate an obstetrical problem or condition exists. Code category Z34 is indexed under "Pregnancy, normal, supervision (of) (for)" in the Alphabetic Index to Diseases.

> **EXAMPLE:**   The patient is a 30-year-old female who is in her 22nd week of her first pregnancy and is seen in the obstetrician's office for her monthly evaluation. No problems were identified, and the patient will be seen in four weeks. The diagnosis for this visit is "first pregnancy, normal supervision visit."
>
> Z34.02, Encounter for supervision of normal first pregnancy, second trimester.

Category Z36, Encounter for Antenatal Screening of Mother

Code Z36, Encounter for **antenatal screening** of mother, describes the testing of the female during pregnancy for a variety of conditions and abnormalities. These codes, which are intended to describe the female, not the fetus, are used to indicate that the screening was planned. Some of these screening procedures have become common during the antepartum period. If the screening test results are returned with abnormal findings or determine that a condition is present, the abnormal finding or condition should be coded as an additional code with the Z36 screening category code. The Z36 code is not used if the testing of the female is to rule out or confirm a suspected diagnosis because the patient has some sign or symptom. That is a diagnostic examination, and the sign or symptom code is used to explain the reason for the test. The Z36 code also indicates that the screening examination was planned. A procedure code is required to confirm that the screening was performed, usually this would be a CPT/HCPCS code as these procedures are routinely performed on an outpatient basis. Code category Z36 is indexed under Antenatal, Encounter, Prenatal, and Screening, in the Alphabetic Index to Diseases.

EXAMPLE: The patient is a 32-year-old female who is in her 12th week of her first pregnancy and is seen in the obstetrician's office for the first ultrasound of the pregnant uterus to screen the patient for Streptococcus B. The patient has no symptoms of any problem. The diagnosis for this visit is "antenatal screening for Streptococcus B"

Z36.85, Encounter for antenatal screening, Streptococcus B

Category Z3A, Weeks of Gestation

Codes from category Z3A are used on the mother's record to indicate the weeks of gestation for the current pregnancy, if known. Codes from this category are not to be used on the newborn record. The coder must first assign the diagnosis codes for the complications of pregnancy and childbirth (O09–O9A) with a few exceptions. Category Z3A codes should not be assigned for pregnancies with abortive outcomes (categories O00–O08), elective termination of pregnancy (code Z33.2), nor for postpartum conditions, as category Z3A is not applicable to these conditions. These codes are used at any time during the patient's pregnancy and not just at the time of the delivery. Code category Z3A is indexed under "Pregnancy, weeks of gestation" in the Alphabetic Index to Diseases.

Category Z37, Outcome of Delivery

A code from category Z37, **Outcome of delivery**, should be included on every maternal record when a delivery has occurred. These codes are not to be used on subsequent postpartum records or on the newborn record. They are always secondary codes on the maternal record at the time of delivery. The Z37 code indicates whether the delivery produced a single or multiple birth and whether the infants were live births or stillbirths. The unspecified code, Z37.9, should not be used because the maternal health record will identify the details of the delivery. Codes in category Z37 are indexed under "Outcome of delivery" in the Alphabetic Index.

EXAMPLE: Spontaneous delivery of full-term live infant: O80, Encounter for full-term uncomplicated; Z37.0, Outcome of delivery, single live birth

Category Z37 codes are only assigned to the mother's health record. These codes should not appear on the baby's health record. Do not confuse the Z37 maternal codes with the Z38 liveborn infant codes that are used to describe the newborn's birth status.

Category Z38, Liveborn Infants According to Place of Birth and Type of Delivery

A code from categories Z38.0 through Z38.8 is used to identify all types of births and is always the first code listed on the health record of the newborn. The Z38 code is used "once in a lifetime" when the infant is born. Codes from the Z38 category are not to be used on the maternal record. The Z38 category code is used as the principal code on the initial record of the newborn infant. If the newborn is transferred to another institution, the Z38 code is not used at the second institution or on the infant's subsequent admissions or outpatient visits to any healthcare provider. The Z38 codes describe single or multiple live births and single or multiple stillborns.

Codes for these categories are indexed under Newborn or Infant in the Alphabetic Index. Using the Alphabetic Index and the main term Newborn, born in hospital or born outside of hospital," the next information to be reviewed is the birth status of the infant: single, twin, triplet, quadruplet, quintuplet, or other multiple liveborn infant born to the same mother. If the infant was a single birth, the next information needed is whether the baby was born in or outside the hospital. If the infant was born inside the hospital, was the birth a vaginal or cesarean delivery? In addition to the Z38 category code, any disease or birth injury should also be coded as additional diagnoses, if applicable, on the infant's record.

EXAMPLES: Single male infant, born in hospital by cesarean delivery
Z38.01, Single liveborn infant, delivered by cesarean

Twin liveborn infant, born in hospital delivered vaginally
Z38.30, Twin liveborn infant, delivered vaginally

Triplet liveborn infant, born in hospital by cesarean delivery
Z38.62, Triplet liveborn infant, delivered by cesarean

Check Your Understanding 24.2

Assign diagnosis codes for the following conditions.

1. Carrier of methicillin-resistant *Staphylococcus aureus*

2. Encounter for insertion of intrauterine contraceptive device

3. Encounter for in vitro fertilization cycle (assisted reproductive fertility procedure)

4. Office visit for prophylactic immunotherapy for respiratory syncytial virus

5. Lack of availability of vaccine, immunization not done

Encounters for Other Specific Health Care (Z40–Z53)

CMS includes the following important note for categories Z40–Z53 at the beginning of this block of codes: "Categories Z40–Z53 are intended for use to indicate a reason for care in patients who may have already been treated for some disease or injury not now present, or who are receiving aftercare or prophylactic care consolidate the treatment or to deal with residual states" (CDC 2019).

Category Z40, Encounter for Prophylactic Surgery

A patient who has a genetic susceptibility to a disease, particularly if it is a malignancy, may request prophylactic removal of an organ to prevent the disease from occurring. These codes can be used to identify encounters for prophylactic organ removal, including breast, ovary, or removal of another organ. A note is included to "use additional code" to identify the risk factor leading to this surgery. Codes in category Z40 are indexed under Admission and Prophylactic in the Alphabetic Index.

EXAMPLES: The patient is a 45-year-old female who has a family history of malignant ovarian neoplasm in her mother, sister, and maternal aunt. She has been found to have genetic susceptibility to ovarian carcinoma. The patient has no symptoms of the disease now. However, for family history and genetic reasons, the patient agreed with her physician that a bilateral salpingo-oophorectomy was indicated, and it was completed as an open surgical procedure.

The patient was discharge on postoperative day two (2.) The codes appropriate for this hospital stay are as follows:

Z40.02, Encounter for prophylactic removal of ovary
Z15.02, Genetic susceptibility to malignant neoplasm of ovary
Z80.41, Family history of malignant neoplasm of ovary

Category Z43, Encounter for Attention to Artificial Openings

Category Z43 describes attention to the artificial opening, which may include the following services:

- Closure of artificial openings

- Passage of sounds or bougies through artificial openings

- Reforming of artificial openings

- Removal or replacement of catheter from artificial openings

- Toileting or cleansing of artificial openings

Category Z43 codes may be first-listed diagnoses or used as additional diagnosis codes. These codes identify encounters for catheter cleaning, fitting, and adjustment services and other care that is distinct from actual treatment. These codes are not used when there is a complication of the external stoma. Codes in category Z43 are indexed under Admission, Attention, Change, and Removal in the Alphabetic Index.

EXAMPLES: Emergency department visit for a patient who needs replacement of a clogged gastrostomy tube: Z43.1, Encounter for attention to gastrostomy

A patient is admitted for a scheduled closure of a colostomy: Z43.3, Encounter for attention to colostomy

Encounter for replacement of cystostomy tube: Z43.5, Encounter for attention to cystostomy

Category Z47, Orthopedic Aftercare

Aftercare visits are for patients who have had the initial treatment of their condition, such as surgery, completed and now the patient requires continued care during their recovery period (CDC 2019). Category Z47 is subdivided to describe particular orthopedic **aftercare**. Subcategory code Z47.1 is used to describe an encounter for aftercare following joint replacement surgery. An additional code is used with Z47.1 to identify the joint (Z96.6-). Subcategory Z47.2, Encounter for removal of internal fixation device, is used to code the reason for the visit when a fixation device, such as a screw, plate, or pin, for example, is removed from the body. Subcategory code Z47.3 is subdivided to identify aftercare following explantation of joint prosthesis, specifically the shoulder joint, hip joint, or knee joint. The intent of these codes is to identify the healthcare encounter for the patient who has had their artificial joint removed, usually because of an infection in the joint or another complication. Other codes in this category identify encounters for orthopedic aftercare following surgical amputation, scoliosis surgery, or other specified orthopedic care. Codes in category Z47 are indexed under Aftercare and Encounter in the Alphabetic Index.

EXAMPLE: The patient is a 16-year-old female who is one week post-op following surgery to correct the scoliosis of her spine. The patient is recovering well from the surgery and has no complaints. The patient's mother will return to the office in two weeks to evaluate the patient's healing and determine when the patient can return to school. The diagnosis documented for this visit was "Follow-up visit to evaluate postoperative status, scoliosis surgery, normal healing in progress."

Z47.82, Encounter for orthopedic aftercare following scoliosis surgery

Category Z48, Encounter for Other Postprocedural Aftercare

Subcategory Z48.0 would be used for an encounter for change or removal of nonsurgical and surgical wound dressing. Typically, these encounters occur in a physician's office, in an ambulatory clinic or center, or during a home healthcare visit. Code Z48.00 is intended to describe the encounter for the change or removal of a nonsurgical wound dressing. The encounter for the change or removal of a surgical wound dressing or packing is code Z48.01. An encounter for the purpose of removing sutures or staples would be reported with code Z48.02.

Broad categories exist for aftercare following organ transplant (Z48.2-) and surgical aftercare following surgery on specified body systems (Z48.8-). The aftercare codes are usually reported outside the acute-care hospital setting to identify the postsurgical treatment after the initial treatment and surgery is completed. This postsurgical care may be received in a long-term care hospital or facility or through home care services. Codes in category Z48 are indexed under Aftercare Attention, Change, and Removal in the Alphabetic Index.

EXAMPLE: The patient is a 50-year-old female who was seen in the surgeon's office five days after being discharged from the hospital following abdominal surgery. The surgeon removed the postoperative drain that was left in the patient and inspected the surgical wound that was healing well. The patient was advised to return to the office in one week. The diagnosis given by the physician for this visit was: Drain removal, postsurgical status.

Z48.03, Encounter for change or removal of drain

Category Z49, Encounter for Care Involving Renal Dialysis

Z49 codes are used to identify the main reason for the encounter, for example, preparatory care for renal dialysis. Specifically, the fitting and adjustment of an extracorporeal dialysis catheter or peritoneal dialysis catheter are included in subcategory Z49.0-. An encounter for adequacy testing for hemodialysis or peritoneal dialysis is coded with a subcategory code from Z49.3-. The note "Code also associated end-stage renal disease (N18.6)" appears under the category heading for Z49. Codes in category Z49 are indexed under Management Preparatory care and Test in the Alphabetic Index.

EXAMPLE: The patient is a 62-year-old male who has end-stage renal disease and is seen in the renal clinic today for cleansing of his renal dialysis catheter completed by flushing with prepared fluids. The diagnosis included by the physician in the daily progress note was "management of renal dialysis catheter."

Z49.01, Encounter for filling and adjustment of extracorporeal dialysis catheter
N18.6, End stage renal disease

Category Z51, Encounter for Other Aftercare

Category Z51 includes codes for admissions or encounters for antineoplastic radiotherapy, antineoplastic chemotherapy, and immunotherapy; encounters for palliative care; and other specified aftercare. Codes in category Z51 are indexed under Admission Aftercare, Care, Chemotherapy, Encounter, Maintenance, Monitoring, Palliative, Radiotherapy, and Radiation in the Alphabetic Index.

Codes Z51.0, Encounter for antineoplastic radiation therapy, and codes from subcategory Z51.1, Encounter for antineoplastic chemotherapy and immunotherapy, are to be first listed, followed by the diagnosis code when a patient's encounter is solely to receive radiation therapy, chemotherapy, or immunotherapy for the treatment of a neoplasm. If the reason for the encounter is more than one type of antineoplastic therapy, code Z51.0 and a code from subcategory Z51.1 may be assigned together, in which case one of these codes would be reported as a secondary diagnosis.

> **EXAMPLE:** Admission for chemotherapy for patient with metastasis to bone; patient has history of breast carcinoma with mastectomy performed eight years ago:
>
> Z51.1, Encounter for antineoplastic chemotherapy;
> C79.51, Secondary malignant neoplasm of bone;
> Z85.3, Personal history of malignant neoplasm of breast. A procedure code would be assigned for the chemotherapy administration.

Code Z51.5 describes an encounter for palliative care. Code Z51.5 is a code for a patient receiving palliative care for a terminal condition or end-of-life diseases. Code Z51.5, would be used as the principal diagnosis when palliative care is the reason for the patient's admission. Code Z51.5 can be used for long-term care facility admissions and home health services where it would be the first-listed diagnosis when the patient's admission is for the purpose of receiving palliative care. This code would not likely be the principal diagnosis in the inpatient hospital setting. In many cases, it would be more appropriate as a secondary diagnosis in the acute care setting. Palliative care may be a decision made in the hospital and then coded as an additional diagnosis when it is determined that palliative care will be initiated and no further treatment for the terminal illness is desired. There is no time limit or minimum for the use of this code assignment. The patient's underlying condition, such as carcinoma, heart failure, COPD, Alzheimer's disease, or AIDS, should also be coded. Code Z51.81, Encounter for therapeutic drug level monitoring, is the correct code to use when a patient visit is for the purpose of undergoing a laboratory test to measure the drug level in the patient's blood or urine or to measure a specific function to assess the effectiveness of a drug. Z51.81 code may be used alone if the monitoring is for a drug that the patient is on for only a brief period, not long term. However, there is a "code also" note under this code to code any long-term (current) drug therapy (Z79.-) to indicate what drug is being monitored.

Category Z52, Donors of Organs and Tissues

Codes from category Z52, Donors, are used for living individuals who are donating blood, tissue, or an organ to be transplanted into another individual. Z52 codes are not used when the potential donor is examined (code Z00.5). Also, these codes are not used for cadaveric donations, that is, when a patient's organ(s) are harvested at the time of death according to the patient's stated wishes. These codes are only for individuals donating for others with the exception of Z52.01- for autologous blood donors. They are not used to identify cadaveric donations. Subcategory codes identify the donor of blood, skin, bone, bone marrow, kidney, cornea, and liver. Codes in category Z52 are indexed under Donor in the Alphabetic Index.

There are also codes for egg or oocyte donors that identify the age of the donor and whether the eggs are intended to be used for anonymous donations or for a designated recipient. Codes Z52.810–Z52.819 identify the age of the egg or oocyte donor (either younger than age 35 years or aged 35 years or older) and specify whether the intended recipient is anonymous or designated.

EXAMPLE: The patient is a 40-year-old healthy female who is donating her left kidney as she is a "match" for her 45-year-old sister who suffers from end-stage renal disease. She was discharged from the hospital five days after the left nephrectomy was performed on her in order to be transplanted into her sister. Her final diagnosis on the inpatient record was "kidney donor."

Z52.4, Kidney donor

Category Z53, Persons Encountering Health Services for Specific Procedures and Treatment, Not Carried Out

Codes Z53.01 and Z53.09 state that a procedure or treatment was not carried out because of a contraindication. A contraindication is any medical condition that renders some form of treatment improper or undesirable (Dorland 2012, 410). For example, the patient may have an infection, cardiac condition, or abnormal diagnostic test that would make performing the surgical procedure unsafe until the contraindication is resolved.

The patient may also decide, sometimes at the last minute before surgery begins, that he or she does not want the surgery or procedure performed at this time and the procedure is cancelled. Codes in subcategories Z53.20–Z53.29 identify when a patient decides not to have a procedure by leaving prior to being seen by healthcare provider or decides against the procedure for some reason. Subcategory codes Z53.3 identify procedures that are converted to open procedures, including, Z53.31, Laparoscopic surgical procedure converted to open procedure; Z53.32, Thoracoscopic surgical procedure converted to open procedure; Z53.33, Arthroscopic surgical procedure converted to open procedure; and Z53.39, Other surgical procedure converted to open procedure. Two other codes, Z53.8 and Z53.9, are available to identify the scenarios where a procedure or treatment is not carried out for another reason or for an unspecified reason. Codes in category Z53 are indexed under Canceled procedure, Procedure, and Refusal in the Alphabetic Index.

EXAMPLE: The patient was a 44-year-old male who arrived at the ambulatory surgery center in the morning for his scheduled right inguinal hernia repair. He checked in at the registration desk, completed the paperwork, and was taken to the surgical preparation area by the nurse. After showing him to his room, the nurse left to gather supplies, and when she returned, the man was gone. Another staff member saw him leave. When the nurse called his cell phone, the patient said he decided not to have the surgery and was going home. The patient called the physician who later documented in the record: right inguinal hernia, surgery canceled by patient's decision, unknown reason.

K40.90, Unilateral inguinal hernia, without obstruction or gangrene, not specified as recurrent
Z53.20, Procedure and treatment not carried out because of patient's decision (for unspecified reason)

Persons with Potential Health Hazards Related to Socioeconomic and Psychosocial Circumstances (Z55–Z65)

Codes from the categories in this section are likely to be used to describe patients who require counseling or other social and supportive services for factors that are not specific health conditions but represent situations that influence physical and emotional health statuses.

Category Z59, Problems Related to Housing and Economic Circumstances

Codes in category Z59 are used primarily as additional diagnosis codes to further explain the socioeconomic factors that may be influencing the patient's need for healthcare services. The codes in this category may be used to describe circumstances that lead to the disruption of the family unit and create the need for specific healthcare services. For example, code Z59.0 identifies the patient as being homeless, which will impact the care and management of the patient by the healthcare provider. Codes in category Z59 are indexed under Counseling, Discord, Economic, Financial, Homelessness Inadequate, Insufficiency, Lack, Low, and Social in the Alphabetic Index.

EXAMPLE: An 88-year-old female was brought to the ED by the police after being asked to conduct a well-being check by neighbors. The police found the lady in an unheated home with structural defects that appeared to make it unsafe for someone to live there. The ED physician found the woman to have heart failure and chronic kidney disease due to hypertension. The patient was admitted to the hospital for treatment and through the efforts of the social worker was able to discharge the patient to an extended care facility. The final diagnoses written by the attending physician are as follows: Heart failure and chronic kidney disease, stage 3 due to hypertension and lack of adequate housing.

I13.0, Hypertensive heart and chronic kidney disease with health failure and stage 1 through stage 4 chronic kidney disease
I50.9, Heart failure
N18.3, Chronic kidney disease, stage 3
Z59.1, Inadequate housing

Category Z62, Problems Related to Upbringing

Codes within this category identify circumstances such as current and past negative life events in childhood as well as current and past problems of a child related to upbringing. These circumstances may lead to counseling or other services for the patient. The personal history of physical and sexual abuse in childhood can be described with subcategory codes Z62.81-. Other problems that can be identified with codes in this category are parental overprotection, child in welfare custody, parent-child conflict, and other parent-child-sibling problems. Codes in category Z62 are indexed under Alteration, Atypical, Conflict, Inadequate, Lack, Loss, Neglect, Problem, and Upbringing in the Alphabetic Index.

EXAMPLE: The patient, a 15-year-old male, and his foster mother were seen by the psychologist in the behavioral health center for ongoing psychological therapy. The documented reason for the therapy visit was "conflict between child and foster family."

Z62.822, Parent-foster child conflict

Category Z63, Other Problems Related to Primary Support Group, Including Family Circumstances

Category Z63 is one of several categories in ICD-10-CM that may be used when a patient or family member receives counseling services after an illness or injury or when support is required to cope with family and social problems. These codes are not used in conjunction with a diagnosis code when counseling is considered integral to the treatment for the condition. Subcategory codes identify family circumstances that occur when a family member is absent, for example, due to military deployment, disappearance, or death of a family member, or disruption of the family due to divorce or separation. Other situations that may lead to counseling or other care include a dependent relative needing care at home, alcoholism and drug addiction in the family, or other family estrangement or inadequate family support. Codes in category Z63 are indexed under Absence, Bereavement, Care, Conflict, Death, Discord, Disruption, Divorce, Estrangement, Incompatibility, and Loss in the Alphabetic Index.

EXAMPLE: The mother of an 11-year-old male child brought him to the pediatrician's office to seek help for her son who is emotionally distraught over the fact his father who is in the US Army was assigned to a military base overseas. The son is not comforted by video chats with his father and has started having disciplinary problems at school and home. The pediatrician recognized the impact of the absent father on the child and arranged for a consultation with a pediatric psychologist. The diagnosis as "absence of father due to military obligations impacting child."

Z63.31, Absence of family member due to military deployment

Do Not Resuscitate (Z66)

This code may be used when it is documented by the provider that a patient is on **do not resuscitate (DNR)** status, that is, has a physician's order to limit emergency treatment or do not resuscitation of the patient at any time during the stay. The DNR code Z66 will most likely be used on inpatient records to identify the decision made by the patient or according to the patient's documented wishes not to pursue resuscitation if the patient suffers a cardiopulmonary arrest. Usually, the patient has a serious or terminal condition with a poor prognosis and may or may not be receiving palliative care at the time the DNR status identified. Codes in category Z66 are indexed under DNR and Status in the Alphabetic Index.

Body Mass Index (Z68)

The **body mass index (BMI)** is the determination of a patient's weight in proportion to height. BMI measures are calculated as kilograms per meters squared. BMI can be used to characterize underweight as well as overweight status (Dorland 2012, 930). For overweight individuals, codes in this category are used in conjunction with a code from category E66, Overweight and obesity, to provide specific information about the patient's status.

The BMI adult codes are for use for individuals 21 years of age and older. The codes for pediatric BMI use the value ranges for children currently represented in the Centers for Disease Control and Prevention (CDC) growth charts (CDC 2019). The age group represented in the published CDC growth charts is 2 to 20 years old. The pediatric codes report percentiles as used on the growth charts.

For coding of the body mass index measurement, code assignments may be based on documentation from clinicians in addition to the patient's physician. Typically, a dietitian will

691

document the BMI number in a nutritional evaluation progress note. However, the dietitian's documentation can only supplement, not replace, the physician's documentation. The physician must document the medical diagnosis of overweight, obesity, or other nutritional problems to be coded. The BMI should only be assigned when there is an associated, reportable diagnosis (such as obesity). Do no assign BMI codes during pregnancy. Codes in category Z68 are indexed under Body, Mass Index in the Alphabetic Index.

The specific BMI values are contained in the following subcategory codes:

Z68.1,   Body mass index [BMI] 19.9 or less, adult
Z68.2-,   Body mass index [BMI] 20 to 29, adult
Z68.3-,   Body mass index [BMI] 30 to 39, adult
Z68.4-,   Body mass index [BMI] 40 or greater, adult
Z68.5-,   Body mass index [BMI] pediatric

Persons Encountering Health Services in Other Circumstances (Z69–Z76)

The block of codes from Z69 to Z76 describe a variety of situations when a patient seeks counseling and other services related to health and lifestyle issues.

Category Z69, Encounter for Mental Health Services for Victims and Perpetrator of Abuse

These codes describe encounters for counseling for victims and perpetrators of abuse. Specific services include encounters for mental health services for victims and perpetrators of parental child abuse (Z69.010–Z69.011) and nonparental child abuse (Z69.020–Z69.021). Other codes identify mental health services for victims and perpetrators of spousal or partner abuse (Z69.11–Z6.12) and other abuse such as rape victim counseling (Z69.81). Codes in category Z69 are indexed under Counseling and Encounter in the Alphabetic Index.

EXAMPLE: The client is a 30-year-old married female, mother of three children, who was referred by a social service agency to the behavioral health center for focused mental health services for victims of spousal abuse. The client has been treated medically for her injuries and is now able to participate in the counseling services provided by the center. The client's registration indicates her reason for services is "spousal abuse victim."

Z69.11, encounter for mental health services for spousal or partner abuse problems.

Category Z71, Persons Encountering Health Services for Other Counseling and Medical Advice, Not Elsewhere Classified

More counseling type services can be identified with codes from category Z71. These can be medical office or community mental health services for patients seeking relief from a dependence or other distress. Codes Z71.41 and Z71.42 are used to describe alcohol abuse counseling and surveillance services for the patient with alcoholism and the family members. Similar codes, Z71.51 and Z71.52, are used for drug abuse counseling and surveillance for the patient and the family members. A patient seeking HIV counseling would have code Z71.7 assigned for the encounter. Code Z71.84, encounter for health counseling related to travel, is to be used for health risk and safety counseling for future travel purposes. Other codes in this category describe an encounter for a patient who has a feared condition that was not found (Z71.1), an encounter for a person who is seeking advice or treatment for another person (Z71.0), and an encounter when a person is seeking dietary counseling and surveillance (Z71.3). Code Z71.3 includes two "use additional code" notes to identify any associated underlying medical condition and body mass index, if known. Codes in category Z71 are indexed under Abuse, Admission, Alcohol, Allergy, Consultation, Counseling, Feared, Problem, and Supervision in the Alphabetic Index.

Category Z74, Problems Related to Care Provider Dependency

Category Z74 identifies the patient who is dependent on others for care on a daily basis. The codes here identify bed confinement status, which means, for example, that the patient is unable to ambulate or is bedridden (Z74.01) or that the patient has reduced mobility and is confined to a chair (Z74.09). Other codes in this category cover when the patient needs assistance with personal care, for example, with bathing, dressing, and meal preparation (Z74.1), and when the patient needs continuous supervision or is unable to be left alone (Z74.3). Codes in category Z74 are indexed under Bed Confinement, Bedridden, Dependency, Impaired, Lack, Loss, Need, Reduced, and Status in the Alphabetic Index.

Category Z75, Problems Related to Medical Facilities and Other Health Care

Category Z75 codes would be used to describe the situation for a patient who needs health services because other medical services are not available to this particular patient. For example, the patient may need to be hospitalized for a brief time because medical services are not available in the home (Z75.0) or the patient is awaiting admission to an adequate facility elsewhere (Z75.1). Other patients may need respite care in a long-term facility for a period of time while family members who usually provide care need a break or are unavailable for a time period (Z75.5). Codes in category Z75 are indexed under Admission, Care, Inadequate, Impaired, Person, Respite, and Unavailability in the Alphabetic Index.

Category Z76, Persons Encountering Health Services in Other Circumstances

The common theme to these codes is the individuals who would be described by these codes are not sick. Instead, the person needs a healthcare service for a specific reason. For example, a patient may simply need to obtain a repeat prescription for a medication, eyeglasses, or a device (Z76.0). Other situations may arise when a baby or child needs supervision and care in an alternative location when there are problems in the home or no one available to care for the child (Z76.1–Z76.2). The code Z76.81 is used for an expectant parent(s)' prebirth or preadoption visit to a pediatrician's office to discuss future care for their child. Finally, a patient may be awaiting organ transplant status and needs to be seen by a provider who may also be providing healthcare for their illness, but the issue of waiting for the transplant surgery is also a concern (Z76.82). Codes in category Z76 are indexed under Boarder, Care, Disorder, Encounter, Feigned, Malingerer, and Status in the Alphabetic Index.

> **EXAMPLE:**   The case worker from the state's child protective services division from the 10-month-old infant to the University Pediatrics Clinic to confirm the child was healthy and able to be placed into a foster home within the next week. The pediatrician confirmed the child was healthy and had no contraindications from being placed in a safe foster home.
>
> Z76.2, Encounter for health supervision and care of other healthy infant and child

---

Check Your Understanding 24.3

Assign diagnosis codes for the following conditions.

1. Encounter for breast reconstruction following mastectomy

2. Aftercare following explantation of knee joint prosthesis

3. Man brought to the emergency department by the local police after the man told the policeman that he was going to kill himself and not to stop him. It was determined the patient was unemployed, homeless, and had no income. The patient was admitted for care of his suicide ideation and for social services to locate resources to help him with his lack of housing and his extreme poverty.

4. Encounter for mental health services for a victim of parental child abuse, one of five children in the home suffering abuse

5. Admitted for respite care due to family member out of town on vacation

---

Persons with Potential Health Hazards Related to Family and Personal History and Certain Conditions Influencing Health Status (Z77–Z99)

Many codes in this section are used on a daily basis for healthcare encounters in both hospital and ambulatory settings to identify common health issues in patients: family history of diseases, personal history of diseases, long-term current drug therapy, allergy status, acquired absence of limbs and organs, transplant status, presence of vascular implants, and grafts to name only a few.

Category Z77, Other Contact with and (Suspected) Exposures Hazardous to Health

Codes within subcategories Z77.01–Z77.9 can be used to describe patients who seek medical care due to exposure or contact with nonmedical substances that pose a threat to their health. Such substances include, for example, arsenic, lead, uranium, and asbestos. Other hazardous substances included here are aromatic amines, benzene, as well as air, water, and soil pollution. Other hazards in the physical environment that may be damaging to a patient can be identified with codes here for exposure to mold, algae toxins, noise, radon, and other naturally occurring radiation. A commonly used code from this category may be Z77.22 for contact with and (suspected) exposure to environmental tobacco smoke, otherwise known as passive smoking, which has been recognized as a health risk for many people. These patients may be without symptoms due to the exposure but have other injuries from the same event. Codes in category Z77 are indexed under Contact, Exposure, Passive, and Smoking in the Alphabetic Index.

EXAMPLE: The patient is a 30-year-old male who works for a building demolition company and was sent to the physician's office by the company's occupational health department for evaluation of suspected mold exposure. The patient worked to demolish a building that was heavily infested with mold and unknown other substances. The patient was examined, and laboratory and sputum specimens were collected for analysis. The physician's diagnosis on the visit progress note was "Suspected contact/exposure to mold on the job."

Z77.120, Contact with and (suspected) exposure to mold (toxic)

Category Z79, Long Term (Current) Drug Therapy

Category Z79, Long term (current) drug therapy, contains status codes that are intended to be used in addition to Z51.81, Encounter for therapeutic drug level monitoring. Category Z79 codes only state that a patient is on a prescribed drug for an extended period of time. There is no official definition or time frame for long term. If a patient receives a drug on a regular basis and has multiple refills available for a prescription, it is appropriate to document long-term drug use. The code indicates a patient's continuous use of a prescribed drug for long-term treatment of a condition or for prophylactic use. Codes in category Z79 are indexed under Long-term drug therapy, Monitoring, and Therapy, drug, long term in the Alphabetic Index.

Category Z79 codes are not used to describe patients who have addictions to drugs. This category also is not used to describe the administration of medications to prevent withdrawal symptoms in patients with drug dependence—for example, methadone maintenance programs. Instead, assign the appropriate code for the drug dependence for this type of visit.

These Z79 codes are used for long-term drug treatment as a prophylactic measure (to prevent the recurrence of deep vein thrombosis), to treat a chronic disease (such as insulin for diabetes), or for treatment of a disease that requires long-term drug therapy (such as arthritis). Codes from category Z79 are not assigned for medications administered for a brief period of time to treat an acute illness or injury or to bring a chronic condition under better control. For example, a type 2 diabetic patient may receive insulin for a period of time when hospitalized to control the blood sugar while the patient is recovering from surgery or another illness. The use of insulin during this hospital stay is not coded with Z79.4.

Code Z51.81, Encounter for therapeutic drug level monitoring, is the correct code to use when a patient visit is for the purpose of undergoing a laboratory test to measure the drug level in the patient's blood or urine or to measure a specific function to assess the effectiveness of a drug. Z51.81 code may be used alone if the monitoring is for a drug that the patient is on for only a brief period, not long term. However, there is a "use additional code" note after code Z51.81 to remind the coder to use an additional code for any long-term (current) drug therapy (Z79.-) to indicate what drug is being monitored. Likewise, under the category Z79 heading is a note to "code also" any therapeutic drug level monitoring with Z51.81.

> **EXAMPLE:** The patient is on anticoagulants and the physician orders a prothrombin time (PT) to be obtained in the outpatient department: Z51.81, Encounter for therapeutic drug level monitoring; Z79.01, Long-term (current) use of anticoagulants and antithrombotics/ antiplatelets

Categories Z80–Z84, Family History of Primary Malignant Neoplasm, Mental and Behavioral Disorders, Certain Disabilities and Chronic Diseases, Other Specified Disorders and Other Conditions

Family history codes in ICD-10-CM, categories Z80–Z84, are used when a patient's family member(s) has a particular disease that puts the patient at higher risk of contracting the same condition. Physicians generally mean the same thing when using the term "family history."

Category Z80 describes a family history of primary malignant neoplasm. This risk factor is an important medical fact about a patient and may be the reason for increased monitoring and diagnostic testing of the patient with a family history of cancer. Specific codes are provided for the primary site of the neoplasm, such as digestive organs (Z80.0), lung (Z80.1), or breast (Z80.3) as well as family history of leukemia and other lymphoid, hematopoietic, and related tissue. The main term to use in the Alphabetic Index is "History, family, malignant neoplasm."

Category Z81 describes a family history of mental and behavioral disorders. Codes within this category identify family history of alcohol abuse and dependence (Z81.1), history of other psychoactive substance abuse (Z81.3), and other mental and behavioral disorders (Z81.8). The main term to use in the Alphabetic Index is "History, family."

Category Z82 describes certain disabilities and chronic diseases leading to disablement. For example, codes are available to identify family history of stroke (Z82.3), family history of sudden cardiac death (Z82.41), and numerous other disabling conditions such as ischemic heart disease, asthma, arthritis, osteoporosis, polycystic kidney disease, and other congenital malformations, deformations, and chromosomal abnormalities. The main term to use in the Alphabetic Index is "History, family."

Category Z83 codes identify a family history of certain other specific conditions that may describe a patient's reason for a healthcare encounter. These may be isolated illnesses or chronic conditions that the family member was diagnosed with; the patient possibly could have inherited the illness or condition or be at risk for developing it. For example, Z83.71, Family history of digestive disorders, colonic polyps, may be the reason a patient has a screening colonoscopy performed at an earlier age or with more frequency than do individuals with average risk. Certain individuals are at greater risk of developing colon polyps if they have a family member in whom colon polyps have been diagnosed.

These Z codes are indexed under "History (personal) of" in the Alphabetic Index. Note the subterm "family" is indented under "History (personal) of" and is the point of reference for familial conditions.

EXAMPLES: A 50-year-old female is at the breast center for a mammogram with the reason for the service written on the physician's order of family history of breast carcinoma:

Z80.3, Family history of malignant neoplasm of breast

The patient is a 60-year-old female who is at her physician's office for a bone density study that the physician ordered because of her family history of osteoporosis.

Z82.62, Family history of osteoporosis

The patient is a 45-year-old male who comes to the hospital outpatient laboratory department for a blood glucose and AIC lab test. The order written for the tests includes the reason for the visit as family history of diabetes.

Z83.3, Family history of diabetes mellitus

Categories Z85–Z87, Personal History of Primary Malignant Neoplasm, Certain Other Diseases and Other Diseases and Conditions

As a reminder, the word "history" as used with all Z codes may not be consistent with the intent of the word "history" when used by a physician to describe a patient's current condition.

Personal history in ICD-10-CM means the patient's past medical condition no longer exists and the patient is not receiving any treatment for the condition. However, the information is important because the condition has the potential for recurrence and the patient may require continued monitoring. A physician may use the word "history" to describe a current condition the patient is being treated for, such as history of diabetes mellitus or history of hypertension. If the patient is receiving treatment for the condition, it would not be classified as a history code in ICD-10-CM.

Personal history codes are frequently used in conjunction with follow-up Z codes and family history Z codes, as well as screening Z codes, to explain the reason for the visit or diagnostic testing. These codes are important information as their presence may alter the type of treatment the patient receives.

Categories Z85 through Z87 include codes for personal and family histories of malignant neoplasms and other health problems.

The personal history of malignant neoplasm (Z85) category includes primary cancer sites only, including leukemia and lymphoid, hematopoietic, and related tissues. According to the *ICD-10-CM Official Guidelines for Coding and Reporting*, Part I.C.2.m, subcategories Z85.0–Z85.07 should only be assigned for the former site of a primary malignancy, not the site of a secondary malignancy. Codes from subcategory Z85.8- may be assigned for the former site(s) of either a primary or secondary malignancy included in this subcategory (CDC 2019). The main term to use in the Alphabetic Index is "History, personal."

The instructional notes listed under each subcategory refer to specific code ranges for primary malignancy categories (categories C00–C96). Secondary and CA *in situ* malignancies are excluded from this range of codes. A patient with leukemia in remission should be classified to the C91–C95 categories with the fifth character identifying "in remission" status instead of the Z codes in this range. The history of leukemia or lymphatic or hematopoietic neoplasms codes in the Z85 subcategories means the patient is completely cured of the disease. Directional notes appear under the category heading of Z85, Personal history of malignant neoplasm to

- Code first any follow-up examination after treatment of malignant neoplasm (Z08)

- Use additional codes to identify:

  ○ Alcohol use and dependence (F10.-)

  ○ Exposure to environmental tobacco smoke (Z77.22)

  ○ History of tobacco dependence (Z87.891)

  ○ Occupational exposure to environmental tobacco smoke (Z57.31)

  ○ Tobacco dependence (F17.-)

  ○ Tobacco use (Z72.)

Categories Z86 and Z87 identify certain other conditions that the patient may have a personal history of that is important to consider for future healthcare needs. Both category headings include the note to "code first any follow-up examination after treatment (Z09)" as these conditions are frequently the reason for follow-up examinations to assure the condition has not recurred in the patient. The main term to use in the Alphabetic Index is History, personal.

There are several conditions in the categories that are frequently documented by the physician in the health record and are used to explain the reason for the health encounter. For example, personal history of such serious health conditions included in category Z86, include the following personal history of certain other conditions:

- In-situ neoplasm of breast (Z86.000) or cervix uteri (Z86.001) and other sites (Z86.002-Z86.008)

- Colonic polyps (Z86.010)

- Methicillin resistant *Staphylococcus aureus* infection (Z86.14)

- Combat and operational stress reaction (Z86.51)

- History of diseases of the circulatory system (Z86.7-) including pulmonary embolism, other venous thrombosis, transient ischemic attack, or cerebral infarction

In the Z87 category, codes are available to identify a patient's past medical condition that may have an impact on the current care or need for future services. For example, personal history of other diseases and conditions are coded as follows:

- Peptic ulcer disease (Z87.11)

- Dysplasia of female genital tract (Z87.410-Z87.412)

- Urinary tract infections (Z87.440)

- Complications of pregnancy, childbirth and puerperium including pre-term labor (Z87.51–Z87.59)

- Nicotine dependence (Z87.891)

A set of subcategory codes, Z87.7, Personal history of (corrected) congenital malformation, is included here to be used to classify the patient with a known history of a congenital condition that has been repaired or corrected. An Excludes1 note appears under this subcategory to remind the coder that these codes would not be used if the congenital malformation has only been partially repaired and the patient still required medical treatment for it. Then, the congenital condition would be coded instead. The congenital conditions in all body systems are included here, for example, malformations of the genitourinary tract, nervous system, digestive system, and heart and circulatory system.

Finally, in subcategory Z87.8, there are codes available for specific conditions that are important to note for a patient's health status. For example, personal history of healed traumatic fracture (Z87.81), traumatic brain injury (Z87.820), and anaphylaxis (Z87.892) are coded here.

Category Z88, Allergy Status to Drugs, Medicaments and Biological Substances and Subcategory Z91.0, Allergy Status, Other Than to Drugs and Biological Substances

The codes in categories Z88 and Z91.0 are considered allergy status codes that describe the fact the patient has a history of an allergy to a known substance. These people have had an allergic reaction to food or a substance and will always be considered allergic to that substance. These Z codes indicate that the person is not currently exhibiting an allergic reaction but, instead, has the potential for a reaction if exposed to the substance in the future. The Z88 codes identify allergy status to drugs and biological substances such as penicillin, sulfonamides, anesthetic agent or serum, and vaccines. The Z91.0 subcategory identifies food allergy status with six-character codes for allergies to peanuts, milk products, and eggs, for example. The other codes in category Z91 describe allergies to nonfood and nonmedicinals such as bee sting allergy and allergies to latex objects and radiographic dye or contrast materials. The main term "history" or "allergy" in the Alphabetic Index has subterms for drug, food, and other substances.

> **EXAMPLE:** The patient is scheduled for hip replacement surgery and reminds her physician that she has had allergic reactions to narcotic drugs in the past after surgery. The physician makes a clear note in the patient's preoperative history and physical that the patient has an allergy to narcotics.
>
> Z88.5, Allergic status to narcotic agent status

Category Z89, Acquired Absence of Limb

Codes within this category identify the status of the patient who has had an amputation of a limb that may be postprocedural or posttraumatic loss of the limb. The codes are specific to the limb and the laterality, for example, acquired absence of the right finger(s) (Z89.021), acquired absence of the left hand (Z89.112), or acquired absence of the right great toe (Z89.411). The acquired absence of the leg below the knee is identified with codes for the right leg, left leg, and unspecified leg (Z89.511–Z89.519). Likewise, the acquired absence of the leg above the knee is identified with codes Z89.611–Z89.619. If a patient had an explantation or removal of a joint prosthesis with or without the presence of an antibiotic-impregnated cement spacer, the specific loss of a joint can be identified for the shoulder (Z89.231–Z89.239), the knee (Z89.521–Z89.529), and the hip (Z89.621–Z89.629). The main term to use in the Alphabetic Index is "Absence (of) (organ or part) (complete or partial)".

EXAMPLE: The patient is an 88-year-old male who is seen in his primary care physician's office for ongoing management of his type 2 diabetic peripheral angiopathy. The patient has already lost his right great toe and two other toes on his right foot due to the diabetic peripheral disease. No new problems were detected today, and the patient will continue on his present diabetic drug management.

E11.51, Type 2 diabetes mellitus with diabetic peripheral angiopathy without gangrene
Z89.411, Acquired absence of right great toe, right foot
Z89.421, Acquired absence of other toe(s), right foot

Check Your Understanding 24.4

Assign diagnosis codes to the following conditions.

1. Family history of elevated lipoprotein(s) or Lp(a)

2. Long-term (current) use of anticoagulants

3. Personal history of colon cancer

4. Personal history of transient ischemic attack without residual deficits

5. Dietary counseling for an adult patient with morbid obesity and a BMI of 45.0

Category Z90, Acquired Absence of Organs, Not Elsewhere Classified

The status of an acquired absence may be postprocedural or posttraumatic loss of a body part; these situations should be classified to this category. Any congenital absence of an organ would be classified elsewhere in ICD-10-CM. Frequently, these codes are used to describe patients who have had a malignant condition and had surgery to remove a diseased organ. For example, acquired absence of breast and nipple (Z90.10–Z90.13), kidney (Z90.5), and prostate (Z90.79). For acquired absence of the pancreas, a use additional note appears to remind the coder to use an additional code to identify any associated insulin use (Z79.4) or postpancreatectomy diabetes mellitus (E13.-). Some of the codes within this category are important for tracking Pap smear necessity. Women who have had a total hysterectomy with removal of the cervix

(Z90.710) no longer require cervical Pap smears but do require vaginal smears to test for vaginal malignancies. Women with a cervical stump (Z90.711) following a hysterectomy still require cervical Pap smears. Code Z90.712 would identify the woman who has a surgically absent cervix but in whom the uterus remains. These conditions can be found in the Index under the main term "Absence," followed by the organ name.

> **EXAMPLE:** The patient is a 68-year-old male who had surgical removal of part of his stomach due to gastric carcinoma that is still undergoing chemotherapy. The patient is being evaluated today as part of his recovery from the partial gastrectomy. The diagnoses listed on the physician's progress note for the visit are carcinoma of the stomach, greater curvature, and status post partial gastrectomy.
>
> C16.6, Malignant neoplasm of greater curvature of stomach, unspecified
> Z90.3, Acquired absence of stomach [part of]

Category Z91, Personal Risk Factors, Not Elsewhere Classified

Other codes in category Z91 identify the fact that the patient has a personal history that presents hazards to health. Examples of commonly used codes in this category are **noncompliance** with medical treatment and regimen. Individual codes are available to describe a patient's noncompliance with dietary regimen (Z91.11). Other codes describe a patient's other noncompliance with medication regimen (Z91.14), a patient's noncompliance with renal dialysis (Z91.15), and a patient's noncompliance with other medical treatment and regimen (Z91.16). Any of these noncompliance activities can be a detriment to a patient's health status. Another risk to the patient can occur when the patient is noncompliant with his or her scheduled medications. Codes exist for the patient who takes less of their prescribed medication, which is identified as underdosing in ICD-10-CM. A patient may intentionally take less of their medication for financial reasons (Z91.120) or intentionally for another reason (Z91.128). In other situations, the patient may take less of the medication unintentionally because of the patient's age-related debility such as forgetfulness or dementia (Z91.130) or unintentionally for other reasons (Z91.138). The codes for these conditions are located in the Alphabetic Index under the main term "Noncompliance."

A patient with a history of fall(s) or identified as at risk for falling can be classified with code Z91.81. This code is used to identify patients at risk for falling or who have a history of falls with or without subsequent injuries. Falls are an important public health problem affecting about one-third of adults aged 65 years and older annually. People who fall may suffer moderate to severe injuries, including hip and other fractures and head trauma. Adults who are aged 75 years or older and fall are more likely to be admitted to a long-term care facility. Code Z91.81 can be used to identify patients who require closer monitoring to prevent falls, to justify specific diagnostic or therapeutic services to identify causes of falling, or to order preventive evaluation or services. In order to locate codes in category Z92, Personal History of Medical Treatment, the main term to be used in the Alphabetic Index is "history, personal" and the treatment that was provided or status such as falling.

Within this category are codes to identify the patient's personal history of antineoplastic chemotherapy (Z92.21), personal history of monoclonal drug therapy (Z92.22), personal history of estrogen therapy (Z92.23), personal history of inhaled steroid therapy (Z92.240), personal history of systemic steroid therapy (Z92.241), personal history of immunosuppressive therapy (Z92.25), and personal history of other drug therapy (Z92.299). Other codes for history of the particular condition for which the patient received chemotherapy or drug therapy could be used with these codes. Other facts about the patient can be described with other codes in this category, for example, the fact that the patient has received therapeutic radiation (Z92.3) or received tPA in a different facility in the past 24 hours (Z92.82) and the fact that the patient has a history of failed moderate or conscious sedation (Z92.83). All of these factors can have an impact on the patient's current and future healthcare needs.

> **EXAMPLES:** Z91.15, Patient's noncompliance with renal dialysis
> Z91.412, Personal history of adult neglect
> Z91.5, Personal history of suicide attempt

Category Z93, Artificial Opening Status

Category Z93 is subdivided to identify the presence of an artificial opening, such as a tracheostomy (Z93.0), ileostomy (Z93.2), colostomy (Z93.3), cystostomy (Z93.5-), and so forth. These codes are indexed under "Status (post), artificial opening" in the Alphabetic Index.

> **EXAMPLE:** The patient is seen in the Stoma Clinic for evaluation of his nephrostomy stoma.
>
> Z93.6, Other artificial openings of urinary tract status (nephrostomy)

The exclusion note at the beginning of category Z93 instructs coders to use a code from subcategory Z43.- when the encounter or admission is for attention to or management of that artificial opening or when there are complications of the external stoma (J95.0-, K94.-, or N99.5-).

Category Z94, Transplanted Organ or Tissue Status

Category Z94 is used for homologous or heterologous (animal or human) organ, bone marrow, cornea, and stem cell transplants among other organs. If there are complications of the transplanted organ or tissue, the Alphabetic Index will direct the coder to the codes for the specific complications. This category of codes does not imply there is a problem with the transplanted organ or tissue.
These codes are indexed under "Transplant(ed) (status)" in the Alphabetic Index.

> **EXAMPLE:** The patient is seen in the Transplant Center for his ongoing recovery from his liver transplant surgery.
>
> Z94.4, Liver transplant status

Another code, Z76.82, Awaiting organ transplant status, is included in another category of ICD-10-CM. Some patients who are on a waiting list for a heart transplant may be hospitalized due to the severity of their illness. Z76.82 is a status code to distinguish patients who are hospitalized while awaiting a new heart from patients who are hospitalized for direct treatment of their heart disease. This code could also be used to indicate that the patient is on any organ transplant waiting list.

Category Z95, Presence of Cardiac and Vascular Implants and Grafts

Category Z95 includes codes for a variety of postprocedural states, such as cardiac pacemaker *in situ* (Z95.0), automatic implantable cardiac defibrillator (Z95.810), aortocoronary bypass graft (Z95.1), presence of prosthetic heart valve (Z95.2), coronary angioplasty implant (stent) (Z95.5), heart assist device (Z95.811), and presence of fully implantable artificial heart (Z95.812). The Excludes1 note under this category reminds the coder that complications of cardiac and vascular devices, implants, and grafts are found in category T82.-. These postprocedural states are located in the Alphabetic Index under the main term Cardiac, Dependence, Presence, Replacement, and Status (post).

EXAMPLE: The patient is seen in the Cardiology Clinic for ongoing management of sick sinus syndrome and to evaluate the presence of his automatic implantable cardiac defibrillator (AICD) with synchronous cardiac pacemaker.

I49.5, Sick sinus syndrome
Z95.810, Presence of AICD with synchronous cardiac pacemaker

Categories Z96, Presence of Other Functional Implants and Z97, Presence of Other Devices

These two categories identify other postprocedural states for the patient that specify what body part has been replaced with an implant or device. Examples of frequently used codes in these categories are presence of the following:

- Z96.1, Intraocular lens or pseudophakos

- Z96.41, Insulin pump (external)(internal)

- Z96.6, Orthopedic joint implant identified by joint and laterality

- Z97.1-, Artificial limb (complete)(partial) identified by limb and laterality

- Z97.5, Contraceptive (intrauterine) device

The presence of an implant or device is identified by a code found in the Alphabetic Index under the main term Presence (of), Pseudophakia, Replacement, and Status.

Category Z98, Other Postprocedural States

Codes in this category identify a postsurgical or postprocedural status of the patient that can be important for future healthcare needs. Examples of frequently used codes in this category are as follows:

- Z98.0, Intestinal bypass and anastomosis status

- Z98.4-, Cataract extraction status

A note appears under this code to use additional code to identify the presence of an intraocular lens implant (Z96.1).

- Z98.5-, Sterilization status for both tubal ligation and vasectomy status

- Z98.84, Bariatric surgery status

- Z98.85, Transplanted organ removal status

An Excludes1 note appears with this code that an encounter for the removal of the transplanted organ should be coded to complication of transplanted organ (T86.-).

These postprocedural descriptions of a patient can be found in the Alphabetic Index under the main term Status (post,) Absence, Postsurgical status, Presence, and Transplant.

Category Z99, Dependence of Enabling Machines and Devices, Not Elsewhere Classified

The last category in ICD-10-CM identifies the patient's dependence or required use of a machine or device to sustain life or function. The presence and dependence on cardiac devices are classified to category Z95. For example, many patients in both inpatient and outpatient settings would be identified for their special needs through the use of these codes:

- Z99.11, Dependence on respirator (ventilator)(mechanical ventilation)

- Z99.2, Dependence on renal dialysis

- Z99.81, Dependence on supplemental oxygen

The main term for use in the Alphabetic Index for these scenarios is Dependence on or Admission.

Check Your Understanding 24.5

Assign diagnosis codes to the following conditions.

1. Personal history of radiation therapy and personal history of malignant neoplasm of the pancreas with acquired partial absence of pancreas

2. Personal history of severe allergy to bee insects

3. Presence of artificial knee joint, left

4. Ventilator dependent

5. Live transplant status

ICD-10-CM Review Exercises: Chapter 24

Assign the correct ICD-10-CM diagnosis codes to the following exercises.

1. This single newborn was born vaginally in the hospital. The baby, with documented type A+ blood, is being treated for Rh isoimmunization with the mother's blood type documented as A–. What is the correct diagnosis code(s)?

_____

2. Encounter for a medical examination of 55-year-old male to determine his physical disability status and issue a medical certificate of incapacity prior to receiving long term disability insurance.

_____

3. The patient seen for fitting of right artificial leg after the patient had below-knee amputation due to a medical condition.

_____

4. Counseling visit for patient with alcohol dependence with alcohol-induced anxiety disorder

_____

(*Continued on next page*)

ICD-10-CM Review Exercises: Chapter 24 (continued)

5. Personal history of lung carcinoma with past history of tobacco dependence

   _____

6. Presence of AICD (automatic cardioverter defibrillator) and status post coronary artery angioplasty

   _____

7. The patient is having a screening colonoscopy and has a family history of colon carcinoma.

   _____

8. The encounter is for a patient to receive antineoplastic chemotherapy to treat giant cell glioblastoma of the brain.

   _____

9. The encounter is for an elective termination of pregnancy.

   _____

10. The patient is a newborn triplet born in the hospital by cesarean delivery. The newborn is premature born during the 35th week of the mother's pregnancy and has a low birth weight of 1,769 grams.

    _____

11. The patient was seen in the physician's office to determine if the patient has acquired an infection after being exposed to the HIV virus that her sexual partner admitted to having just been diagnosed.

    _____

12. The patient requests permanent sterilization because of the patient's grand multiparity status and she does not want any more children.

    _____

13. The patient was admitted to the hospital to donate her left kidney for a relative who needs a kidney transplant for end stage kidney disease.

    _____

14. The patient was seen in the gynecologist's office for a routine gynecological examination with a cervical Papanicolaou smear.

    _____

15. The patient was seen in her oncologist's office for follow-up examination after the completion of her chemotherapy treatment for a primary carcinoma of the breast that is stated to no longer be present.

    _____

16. The male patient, age 25, was brought to the emergency department after a motor vehicle crash that involved several vehicles and trucks and the patient had to be extricated from the vehicle but insisted he was not injured. The ambulance personnel convinced him to go to the hospital as a precaution. After examination, the patient was found not to have any injury from the crash.

    _____

ICD-10-CM Review Exercises: Chapter 24 (continued)

17. The patient was treated 10 days after an accident in which he was injured while cleaning windows at home when a glass windowpane broke. The patient had lacerations that were repaired. At this time, the patient's arm was reexamined and a small piece of glass was found imbedded in soft tissue that was not previously found. The patient's primary care physician made a small incision and removed the sliver of glass. Code only the diagnosis for the condition of retained glass fragment but do not code the external cause of injury or the procedure code for removal of glass.

18. The 2-year-old female patient was brought to the pediatrician's office by her mother and grandmother because the grandmother was concerned that the child had not received all of her immunizations because the patient's mother feared the vaccines would cause the child to develop a reaction. The physician counseled the mother about the risks and benefits of immunization and reassured her of the safety of the vaccines for children. The mother agreed to think about it and bring the patient back to the physician's office the following week for possible vaccine administrations. The physician describes the patient in her record as being delinquent with her immunization status.

19. The patient is a 45-year-old female who made an appointment with a psychologist to discuss the problems she is having with two family members, one with alcoholism and another person with drug addiction.

20. The patient is a 30-year-old female who is being seen by her obstetrician for normal prenatal care during the third trimester of her first pregnancy. The patient has not had any complications of pregnancy and is expected to deliver in the next three weeks.

References

American Cancer Society (ACS). 2017. Hormone Therapy for Breast Cancer. http://www.cancer.org/cancer/breastcancer/detailedguide/breast-cancer-treating-hormone-therapy.

American Hospital Association (AHA). 2009. *Coding Clinic for ICD-9-CM*. Fourth Quarter.

Centers for Disease Control and Prevention (CDC), National Center for Health Statistics (NCHS). 2019. *ICD-10-CM Official Guidelines for Coding and Reporting*, 2020. http://www.cdc.gov/nchs/icd/icd10cm.htm or https://www.cdc.gov/nchs/data/icd/10cmguidelines-FY2020_final.pdf.

Centers for Disease Control and Prevention (CDC). 2017. Clinical Growth Charts. http://www.cdc.gov/growthcharts/clinical_charts.htm.

Dorland, W.A.N., ed. 2012. *Dorland's Illustrated Medical Dictionary*, 32nd ed. Philadelphia: Elsevier Saunders.

Chapter 25

Coding and Reimbursement

Learning Objectives

At the conclusion of this chapter, you should be able to do the following:

- Explain how the Medicare Severity Diagnosis-Related Groups (MS-DRGs) identify the levels of severity differences in a patient's condition

- Briefly describe the hospital inpatient prospective payment system, including how base payment rates are determined and the formula for computing the hospital payment

- Describe the purpose and activities of quality improvement organizations, comprehensive error testing programs, and recovery audit contractors

- Define medical necessity and its relationship to ICD-10-CM diagnosis codes

- Summarize the purpose of advance beneficiary notice

Key Terms

Advance beneficiary notice (ABN)
Case Mix Index (CMI)
Complication
Comorbidity
Comprehensive Error Rate Testing (CERT)
Diagnosis-related group (DRG)
Direct graduate medical education (DGME)
Discharge disposition
Disproportionate share hospital (DSH)
Hospital acquired condition (HAC)
Hospital inpatient prospective payment system (IPPS)
Hospital's base rate
Hospital's payment rate
Indirect medical education (IME)
Local Coverage Determinations (LCD)

Medical necessity
Medicare Administrative Contractor (MAC)
Medicare-dependent hospital (MDH)
Medicare Severity Diagnosis-Related Groups (MS-DRGs)
National Coverage Determinations (NCD)
Office of Inspector General (OIG) Workplan
Outlier
Post–acute-care setting
Present on Admission (POA)
Quality Improvement Organization (QIO)
Recovery Audit Contractor (RAC)
Relative weight
Severity of illness
Sole community hospital (SCH)
Value Based Purchasing (VBP)

This text has included a thorough review of the characteristics and conventions of ICD-10-CM. Classification systems are established for statistical comparison and research, and in the case of the ICD-10-CM classifications, the codes are used for reimbursement and other important purposes such as quality tracking and improvement. This chapter includes a brief discussion of some of the reimbursement purposes for coding; the hospital inpatient prospective payment system, Medicare payment review programs, present on admission, and medical necessity.

Hospital Inpatient Prospective Payment System

The **hospital inpatient prospective payment system** (IPPS) is a method of payment undertaken by the Centers for Medicare and Medicaid Services (CMS) to control the cost of inpatient acute-care hospital services to Medicare recipients. Title VI of the Social Security Amendments of 1983 established the prospective payment system (PPS) to provide payment to hospitals for each Medicare case at a set reimbursement rate, rather than on a fee-for-service or per-day basis (CMS 2019a). Under CMS, Medicare recipients must be over the age of 65 and/or identified with certain disabilities or end-stage renal disease. Medicare includes the following coverage:

- Part A: inpatient hospital, skilled nursing, some home health

- Part B: medical insurance premium, physician services, outpatient hospital services, some home health, durable medical equipment

- Part C: Medicare + Choice (Medicare as an HMO product), or Medicare Advantage Plan

- Part D: Prescription drug coverage (Medicare Interactive 2018)

Medicaid is another type of coverage administered by the state governments under CMS and is based on income and resource shortfalls. Both Medicare and Medicaid include quality and medical necessity provisions. It is important to note that third-party payers and private insurance companies follow CMS's lead in reimbursement; however, the major difference is using negotiated versus set base rates for hospitals. Base rates will be explained in detail below.

Inpatient hospital payment rates are established before services are rendered and are based on **diagnosis-related groups (DRGs)**. For fiscal year 2008, Medicare adopted a severity-adjusted diagnosis-related group system called **Medicare Severity Diagnosis-Related Groups (MS-DRGs)**. This was the most drastic revision to the DRG system in 24 years. The goal of the new MS-DRG system was to significantly improve Medicare's ability to recognize severity of illness in its inpatient hospital payments. The intent is to increase payments to hospitals for services provided to the sicker patient and decrease payments for treating less severely ill patients. There are up to three levels of severity in the MS-DRGs that reflect the differences in the patient's condition based on additional diagnoses codes assigned:

- MS-DRGs with major complication or comorbidity (MCC), which reflect the highest level of severity. This level reflects the sickest patient with the highest level of severity and requires a significant amount of resources to treat both the principal diagnosis and the additional conditions the patient has.

- MS-DRG with complication or comorbidity (CC), which is the next level of severity. This is a mid-level degree of severity based on these secondary diagnoses and requires additional resources for treating the principal and additional diagnoses.

- MS-DRGs with no complication or comorbidity (non-CC), which do not significantly affect severity of illness and resource use. This means the patient did not have an additional condition that required significant additional resources other than what was needed to treat the condition the patient had (CMS 2017a).

Both medical and surgical MS-DRGs may be influenced by a secondary diagnosis code (CMS 2019a). For example, if a patient had the principal diagnosis of heart failure, then the presence or the absence of a secondary diagnosis would determine the MS-DRG assigned. See table 25.1 for examples of the medical MS-DRGs for Heart Failure and Shock.

Table 25.1. **Medical MS-DRGs for heart failure and shock**

MS-DRG	Principal diagnosis	Secondary diagnosis	Is the secondary diagnosis an MCC, CC, or Neither?
291	Heart failure and Shock	Pneumonia due to *Haemophilus influenza*	MCC
292	Heart failure and Shock	Primary pulmonary hypertension	CC
293	Heart failure and Shock	Type 2 diabetes	Neither

Source: CMS 2019a

Another example describes a surgical MS-DRG and the influence of secondary diagnoses codes if the secondary diagnoses contained an MCC or a CC. For example, if a patient had the principal procedure of a cardiac valve procedure and a secondary procedure of a cardiac catheterization, the presence of a secondary diagnosis would determine the MS-DRG assigned. See table 25.2 for examples of the surgical MS-DRGs for cardiac valve procedures.

Table 25.2. **Surgical MS-DRGs for cardiac valve procedures**

MS-DRG	Principal procedure	Secondary diagnosis	Is the secondary diagnosis an MCC, CC, or Neither?
216	Cardiac valve and other major cardiothoracic procedures with cardiac catheterization with MCC	Acute pulmonary edema	MCC
217	Cardiac valve and other major cardiothoracic procedures with cardiac catheterization with CC	Acute respiratory distress	CC
218	Cardiac valve procedure with cardiac catheterization	COPD	Neither

Source: CMS 2019a

There are a few MS-DRGs that are not influenced by the presence of an MCC or a CC. See table 25.3 for examples of medical and surgical MS-DRGs that are not influenced by the presence or absence of the secondary diagnosis that is identified as an MCC, a CC, or neither.

Table 25.3.   **Examples of medical and surgical MS-DRGs that are not influenced by the presence or absence of the secondary diagnosis as a MCC, CC, or neither**

MS-DRG	Principal diagnosis or principal procedure	Explanation
313 Medical MS-DRG	Chest pain	There is one medical MS-DRG (313) for the principal diagnosis of "chest pain." This MS-DRG is not influenced by the presence of any secondary diagnoses that are MCCs or CCs. If there was only one diagnosis present, the principal diagnosis of chest pain, the MS-DRG would be the same 313.
189 Medical MS-DRG	Pulmonary edema and respiratory failure	There is one medical MS-DRG (189) for pulmonary edema and/or respiratory failure that is not treated with mechanical ventilation or respirator. This MS-DRG is not influenced by the presence of a secondary diagnosis.
215 Surgical MS-DRG	Other heart assist system implant	There is one surgical MS-DRG (215) assigned based on the presence of ICD-10-PCS procedure codes for the insertion or revision of certain external or implantable heart assist systems. No secondary diagnosis will change the MS-DRG when one of the identified ICD-10-PCS procedure codes is present.
483	Major joint/limb reattachment procedure of upper extremities	There is one surgical MS-DRG (483) assigned based on the presence of an ICD-10-PCS procedure code for an upper extremities joint replacement or limb reattachment, for example, a replacement of a shoulder joint. No secondary diagnosis will change the MS-DRG when one of the identified ICD-10-PCS procedure codes is present.

Source: CMS 2019a

MS-DRGs represent an inpatient classification system designed to categorize patients who are medically related with respect to diagnoses and treatment and who are statistically similar in their lengths of stay. Each DRG has a preset reimbursement amount that the hospital receives whenever the MS-DRG is assigned. Acute-care hospitals receive Medicare IPPS payments on a per discharge basis for Medicare beneficiaries—one payment per one inpatient hospital stay. All outpatient diagnostic services and admission-related therapeutic services provided by the same hospital on the day of the patient's admission or within three days preceding the date of inpatient admission must be included on the inpatient hospital claim to Medicare and are paid as part of the MS-DRG payment. No separate payment is made for these outpatient services.

The Medicare patient's principal diagnosis and up to 24 additional diagnoses that include diagnoses that are recognized as major or other complication or comorbidity will determine the medical MS-DRG. If the patient had surgery or a significant procedure, this will impact the MS-DRG assignment as well. Up to 25 procedure codes may be reported on the inpatient claim to Medicare, and these will likely cause a surgical MS-DRG to be assigned. Each fiscal year, the Centers for Medicare and Medicaid Services (CMS) evaluates the composition of the MS-DRGs to determine if the DRG still includes clinically similar conditions that require similar amounts of resources to care for the patients. When the clinical and financial information about a particular MS-DRG proves that the group contains significantly different amounts of resources, CMS has the option to assign diagnosis and procedure codes to a different MS-DRG or create a new MS-DRG for a particular set of diagnoses or procedures.

The base payment rates for each MS-DRG are determined from two basic sources. First, each MS-DRG is assigned a relative weight. The **relative weight** represents the average resources required to care for cases in that particular MS-DRG relative to the national average of resources used to treat all Medicare cases. For example, consider how the relative weight of an MS-DRG represents the average resources required to care of a patient within a particular MS-DRG. MS-DRG 343, Appendectomy without complicated diagnosis, without CC/MCC, has an FY 2019 weight of 1.0853. In comparison, MS-DRG 005, Liver Transplant with MCC or Intestinal Transplant, has an FY 2019 weight of 10.2545. A liver transplant patient would take more than 9 times the resources to care for compared to the patient who had an appendectomy without a complicated diagnosis. On the other hand, if a patient was discharged with the final diagnosis of abortion and assigned to MS-DRG 776, Abortion, with a weight of 0.7543, it is expected that this patient would likely be treated medically for a short day and would require half the resources as the appendectomy patient. Each year, the relative weights of the MS-DRGs are updated to reflect changes in treatment patterns, technology, and any other factors that may change the relative use of hospital resources.

The second source that determines MS-DRG payment rate is the individual **hospital's payment rate** per case. This payment rate is based on a regional or national adjusted standardized amount that considers the type of hospital; designation of the hospital as large urban, other urban, or rural; and a wage index for the geographic area in which the hospital is located. This is called the base payment rate or standardized rate and is a dollar amount that includes a labor-related and non–labor-related portion. The labor-related portion is adjusted by the wage index for a geographic area to reflect the differences in the cost of employing individuals to work in the hospitals. The nonlabor rate accounts for capital expenses and operating expenses that determine the cost of providing hospital services other than paying employees. The two factors together are called the hospital's wage-adjusted standard payment rate or the **hospital's base rate**. By submitting a claim for the inpatient services with the financial charges and the diagnoses and procedure codes to the Medicare contractor responsible for processing claims, the payment process begins. Based on the coded data on the claim, the Medicare contractor assigns each case to a specific MS-DRG.

Thus, the actual amount the hospital is reimbursed for each Medicare inpatient is determined by multiplying the hospital's individual base rate by the relative weight of the DRG, less any applicable deductible amount.

The formula for computing the hospital payment for each MS-DRG is as follows:

MS-DRG Relative Weight × Hospital Base Rate = Hospital Payment

For example, a hospital patient was assigned MS-DRG 236, Coronary bypass without cardiac catheterization without MCC. MS-DRG 236 has a relative weight of 3.9263. This hospital had a hospital base rate of $6,000. The hospital could expect the total payment for this patient to be $23,557.80.

For any given patient in an MS-DRG, the hospital knows, in advance, the amount of reimbursement it will receive from Medicare. It is the responsibility of the hospital to ensure that its resource use is reasonably in line with the expected payment. In addition to the basic payment rate, Medicare provides for an additional payment for other factors related to a particular hospital's business. If the hospital treats a high percentage of low-income patients, it receives a percentage add-on payment applied to the MS-DRG–adjusted base payment rate. Another scenario that qualifies a hospital to receive this additional payment is when a hospital is located in an urban setting with 100 or more beds and receives more than 30 percent of the hospital's net revenue from state and other local government sources for indigent care. This add-on payment, known as the **disproportionate share hospital (DSH)** adjustment, provides for a percentage increase in Medicare payments to hospitals that qualify under either of two statutory formulas designed to identify hospitals that serve a disproportionate share of low-income patients.

Teaching hospitals with residents in approved residency programs receive what are called **direct graduate medical education (DGME)** payments that represent the direct costs of operating a residency program, including paying the residents' salaries and supervising physicians. In addition, an approved teaching hospital receives a percentage add-on payment for each Medicare discharge paid under IPPS. This is known as the **indirect medical education (IME)** adjustment. This percentage varies, depending on the ratio of residents to the inpatient beds.

Sole community hospitals (SCHs) can receive an additional operating payment. SCHs are hospitals that are

- located at least 35 miles from another similar acute-care IPPS hospital;

- located in a rural setting located between 25 and 35 miles for another similar hospital and must meet one other criterion related to the admission patterns of the community residents;

- located in a rural setting but because of local topography or periods of prolonged severe weather conditions, the other like hospitals are inaccessible for at least 30 days in each of two out of three years; or

- located in a rural setting and because of distance, posted speed limits, predictable weather conditions, the travel time between the hospital and the nearest like hospital is at least 45 minutes.

As the name of these hospitals implies, these hospitals are the sole source of healthcare in their area (CMS 2017b). The defining legislation for Sole Community Hospitals is Section 1886(d)(5)(D)(iii) of the Social Security Act.

Medicare-dependent hospitals (MDHs) receive additional operating payments. An MDH is a rural hospital with 100 or fewer beds, is not a sole community hospital (SCH), and at least 60 percent of their discharges are Medicare patients as documented in at least two out of the last three most recent audited Medicare cost reporting periods for which there is a settled cost report (CMS 2017c). These hospitals are a major source of care for Medicare beneficiaries in their area. Together with SCHs, MDHs are afforded this special payment in order to maintain access to services for Medicare beneficiaries.

To assure the Medicare beneficiaries have access to high quality, but expensive healthcare, additional payments are made for what is called an **outlier** or extremely costly care. The costs incurred by a hospital for a Medicare beneficiary are evaluated to determine whether the hospital is eligible for an additional payment as an outlier case. A fixed loss amount is set each year. Hospitals are paid 80 percent of their costs above the fixed loss threshold and 90 percent of costs above the outlier threshold for burn patients (CMS 2017c). This additional payment is designed to protect the hospital from large financial losses due to unusually expensive cases. Any outlier payment due is added to the MS-DRG–adjusted base payment rate, plus any DSH, IME, and medical service add-on adjustments.

MS-DRG assignment is based on information that includes the following:

- Diagnoses (principal and secondary)

- Surgical procedures (principal and secondary)

- Discharge disposition or status

- Presence of major or other complications and comorbidities (MCC or CC) as secondary diagnoses

The **discharge disposition** of a patient, or where the patient goes after discharge from the hospital, has an impact on the hospital's payment for the inpatient admission. MS-DRG payments are reduced if the patient is transferred to another acute-care hospital that receives IPPS payments or, for certain MS-DRGs, is transferred to another healthcare setting where Medicare payments are made for the patient's continued care. These **post–acute-care settings** are healthcare settings where a patient receives healthcare services after his or her discharge from an acute-care hospital including long-term care hospitals, rehabilitation or psychiatric hospitals, units in acute-care hospitals, skilled nursing facilities, home health agencies, cancer hospitals, or children's hospitals. Hospitals receive a reduced payment for an IPPS patient who is transferred to another acute-care hospital or to one of the post–acute-care settings.

Additional payment adjustments occur with higher cost outlier cases and for new medical services and technologies. For higher cost outlier cases, an additional payment that is equal to 80 percent of the difference between the hospital's cost for the encounter and the DRG payment plus the threshold amount. Additionally, when new medical services or technologies are provided to Medicare beneficiaries, an additional amount is provided of the DRG payment plus 50 percent of the technology or service cost once established.

CMS evaluates the Medicare IPPS annually. CMS's Notice of Proposed Rulemaking is published in the *Federal Register* in late April or early May each year. This notice, on which the public may comment, will announce proposed ICD-10-CM/PCS code changes after October 1st, as well as proposed revisions to the MS-DRG system each year. CMS's Final Rule announcing final revisions to the IPPS, including the MS-DRG system, is published in the *Federal Register* in July or August and the changes become effective October 1 each year.

Reimbursement

Now that we know that MS-DRGs are divided into Major Diagnostic Categories (MDCs), it is import to make a closer connection to ICD-10-CM. When coding for ICD-10-CM, the principle diagnosis determines the MDC (remembering that if the service was for a procedure, the procedure determines either the medical or surgical MS-DRG). The use of electronic health records has allowed for grouper software or the use of Encoders with grouper software to assign an MS-DRG based on the code selection. In order to properly code, and ultimately get to the correct MS-DRG for reimbursement, the coder should rely on the *Coding Clinic* and coding guidelines as tools to remain current with changes to the MS-DRG system. Changes are published in the *Federal Register* and can include new, deleted, or revised codes, changes to MS-DRG relative weights, and average length of stay definitions and criteria. Another important impact on MS-DRGs includes the complications and comorbidities as described above.

A good rule of thumb is to remember that a complication includes a condition that arises during hospitalization, making it not present on admission (POA). On the other hand, a comorbidity is a pre-existing condition and would be considered POA. The Deficit Reduction Act identified that diagnoses that are considered POA must be identified for reimbursement purposes. According to CMS (2017c), POA general reporting requirements include:

- All claims involving inpatient admissions mandate the collection of POA

- POA must be present at the time of an inpatient admission; including conditions that develop during an outpatient encounter (ED, observation, or outpatient surgery)

- POA is assigned to the principle and secondary diagnosis

- Issues with unclear documentation for POA must be resolved by the provider

A condition that is not POA on admission, but manifests during the stay is considered a hospital-acquired condition (HAC). HACs are considered to be preventable conditions by CMS. In these cases, the hospitals do not receive the higher payment for cases when conditions were acquired during the hospitalization. The case gets paid as though the secondary diagnosis is non-existent.

Additionally, an adjustment is made for MS-DRG payment when excess readmissions are identified. A readmission ratio measures readmissions compared to the national averages of the same conditions. For example, as part of the Hospital Readmissions Reduction Program (HRRP) list of annual conditions for fiscal year 2017, coronary artery bypass graft surgery was included in the program. According to CMS (2017c), a readmission refers to an admission, paid via IPPS, within 30 days of a discharge from the same or other acute care hospital.

The MS-DRG system also allows inpatient hospitals to measure their case-mix index. In other words, a hospital's case-mix is a direct measure of the resource consumption or cost of providing care (CMS 2019b). A complex case mix identifies that the hospital patients are consuming more resources, and thus require a higher cost of care. However, just because the case mix is complex does not mean that the hospital treats patients having a greater severity of illness (SI). SI must be included on the hospitals case mix via the inclusion of CCs and MCCs.

The case mix index can ultimately be impacted by the accuracy of a provider's clinical documentation to validate each inpatient service day medical necessity. Reimbursement may only be provided for services that meet the criteria of medical necessity. Medically necessary services include those that are "proper and needed for the diagnosis or treatment of medical conditions, are provided for the diagnosis, direct care, and treatment of the medical condition, and meet the standards of good medical practice in the area" (CMS 2019c). Policies that outline the criteria for what is deemed medically necessary include both National Coverage determinations (NCDs) and Local Coverage determinations (LCDs). Improved clinical documentation and response rates to coder queries can result in a positive increase of CMI.

Coding for Medical Necessity

Three factors help define the **medical necessity** of a diagnostic test, procedure, or treatment (42 CFR 405.500 1995):

1. The likelihood that a proposed healthcare service will have a reasonable beneficial effect on the patient's physical condition and quality of life at a specific point in his or her illness or lifetime.

2. Healthcare services and supplies that are proven or acknowledged to be effective in the diagnosis, treatment, cure, or relief of a health condition, illness, injury, disease, or its symptoms and are consistent with the community's accepted standard of care. Under medical necessity, only those services, procedures, and patient care warranted by the patient's condition are provided.

3. The concept that procedures are only reimbursed as a covered benefit when they are performed for a specific diagnosis or specified frequency.

Accurate ICD-10-CM diagnosis coding is essential to establishing the medical necessity of a particular service as required by Medicare's reasonable and necessary medical coverage policies. Other third-party payers also want to know the reason for the service before payment is determined. MACs that process Part A and Part B Medicare claims may develop local coverage decisions (LCDs). These policies ensure that claims submitted for certain services—typically outpatient services—have been deemed reasonable and necessary for the patient's condition. National coverage determinations (NCDs) also exist for other diagnostic and therapeutic services including many laboratory tests, for which Medicare payment is contingent on a particular condition being established as the reason the test was ordered.

The coder must be certain that documentation contains all of the reasons why the physician ordered a diagnostic or therapeutic service. Then the coder must assign all of the appropriate ICD-10-CM diagnosis codes for the claim to be reviewed accurately for medical necessity and paid appropriately. The requirements for determining medical necessity have moved the coding personnel outside the traditional HIM department into hospitals' emergency departments, admitting or registration or access departments, central scheduling centers, and a variety of clinical departments performing many outpatient services, such as radiology and laboratory.

The need to know if a patient's condition meets the medical necessity requirements of a particular service is essential prior to issuing an **advance beneficiary notice (ABN)** (CMS 2019d). An ABN is a statement signed by the patient when he or she is notified by the provider, prior to a service or procedure being performed, that Medicare may not reimburse the provider for the service, whereupon the patient indicates that he or she will be responsible for any charges. Medical necessity processing has brought the coding function closer to the point of care and, in some institutions, improved the documentation related to the reasons for outpatient therapy and testing services.

Value-Based Purchasing (VBP) Adjustment

Beginning in 2012, some IPPS payments reflect applicable adjustments based on overall performance on a set of quality measures. The Hospital VBP Program allows organizations to earn back more than, all of, or less than the applicable percent reduction for a given year (CMS 2017d). The VBP program applies to participating acute IPPS hospitals with a few exceptions. The incentive adjustments are paid on a claim-by-claim basis with the adjustment factor based on the hospital's Total Performance Score. The measure set includes clinical process of care, patient experience of care, outcome, and efficiency. According to CMS (2017d), the estimated available funding pool for 2017 was equal to 2 percent of the estimated annual base operating DRG payment amounts for all acute inpatient hospitals eligible for the VBP program, which totals $1.8 billion. The hospital VBP program adjusts payments to hospitals under the IPPS based on the quality of care they deliver.

Check Your Understanding 25.1

Answer the following questions about the hospital inpatient prospective payment system.

1. What is the intent of the CMS Inpatient Prospective Payment System (IPPS) and why did CMS change the reimbursement program?

2. Other than the payment for the inpatient hospital services, what other type of hospital services are included in the MS-DRG payment?

3. How many final diagnosis and procedure codes may be included on the hospital electronic claims submission for hospital inpatient services that are used to determine the MS-DRG assignment?

4. Case scenario: A patient was admitted to the hospital with acute abdominal pain that was determined to be due to acute appendicitis, and the surgeon performed an open appendectomy on the patient. During the recovery period, the patient experienced two episodes of urinary retention that required the placement of a temporary urinary catheter. Would the second diagnosis of urinary retention be reported with a "yes" or a "no" as present on admission?

5. MS-DRG assignment is based on the information include in what four (4) elements?

Medicare Review Programs

CMS reviews acute IPPS and long-term care hospital (LTCH) records for payment purposes. Documentation and code assignment must be accurate and specific. CMS contracts with Medicare Administrative Contractors (MACs) to conduct medical and coding reviews to prevent improper payment of inpatient hospital claims. This review is done to ensure that billed items or services are covered and are reasonable and necessary as specified in section 1862(a)(1)(A) of the Social Security Act (CMS 2019e).

Quality Improvement Organizations

CMS contracts with one or more organizations in each state or region to serve as that area's **Quality Improvement Organization (QIO)**. QIOs are not-for-profit private organizations staffed by health quality experts, clinicians, and consumers organized to improve the care delivered to people with Medicare. QIOs' focus is on improving the quality of healthcare by working with medical providers through quality improvement activities. Originally CMS contracted with a QIO for a three-year period of time with an agreement called a scope of work as to what services the QIO will provide to Medicare beneficiaries or on their behalf (CMS 2019f).

Medicare contracts with QIOs to promote better patient care, better population health, and lower healthcare costs through improvement in the delivery of healthcare services. As a result, QIOs focus their work on the following:

- Improving quality of care for beneficiaries;

- Protecting the integrity of the Medicare Trust Fund. Ensure that Medicare only pays for services that are reasonable and necessary for the Medicare beneficiary and is provided in the most appropriate setting;

- Protecting beneficiaries by performing expedited coverage reviews of appeals or requests, such as beneficiary complaints; provider-based notice appeals; violations of the Emergency Medical Treatment and Labor Act (EMTALA); and other related responsibilities as articulated in QIO-related law. An expedited coverage review is usually a request from the Medicare patient to extend their hospital stay when their physician and hospital has determined the patient should be discharged from the hospital and the patient disagrees with the discharge. The QIO attempts to resolve these discharge disputes between the patient and the physician and hospital.

- Reviewing beneficiaries' appeals in response to provider-based notices;

- Reviewing allegations of violations of the Emergency Medical Treatment and Labor Act (EMTALA) (CMS 2019f)

CMS has restructured its QIO Program over the last several years to enhance its ability to improve the quality of medical services provided to Medicare beneficiaries. The new program maximizes learning and collaborating in improving care by spreading new effective practices and models of care among clinicians. The QIOs are focused on partnering with CMS to meet the goals of the CMS quality strategy and deliver program values to the Medicare population and taxpayers. In the redesign of the QIO programs, CMS separated case review from quality improvement activities. The prior three-year contracts were extended to five-year contracts. CMS removed the restriction of only one QIO entity in each state or region and broadened

CMS considerations of the type of entities that could perform the work. The result has been that two groups of QIO organizations exist in a state or a region. The first type are called Beneficiary and Family-Centered Care (BFCC) QIOs and handle beneficiary complaints, quality of care reviews, EMTALA reviews, and other types of case reviews. The second group of QIOs, Quality Innovation Network (QIN) QIOs, partner with healthcare providers on data-driven projects to improve patient safety, reduce harm, and improve clinical care at the local community level. In addition, CMS established a website, QualityNet, to provide healthcare quality improvement news, references, reporting tools, and data resources used by healthcare providers and only. QualityNet provides secure communication and healthcare quality data exchange between QIOs and clinicians (CMS 2019g).

Medicare Administrative Contractors

Ever since Medicare started in 1966, CMS has contracted with private healthcare insurance companies to process medical claims for Medicare beneficiaries. For many years, these entities were known as Part A Fiscal Intermediaries (FI) and Part B carriers. The Medicare Prescription Drug, Improvement, and Modernization Act (MMA) of 2003 directed CMS to replace the Part A FIs and Part B carriers with MACs (CMS 2019h).

Starting in 2012, CMS awarded Medicare claims processing contracts through a competitive bidding process to replace the claims contractors (fiscal intermediaries and carriers) with new contracted business called **Medicare Administrative Contractors (MACs)**. As of December 2015, there were 12 Part A and Part B MACs and 4 durable medical equipment (DME) MACs that processed Medicare fee-for-service (FFS) claims for the great majority of the total Medicare beneficiary population (CMS 2019i).

MACs process Part A and Part B Medicare FFS claims to make payments to providers. They also enroll physicians and others as providers into the Medicare FFS program. The MACs work with providers, both hospitals and clinicians, to handle reimbursement issues, audit provider cost reports, respond to providers questions, and educate the providers about Medicare FFS billing requirements. In addition, the MACs establish local coverage determination (LCD) policies to determine when an outpatient service is reasonable and necessary for a Medicare beneficiary's medical condition. The MACs perform reviews of medical records on selected claims for coding, billing, and medical necessity requirements.

Comprehensive Error Rate Testing Program

The **Comprehensive Error Rate Testing (CERT)** contractor reviews claims for the purpose of producing a national Medicare fee-for-service payment error rate. There is a rate calculated for inpatient hospitals, durable medical equipment, physicians, labs, ambulance, and noninpatient hospital facilities. The CERT contractor performs reviews on a postpayment basis. In order to determine the error rate by which Medicare MACs are paying acute IPPS hospital and LTCH claims appropriately, the review is conducted in accordance with coverage, coding, and medical necessity guidelines. In order to produce a national Medicare fee-for-service payment error rate, the CERT contractor's clinical staff review the claim with the submitted medical record to determine if the Medicare claim submitted was coded correctly, met medical necessity requirements, and was paid appropriately. A statistically valid random sample of Medicare claims are reviewed on a postpayment basis (CMS 2017d).

Each hospital is notified when a claim has been selected for review in slightly different ways, depending on the review entity. The CERT contractor notifies providers that a claim is selected for CERT review via letter. The hospital provides copies of the selected reviews by mail or as directed to the CERT contractor. The provider must submit a copy of the record by the date requested. The MAC reviews the claim and makes any necessary payment adjustments based on the review. The provider has the right to appeal the decision made by the CERT contractor through an established procedure. The CERT program provides Medicare with two measurements: how well the provider codes and submits the claim and how well the MAC educates the provider community on how to submit claims correctly (CMS 2019e).

Recovery Audit Program Contractors

Despite the efforts of QIOs and other initiatives that CMS has undertaken, there are concerns that the Medicare Trust Fund may not be adequately protected against improper payments. Congress passed the Medicare Prescription Drug, Improvement, and Modernization Act of 2003 (MMA), which was designed to enhance and support Medicare's current efforts (MMA 2003).

Congress directed the Department of Health and Human Services (HHS) to conduct a three-year demonstration project using **Recovery Audit Contractors (RACs)** to detect and correct improper payments in the traditional Medicare fee-for-service program. Section 302 of the Tax Relief and Health Care Act of 2006 made the PAC program permanent and required the program be expanded to all 50 states (CMS 2019b).

The demonstration project began in 2005 and ended in 2008 with three contractors focusing on Medicare beneficiaries' healthcare claims in three states with large numbers of Medicare beneficiaries: New York, Florida, and California. The demonstration project allowed Medicare to evaluate the efficiency and effectiveness of the program in order to make improvements in the RAC program. Congress made the program permanent and CMS expanded the program to all states in 2010. The types of services included in RAC reviews are hospital inpatient admission, outpatient hospital visits, physician visits, skilled nursing facility admissions, home health services, and durable medical equipment provided.

The RACs performed reviews of medical records with the corresponding Medicare claims to

- Detect improper Medicare payments, including both underpayments and overpayments
- Correct improper Medicare payments

The types of errors found by the RACs that resulted in improper payments may result from

- Incorrect payment amounts calculated by the payer (MAC, FI, or Carrier)
- Noncovered services including services that are not reasonable and necessary under Section 1862(a)(1)(A) of the Social Security Act, often referred to as not "medically necessary."
- Incorrectly coded services that result in incorrect DRGs
- Duplicate services billed by and paid to a provider

To be more specific, the RACs attributed the improper payments to six reasons as a result of their reviews:

- Medically unnecessary services paid for (74 percent)
- Insufficient documentation to justify payment (12.2 percent)

- Underpayment due to incorrect coding (7.1 percent)

- Overpayment due to incorrect coding (5.1 percent)

- No documentation to justify payment (1.2 percent)

- Other reasons (0.5 percent) (CMS 2012)

Each RAC is responsible for identifying overpayment and underpayments in approximately one-quarter of the country (CMS 2019b).

RAC contractors review claims on a post-payment basis for potential overpayments and underpayments by the MAC. The reviews are based on the CMS regulations for billing, medical necessity, coverage determinations, and coding guidelines. The RAC contractors do not develop their own billing and coding policies. The claims are selected based on focused areas of review for both inpatient and outpatient records. Inpatient records are selected based on the specific MS-DRGs targeted for review based on the RAC contractor's past experience with coding and sequencing errors. The inpatient record reviews are referred to as complex reviews. Outpatient records are selected based on experience primarily with billing errors using CPT/HCPCS codes. Each hospital is notified when a claim has been selected for review with an "Additional Documentation Request" sent to the RAC coordinator at the hospital. The hospital must submit the record for each case identified for a review within a specified period of time. If the record is not submitted on a timely basis, the claim will be delayed and the payment made previously will be collected. The RAC contractor also performs what is called automated reviews strictly on the submitted outpatient claims based on experience with the use of CPT/HCPCS codes and the number of units charged for a particular procedure code using proprietary software. The RAC can only review claims submitted in the past three years.

If a particular record has been reviewed by another entity, such as the QIO or CERT contractor, the RAC contractor will not review the same case. When the RAC concludes that a billing or coding error has been made with an improper payment made, it will notify the FI/MAC to adjust the claim and recoup the payment from the providers. The error may be either an overpayment or an underpayment to the provider. The provider is notified of the finding and has the opportunity to appeal following an established appeal process that involves submitting documentation to support the provider's disagreement with the RAC decision. The appeals process used for the RAC is the same for all providers who want to appeal a Medicare's claim decision (CMS 2017a). There are five levels of appeals:

1. First level of appeal is submitted to the claims processing contractors such as a Medicare carrier, fiscal intermediary (FI), or Medicare Administrative Contractor (MAC).

2. Second level of appeal is submitted to a qualified independent contractor (QIC).

3. Third level of appeal is submitted to an administrative law judge (ALJ) in the Office of Medicare Hearings and Appeals.

4. Fourth level of appeal is submitted to the Medicare Appeals Council.

5. Fifth level of appeal is submitted for a judicial review through the Federal District Court review process.

The examination of ICD-10-CM coding has been a major area of focus for the RACs because the diagnosis and procedure codes create the MS-DRGs, which are the basis of payment for acute-care hospitals. When ICD-10-CM coding is implemented, the examination of these codes will be the focus of RAC reviews for reimbursement purposes. ICD-10-CM/PCS and CPT coding in other healthcare organizations, such as rehabilitation hospitals and units and physician offices, determine reimbursement to the providers and therefore are a focus of attention during these providers' reviews. Certified coders are employed by RACs to perform coding reviews.

The mission of the RAC program is to identify and correct Medicare and Medicaid improper payments. Since the program's inception, improper payments have been found for items and services that do not meet Medicare's coverage and medical necessity policies. Other payments were made in error based on the record being incorrectly coded. Finally, payments for services were found to be made in error based on the supporting documentation submitted that did not support the ordered service. An overpayment results in money collected from the provider paid by Medicare. An underpayment is made to the provider when the review determines the provider was owed additional money. CMS is obligated to provide a summary report to Congress each year about the RAC activities. The "Recovery Auditing in Medicare for Fiscal Year 2014, FY 2014 Report to Congress as Required by Section 1893(h) of the Social Security Act" provides a comprehensive review of the performance of the RACs in identifying the savings to the Medicare program that were accomplished (CMS 2017c).

Check Your Understanding 25.2

Answer the following questions about Medicare coding reviews.

1. What is the intent of Medicare's contracts with Quality Improvement Organizations (QIOs)?

2. What is an "expedited (coverage) review" performed by the Quality Review Organizations?

3. What is the primary purpose of the Medicare Administrative Contractors (MACs)?

4. How do the CERT contractors determine the Medicare fee-for-service payment error rate?

5. What are the five (5) levels of appeals used for RAC claim decisions?

OIG Work Plan

The Office of the Inspector General (OIG) has the mission to protect DHHS program integrity as well as protect the program beneficiaries. The OIG releases annual plans to set priorities and emerging issues which include projects, evaluations, and audits to be addressed during the fiscal year by the OIG's Office of Audit Services and Office of Evaluation and Inspections (OIG 2019). A more recent care delivery and Medicare financing model is the Accountable Care Organization (ACO). A few of the ACO programs included in the Medicare Shared Savings Program (MSSP) are the Medicare shared savings program, advance payment ACO model and pioneer ACO model (OIG 2001). These models form networks that coordinate patient care. When care is provided more efficiently, the organizations become eligible for bonuses and make more when they keep their patients healthy. These networks share both the financial and medical responsibility of providing high quality and coordinated care to patients.

Review Exercises: Chapter 25

Answer the following questions in the space provided.

1. What was the goal of the MS-DRG system that replaced the DRG system?

2. What is the basic formula for calculating each MS-DRG hospital payment?

3. What are possible "add-on" payments that a hospital could receive in addition to the basic Medicare MS-DRG payment?

4. What additional factor is involved in the assignment of MS-DRGs beside principal and secondary diagnoses including the presence of major or other complications or comorbidities and discharge disposition or status?

5. What are the QIO's programs designed to accomplish?

6. Describe what a hospital-acquired condition (HAC) is considered and how it impacts reimbursement.

7. How does Medicare or other third-party payers determine whether the patient has medical necessity for the tests, procedures, or treatment billed on a claim form?

8. How does a hospital qualify for a disproportionate share adjustment from Medicare?

9. What are the factors that help to define the medical necessity of a diagnostic test, procedure, or treatment?

10. What is the role of a CERT contractor?

References

42 CFR 405.500. 60 FR 63175, Dec. 9, 1995. http://www.ecfr.gov.

Centers for Medicare and Medicaid Services (CMS). 2019a. ICD-10-CM/PCS MS-DRGv33 Definitions Manual. https://www.cms.gov/ICD10Manual/version33-fullcode-cms/fullcode_cms/P0001.html.

Centers for Medicare and Medicaid Services (CMS). 2019b. Case Mix Index. https://www.cms.gov/Medicare/Medicare-Fee-for-Service-Payment/AcuteInpatientPPS/Acute-Inpatient-Files-for-Download-Items/CMS022630.html.

Centers for Medicare and Medicaid Services (CMS) 2019c. Glossary. https://www.cms.gov/apps/glossary/.

Centers for Medicare and Medicaid Services (CMS). 2019d. Medicare Review and education. https://www.cms.gov/Research-Statistics-Data-and-Systems/Monitoring-Programs/Medicare-FFS-Compliance-Programs/Medical-Review/.

Centers for Medicare and Medicaid Services (CMS). 2019e. Quality Improvement Organizations. https://www.cms.gov/Medicare/Quality-Initiatives-Patient-Assessment-Instruments/QualityImprovementOrgs/index.html?redirect=/qualityimprovementorgs/.

Centers for Medicare and Medicaid Services (CMS). 2019f. QualityNet. QIO Directories. http://www.qualitynet.org/dcs/ContentServer?c=Page&pagename=QnetPublic%2FPage%2FQnetTier2&cid=1144767874793.

Centers for Medicare and Medicaid Services (CMS). 2019g. Who are the MACs? https://www.cms.gov/Medicare/Medicare-Contracting/Medicare-Administrative-Contractors/Who-are-the-MACs.html.

Centers for Medicare and Medicaid Services (CMS). 2019h. Recovery Audit Program. https://www.cms.gov/research-statistics-data-and-systems/monitoring-programs/medicare-ffs-compliance-programs/recovery-audit-program/.

Centers for Medicare and Medicaid Services (CMS). 2019i. Recovery Auditing in Medicare for Fiscal Year 2015. https://www.cms.gov/Research-Statistics-Data-and-Systems/Monitoring-Programs/Medicare-FFS-Compliance-Programs/Recovery-Audit-Program/.

Centers for Medicare and Medicaid Services (CMS). 2017a. Medicare Administrative Contractors. https://www.cms.gov/medicare/medicare-contracting/medicare-administrative-contractors/medicareadministrativecontractors.html.

Centers for Medicare and Medicaid Services (CMS). 2017b. Medicare Advance Beneficiary Notices. ICN 006266. https://www.cms.gov/Outreach-and-Education/Medicare-Learning-Network-MLN/MLNProducts/Downloads/ABN-Booklet-ICN006266TextOnly.pdf.

Centers for Medicare and Medicaid Services (CMS). 2017c. Hospital-Acquired Conditions and Present on Admission Indicator Reporting Provision. https://www.cms.gov/Outreach-and-Education/Medicare-Learning-Network-MLN/MLNProducts/Downloads/wPOA-Fact-Sheet.pdf.

Centers for Medicare and Medicaid Services (CMS). 2012. Medicare Fee-for-service Recovery Audit Program Myths. https://www.cms.gov/Research-Statistics-Data-and-Systems/Monitoring-Programs/Recovery-Audit-Program/Downloads/RAC-Program-Myths-12-18-12.pdf.

Medicare Prescription Drug, Improvement and Modernization Act of 2003 (MMA). Public Law No: 108-173.

Medicare Interactive. 2018. What does Medicare cover (Parts A, B, C, and D). https://www.medicareinteractive.org/get-answers/introduction-to-medicare/explaining-medicare/what-does-medicare-cover-parts-a-b-c-and-d.

Office of the Inspector General (OIG). 2001. Medicare Hospital Prospective Payment System How DRG Rates Are Calculated and Updated. https://oig.hhs.gov/oei/reports/oei-09-00-00200.pdf.

Office of the Inspector General (OIG). 2019. Work Plan. https://oig.hhs.gov/reports-and-publications/workplan/index.asp.

Coding Self-Test

Assign the appropriate ICD-10-CM and ICD-10-PCS codes (include procedure codes, external cause codes, and Z codes, where applicable) to the following:

1. Abnormal partial thromboplastin time (PTT) and abnormal prothrombin time (PT), cause to be determined

2. Peptic ulcer of the lesser curvature of the stomach, acute, with hemorrhage; esophagogastroduodenoscopy (EGD) with closed biopsy of stomach

3. Adenocarcinoma of descending colon with extension to mesenteric lymph nodes; permanent descending colon colostomy, open procedure with colostomy brought to the skin level

4. Chronic kidney disease, ESRD, dependence on renal dialysis; patient received intermittent type hemodialysis, single session that was performed for 4 hours on one day

5. Encounter for complete elective abortion at eight weeks, due to maternal rubella (no longer active virus), with suspected damage to fetus affecting management of pregnancy; abortion by laminaria

6. Rapidly progressive glomerulonephritis with minor glomerular abnormality; percutaneous renal biopsy, right kidney

7. Acute exacerbation of COPD with acute bronchitis

8. Patient with a history of bladder carcinoma seen for a follow-up examination related to his past partial cystectomy treatment; no recurrence found; preprocedure lab results found idiopathic hypercalciuria, cause to be determined. Cystoscopy with biopsy of bladder

9. Degenerative joint disease, bilateral knees with left knee most bothersome for the patient. Total knee replacement using oxidized zirconium polyethylene prosthesis cemented, left knee

10. Partial intestinal obstruction due to adhesions

11. Contusion of the cerebellum with loss of consciousness for 45 minutes due to motor vehicle collision with another vehicle (patient was driving his vehicle) initial encounter

12. Malignant lymphoma, undifferentiated Burkitt type, Intrathoracic; percutaneous bone marrow biopsy, iliac

13. Left heel ulcer with gangrene of skin and necrosis of muscle due to uncontrolled type 1 diabetes with hyperglycemia

14. Recurrence of Clostridium difficile enterocolitis infection

15. Group 2 pulmonary hypertension, due to left heart disease, that is, rheumatic mitral valve stenosis

16. Coronary artery disease in previous autologous vein bypass grafts in the left anterior descending, left circumflex, and right posterior descending arteries. Procedures performed are coronary artery bypass grafts with double (left and right) internal mammary bypass to the left anterior descending and the left circumflex, and a single aortocoronary bypass to the right posterior descending artery using saphenous vein graft, left leg, harvested under an open approach with cardiopulmonary bypass.

17. Postprocedural stricture of urethra with urinary retention; cystoscopic release of urethral stricture (female patient)

18. Hypertensive heart and kidney disease with chronic kidney disease, stage 3; elevated lipoprotein(a) level

19. Inflamed seborrheic keratosis, multiple lesions, of right face; cryotherapy of multiple (3) lesions on right temple

20. Secondary thrombocytopenia due to hypersplenism; total splenectomy, open

21. Iron deficiency anemia due to chronic blood loss

22. Pneumonia due to *Staphylococcus aureus*; Fiberoptic bronchoscopy, tracheobronchial tree

23. Type 1 diabetes with ketoacidosis and coma with long term use of insulin for control

___

24. Pregnancy, preterm labor with preterm delivery at 35 weeks, single liveborn infant; postpartum fever of unknown origin; patient with known continuous marijuana drug dependence; spontaneous vaginal delivery

___

25. Lyme disease with associated arthritis

___

26. Infiltrating duct breast carcinoma, right upper outer quadrant, with metastases to bone (female patient.) Lump in left breast, in overlapping quadrants.

___

27. Newborn twin, male, delivered by cesarean delivery (in hospital) with syndrome of infant of diabetic mother and neonatal hypomagnesemia

___

28. Obstructive hydrocephalus; cerebral ventricle to atrium shunt using synthetic substitute by open approach

___

29. Chlamydial vaginitis

___

30. Traumatic arthritis of left wrist secondary to old fracture-dislocation of lower end of radius, left

___

31. Organic brain syndrome due to cerebral arteriosclerosis

___

32. Gunshot wound of chest with massive intrathoracic injury to right lung with laceration; shot by another person with a handgun who was charged with attempted homicide; injury occurred on a local residential street; patient died during an exploratory thoracotomy to examine right lung

___

33. Ovarian retention cyst; laparoscopic partial oophorectomy, left side

___

34. Paranoid schizophrenia; cannabis dependence with withdrawal

___

35. Internal derangement of lateral meniscus, old tear, posterior horn, right knee; right knee arthroscopic meniscecetomy

___

36. Parkinsonism secondary to haloperidol neuroleptic drug therapy, initial encounter; drug was discontinued at the conclusion of this encounter. The patient had been taking the drug as directed by her physian.

___

37. Moderate mental retardation as the sequela of acute bacterial meningitis 10 years ago

___

38. Chronic hidradenitis suppurative, subcutaneous tissue, right axilla; two procedures are performed: wide excision of hidradenitis of right axilla and partial-thickness skin graft. Patient's own skin excised and grafted from patient's back to right axilla.

39. Postpartum abscess of breast; postnatal depression; (Patient discharged five days ago following spontaneous delivery of live newborn son)

40. Pituitary-dependent Cushing's syndrome; screening for depression also occurred during this visit

41. Ingestion of 30 doxepin (Sinequan) [Doxepin is a tricyclic antidepressant drug] tablets resulting in an overdose, determined to be a suicide attempt; tachycardia, initial episode of care

42. Fracture, right shoulder, humerus upper end (head), as the result of a fall from a chair she was standing on to reach a high shelf, occurred at her single family residence, in her kitchen while cooking. The procedure performed was a closed reduction of the right humeral head. This was the initial episode of care. Patient is retired.

43. Unexplained dizziness; fainting; personal history of falls

44. Congenital hypertrophic pyloric stenosis in a four-week-old infant, corrected by open pyloromyotomy when the physician made an anterior incision in the muscle of the pylorus to restore it to its normal function and allow food to pass from the stomach to the small intestine

45. Third-degree burn of chest and second-degree burn of right leg, initial encounter

46. Newborn delivered in community hospital transferred to university medical center. Code for the infant at the university medical center treated for hypoplastic left heart syndrome.

47. Positive tuberculin skin test with prior contact or exposure to tuberculosis, no evidence of active disease

48. Coronary arteriosclerosis of autologous vein bypass grafts with unstable angina; family history of familial combined hyperlipidemia

49. Heroin poisoning, accidental overdose resulting in acute lung edema; multiple drug dependence including heroin and barbiturates, initial encounter

50. Acute idiopathic pancreatitis with an additional problem of primary sclerosing cholangitis

51. History of allergic reaction to flu vaccination

---

52. Infiltrative tuberculosis of both lungs with tuberculous pleurisy

---

53. Diabetic hypoglycemic coma in a patient with type 1 diabetes

---

54. Spinal stenosis of the lumbar region with neurogenic claudication

---

55. Trichorionic, triamniotic triplet pregnancy, 32 weeks of gestation in the third trimester (each fetus with its own placenta and amniotic sac)

---

56. Accidental overdose by Ecstasy, emergency department evaluation. (The proper drug name of 3,4-Methylenedioxymethamphetamine, also known as MDMA.)

---

57. Brow ptosis of both eyes

---

58. Superficial incisional wound infection of obstetrical wound

---

59. Cerebral infarction due to occlusion of small artery (Lacunar infarction)

---

60. Patient admitted for her first round of antineoplastic chemotherapy after a total abdominal hysterectomy and bilateral salpingo-oophorectomy (performed four weeks ago) for right ovarian carcinoma with known metastases to intrapelvic lymph nodes; administration of antineoplastic chemotherapy by central vein infusion.

---

61. The patient is a 15-year-old male who was attacked by an unknown male with a knife while the patient was riding his bicycle home from high school on a residential street near his home. The knife created a deep gaping laceration of his left external ear that was sutured in multiple layers in the emergency department where he was brought by paramedics. The patient was also found to have acute blood loss anemia from the loss of blood from the wound.

---

62. The patient is a 70-year-old female who is being seen in the Ophthalmology Clinic at the university hospital to be re-evaluated for her bilateral glaucoma. The patient has mild stage primary open-angle glaucoma in the right eye and moderate stage primary open-angle glaucoma in the left eye. The physician documents that the right eye appears to be stable but the left eye glaucoma is worsening. The physician renews the patient's medication prescriptions and requests the patient return in three months for another examination.

---

63. The patient is a 29-year-old male who is being seen in the psychiatrist office at the request of his parents because he keeps relapsing on alcohol. The patient has been in and out of different treatment centers over the past 15 years for a variety of problems related to school, family, and work situations. The issues were behavioral problems, court-ordered anger management therapy, anxiety, and alcoholism. At this time, the patient is visibly nervous and unable to sit still in a chair during the interview. He admits to drinking daily for the past month but thinks he can stop whenever he wants to. The patient has no evidence of psychosis and denies being depressed, but the patient is in denial about the extent of his drinking problems. The patient agrees to be hospitalized in the alcohol treatment unit at the local hospital and will be transported to the unit by a counselor from the physician's office. The physician lists the diagnoses of alcohol dependence, generalized anxiety disorder, and Asperger's syndrome.

64. The patient is a 74-year-old female who claims she "bumped" her left ankle on her husband's wheelchair two months ago and suffered a tear of her skin that over time seemed to deepen and did not heal. The patient is seen in the outpatient Wound Clinic today to evaluate the wound on her near her left ankle. The area is ulcerated and measures 0.8 cm × 0.5 cm × 0.1 cm with the base of the ulceration being 50 percent granulated tissue and 50 percent slough. The patient was seen last month and underwent a nonexcisional debridement, but the ulcer today does not look much better. The patient agreed to schedule an excision debridement that will be performed in the outpatient surgery department three days after this visit. In addition, because of no improvement in the ulceration that is limited to skin breakdown only, the physician ordered laboratory tests as part of a workup for underlying conditions. The wound was treated with collagen and covered with gauze and Medifix tape. The final diagnosis for the patient's visit is nonpressure ulcer, lower limb, left ankle.

65. The parent of a 10-year-old male child brought him to the emergency department (ED) of the hospital after they were unable to stop a nosebleed that occurred at home. The parent gives a history of the child having frequent nose bleeds at home and at school. The child has had his nose cauterized in the ED on two occasions. The parent has a nose clamp at home that they apply when a nose bleed starts and that frequently stops the bleeding. On this occasion, the bleeding would not stop. However, by the time the parent and child arrived at the ED, the bleeding had stopped, and there was no need on this visit to perform any cauterization. Upon examination, the ED physician noted the patient had bilateral acute otitis media. The mother stated the child had recovered from a mild upper respiratory infection last week but was not complaining about his ears. The child agreed with these statements. The ED physician recommended the mother to use saline nasal spray as directed for moisturization and to continue to use the humidifier in the child's bedroom at night. The ED physician did not prescribe medications for the child's ear infections as the mother agreed to take the child to his pediatrician the next day. The final diagnoses for this visit were (1) epistaxis and (2) bilateral acute otitis media.

66. A 59-year-old male came to the emergency department (ED) complaining of a "funny feeling" in his left upper chest. He claimed it was not painful, just a sensation he had not experienced before. He first felt it this morning and thought perhaps he had slept in an unusual position overnight. But today, after he changed a tire on a car, he thought the feeling intensified, and his wife insisted he come to the ED. The patient is under treatment for hypertension that appeared to be controlled with his current medications. He had a family history of ischemic heart disease with his parents having heart attacks. The ED physician went forward with a workup to rule out acute coronary syndrome, aortic dissection, pulmonary embolism with EKG, chest x-ray, and standard labs. After all the tests were completed, the physician met with the patient to review the findings. The EKG showed some minor abnormalities, but there was no clear evidence of ischemia. The chest x-ray was normal. The only abnormality found in the lab work was mild hypokalemia. Given the patient's pain had been present since morning, an elevation in troponin

would have been expected by now if the patient had acute coronary syndrome. The patient agreed to be discharged home and agreed to return to the ED if the pain worsened and agreed to make an appointment with a primary care physician within the next three days. The patient did not have a physician but was given a referral to a local medical group. The ED physician documented the following as final diagnoses: Musculoskeletal chest pain; abnormal EKG; hypokalemia; and hypertension.

67. The patient is a 25-year-old male presenting to the occupational therapy services for continued therapy. The medical diagnosis provided by the patient's physician for therapy is multiple right forearm and wrist lacerations involving tendons. The treatment objective was to aid in the recovery of the right upper extremity lacerations and muscle weakness involving the tendons of the forearm and wrist. The patient had decreased range of motion of his fingers. The patient's grip is decreased. After the series of treatment, the patient's sensation is improving in all his fingers. The patient will return for continued skilled OT to increase range of other and strength to increase functional use of his right hand. The patient's rehabilitation potential is good. The facility's coding guidelines state to code the medical diagnosis and the treatment objective for all occupational therapy visits.

68. The patient is a 65-year-old male who is seen today for a CT of the abdomen and pelvis without contrast. The diagnosis provided on the order for the CT exam is right low back pain and microscopic hematuria. The impression written by the radiologist on the CT report is nonobstructive right renal calculi and enlarged prostate gland. A third impression was a cyst in the right hepatic lobe that was not present in the last exam in 2009, and the type of cyst is undetermined, and the radiologist recommended further evaluation with a dedicated liver ultrasound or liver CT. The facility's coding guideline is to code both the diagnosis provided on the order for an imaging examination as well as the impression written by the radiologist.

69. The patient is a 40-year-old male seen in his primary care physician's office prior to nasal surgery. The patient is scheduled for inferior turbinate reduction in one week. He has sinus congestion and uses Afrin once a week. His active problems are allergic rhinitis, epistaxis, hypertrophy of nasal turbinates, and hypertension. He is a former smoker and is currently employed full time. Other than his sinus congestion, his physical examination is normal. Based on preoperative laboratory results, the patient is also diagnosed with elevated serum cholesterol. The final diagnoses included on the preoperative H&P submitted for the nasal surgery are allergic rhinitis, hypertrophy of nasal turbinate, epistaxis, elevated serum cholesterol, hypertension, and history of nicotine dependence.

70. The patient is a 50-year-old female with postmenopausal bleeding. The physician was previously unable to perform an endometrial biopsy in the office secondary to cervical stenosis. Today, the patient was taken to the operating room for an examination under anesthesia and cervical dilation. Despite 25 minutes of attempts of dilating the cervix through the vagina, the physician states that she was unable to locate the axis of the endocervical canal despite the usage of lacrimal duct probes, pediatric dilators, and normal dilators. The physician documented she was unable to ascertain the correct axis of the patient's anatomy; therefore, any additional procedures were deferred until the physician was able to talk to the patient in the office about additional options. The postoperative diagnosis is postmenopausal bleeding and cervical stenosis. The procedure was attempted cervical dilation, failed.

71. Operative report

    Pre- and Post-Operative Diagnosis: Symptomatic sick sinus syndrome

    Procedure performed: Dual-chamber Medtronic pacemaker placement with active atrial and active ventricular leads using intraoperative fluoroscopy.

    History: The patient is a 69-year-old female with sick sinus syndrome admitted to the hospital with symptoms of shortness of breath and lightheadedness. Due to her multiple episodes of significant bradycardia while being treated due to her symptoms, we recommended and the patient agreed to the placement of a dual chamber pacemaker.

    Procedure in detail: The patient was brought to the operating room, placed in supine position, and general anesthesia was administered without complication. The neck and chest were prepped and draped in sterile fashion. Approximately 20 mL of 1% lidocaine was used to infiltrate the skin in the left upper outer quadrant of the chest. A 4-cm incision was then carried out. The skin incision was carried from the skin down through the subcutaneous tissue to the pectoralis fascia. A 6 cm × 6 cm subfascial pocket was then created in preparation for placement of pacemaker generator. Access to the left subclavian vein was achieved via Seldinger technique under direct fluoroscopy guidance. Subsequently, the sheath was placed over the wire and directed into the left subclavian vein. An active Medtronic ventricular pacemaker lead model #9999 with serial number BBL123455 was placed over the peel-away sheath and directed into the right ventricular appendage. The lead was then deployed into position. Testing of the ventricular lead revealed threshold voltage of 0.7 V and impedance of 752 ohms and R wave of 19 mV. The lead was then secured at two positions to the pectoralis fascia. Similarly, an active right atrial lead, model #8888 and serial number AAL456788, was placed over the peel-away sheath and directed into the right atrial appendage. The atrial lead was then deployed into position. Testing of the atrial lead revealed a threshold voltage of 1.0 V with impedance of 702 ohms and a P wave of 4.8 mV. It was then secured at two positions to the pectoralis fascia. Hemostasis was achieved. The leads were then connected to a Medtronic pacemaker, model #2222, serial number 987665. It was then placed into the subfascial pocket and secured one position to the pectoralis fascia. Hemostasis was achieved, and copious irrigation using antibiotic saline was then carried out. The leads were then tested at 10 mV revealing no evidence of diaphragmatic involvement. Postplacement fluoroscopy revealed no evidence of hemo- or pneumothorax. The incision was then reapproximated in three-layer fashion using absorbable suture for the deep fascia, subcutaneous and subcuticular. Dermabond was applied. The patient tolerated the procedure well. All sponges and needles were accounted for.

72. The patient is a 58-year-old male with a history of ulcerative colitis in remission who is two weeks status post total colectomy with ileostomy in place. The patient has had two episodes of bleeding from the ileostomy sites that were treated in the emergency department (ED). On this date, the hemorrhage is more active than the previous occasions, the site was inspected in the ED and pressure was applied, and the patient was placed in the observation unit at the hospital. The ileostomy was inspected the next morning, and there was no bleeding. Laboratory tests identified the presence of acute on chronic anemia from acute blood loss secondary to the bleeding ileostomy, and the patient's glucose is elevated at 350 mg/dL. The patient's creatinine is also elevated at 1.45 and BUN at 35. The patient is also known to have type 2 insulin dependent diabetes with nephropathy, coronary artery disease, and hypertension. The patient is discharged home to resume her regular medications and will report to the primary care physician's office in three days. The final diagnoses are (1) hemorrhage complicating the existing ileostomy, (2) acute on chronic blood loss anemia, (3) diabetic nephropathy, (4) coronary artery disease, (5) hypertension, and (6) status postcolectomy with absence of large intestine.

73. The patient is seen in the outpatient radiology department to have an MRI of the brain without contrast. The clinical indications for the test are simple partial seizure and right lower extremity muscle weakness. Findings of the exam show two masses in the left frontal lobe of the brain and in the left cerebellar hemisphere. There is no evidence of an acute infarct or stroke and no shift of the midline structures or hydrocephalus. The radiologist's conclusion is documented as space-occupying tumors in the left frontal lobe and left cerebellar hemisphere that are evidence of intracranial metastatic disease in a patient with no known primary malignant neoplasm. The radiologist recommends further radiological evaluation with contrast. The facility's coding guideline is to code both the diagnosis provided on the order for an imaging examination as well as the impression written by the radiologist.

74. Operative Report

Pre- and Post-operative diagnosis: Right proximal humerus, glenohumeral joint dislocation

Procedure performed: Closed reduction, right proximal humerus, glenohumeral joint dislocation under general anesthesia

Indications: The patient is a 60-year-old female who sustained this injury to her shoulder and had two attempts at reduction in the emergency department (ED) per the ED physician which were unsuccessful. The ED physician felt that the shoulder kept coming out of every time he put it in. The patient was therefore brought to the operating room for closed reduction, possible open reduction, and internal fixation.

Description of procedure: After appropriate consent was obtained, the patient was administered mask anesthesia. When the patient was sufficiently relaxed, gentle traction counter traction on the arm with internal rotation allowed for a closed reduction of the glenohumeral joint. An open reduction of the joint was not necessary. There was a stable reduction confirmed with intraoperative AP and lateral fluoroscopic x-rays. Passive internal and external rotation of the shoulder maintained the glenohumeral reduction. She was placed in a sling and swathe. She was awakened from the anesthetic and brought to recovery room in stable condition. There were no complications.

75. The patient is a 62-year-old female who was given a same-day appointment in the ophthalmologist office. This morning she had abrupt decreased vision with blurring of what little vision she had in her left eye. She denies flashes, floaters, or other eye complaints prior to today. She has a history of bilateral cataract extractions over the past two years, and she has a family history of retinal detachment. After a thorough eye exam, the physician concluded the patient had a rhegmatogenous retinal detachment with a retinal break that is suspected to be a giant break. The patient is scheduled for urgent pars plana vitrectomy, endolaser, and air-fluid exchange tomorrow.

Index

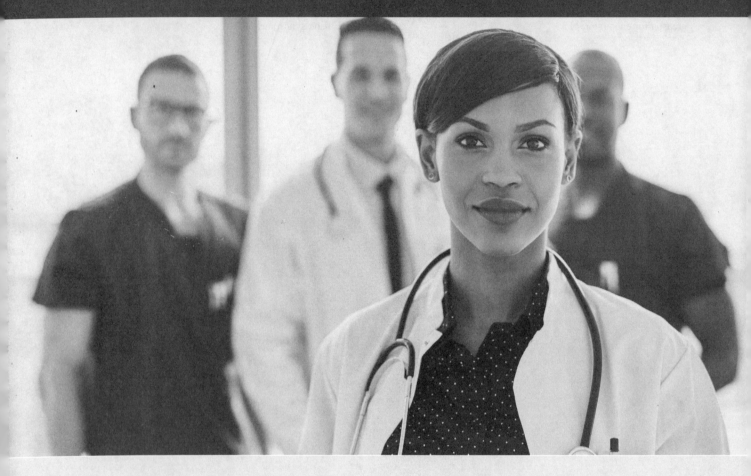